Biochemistry and Biology of Plasma Lipoproteins

THE BIOCHEMISTRY OF DISEASE

A Molecular Approach to Cell Pathology

A Series of Monographs

SERIES EDITORS

Emmanuel Farber
Department of Pathology
University of Toronto
Toronto, Ontario, Canada

Henry C. Pitot
McArdle Laboratory for Cancer Research
University of Wisconsin
Madison, Wisconsin

Volume 1 The Cell Cycle and Cancer
Edited by Renato Baserga

Volume 2 The Pathology of Transcription and Translation
Edited by Emmanuel Farber

Volume 3 Molecular Pathology of Connective Tissues
Edited by Ruy Pérez-Tamayo and M. Rojkind

Volume 4 Chemical Carcinogenesis (in two parts)
Edited by Paul O. P. Ts'o and Joseph A. DiPaolo

Volume 5 The Liver: Normal and Abnormal Functions (in two parts)
Edited by Frederick F. Becker

Volume 6 Multiplication and Division in Mammalian Cells
by Renato Baserga

Volume 7 The Biochemistry of Atherosclerosis
Edited by Angelo M. Scanu, Robert W. Wissler, and Godfrey S. Getz

Volume 8 Polyamines in Biology and Medicine
Edited by David R. Morris and Laurence J. Marton

Volume 9 Vascular Injury and Atherosclerosis
Edited by Sean Moore

Volume 10 Nutritional Pathology: Pathobiochemistry of Dietary Imbalances
Edited by Herschel Sidransky

Volume 11 Biochemistry and Biology of Plasma Lipoproteins
Edited by Angelo M. Scanu and Arthur A. Spector

Other Volumes in Preparation

Biochemistry and Biology of Plasma Lipoproteins

edited by

Angelo M. Scanu
The Pritzker School of Medicine
The University of Chicago
Chicago, Illinois

Arthur A. Spector
University of Iowa
Iowa City, Iowa

MARCEL DEKKER, INC. New York • Basel

Library of Congress Cataloging-in-Publication Data

Biochemistry and biology of plasma.

(The Biochemistry of disease ; v. 11)
Includes index.
1. Blood lipoproteins. I. Scanu, Angelo M., [date].
II. Spector, Arthur A., [date].
[DNLM: 1. Lipoproteins--blood. W1 BI64F v.11 /
QU 85 B6147]
QP99.3.L52B56 1986 612'.116 86-1464
ISBN 0-8247-7529-5

MARCEL DEKKER, INC.
270 Madison Avenue, New York, New York 10016

Current printing (last digit):
10 9 8 7 6 5 4 3 2 1

PRINTED IN THE UNITED STATES OF AMERICA

Preface

More than 50 years ago a French biochemist, Macheboeuf, working at the Pasteur Institute in Paris, established experimentally that plasma lipids are associated with proteins to form water-soluble complexes that have distinct physical and chemical properties. He was working with horse serum and we now know that the lipoprotein species that he precipitated in half-saturated ammonium sulfate under acidic conditions was a high-density lipoprotein, particularly abundant in this animal species. This was a historical event in the field of lipoprotein research since it came at a time when there was much skepticism about the existence of specific lipoprotein complexes in the circulation. Although the earliest application of the ultracentrifuge to the study of plasma lipoprotein was carried out in 1947 by Pedersen at the Karolinska Institute in Uppsala, it was the classic work carried out at the Donner Laboratory in Berkeley by Gofman and his colleagues in the late 1940s that established the power and the versatility of the ultracentrifugal method for study of the serum lipoproteins. That work generated the nomenclature of the main lipoprotein classes based on their flotational properties. It also described the main features of the lipoprotein distribution in the serum of normal and dyslipoproteinemic subjects. For the first time an attempt was made to establish a relationship between plasma lipoprotein and cardiovascular disease, and an atherogenic value was assigned to certain low-density lipoprotein classes occurring in serum at high concentrations. During this period, the metabolic importance of the plasma free fatty acid and the role of albumin in this process was discovered. Therefore, sufficient information was beginning to emerge to provide a rudimentary understanding of plasma lipid transport and how abnormalities in this system might predispose to atherosclerotic cardiovascular disease.

In the early 1950s, methods for the separation of serum lipoproteins by preparative ultracentrifugation were described, and with some modifications they still remain the basis for much of the work in the lipoprotein field. Electrophoretic methods in their various modes (free boundary, zonal, starch block, paper, agarose, and other supporting media) were also applied to the study of serum lipoproteins, as well as chemical procedures such as polyanion precipitation, Cohn's fractionation, and so on. In an unfortunate turn of events the atherogenic index proposed by Gofman failed to win the general approval of the experts at that time, who felt that levels of total serum cholesterol were as good predictors of cardiovascular disease as lipoproteins. This led to a temporary decline in interest in lipoprotein research essentially until the clinical studies of Fredrickson and his colleagues at the National Institutes of Health. They combined electrophoretic and chemical techniques to develop a classification of lipoprotein disorders based on given sets of phenotypes, which improved considerably our understanding of lipid disorders and also facilitated the dialogue among investigators and clinicians.

In chemical terms, the early work was directed at defining the lipid components of the various lipoprotein classes, whereas the apolipoproteins received comparatively less attention. It was only in the late 1950s that delipidation techniques were developed, and they marked the birth of the apolipoprotein field, which has progressively emerged as one of the most fascinating areas of lipoprotein research. Without their lipid complement, the apolipoproteins became amenable to fractionation. Pure polypeptides were obtained and work on their primary structure led to the important realization that amphiphilic structures are predominant in apolipoproteins and that these structures are involved in lipid binding. These studies also led to an understanding of the chemical basis of the apolipoprotein polymorphism and to the definition of the functional significance of polymorphic forms in terms of lipid binding, enzyme activation, or interaction with cell membrane receptors. Specific polyclonal antibodies have been raised against each of the known apolipoproteins, and they continue to be used widely to quantify these proteins in various body fluids through a series of immunoassay techniques. More recently, monoclonal antibodies have also entered the field of lipoprotein research. Although their true impact is yet difficult to measure, they have already seen important applications that have taken advantage of their high specificity and relative ease of preparation.

Like many other research areas, progress in the field of plasma lipoproteins has been dependent on the development of new techniques. The latest to enter this field have been those of cell and molecular biology. Through the exciting work by Goldstein and Brown we have learned about the role played by low density lipoproteins in regulating cellular cholesterol metabolism and its dependence on what is now known as the apo B,E receptor. This has generated a large volume of research activities. A second receptor, that for apo E, has also been isolated although its properties are not yet as well established; other receptors are being actively investigated. Equally exciting have been the advances in the studies directed at the clarification of the co- and posttranslational proteolytic events attending the biosynthesis of the plasma apolipoproteins. The cDNA clones of most of the apolipoproteins are now available and the chromosomal localization of most of the apolipoprotein genes has been determined. Clones for the apo B,E receptor and HMGCoA reductase also have recently been identified. The tools for analyzing the genetic basis of lipoprotein disorders are now in hand and soon we may be able to unravel the role that genetic factors play in the pathogenesis of atherosclerotic cardiovascular disease. About 60 years after Macheboeuf's pioneering work, the lipoprotein field is enjoying a period of extensive and exciting productivity that is unlikely to abate in future years. We now know that proteins, whether apolipoproteins, enzymes, or receptors, play an important role in lipid metabolism and they are expected to continue receiving attention at various levels of endeavor.

The topics mentioned in the preceding overview were covered in a series of lectures given to graduate students in Biochemistry at the University of Chicago during the spring of 1983. With suitable updating, they are now presented in this book. Its preparation was prompted by the need for ready access to background material as an aid to students in the classroom, in the library, and at the laboratory bench. We have attempted to provide a selective coverage of important subjects in the lipoprotein field but not to produce an exhaustive treatise. In consequence, the reader will find inevitable omissions that should be viewed not as a lack of appreciation of significant work by highly qualified investigators but as a need to distill and condense much valuable information into a volume of a manageable size. The authors have responded well to our request for conciseness and clarity and we wish to thank them for their fine and timely contributions.

Angelo M. Scanu
Arthur A. Spector

Contributors

Ann L. Akeson University of Cincinnati College of Medicine, Cincinnati, Ohio

Jan L. Breslow, M.D. Laboratory of Biochemical Genetics and Metabolism, The Rockefeller University, New York, New York

Veneracion Cabana, M.D. Department of Medicine, The Pritzker School of Medicine, The University of Chicago, Chicago, Illinois

Gerhard A. Coetzee, Ph.D. Department of Medical Biochemistry, MRC/UCT Muscle Research Unit, University of Cape Town Medical School, Observatory, South Africa

Glyn Dawson, Ph.D. Departments of Pediatrics, Biochemistry, and Molecular Biology, The Pritzker School of Medicine, The University of Chicago, Chicago, Illinois

Donna Driscoll, Ph.D.* Department of Pathology, The Pritzker School of Medicine, The University of Chicago, Chicago, Illinois

Celina Edelstein Department of Medicine, The Pritzker School of Medicine, The University of Chicago, Chicago, Illinois

Jamal Farooqui, Ph.D. Department of Medicine, The Pritzker School of Medicine, The University of Chicago, Chicago, Illinois

---

**Current affiliation:* Laboratory of Developmental Gene Expression, Imperial Cancer Research Fund, Mill Hill Laboratories, London, England

Gunther M. Fless, Ph.D. Department of Medicine, The Pritzker School of Medicine, The University of Chicago, Chicago, Illinois

Godfrey Getz, M.D., Ph.D. Department of Pathology, The Pritzker School of Medicine, The University of Chicago, Chicago, Illinois

Wieland Gevers, Ph.D. Department of Medical Biochemistry, MRC/UCT Muscle Research Unit, University of Cape Town Medical School, Observatory, South Africa

Stephan A. Grupp, M.D. University of Cincinnati College of Medicine, Cincinnati, Ohio

Issam A. Haddad, M.D. Laboratory of Molecular and Cellular Cardiology, Children's Hospital and Department of Pediatrics, Harvard Medical School, Boston, Massachusetts

Judith A. K. Harmony, Ph.D. Department of Medicine, Pharmacology and Cell Biophysics, University of Cincinnati, College of Medicine, Cincinnati, Ohio

Rick Hay, Ph.D., M.D. Department of Pathology, The Pritzker School of Medicine, The University of Chicago, Chicago, Illinois

Andrew A. Kandutsch, Ph.D The Jackson Laboratory, Bar Harbor, Maine

Sotirios K. Karathanasis, M.D. Laboratory of Molecular and Cellular Cardiology, Children's Hospital and Department of Pediatrics, Harvard Medical School, Boston, Massachusetts

Yvonne Lange, Ph.D. Departments of Pathology and Biochemistry, Rush-Presbyterian-St. Luke's Medical Center, Chicago, Illinois

Becky M. McCarthy, M.D. University of Cincinnati, College of Medicine, Cincinnati, Ohio

Randall E. Morris University of Cincinnati College of Medicine, Cincinnati, Ohio

Elizabeth Salmon Boston University Medical Center, Boston, Massachusetts

Angelo M. Scanu, M.D. Department of Medicine, Biochemistry and Molecular Biology, The Pritzker School of Medicine, The University of Chicago, Chicago, Illinois

James R. Schreiber, M.D. Department of Obstetrics-Gynecology, The Pritzker School of Medicine, The University of Chicago, Chicago, Illinois

David W. Scupham, M.D. University of Cincinnati College of Medicine, Cincinnati, Ohio

Arthur A. Spector, M.D. Departments of Biochemistry and Internal Medicine, College of Medicine, University of Iowa, Iowa City, Iowa

Theodore L. Steck, M.D. Department of Biochemistry and Molecular Biology, The Pritzker School of Medicine, The University of Chicago, Chicago, Illinois

David B. Weinstein, Ph.D. Department of Atherosclerosis Research, Sandoz Corporation, East Hanover, New Jersey

Karl H. Weisgraber, Ph.D Gladstone Foundation Laboratories for Cardiovascular Disease, Cardiovascular Institute, Department of Pathology, University of California, San Francisco, California

Deneys R. van der Westhuyzen, Ph.D. Department of Medical Biochemistry, MRC/UCT Muscle Research Unit, University of Cape Town Medical School, Observatory, South Africa

Vassilis I. Zannis, M.D. Boston University Medical Center, Boston, Massachusetts

Contents

Preface iii

Contributors vii

1. Plasma Lipoproteins: An Overview 1
   Angelo M. Scanu

2. The Biogenesis of Lipoproteins 11
   Rick Hay, Donna Driscoll, and Godfrey Getz

3. Extracellular Posttranslational Proteolytic Processing of Apolipoproteins 53
   Celina Edelstein and Angelo M. Scanu

4. Lipoprotein(a): Biochemistry and Biology 73
   Gunther M. Fless and Angelo M. Scanu

5. Genetics of the Human Apolipoproteins 85
   Jan L. Breslow

6. Biological Membranes 145
   Theodore L. Steck

7. Membrane Cholesterol 179
   Yvonne Lange

8. Glycolipid Dynamics in Serum Lipoproteins 201
   Glyn Dawson

9. Lecithin Cholesterol Acyltransferase and Cholesteryl Ester Transfer/Exchange Proteins 223
Jamal Farooqui and Angelo M. Scanu

10. Plasma Albumin as a Lipoprotein 247
Arthur A. Spector

11. Apo B-Dependent and -Independent Cellular Cholesterol Homeostasis 281
Andrew A. Kandutsch

12. The Role of Apo E in Cholesterol Metabolism 301
Karl H. Weisgraber

13. Biological and Clinical Implications of LDL Receptors 331
Wieland Gevers, Gerhard A. Coetzee, and Deneys R. van der Westhuyzen

14. Lipoprotein Receptors in Steroidogenesis 359
James R. Schreiber and David B. Weinstein

15. Immunoregulation by Plasma Lipoproteins 403
Judith A. K. Harmony, Ann L. Akeson, Becky M. McCarthy, Randall E. Morris, David W. Scupham, and Stephan A. Grupp

16. Lipoprotein Disorders: Defects of Apolipoproteins, Enzymes, and Receptors 453
Angelo M. Scanu, Veneracion Cabana, and Arthur A. Spector

Appendix 1: Nucleotide and Corresponding Amino Acid Sequences of Human Apo A-I, Apo A-II, Apo C-I, Apo C-II, Apo C-III, and Apo E cDNA Clones 475
Sotirios K. Karathanasis, Issam A. Haddad, Elizabeth Salmon, and Vassilis I. Zannis

Appendix 2: General Properties of Plasma Lipoproteins and Apolipoproteins 495
Celina Edelstein

Index 507

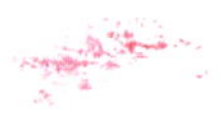

1

Plasma Lipoproteins: An Overview

ANGELO M. SCANU The Pritzker School of Medicine, The University of Chicago, Chicago, Illinois

INTRODUCTION

The plasma lipoproteins are water-soluble complexes containing specific proteins, apolipoproteins, and lipids, free cholesterol and esters, phospholipids, and triglycerides (1). These lipoproteins all recognize a common structural organization that is characterized by a hydrophobic core composed of cholesteryl esters and triglycerides surrounded by a relatively more hydrophilic shell comprised of proteins, phospholipids, and unesterified cholesterol projecting their hydrophilic domains into the aqueous environment. A model for high-density lipoproteins proposed in 1977 by Shen et al. (2) is shown in Fig. 1. The most commonly adopted classification of plasma lipoproteins is based on their behavior in the ultracentrifuge in high-salt media (Fig. 2). According to their flotational characteristics, the lipoproteins have been classified as very low density (VLDL), low density (LDL), and high density (HDL), each exhibiting density heterogeneity and differences in size and protein lipid distribution (2). This property is exploited in their separation by isopycnic density gradient ultracentrifugation, where each lipoprotein bands in an equilibrium region where its buoyant density spent coincides with that of the salt medium. Chylomicrons, which accumulate in the plasma after a fatty meal, are usually not classified according to their hydrated density; they have a very high flotational rate and thus move rapidly to the top of the collection tube even in the absence of a gravitational field.

Plasma lipoproteins can also be separated by electrophoretic methods in various supporting media. According to their electrophoretic migration, they can be classified as pre-beta- (VLDL), beta- (LDL), and alpha-lipoproteins (HDL) (Fig. 3). Chylomicrons stay at the origin.

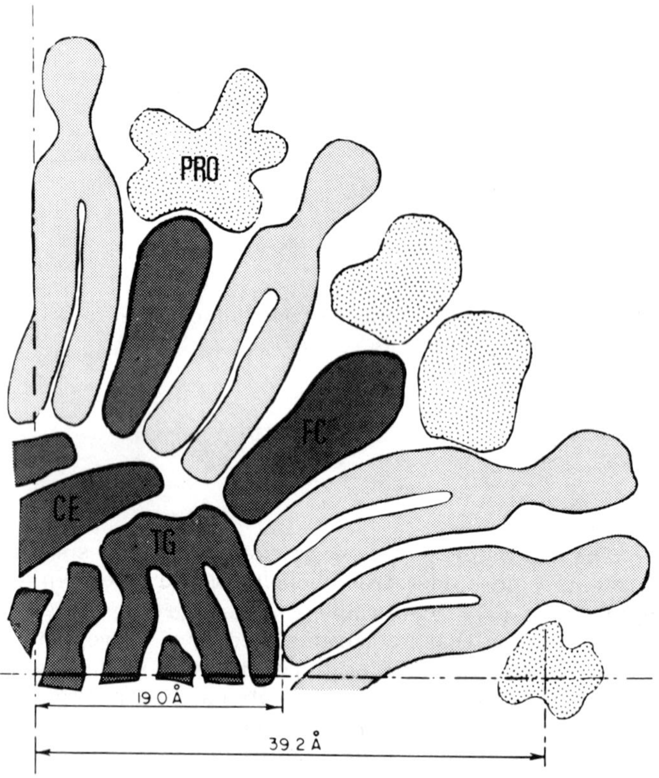

Fig. 1 Structural model of HDL_3 according to Shen et al. (2). PL, phospholipids; FC, free cholesterol; PRO, protein, CE, cholesteryl esters; TG, triglycerides.

Several subspecies comprise each liproprotein class. For some of them there are questions whether they are real or artifactual, but in general they appear to have distinct functions. Plasma lipoproteins represent dynamic structures subject to exchange and transfer processes as well as remodeling; however, as ultracentrifugal isolates they can be considered discrete entities. Each of them is associated with apolipoproteins in varying concentrations and distribution (Fig. 4).

The main characteristics of each main lipoprotein class are outlined below.

CLASS	SIZE Å	DENSITY gm/ml	S_f (1.063)	PLASMA CONC. mg/100ml	APPROXIMATE COMPOSITION (% WEIGHT) 10 30 50 70 90
CHYLO-MICRONS				0 to 50	
VLDL	700	0.96	400		
LDL_1	400	1.019	12	225	
LDL_2	200	1.063	0	350	
HDL_2	120	1.125		100	
HDL_3	75	1.21		200	
$VHDL_1$		1.25		10	
$VHDL_2$	?	>1.25		?	

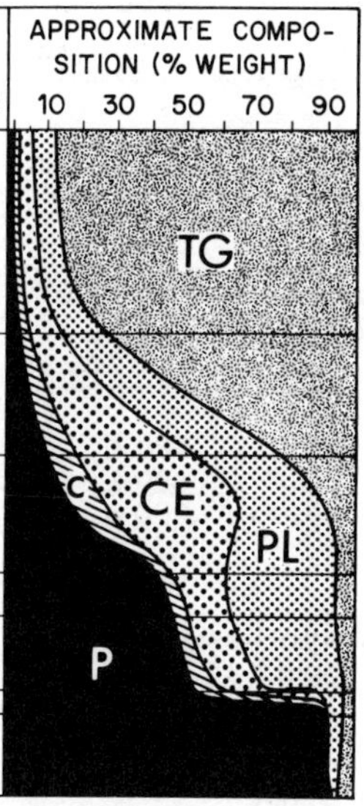

Fig. 2 Schematic distribution of the major classes of plasma lipoproteins according to their flotation in the analytical ultracentrifuge. For each lipoprotein class, the apolipoprotein components are listed.

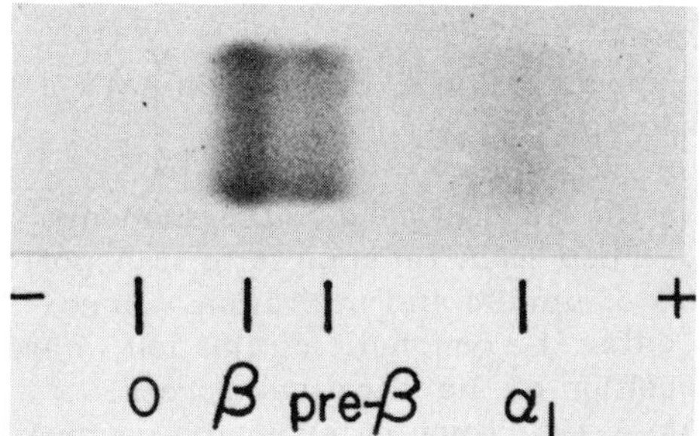

Fig. 3 Agarose gel electrophoretic protein of a human serum. Staining with Sudan black. The chylomicrons, if present, would remain at the origin.

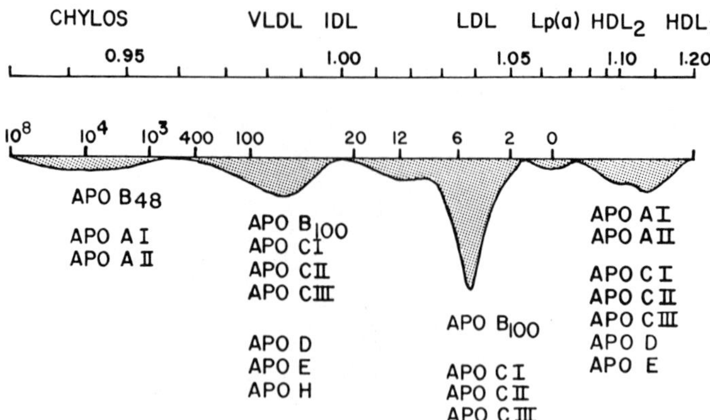

Fig. 4 A synthesis of the physical and chemical properties of the major plasma lipoproteins.

CHYLOMICRONS

Source: intestine
Density: <0.95 mg/ml
Size: 800–1000 A
Total lipid, % total particle mass: 98
  Lipid classes, % total lipids:
    Triglycerides ∿90
    Phospholipids ∿8
    Cholesterol ∿5
Protein, % total particle mass: 2
  Major components: apo B48, apo A-I, apo A-II, and apo A-IV
  Minor components: apo Cs and apo E

The chylomicrons are synthesized in the mucosal cells of the duodenum and jejunum during fat absorption. Their main function is to transport the triglycerides to the cellular sites of uptake and utilization. Once synthesized by the intestine, they enter the lymphatic circulation where they retain the apolipoprotein composition of the intestinal mucosa: apo B48, apo A-I, apo A-II, and apo A-IV. Upon entering the general circulation via the thoracic duct, they acquire additional apolipoproteins, namely apo Cs and apo E, from their interaction with other lipoproteins. By acquiring apo C-II, they become suitable for attack by the enzyme lipoprotein lipase at the levels of the endothelial cell surface; within minutes they are transformed into remnants which are structures impoverished in triglycerides through lipolysis and enriched in apo Cs and cholesteryl esters through the action of the cholesteryl ester exchange/transfer protein. These remnants are taken up by the liver via the apo E receptor whereas the surface components, mostly apo A-I and phospholipids, are transferred to HDL_3, contributing to the transformation of this lipoprotein subspecies into HDL_2. Thus, chylomicrons enter in the process of remodeling plasma HDL.

Scheme of Metabolism of Plasma Chylomicrons

Chylomicrons —Lipoprotein lipase / Apo C-II→
- Chyl remnants → apo E receptor, liver
- Phospholipids / Apo A-I → HDL_3 → HDL_2

From the above it is apparent that once they reach the general circulation, chylomicrons undergo restructuring by partial lipolysis and then reenter the cell for degradation. This explains why in familial disorders where either lipoprotein lipase or its cofactor apo C-II is absent, very high levels of chylomicrons accumulate in the plasma.

VERY-LOW-DENSITY LIPOPROTEINS

Source: liver
Density: 0.95–1.006 g/ml
Size: 280–800 A
Lipid content, % particle mass: 90
  Lipid class, % total lipids:
    Triglycerides ∿60
    Cholesterol ∿17
    Phospholipid ∿20
Protein content, % particle mass: 10–12
  Major apolipoproteins: apo B100, apo Cs, and apo E
  Minor apolipoproteins: apo A-I, apo A-II, and apo B48

The liver synthesizes and secretes essentially all of the VLDL particles present in the fasting plasma. VLDL are heterogeneous in size and density; each subspecies differs in chemical composition and likely metabolic fate. All of the VLDL particles undergo hydrolysis by lipoprotein lipase and are transformed first into intermediate-density lipoproteins (IDL) and then into LDL. The role of hepatic lipase in this lipolytic cascade has not been clearly established. There is no loss of apo B during these conversions, whereas the minor apolipoproteins together with some phospholipids and unesterified cholesterol are transferred to the HDL class. Thus, following lipolysis there are two avenues of degradation for plasma VLDL: uptake as remnants via the apo B,E receptor in the liver cells, and transfer of surface components to heavier lipoproteins.

Scheme of VLDL Metabolism in the Plasma

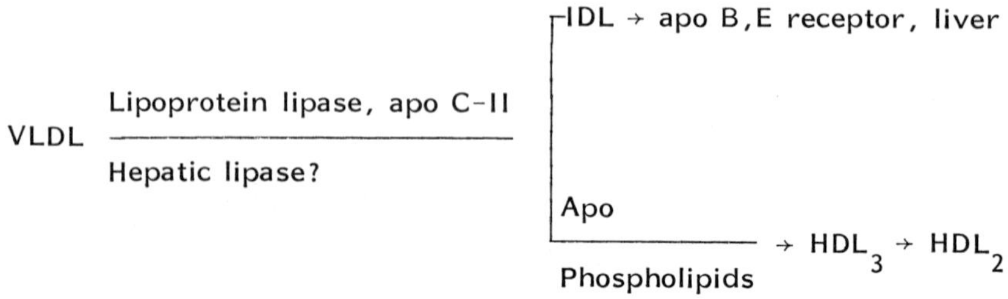

IDL → apo B,E receptor, liver

VLDL —Lipoprotein lipase, apo C-II / Hepatic lipase?—

Apo / Phospholipids → HDL_3 → HDL_2

The VLDL particles are known to migrate electrophoretically in the pre-B position. However, in man following a diet rich in cholesterol and also in experimental animals, a VLDL class with β-migration appears in the circulation. Patients with familial type III hyperlipoproteinemia or dysbetalipoproteinemia also exhibit a β-migrating VLDL. These VLDL species contain about 40% triglycerides and 35% cholesterol, mostly cholesteryl esters, apo B (both apo B100 and apo B48), and apo E; they are taken up by the cells by a dual mechanism—the apo E and the apo B,E receptors.

LOW-DENSITY LIPOPROTEINS

Source: plasma
Density: 1.006–1.063 g/ml
Size: 200–250 A
Lipid content, % particle mass: 75
  Lipid classes, % total lipids:
    Cholesterol ∿60
    Phospholipids ∿30
    Triglycerides ∿10
Protein content, % particle mass: 25
  Major protein: apo B100
  Minor proteins: apo Cs and apo E

Two main subclasses of LDL are recognized: LDL-1, d 1.006–1.019 g/ml, and LDL-2, d 1.019–1.063 g/ml. Additional LDL subclasses can be isolated by density gradient ultracentrifugation. The question as to whether all of these subspecies represent products of the degradation cascade of VLDL or are distinct metabolic entities has not yet been clearly resolved (3). It is apparent, however, that apo B_{100} is the main component in the plasma. In pathological conditions such as homozygous familial hypercholesterolemia there is evidence to suggest that LDL may be secreted directly from the liver. Additional LDL-related particles, Lp(a), are also present in the plasma in different levels. These particles are characterized by the presence of apo B and apo(a) covalently linked to each other by disulfide bridges. The physiological significance of this lipoprotein class is unknown. For details, see Chapter 2.

In terms of LDL catabolism, the work by Goldstein and Brown (4) has established that many peripheral cells as well as the hepatocytes have a receptor which by interacting with LDL via apo B promotes the specific internalization of this lipoprotein particle followed by its hydrolysis in the lysosomes. This internalization process is attended by a set of events: increase in the free cholesterol levels in the cell, decrease in cholesterol production through the inhibition of the enzymes 3-hydroxy-3-methylglutaryl CoA (HMGCoA reductase), and increase in cholesteryl ester formation through the activation of the acyl CoA: cholesterol acyl transferase (ACAT). The synthesis of the LDL receptors is also down-regulated to prevent cholesterol from entering the cell (for details see Chapter 13). When the LDL receptors (also referred to as apo B,E receptors because they interact with both apo B and apo E) are saturated, the entry of the LDL particles into the cell occurs via the independent receptor pathway, which is not subject to regulation. The cholesterol entering through this route accumulates in the cell (see Chapter 13). This scavenger mechanism is prevalent in patients with homozygous familial hypercholesterolemia who lack functional apo B,E receptors. This may be responsible for the development of premature atherosclerosis in these subjects.

Scheme of LDL Metabolism in the Plasma

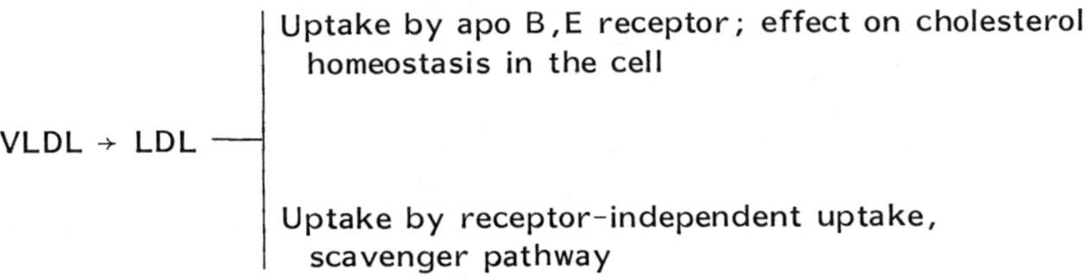

Other receptors have been described for the uptake of modified LDL particles. They are discussed in Chapter 13.

HIGH-DENSITY LIPOPROTEINS

Source: intestine, liver, chylomicrons, others?
Density: 1.063–1.21 g/ml
Size: 50–150 A
Lipid content, % particle mass: 50
  Lipid classes, % total lipids:
    Cholesterol ∿32
    Phospholipids ∿50
    Triglycerides ∿10 5%
Protein content, % particle mass: 50
  Major proteins: apo A-I and apo A-II
  Minor proteins: apo Cs, apo D, and apo E

There are two major subclasses of HDL: HDL2, d 1.063–1.125 g/ml, and HDL3, d 1.125–1.21 g/ml. They also differ in size (HDL_2, average 85–90 Å, HDL_3, 70–75 Å) and in apoprotein distribution, and probably represent lipoproteins in a different stage of maturation and remodeling (5). The third subclass of HDL, referred to as HDL_1 (d 1.03–1.10 g/ml), has the same characteristics of HDLc, a lipoprotein which increases in animals or men fed a high cholesterol diet. The size of this lipoprotein is between 130 and 250 Å in diameter, and it contains mainly apo E and apo A-I and is taken up by the cells via the apo E and the apo B,E receptors. From the functional standpoint it is unclear whether HDL_1 and HDLc are comparable. In general, the actual interrelationships among HDL_1, HDL_2, and HDL_3 have not been clearly established. An attractive postulate is that HDL_3 is transformed into HDL_2 following integration of the surface components liberated from the hydrolysis of the triglyceride-rich particles by lipoprotein lipase. HDLc would result from the incorporation of apo E and some cholesterol into HDL_2 in the plasma. The molecular details of the interconversion among HDL particles have not been worked out, but these processes appear to require the action of the enzymes lipoprotein lipase, lecithin-cholesterol acyl transferase (see Chapter 9), and hepatic lipase. The latter has been suggested to have specificity of action for HDL_2 and to cause this lipoprotein to revert to HDL_3. However, the role of the cholesteryl ester exchange/transfer proteins in these processes (see Chapter 9) cannot be ruled out. Overall we may be dealing with a complex set of equilibria influenced by the rate of entry of nascent HDL into the plasma, the plasma levels of triglyceride-rich particles, the activity of the various lipid-modifying enzymes, and the rates of lipoprotein uptake and degradation by the cells. Although it is established that apo A-containing particles are taken up by several organs like the liver, steroidogenic tissues, and the kidney, comparatively little is known of the exact molecular mechanism of this uptake (6). Some have postulated the existence of an apo A-I receptor, while others have questioned its specificity and, in fact, its existence.

This is an issue that is likely to remain unresolved until the putative receptor is isolated. A more unanimous support has received the concept that HDLs are involved in the mechanism of reverse cholesterol transport, i.e., the movement of cholesterol from the peripheral tissues to the liver. The factors involved in the regulation of cholesterol efflux and transport have not been clearly established (see Chapter 7). Some have postulated the occurrence of a receptor regulation involving apo A-I-containing particles, some a simple cholesterol gradient effect, some a diffusion process regulated by the solubility of free cholesterol in solution, and some have stressed the need of having an active LCAT system and a suitable cholesterol acceptor. It is reasonable to postulate that the reverse cholesterol transport mechanism recognizes multiple regulatory factors and that, depending upon the conditions of the system, cholesterol in its unesterified form either enters or exits the cells. The number of HDL species and their multiple functions appear to be in keeping with the structural flexibility of the HDL class. Their important role in lipoprotein metabolism is well exemplified by the knowledge of disturbances attending the deficiency states of these lipoproteins or by the presence of abnormal apolipoprotein variants (for details see Chapter 16). For many years our thoughts in terms of lipoprotein metabolism have been largely influenced by the notion of lipoprotein complexes isolated by physical methods, particularly the ultracentrifuge. The explosive developments in the apolipoprotein field have led to technical and conceptual changes also favored by the recent studies on the biosynthesis of these apolipoproteins and their mechanism of integration into the mature lipoproteins (see Chapters 2 and 3). Through the use of immunoaffinity columns (7,8), rapid progress is being made in the isolation of lipoproteins containing a single apolipoprotein species, and this is paving the way to the understanding of their structural and functional relationships. LDL particles containing only apo B can readily be prepared; unfortunately, progress in this area has been hampered by the lack of knowledge of the properties of apo B in spite of the information that has rapidly been gathered on its role in cellular cholesterol homeostasis via the apo B,E receptor (see Chapter 13). Apo A-I-containing lipoproteins have been identified but their functional significance is still undetermined. Lipoproteins containing predominantly but not exclusively apo E have been isolated under pathological conditions (cholesterol feeding, type II hyperlipoproteinemia), but their physiological significance has not been established. Immunoaffinity techniques are not free of potential artifacts and must be considered to be at least at the same level as those occurring when the more "established" techniques of lipoprotein analysis and preparation are utilized. There is a need for reexamining the old scheme of classification and for introducing new concepts and technologies so that lipoprotein particles in their nascent state and in their various stages of maturation are identified. There is also a need for assessing the specificity of lipid association of each apolipoprotein and its isoform. The use of monoclonal antibodies should aid in this regard and the recent published results are reason for optimism in this direction.

REFERENCES

1. Assmann, G., *Lipid Metabolism and Atherosclerosis*, Schattauer, Verlag, Stuttgart, Germany, pp. 1-246 (1982).

2. Shen, B. W., Scanu, A. M., and Kezdy, F. J., *Proc. Natl. Acad. Sci. U.S.A.*, *74*:837–841 (1977).

3. Havel, R. J., *J. Lipid Res.*, *25*:1570–1576 (1984).

4. Goldstein, J. L., and Brown, M. S., *J. Lipid Res.*, *25*: 1450–1461 (1984).

5. Scanu, A. M., Edelstein, C., and Gordon, J. I., *Clin. Phys. Biochem.*, *2*:111–122 (1984).

6. Pittman, R. C., and Steinberg, D., *J. Lipid Res.*, *25*:1577–1585 (1984).

7. Kanitake, S. T., and Kane, J. P., *J. Lipid Res.*, *23*:936–940 (1982).

8. Cheung, M. C., and Albers, J. J., *J. Biol. Chem.*, *259*: 12,201–12,209 (1984).

2

The Biogenesis of Lipoproteins

RICK HAY, DONNA DRISCOLL,* and GODFREY GETZ
The Pritzker School of Medicine, The University of Chicago, Chicago, Illinois

OVERVIEW

Plasma lipoproteins are assemblies of lipid and protein components associated by noncovalent bonds. These particles can be found circulating in the extracellular space in the bloodstream, in the lymph, and in the cerebrospinal fluid. All plasma lipoproteins are similar in their basic structure, each having a hydrophobic core of neutral lipid (cholesteryl ester, triglyceride) and a surface of polar lipids (phospholipid, free cholesterol) and amphipathic apolipoproteins. However, they comprise a complex mixture of macromolecular structures heterogeneous in their origin, their detailed biochemical structure, and their function; they are also subject to considerable metamorphosis between the time they appear in the circulation and the time they are degraded.

The purposes of this chapter are to review what is known about the production of the different plasma lipoprotein classes in a systematic fashion and then to present what we think are the important unknown facets of lipoprotein production and to suggest avenues for future research.

Production of plasma lipoproteins in higher eukaryotes is one of the most intricate of secretory pathway functions. As in the case of simpler, "soluble" secretory products, individual apolipoproteins are translated in a structural or conformational precursor form, segregated into the lumen of the rough endoplasmic reticulum (RER), modified posttranslationally in the RER and in the Golgi apparatus, and then released from the cell by exocytosis. In sharp contrast to the soluble secretory products, individual apolipoproteins combine with lipids as well as with molecules of other, nonidentical apoprotein species to form the particles we recognize as mature lipoproteins.

**Current affiliation:* Imperial Cancer Research Fund, Mill Hill Laboratories, London, England

In addressing the topic of plasma lipoprotein production, then, the following parameters must be considered: (1) cellular acquisition of substrates for the synthesis of individual lipid, protein, and carbohydrate moieties of plasma lipoproteins; (2) biosynthesis of these individual components and their distribution to elements of the secretory pathway; (3) coalescence of the lipid and protein components into particles; (4) maturation of both particles and nonparticulate components as they move transcellularly; (5) secretion of particles and nonparticulate components; and (6) modification of the newly secreted particles and nonparticulate components after they enter the extracellular compartment.

It was originally thought that lipoproteins are fully formed within the cell and that lipoprotein particles leaving the cell are essentially identical to their circulating counterparts. Research from many laboratories has forced a reexamination of this notion. The most significant new findings are (1) that some apolipoproteins may be secreted initially in lipid-deficient form, (2) that extensive redistribution of apolipoproteins among different particulate forms and between particulate and nonparticulate pools begins shortly after their arrival in the circulation, and (3) that the apoproteins themselves continue to be covalently modified after release from the cell.

Some apoproteins can be synthesized and secreted by a variety of cell and tissue types, given the proper physiologic stimulus. Nevertheless, it still seems to hold true that the *nascent* forms of particles we designate very-low-density lipoproteins (VLDL), high-density lipoproteins (HDL), and chylomicrons derive predominantly from liver and intestine, even if some of the components found in *mature* circulatory particles may be appended from other tissue sources once the primary particles have been secreted.

Lipoprotein biosynthesis is only one of many factors that determine the steady-state concentrations of lipoproteins in the plasma. The lipoprotein system of the plasma and extracellular fluid is a complex one depending upon the production of lipoprotein particles and components, upon lipoprotein processing within the plasma, upon component interchange among lipoproteins within the plasma, and finally upon the tissue uptake of intact lipoproteins and lipoprotein components. Most of these processes are considered in detail elsewhere in this volume. Although many of these processes can be broadly considered aspects of lipoprotein production, inasmuch as they help to determine the formation of major classes of lipoproteins found in the plasma, they will be reviewed here only in the brief outline needed for coherence in our discussion. Reference will be provided to specific treatises on these issues where appropriate. Because it is generally held that the structural and metabolic uniqueness of an individual lipoprotein class is a function of its apoprotein content and conformation, this chapter will focus on the production, processing, and distribution of apoproteins among lipoprotein components.

The plasma lipoproteins can be classified into four classes based on their flotational density in the ultracentrifuge. Each class of lipoproteins displays a broad characteristic lipid and apolipoprotein profile, although there is a great deal of heterogeneity even within a single lipoprotein class. The intestine secretes chylomicrons and VLDL, large triglyceride-rich particles that transport dietary triglyceride to extrahepatic tissues for energy or storage (1). Triglyceride-rich VLDL are also synthesized by the liver and carry endogenously synthesized lipid to extrahepatic tissues for energy or storage. The third class of lipoproteins, low-density lipoproteins (LDL), are probably not secreted by either organ, but instead are generated by the intravascular catabolism of VLDL (2). LDL that are rich in cholesteryl ester deliver cholesterol to peripheral cells for membrane or steroid synthesis (3). High-density lipoproteins contain phospholipid and cholesterol and are secreted by both the liver and intestine, although the hepatic and intestinal particles differ somewhat in their structure and composition (4).

NASCENT LIPOPROTEINS ARE REMODELED TO FORM MATURE LIPOPROTEINS

Nascent Lipoproteins (Fig. 1)

In attempting to define "nascent" lipoproteins, i.e., precursors to mature lipoproteins as they are secreted from the cell of origin, the high potential for postsecretory modification of these particles beginning shortly after their secretion has to be kept in mind. Because of this, many of the systems used for the study of lipoproteins are inappropriate for the true characterization of nascent lipoproteins. Only the isolation of these latter particles from a presecretory organelle (Golgi apparatus or secretory granule) or from a nonrecirculating perfusate of liver or intestine is likely to yield reliable information on the nature of such particles.

Lipoproteins collected in much more frequently employed systems, such as recirculating liver perfusion and hepatocytes in culture, are subject to the effects of extracellular lipoprotein modification and interactions. All perfusion systems and culture systems also suffer potential difficulties related to maintaining the health of tissue and of cells, and to simulating the nutritional and neuroendocrine influences that normally operate on the systems in vivo. Moreover, lipoproteins secreted in these systems are much more dilute than in vivo, a situation that may create problems for particle stability. These kinds of problems have to be kept in mind in interpreting the results obtained with these systems and in applying conclusions from them to the situation in vivo. These attendant artifacts notwithstanding, the study of lipoprotein production in isolated cell and organ systems has given us insight into a complex process that is simply not attainable through intact animal studies alone.

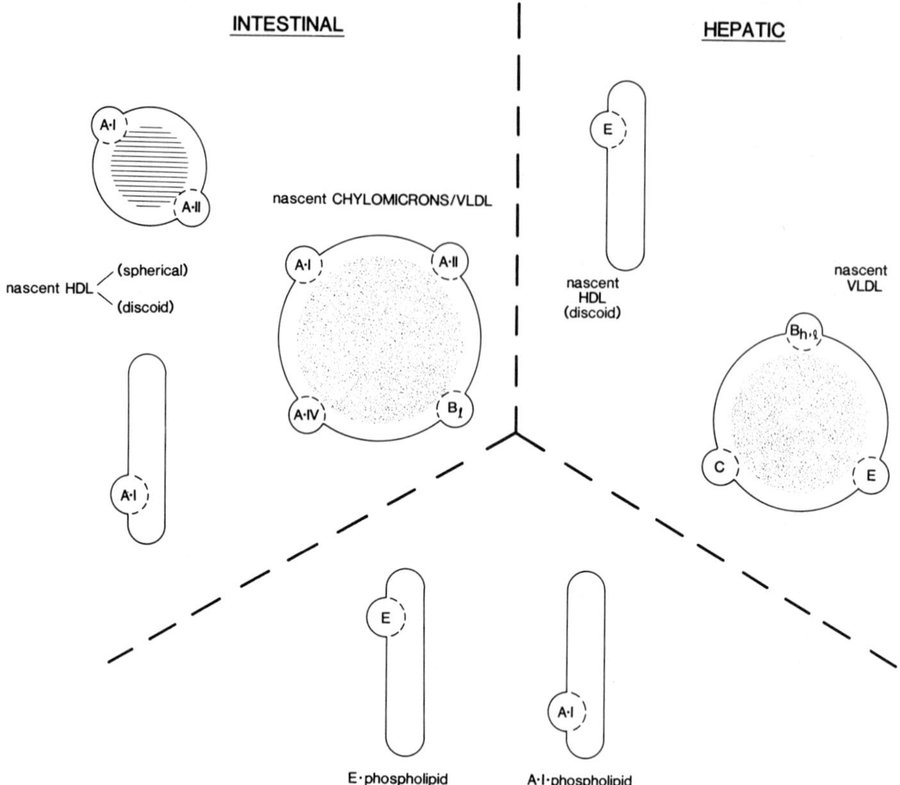

Fig. 1 Nascent lipoproteins. Primary secretory products shown or inferred to be produced by intestinal epithelium, hepatocytes, and other tissues are depicted in schematic form. In this and subsequent figures, the major apolipoproteins of each particle are represented as small circles occupying the polar lipid surface. The neutral lipid cores of the spherical particles are shown as being either predominantly triglyceride (speckled) or predominantly cholesteryl ester (hatched). The extrasplanchnic A-I:phospholipid complex has so far been detected only in avians. Please see text for apolipoprotein designations.

Intestinal Lipoproteins

Fat Absorption and Triglyceride-Rich Particles

The small intestine, predominantly the proximal portion, absorbs dietary fat as well as fats delivered into the gastrointestinal lumen in the bile. Dietary fat (mostly triglyceride) is hydrolyzed in the gastrointestinal lumen to smaller components such as free fatty acids, monoglycerides, and free cholesterol. These components are absorbed into the apical regions of the villus tip enterocytes. Here triglycerides are resynthesized, coupled with the apoproteins and other lipid components of the nascent triglyceride-rich lipoproteins, packaged in the Golgi apparatus, and secreted from the cell across the basolateral plasma membrane into the lateral intercellular space (5). Very soon after contact with other plasma lipoproteins in the blood or with those that have reached the lymph by filtration, the surface of the nascent triglyceride-rich particles is remodeled by the acquisition and exchange of surface components, i.e., phospholipid, free cholesterol, and apoproteins.

Chylomicrons

The triglyceride-rich lipoproteins produced by the intestine are chylomicrons or VLDL particles ranging in diameter from about 30 to several hundred nanometers. These two types of particles resemble one another in surface composition, but differ in size and surface-to-core ratio, mainly as a function of the flux of triglyceride through the enterocytes. Intestinal nascent VLDL particles, although behaving in the ultracentrifuge-like hepatogenous VLDL, differ significantly from the latter in apoprotein composition and have been designated by some as small chylomicrons (6). It seems that the capacity of the enterocytes to synthesize and package chylomicron surface constituents is limited. To conserve these elements, the diameter of the triglyceride-rich intestinal lipoproteins expands as the flux of the triglyceride through the enterocyte increases. Because of the rapid remodeling that occurs upon exocytosis of chylomicrons, it is difficult to characterize truly nascent particles. It is clear, however, from ancillary studies on the synthetic capacity of absorptive enterocytes (1,7) and the known interchanges in surface constituents that follow particle secretion (8), that the surface apoproteins of intestinal triglyceride-rich particles are largely apoproteins B_l, A-I, A-IV, and, in the case of humans, A-II.* Only small quantities of C apoproteins, and little or no apoprotein E,

---

*In this chapter the two major isoforms of apolipoprotein B are designated B_h (the form of greater M_r) and B_l (the form of lesser M_r). These correspond, respectively, to the forms designated B-100 and B-48 by some authors.

are present in primary secretory products of enterocytes. This conclusion has been reinforced by the demonstration that particles obtained from rat enterocyte Golgi fractions also contain predominantly apoproteins B, A-I, and A-IV (9) with very little C peptides and no detectable apoprotein E. The overall composition of the VLDL-type particle isolated from intestinal Golgi of fasting rats, 30 to 75 nm in diameter, is 12% protein, 72% triglyceride, 5% cholesteryl ester, 1% free cholesterol, and 9% phospholipid. Chylomicrons as larger particles contain much more triglyceride (86 to 92%) and much less protein (1 to 1.5%) (1). In this case the triglyceride fatty acids closely resemble those of the diet; in contrast, the phospholipids (largely lecithin) have a fatty acid composition different from that of the diet. Phospholipid and protein are present in sufficient amounts to cover the entire surface of these particles.

The protein of the mesenteric lymph chylomicrons comprises 10% apoprotein B, 50% apoprotein A-I, and 7 to 13% apoprotein A-IV with the remainder as apoprotein C (6). Following pulse labeling of enterocytes in situ, protein-associated radioactivity was distributed into apoprotein B (27%), apoprotein A-IV (12%), and apoprotein A-I (62%) of nascent Golgi VLDL (9). The B apoprotein in these particles was exclusively B_l (B-48). There was no evidence of B_h (B-100). Much of the apoprotein A-I present in mesenteric lymph lipoproteins is in the form of proapoprotein A-I (10), perhaps accounting for its ability to associate with large triglyceride-rich lipoproteins (11).

Upon entry into the venous circulation via the thoracic lymph duct, chylomicrons lose apoprotein A-IV and acquire apoprotein E and a relatively large amount of apoprotein C, mainly from plasma HDL (6) (Fig. 2). Thus, though the intestine appears to contribute little if any apo E, some of this apoprotein is essential for the subsequent metabolism of chylomicrons. Although the proportion of chylomicron mass made up of protein is small, the total flux of protein in the form of chylomicrons in the average man (corresponding to a daily absorption of 100 g of fat) is high.

Chylomicrons are rapidly removed from the plasma. The core triglycerides are hydrolyzed by capillary lipoprotein lipase, liberating free fatty acid for tissue storage or metabolism. Acquisition of cofactor apoprotein C-II is critical for this process. Removal of a large proportion of the core lipid creates a redundant surface, leading to redistribution of surplus apoprotein A-I and C apoproteins, as well as phospholipid, free cholesterol, and probably even some triglyceride to HDL. The residual particles, or chylomicron remnants, retain much of their previously acquired apoprotein E, which serves as ligand for the hepatic chylomicron remnant receptor. This high affinity receptor is responsible for the rapid and efficient removal of chylomicron remnants from the plasma. By mediating the partitioning of dietary cholesterol into the hepatocyte, this receptor regulates hepatic cholesterologenesis.

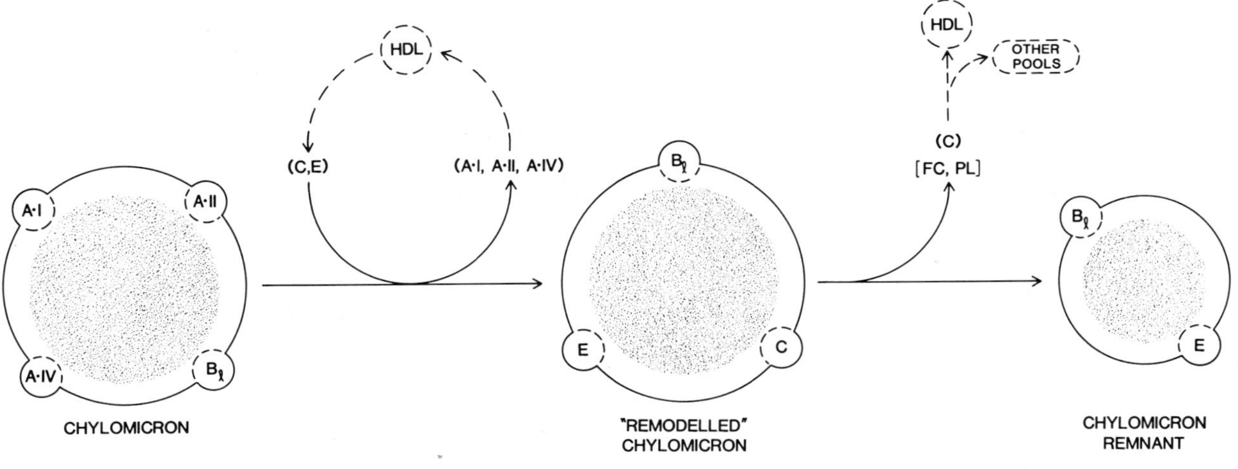

Fig. 2 Postsecretory transformations of chylomicrons. Here and in subsequent figures, transfers among particles of apolipoproteins are indicated within parentheses, while transfers of lipid components are indicated within brackets. FC, free cholesterol; PL, phospholipid. Note that apo A-IV is transferred to HDL in rats, but probably to a nonlipoprotein pool in humans. Also, some apo A-I remains on chylomicron remnants in rats.

Apoprotein B_1 does not appear to be a positive effector of this uptake mechanism (12,13), nor does the absolute ratio of apoproteins E and C on the surface of these particles (14). The intravascular remodeling of chylomicrons or their remnants does not result in the production of plasma LDL (15).

LDL

Few if any particles in the LDL density range arise from the intestine. The small amounts of LDL found in mesenteric or thoracic duct lymph probably represent LDL filtered from the plasma.

Nascent HDL

Apoprotein A-I is distributed among the lipoproteins originating from the intestine as a major component of chylomicrons and at least two particles in the HDL density range. Two estimates have been given for the distribution of apoprotein A-I between triglyceride-rich lipoproteins and denser lipoproteins. In one study 85% of apo A-I was in the dense fraction of lymph of fasting rats and 50% in the lymph of fed rats (16); the corresponding figures were 30 to 40 and 4 to 18%, respectively, in a second study (8). Examination of the HDL-containing apoprotein A-I revealed at least two entities. One is a discoid particle containing predominantly apoprotein A-I, rather than apoprotein E, and with a 7:1 phospholipid-to-free-cholesterol ratio. These particles represent a larger proportion by mass (50%) of HDL-type particles in the lymph of fasted rats than in fed rats (17). The difficulty of ascertaining the origin of lymph HDL is compounded by the filtration of some plasma HDL. However, a second smaller unique spherical HDL particle has also been described in the lymph of rats (4). Its cholesteryl ester appears to result from the activity of intestinal acylcoenzyme A:cholesterol acyltransferase (ACAT), distinguishing it from plasma HDL. Apoprotein A-I has also been reported to be secreted by pig intestinal organ cultures in forms not associated with lipid (18).

The significance of discoid lymphatic particles is not clear. Although these are generally assumed to be nascent lipoprotein forms, some reservations about this interpretation have been expressed recently by Eisenberg (11). An alternative possible origin is the redundant surface of recently secreted triglyceride-rich particles that had undergone particle lipolysis, perhaps mediated by intestinal macrophage lipases.

Hepatic Lipoproteins

VLDL

Unlike chylomicrons and HDL, newly secreted hepatogenous VLDL bears a striking resemblance to mature plasma VLDL. Indeed, this similarity also holds true for nascent VLDL isolated from the hepatocytic

Golgi apparatus. Newly secreted VLDL is rich in triglyceride. Its cholesteryl esters are probably formed by intrahepatic ACAT. Its apoprotein components are similar to those of plasma VLDL both in kind and in relative amounts, except that apo E is lower and apo C is proportionally higher in mature plasma VLDL. The normal hepatogenous VLDL of most species so far examined contains B_h as its exclusive apoprotein B isoform, a fact that distinguishes these particles from small chylomicrons. Rat liver, however, is unlike the liver of other species, and produces both apo B_h and apo B_l (although the identity of apo B_l of hepatic and intestinal origin has not yet been firmly established).

The composition of VLDL can be modified by dietary treatment. The diameter of VLDL particles produced by perfused rat liver and rhesus monkey liver can be modulated by the amount and class of fatty acid furnished in the perfusate (19; T. Teramoto, unpublished observations). The feeding of cholesterol to rats results in production of a hepatic VLDL species enriched in cholesteryl ester and having some of the properties of beta-VLDL (20–23). Baboons and rhesus monkeys produce a cholesteryl-ester-rich VLDL after prolonged cholesterol feeding. Although it has fast pre-beta rather than beta electrophoretic mobility, this VLDL from some animal livers nevertheless has the capacity to stimulate cholesteryl ester production in macrophages (S. Bates and P. Soltys, unpublished observations). Recirculating perfusates of livers derived from responding rhesus monkeys fed high cholesterol and peanut oil ration contain a VLDL apoprotein having the electrophoretic mobility of B_l, although its identity with this apoprotein is yet to be established (P. Soltys, unpublished observations).

The major conclusion to be drawn from these observations is that the structure of "mature" plasma VLDL is largely determined at the time its nascent VLDL precursor is released from the hepatocyte, and relatively little particle remodeling occurs at this step.

VLDL Is Converted to LDL (Fig. 3)

VLDL is known to be metabolized by capillary lipoprotein lipase to yield lipolysis intermediates. This continuing process leads to the formation of intermediate-density lipoprotein (IDL). A proportion of these particles is ultimately converted by further lipolysis to LDL, in the course of which IDL surface components (phospholipid, free cholesterol, and apoproteins E and C) are lost, mainly to HDL. The proportion of VLDL converted to LDL varies considerably among species. In rats (24), rabbits (25,26), and guinea pigs (27), about 90% of VLDL is removed from the plasma prior to LDL formation. In contrast, this proportion is less than 50% in humans (28). The basis for these differences is not entirely clear. However, the hepatic LDL receptor [(B,E) receptor] is thought to be involved in the removal of IDL particles from the plasma, prior to their conversion to LDL, by the so-called

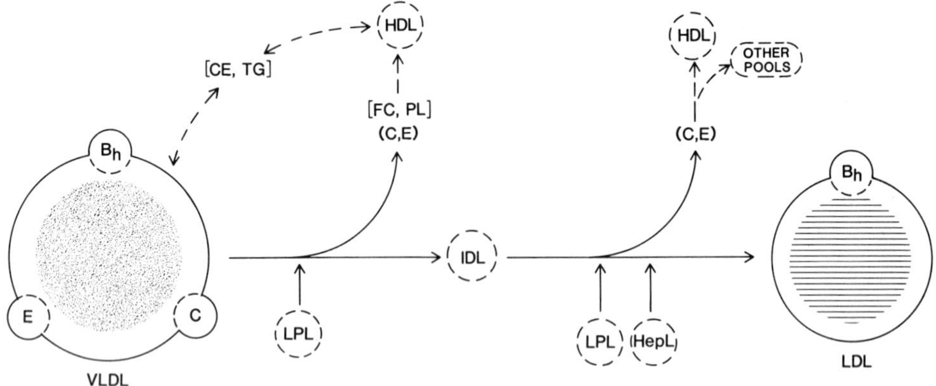

Fig. 3 VLDL is converted to LDL. This conversion is thought to take place through an intermediate-density lipoprotein particle (IDL). In addition to this major pathway, VLDL and HDL may directly exchange cholesteryl ester (CE) via cholesteryl ester transfer protein, as well as some triglyceride (TG). LPL, lipoprotein lipase; HepL, hepatic lipase.

"shunt pathway" (28). In (B,E) receptor-negative familial hypercholesterolemic humans and Watanabe hypercholesterolemic rabbits (28), there is a more substantial conversion of VLDL to LDL.

Not all VLDL subclasses are equally likely to be converted to LDL. It has recently been suggested that large "nascent" VLDL particles are very rapidly removed from the plasma without being transformed to LDL (29). Indeed, size may be one of the determinants of the conversion rate. Those animal species that rapidly clear most of their VLDL have larger VLDL particles than the average human VLDL. Intestinal triglyceride-rich particles containing apo B_l are not converted into LDL (15; R. Padley, unpublished observations). Prior determinations of the proportions of VLDL converted to LDL depend upon the tracer VLDL employed. Few of these studies have taken account of the structural and functional heterogeneity of VLDL as a precursor of LDL, suggesting that these earlier estimations may have to be revised. As we have mentioned above, the rat is exceptional among species in producing hepatogenous VLDL containing apo B_h and apo B_l. Subclasses of these particles containing only apo B_l are more rapidly removed from rat plasma than VLDL containing apo B_h (30). However, small proportions of apo B_l containing VLDL are apparently converted to LDL, as 7% of normal rat LDL apo B is apo B_l.

Can LDL Be Produced de Novo?

The vast majority of LDL is derived from VLDL. Whether LDL can be produced as a primary secretory product of the liver is not clear. Claims to this effect have been made based upon VLDL and LDL turnover experiments in whole animals and upon liver perfusion experiments. Quantitation of the results in the turnover experiments may have been complicated by the heterogeneity of VLDL. The particles within the density fraction normally encompassing plasma LDL have not always been carefully characterized. Several questions emerge in the few perfusion experiments addressing this issue. Is the material in the LDL fraction newly synthesized, i.e., does it become labeled with amino acid precursors during perfusion? Has trapped LDL or VLDL taken up radioactive amino acid in noncovalent form (31)? Is the labeled protein largely apoprotein B? Is it the result of postsecretory modification of secreted VLDL, i.e., is the "LDL" apoprotein B material present in nonrecirculating perfusates? Has account been taken of the likely effects of washout of trapped plasma LDL during the early period of perfusion? Experience with perfusions of rhesus monkey livers reveals that most material isolated in the LDL density fraction (1.006 to 1.063 g/ml) results from washout of unlabeled pools of presynthesized or trapped plasma LDL, and that most of the isotope incorporation in this fraction is into apoprotein E rather than apoprotein B. The small amount of labeled apoprotein B_h found in this fraction is associated with material that bands at the lightest end of an equilibrium gradient (0 to 10% sodium bromide), suggesting that it may result from the partial processing of secreted VLDL (32). It is, however, possible that small amounts of LDL are formed in the liver, especially in animals fed cholesterol. Swift et al. (22) have found particles of the size and apparent composition of LDL in the Golgi apparatus of cholesterol-fed rats; these particles are cholesteryl-ester-rich and may be precursors to plasma IDL (23).

The origin of Lp(a), a cholesterol-rich lipoprotein more dense than conventional LDL, is not known. This lipoprotein contains both apo B_h and the (a) antigen (33) whose site of synthesis has not been identified.

Nascent HDL Differs Markedly from Plasma HDL (Fig. 4)

Unlike VLDL and LDL particles that can be marked by their nonexchangeable apoprotein B components, HDL possesses no immobile components that permit the history of these particles to be mapped. Each of the HDL components is apparently capable of independent movement among lipoproteins and between HDL and cells. Thus the origin of plasma HDL is difficult to define in a simple fashion. Since the recognition that lecithin cholesterol acyltransferase (LCAT) plays an important role in the intraplasmatic formation of HDL cholesteryl ester, it has been assumed that particles accumulating either in the plasma or

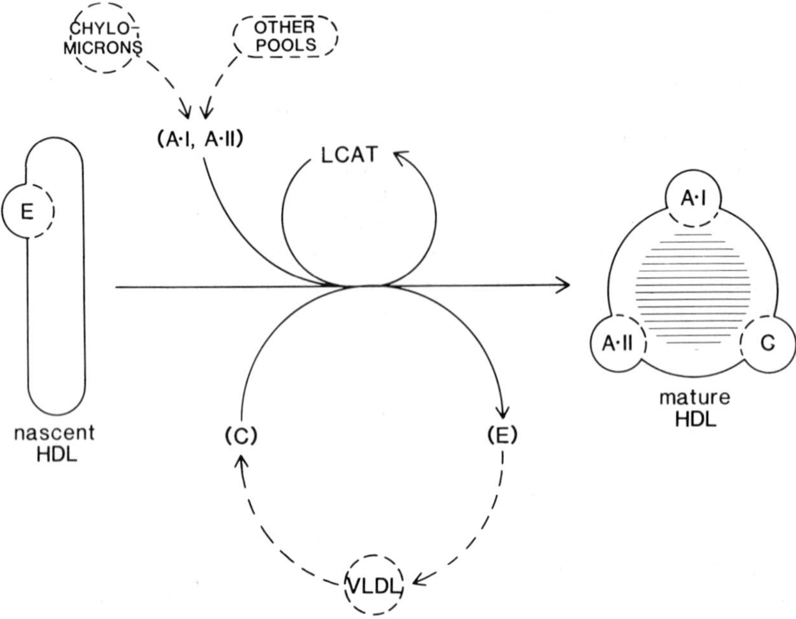

Fig. 4 Maturation of hepatic HDL. The conversion of discoid HDL to spherical HDL is thought to involve the coordinate acquisition of apo A-I (and apo A-II) and action of lecithin:cholesterol acyltransferase (LCAT); the transfer of apo E to VLDL; and the acquisition of apo C species from VLDL. Possible sources of apo A-I and apo A-II besides chylomicrons include A-I:PL complexes and lipid-free apo A-I. Certain species such as the rat retain some apo E in the mature HDL particles.

in liver perfusates in the absence of LCAT activity are related to nascent HDL. Discoid particles rich in lecithin, free cholesterol, and apoprotein E have been isolated from the plasma of patients having genetic LCAT deficiency (34) or acquired LCAT deficiency as in alcoholic hepatitis (35), as well as from perfusates in which LCAT either exhibits low activity or is intentionally inhibited (36). It is thought that these discoid particles are converted to spherical HDL particles by LCAT-catalyzed esterification of discoid-free cholesterol at the expense of the beta fatty acid of lecithin. The addition of LCAT to the plasma of LCAT-deficient patients results not only in the esterification of discoid cholesterol, the decrease in the numbers of discoid particles, and the appearance of increased apoprotein A-I in the HDL fraction, but also in the apparent displacement of HDL apoprotein E to the VLDL fraction. While discoid precursors may be converted to spherical HDL, it is not clear that all discoid lipoprotein precursors are primary secretion products of the liver or intestine. Eisenberg (11) has suggested that they may be surface products of chylomicron lipolysis, mediated perhaps by intestinal macrophage lipoprotein lipase or derived from hepatic VLDL by the action of hepatic lipase. Consistent with this conclusion are the observations that discoid particles have not been found in the secretory apparatus of either liver or intestine, and that the discoid particles of liver and intestine are associated with the major soluble transferable apoproteins E and A-I, respectively. These apoproteins and their complement of phospholipid could be derived from the triglyceride-rich lipoproteins produced by each of these tissues. Even if discoid particles can originate as the products of triglyceride-rich lipoprotein lipolysis, it is unlikely that this mechanism totally accounts for their origin. Macrophages, cultured in a serum-free medium, can produce discoid particles rich in phospholipid and apoprotein E despite the absence of triglyceride-rich particles from the medium in which they are cultured (37).

While the pathway from discoid lipoprotein precursors to plasma HDL is eminently plausible, it is by no means clear that this pathway is obligatory for the de novo synthesis of HDL. The HDL of LCAT-deficient plasma is heterogeneous and includes an HDL subfraction that is spherical but smaller than normal plasma HDL (34). In rhesus monkey liver perfusions possessing little ability to esterify cholesterol, small spherical HDL containing apoproteins A-I and A-II are observed, even in the absence of detectable concentrations of discoid apoprotein-E-rich nascent HDL (32). It is possible that this small spherical HDL is a newly secreted HDL precursor. On the other hand, discoid HDL particles rich in apoprotein E abound in the perfusates of African green monkey livers (38,39).

Mature HDL contains predominantly apoproteins A-I and (in many species) A-II. The evolution of discoid apoprotein-E-rich precursors to mature HDL involves not only esterification of free cholesterol and the loss of apoprotein E to VLDL, but also acquisition of apoprotein A-I (Fig. 4). The source of the latter apoprotein has not been clarified. Several potential sources exist. The first of these is from the surface of chylomicrons, either coupled with chylomicron phospholipid and free cholesterol or as free apoprotein. An alternative source is the new synthesis of apoprotein A-I by the liver.

The form in which apoprotein A-I leaves the liver is presently under investigation. Apoprotein A-I is secreted as a proapoprotein containing an aminoterminal extension of six amino acid residues. The hepatocytic production of proapoprotein A-I has been shown in human hepatoma cells (G2) in culture (40), in perfused rat liver (41), and in perfused rhesus monkey liver (32) and perfused baboon liver (P. Soltys, unpublished observations). However, it is not clear how much of this proapoprotein is secreted in association with lipid and how much might be secreted as lipid-free apoprotein. The secretion of proapoprotein A-I unassociated with lipid is very difficult to establish, since the possibility always exists that procedures used to fractionate lipoproteins may strip apoprotein A-I from nascent HDL. In experiments with rat liver perfusion (42) when LCAT was inhibited with dithionitrobenzene, as much as 33% of the apoprotein A-I in the perfusate was recovered in the fraction of density greater than 1.21 g/ml. With perfusion of the rhesus monkey liver, as much as 90% of the secreted apoprotein A-I may be found unassociated with lipoprotein. Many procedures, including ultracentrifugation, gel filtration (43), and nondenaturing polyacrylamide gel electrophoresis, all yield essentially similar results (32). This last technique involves no prior separation of lipoproteins and so is probably least complicated by preparative artifacts. The appearance of apoprotein A-I free of lipoprotein seems to be related to a lack of activity of LCAT. In the perfusion system it remains to be established whether cholesterol esterification is the factor limiting association of newly synthesized and secreted apoprotein A-I with HDL, or whether conversion of proapoprotein A-I to apoprotein A-I is the critical determinant. The plasma of patients with familial LCAT deficiency has an abnormal distribution of apoprotein A-I: 70 to 80% is found in the lipoprotein-free "bottom fraction" (44,45). How much of this apoprotein A-I is mature and how much is proapoprotein A-I is not yet defined. In Tangier disease, a large proportion of the small amount of apoprotein A-I in the plasma is proapoprotein A-I apparently in a lipoprotein-free state. It has recently been reported that Tangier proapoprotein A-I associates with lipid less effectively than mature normal apoprotein A-I (46). Nevertheless, the small amount of newly synthesized apoprotein A-I associated with small HDL particles in the perfusate of rhesus monkey liver is proapoprotein A-I. The role of proapoprotein A-I to apoprotein A-I conversion in the formation and maturation of HDL is not clear.

Apoprotein A-II, like apoprotein A-I, is generated and secreted as a proapoprotein with an aminoterminal extension of five amino acid residues (47). Like apoprotein A-I, newly secreted apoprotein A-II is found in the lipoprotein-free fraction (32,43) of rhesus monkey and baboon liver perfusates.

Another apoprotein associated with HDL is serum amyloid protein A (SAA), an acute phase protein inducible in mice, humans, and several other species. At least in mice SAA is synthesized in the liver; upon secretion it associates with a heavy subfraction of HDL (48).

The fate of HDL is not well understood. Transformations of HDL_3 to HDL_2, of HDL_2 to HDL_1, and of HDL_2 to HDL_3 have been described (11). It has recently been demonstrated that HDL does not necessarily disappear from the plasma as an intact particle. The rates of clearance of apoprotein A-I and of the cholesteryl ester of HDL are dissimilar, at least in relation to uptake by the liver and the adrenal (49). Moreover, HDL containing apoprotein E (HDL_1 or HDL_c) may be taken up by cells possessing either the (B,E) receptor or the E receptor (50). In humans with abetalipoproteinemia, HDL_1 is increased in amount; it is the only lipoprotein in these patients' plasma capable of being internalized by the (B,E) receptor and of regulating cellular cholesterol homeostasis and endogenous synthesis (51).

Extrahepatic Synthesis of Lipoproteins

Until very recently it was thought that only the liver and the intestine are capable of contributing to plasma lipoproteins. Several recent reports suggest that particles resembling nascent hepatic lipoproteins may be generated in the periphery. Macrophages secrete apoprotein E in the form of discoid phospholipid-containing particles (37). In cholesterol-fed dogs, discoid HDL particles containing phospholipid, apoprotein E, and free cholesterol accumulate in the peripheral lymph, which has very low LCAT activity. The addition of LCAT to this lymph results in redistribution of these components. Some apoprotein E moves to lower density lipoprotein, an event associated with the esterification of HDL cholesterol (52). Celite-loaded cholesterol or cholesterol-loaded macrophages can stimulate the conversion of HDL_3 to HDL_c (53).

Apoprotein A-I may also be synthesized in peripheral tissues of birds, especially muscle, at the time of hatching (54). Some of this apoprotein A-I seems to be secreted in association with lipid.

THE CELL BIOLOGY OF APOLIPOPROTEIN SYNTHESIS AND SECRETION

The general topic of protein synthesis and secretion has been reviewed extensively (55). Salient features of this pathway as they apply to the plasma apolipoproteins have been described in detail elsewhere (56) and may be summarized here as follows.

Expression of many proteins is regulated at the level of gene transcription. Initial transcripts of structural genes are larger than the actual coding sequences. Intervening sequences present in the initial transcripts are excised in the nucleus, in some cases by rather exotic mechanisms, in the process of RNA splicing (57). Transcripts also undergo capping at the 5' end, and poly (A) addition at the 3' end. The result of this process is a messenger RNA molecule (mRNA) that is subsequently transported to the soluble cytoplasm, probably via nuclear pores.

The detailed structures of genes coding for several apolipoprotein species have been determined during the past few years (Chapter 5). Two human apolipoprotein genes are colinear on chromosome 11 (apo C-III and apo A-I). Apolipoprotein transcripts range from about 0.1 to 1.0% of total cellular mRNA, depending upon the tissue and the species examined, making them moderate- to high-abundance mRNA species. Transcripts for apo E have not been found in intestinal epithelium under most conditions. The steady-state levels of some apolipoprotein gene transcripts have been found to change in response to metabolic and dietary perturbations. However, it is by no means clear whether these altered levels reflect changes in transcript production or in transcript turnover.

Translation of all nuclear-encoded molecules begins in the cytosol. Those nascent chains possessing the appropriate aminoterminal structure for targeting to the secretory pathway are recognized by the signal recognition particle (SRP), a ribonucleoprotein complex consisting of a 7S RNA molecule and six distinct proteins (58). While it is not known exactly how the SRP binds to a ribosome-nascent polypeptide complex, the SRP accurately discriminates between polysomes synthesizing secretory proteins-to-be and those synthesizing proteins destined to remain in the extramembranous cytoplasm or destined for nonsecretory membranous organelles (59,60). Association of SRP with the ribosome-nascent chain complex results in arrest of translation. This SRP-ribosome-nascent chain complex then binds to an SRP-receptor protein, also called docking protein, on the cytoplasmic face of the rough endoplasmic reticulum (58,61). Formation of this complex results, by mechanisms unknown, in release of the translation arrest and vectorial discharge of the elongating nascent chain across the membrane bilayer. The molecular mechanisms by which some newly synthesized proteins remain in a transmembranous state (such as viral proteins and intrinsic membrane proteins) while others are released into the RER cisternae are not fully understood (62). It is presumed, but by no means yet proven, that the plasma apolipoproteins fit into the latter class of proteins.

Soon after their entry into the RER, newly synthesized proteins undergo a series of co- and posttranslational modifications. In some instances it is not agreed whether a given modification is exclusively post- or cotranslational, so they are presented here together. The most common covalent modification is that of cleavage of the "signal peptide," the aminoterminal extension usually comprising about 20 amino acids whose primary purpose is thought to be association with SRP in the cytoplasm. The primary translation products of apo A-I, apo A-II, apo A-IV, apo C-II, apo C-III, and apo E have so far been shown or inferred to contain cleavable aminoterminal extensions (63–69). There are no structural features of these signal pieces that distinguish them from those of other secretory proteins. Nevertheless, there are some interesting homologies that await explanation.

All known signal peptides contain a polar aminoterminus, a central hydrophobic core and a charged carboxyterminus often composed of small side chain amino acids, although precise amino acid homologies are not common among signal peptides. On the other hand, it is notable that there is a high degree of homology between the signal peptides of rat apoprotein A-I and apoprotein A-IV on the one hand, and human and rat apoprotein A-I and apo E on the other (66,70). These relationships suggest that nucleotides encoding the signal peptides of the three apoproteins originate from a common ancestral exon (70). However, the precise pattern of amino acid homologies among these three apoproteins raises other possibilities. The signal peptides of apo A-I and apo A-IV are highly homologous in their core regions (63,64). In contrast, the apo A-I and apo E signal peptides, although not especially homologous in their core regions, do exhibit a high degree of homology at both termini with five of six carboxyterminal amino acids identical (66). The meaning of these unusual homologies in the signal peptides is not clear.

In addition to a signal peptide, the intracellular precursors of apo A-I and apo A-II also contain aminoterminal propeptides that are not cotranslationally removed by the signal peptidase. The five-amino-acid propeptide of human apo A-II is structurally similar to other known propeptides in that it ends with paired basic amino acids. Nevertheless, using HepG2 cells capable of accurately and efficiently removing the prosegment from proalbumin prior to secretion, Gordon et al. have shown that most of the apo A-II propeptide is first secreted prior to cleavage extracellularly to generate the mature protein (47). Both human and rat proapoprotein A-I contain a six-amino-acid propeptide that ends in paired glutamine residues, an unusual carboxyterminus for a propeptide (40,63). Like the proapo A-II, the propeptide of apo A-I is also not removed intracellularly and is secreted from the liver and intestine mostly in the propeptide form.

The second most common modification is glycosylation, which may begin before elongation of the nascent chain on the polyribosome is completed. Proteins may be glycosylated via either N- or O-linkages. N-glycosylation begins in the RER involving dolichol-linked oligosaccharide intermediates and is completed during passage of the molecules through the Golgi apparatus (71). Apo E, apo B, and apo C-III are glycosylated. Apo E does not appear to undergo N-glycosylation, despite a report to the contrary (72): not only is its glycosylation not inhibited by tunicamycin (73), but its primary structure does not include the target tripeptide (asn-x-ser[thr]) requisite for N-glycosylation (74). Apo E does undergo terminal sialylation within the Golgi, an event that partially determines the heterogeneity of circulating apolipoprotein E (75). Apo C-III, found in carbohydrate-deficient form within the rough endoplasmic reticulum of rats fed orotic acid (76), presumably acquires its full complement of O-linked sugars during its passage through the Golgi apparatus. Apo B appears to undergo N-glycosylation at two sites, at least one of which can be converted to a complex type oligosaccharide (77). Neither of the two glycosylation events is required for apoprotein synthesis, for insertion of apoprotein into nascent VLDL (nVLDL), or for particle secretion (78). Phosphorylation may also take place within the lumen of the RER. Of the apolipoproteins, only apo B has been found to be phosphorylated (79).

After traversing the RER membrane, proteins are moved along the secretory pathway to their ultimate destinations at different rates, and probably not all by an identical route through the pathway. Although there is not yet a complete model accounting for these observations, the rate-limiting step for the transcellular movement of many secretory and membrane proteins is their rate of movement out of the ER and into the Golgi apparatus (80). This process is energy dependent and requires some extramembranous cytosolic protein factors (81). Different proteins may take different routes through or around the Golgi apparatus as well, and the post-Golgi steps in secretion can be considered to constitute at least two independent pathways (82). This entire process is exceedingly complex: It has been demonstrated by Schekman and colleagues that protein secretion in yeast requires the participation of at least 23 separate genetic loci (83)! Three groups have published evidence to suggest that different classes of nascent lipoprotein particles may take different routes through the hepatocyte, specifically at the level of the Golgi apparatus (84–86). A recent report (47) provides evidence for different rates of secretion of proapo A-I and proapo A-II, and raises the possibility that these two apoproteins may traverse different limbs of the secretory pathway.

Once directed to the secretory system, secretion of a given protein seems to be the most primitive of options afforded it by the secretory organelles. That is, only proteins with specific signals for nonsecretion (direction to lysosomes, direction to remain within a specific secretory organelle) seem to be retained by the secretory apparatus of the cell; proteins having no specific indicator that they should be held up or diverted from the mainstream of membrane flow and cisternal flow are simply secreted. This notion has been reinforced by observations of the secretion of lysosomal proteins lacking the requisite mannose-6-phosphate recognition site for diversion to the lysosome, or in normal cells whose receptors are immunologically blocked (87,88; W. Brown, personal communication): the proteins produced in excess of or unable to interact with available binding sites are secreted instead. Whether similar mechanisms regulate either the assembly or the movement of lipoprotein particles is an open question.

The biosynthesis and secretion of apolipoprotein B is a complex process that is poorly understood. Two major variants of apo B are found in the plasma. There are B_h (M_r = 335 to 590 kDa) and B_l (M_r = 240 to 260 kDa) (89–91). Although it was initially believed that B_h is synthesized by the liver and B_l exclusively by the intestine, studies with intact animals and liver perfusions have demonstrated that the normal rat liver can synthesize both B_h and B_l (92,93), although the identity of B_l of hepatic origin and of intestinal origin has not yet been proved. Recent experiments with primate liver perfusions suggest that even the primate liver may be capable of synthesizing small amounts of a protein having the electrophoretic mobility of apoprotein B_l (94).

The biochemical relationship between apoproteins B_h and B_l is not clear. Although the two variants are immunologically cross-reactive and share most peptides on peptide maps (91), there are some monoclonal antibodies that recognize B_h but not B_l (95–97). Apoproteins B_h and B_l are differently modified by posttranslational processes: Apoprotein B_h contains four times as much sialic acid (per unit mass of protein) as apo B_l (G. Getz, unpublished observations); apo B_l is heavily phosphorylated (79), while apo B_h is probably not phosphorylated. These structural differences have to be taken into account in evaluating immunochemical differences between the isomorphs. The ability of at least one human subject to synthesize and secrete apo B_l even when apo B_h is absent suggests that apolipoproteins B_h and B_l may be products of different genes (98). Only apo B_l is found in enterocyte Golgi VLDL particles (9), and only apo B_l is apparently synthesized by isolated enterocytes (W. Gevers, unpublished observations). These two observations are most compatible with the two-gene hypothesis. Alternatively, the apolipoproteins B as recognized on electropherograms may be assemblies of smaller subunits, one or more of which is shared between apo B_h and apo B_l. In this model, apo B_h would have at least one unique subunit. Apolipoproteins B_h and B_l may be encoded in a single gene and the isomorphs result from the differential processing of the primary mRNA transcript. It is also possible that these two forms arise from a single primary translation product that is proteolytically processed to yield apo B_l. Indeed, kinetic data consistent with a precursor-product relationship between apo B_h and apo B_l have been generated in studies of rat liver (99): intracellular apo B_h isolated from the Golgi apparatus labels much more rapidly than intracellular apo B_l.

Whatever physiological role these two apo B isomorphs have for the assembly of lipoproteins, it is clear that they are functionally distinct. Lipoproteins containing apo B_l and not apo B_h are not readily recognized by the (B,E) receptor unless they also contain significant quantities of functionally active apoprotein E. In contrast, apo B_h-containing lipoproteins are bound and endocytosed by this same receptor (13). As we have already mentioned, lipoproteins containing apo B_l are either not processed or are very poorly processed to LDL.

In addition to these two major isoforms of apoprotein B, other isoforms have been described, most particularly isoforms designated B-74 and B-26 which can be generated by proteolytic enzymes such as kallikrein present within the plasma (100). Whether these apoproteins occur in vivo or have physiologic significance remains to be established.

SOME APOLIPOPROTEINS ARE SYNTHESIZED IN PERIPHERAL TISSUES

Recently it has become evident that many of the apolipoproteins may be synthesized by tissues other than the liver and the intestine, perhaps not necessarily involved in lipoprotein production.

In the rooster, apoprotein B is synthesized by the kidney and apoprotein A-I by the kidney, artery, vein, and skeletal muscle (101,102). Apo A-I is secreted from cultured myotubes and fibroblast cells as part of a lipid-protein complex, suggesting that apo A-I synthesized by peripheral tissues may promote cholesterol efflux from such cells (102). There is a burst of apo A-I synthesis in chicken breast muscle about the time of hatching which coincides with the hepatic accumulation of lipid from the yolk (54). The apo A-I synthesized by breast muscle may play a role in the transport, storage, or uptake of yolk lipid.

Apo E is synthesized by a broad spectrum of tissues not generally thought to be involved in lipoprotein production in humans, monkeys, marmosets, rats, mice, and guinea pigs (103–107). Apo E is fairly abundant in extrahepatic tissues representing between 0.1 and 1.0% of total protein synthesized. Tissues involved include kidney, spleen, adrenal, ovary, and brain. In the brain, astrocytes seem to be the major cell type engaged in apo E synthesis (108). Based on quantitation of messenger RNA content for apo E in each of the tissues capable of synthesizing it, as much as 35% of the total synthetic capacity for apo E appears to be situated outside the liver (109). Interestingly, very little apo E is synthesized by the intestinal mucosa, which is compatible with the finding that the rat apo E gene is more highly methylated in the intestine than in the liver or in other extrahepatic tissues (104). The fact that macrophages can synthesize apo E in vitro suggests that tissue macrophages may contribute at least in part to the extrahepatic synthesis of apo E (37). However, the magnitude of apo E synthesis in these tissues argues that other cell types are likely to be involved. Among the tissues that are fairly active in the synthesis of extrahepatic apo E are the steroidogenic organs whose synthesis may be under hormonal control.

INTRACELLULAR FORMATION OF LIPOPROTEIN PARTICLES

The complexing of lipid and protein, a process which distinguishes the secretion of apolipoproteins from virtually all other secretory products, remains an enigma despite several years of effort. Even though we do know that lipoproteins emerge from the hepatocyte and the intestinal epithelial cell as lipid and protein complexes of a more or less defined structure, we do not yet fully understand where or how in the cell the marriage of lipid and apolipoproteins takes place.

The transhepatocytic movement of spherical osmiophilic particles, presumed to be precursors to plasma VLDL, has been analyzed in detail by electronmicroscopy. Glaumann et al. (110) concluded that the initial complexing and lipidation of nVLDL apolipoproteins occur in the rough ER, and that triglyceride and phospholipid are added in stepwise fashion as the forming particles traverse the smooth ER (SER) and the Golgi apparatus. However, neither Claude (111) nor Morré and Ovtracht (84) found lipidated particles within the rough ER. Alexander et al. (112) reported that the osmiophilic nVLDL-like particles of the smooth ER do not contain immunodetectable amounts of apolipoprotein B, and therefore postulated that triglyceride-rich lipid particles originate in the SER, acquire apo B first at the RER-SER junction, and then pass directly to the Golgi apparatus. A similar VLDL assembly sequence seems to occur in the enterocyte (113).

Mahley et al. (114) isolated lipid-rich particles from a Golgi-enriched membrane fraction from hepatocytes. These particles contained all the major apoproteins of serum VLDL. Pottenger et al. (76) observed that both apo E and apo C are present as carbohydrate-deficient molecules within the distended endoplasmic reticulum of rats fed orotic acid; however, the state of protein-lipid interaction in these organelles was not rigorously defined (115). From radiolabeling studies, Nestruck and Rubinstein (116) concluded that the VLDL-like particles of the Golgi apparatus are deficient in apo C, but progressively acquire apo C during their passage through the Golgi, the secretory vesicles, and also during or after secretion into the space of Disse. Dolphin (117) found an increase in immunoassayable apo E among VLDL-like particles during movement from the Golgi cisternae to secretory vesicles, suggesting that the acquisition of a full complement of apo E by nVLDL is also a late event in particle assembly.

An obligate role for apo B in nVLDL assembly and secretion can be inferred from several observations. Humans genetically defective in apo B synthesis cannot mobilize cholesterol or triglyceride from enterocytes (118). Intestinal nVLDL can be secreted lacking apo E and apo C, but it always contains apo B. Apo B has only been detected in lipid-associated forms, whereas apo E and apo C appear to utilize a number of modes of secretion. Such data indicate that apo B plays an essential role in VLDL particle assembly and secretion, and that it is the only essential apoprotein in this respect.

The transcellular movement of particle precursors to plasma HDL has not been studied as extensively as that of precursors to VLDL, mainly because of the greater difficulty in identifying HDL particles morphologically within the cell. Howell and Palade (85) recently found that the light Golgi fraction of rat liver contains particles of the appropriate diameter and density for HDL, including apoproteins A-IV, E, A-I, C, and even B_1. Banerjee and Redman (86) also found that the apo A-I present in chicken liver Golgi apparatus displayed a density fitting for HDL, but that the apo A-I and osmiophilic particles resembling nVLDL were distributed differently among Golgi subfractions separated on the basis of their buoyant densities. Thus it appears that the subfraction of Golgi harboring newly formed nVLDL and that containing particles associated with apo A-I, which may be related to HDL, may not be identical.

The details of apolipoprotein and lipid association at the molecular level are sketchy. Even though we do not know precisely where in the

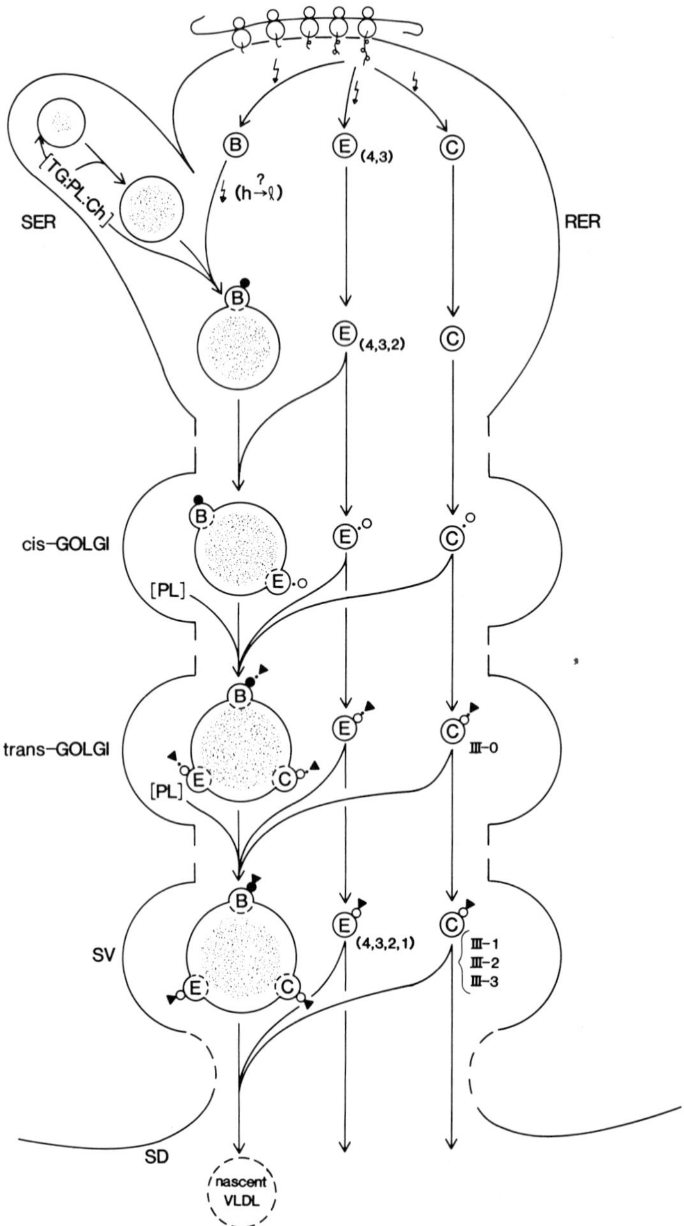
B
E (4,3)
C
[TG:PL:Ch]
(h→ℓ)
SER
RER
B
E (4,3,2)
C
cis–GOLGI
B
E
E
C
[PL]
trans–GOLGI
B
E
C
E
C
III–0
[PL]
SV
B
E
E (4,3,2,1)
C
C
III–1
III–2
III–3
SD
nascent
VLDL

Fig. 5 Proposed model of intrahepatocytic VLDL assembly. Various segments of the hepatocyte secretory pathway and their respective proposed apolipoprotein and particle contents are depicted here. Transition states indicated between organelles (----) may involve either columinal particle and apoprotein movement or interorganellar transport vesicles. Triglyceride (TG), phospholipids (PL), and cholesterol (Ch) are synthesized in the smooth endoplasmic reticulum (SER) and combined into micelles having a central core of neutral lipid, mostly triglyceride (speckled) surrounded by a layer of charged lipid (clear). Precursors to apolipoproteins B, E, and C are translated on membrane-bound polysomes of the rough endoplasmic reticulum (RER) and cleaved (⸙) by the microsomal signal peptidase to their respective intraluminal forms. Apo B undergoes core N-glycosylation (●) during or shortly after completion of translation, and proteolytic conversion of apo B_h to apo B_l may take place either in the RER or during subsequent movement of the apoproteins. Apo E is found initially as isomorphs designated 4 and 3; the more acidic isomorph 2 is generated within the RER by an as yet unknown covalent modification step, probably proteolysis (⸙). Apo C-I, apo C-II, and apo C-III are produced and probably incorporated into the nascent VLDL particle concomitantly; however, since neither apo C-I nor apo C-II is glycosylated, only the proposed pathway of apo C-III modification and insertion is shown here. At the RER-SER junction, apo B is incorporated into the mixed lipid micelle to form a primary nascent VLDL particle. First apo E, and later apo C, is added to this primary particle as it passes to and through the Golgi. Somewhere within the Golgi, additional phospholipid is added to the particle, and the particle progressively acquires more apo E and apo C molecules as it moves distally. Both free and particle-associated apo E undergo O-glycosylation (O), followed by terminal glycosylation (sialylation, ▾) within the Golgi; these modifications lead to the appearance of apo E isomorph 1. O-glycosylation of apo C-III to form apo C-III-O is followed by the addition of 0, 1, 2, or 3 molecules of sialic acid residues to form a mixture of apo C-III-0, -1, -2, and -3. At least some of the oligosaccharides of apo B are sialylated. The nascent VLDL particle found within a secretory vesicle (SV) may acquire additional apo E and apo C before or during release into the space of Disse (SD). Apo E and apo C can also be secreted as lipid-free forms or in association with nascent HDL. Incipient glycosyl linkages are indicated by a dot (●·◂) between the adduct and the acceptor molecules; formed linkages are indicated by juxtaposition of the two molecules (●◂).

cell an apoprotein *does* acquire its complement of lipid, several lines of evidence argue that apoproteins *can* associate with lipid very early in the secretory pathway. First, either postnuclear supernatant fraction, microsomes, or isolated ribosomes from rat liver homogenates can synthesize proteins with many features of apoproteins, including the ability to bind exogenously added lipid (119,120). Second, puromycin-discharged molecules of apolipoprotein B can be secreted as part of the VLDL particle (121). Finally, Pottenger and Getz (115) found a protein-lipid complex in the apoprotein-rich RER liposomes of fatty livers from rats fed orotic acid after partial detergent solubilization, but the protein composition of this complex was not examined. By using sodium carbonate rather than detergents to release organelle contents from the enveloping membranes, we have recently shown that liposomal proteins corresponding electrophoretically to apolipoproteins E, B_h, B_l, and C can be recovered in a rapidly floating lipid-rich fraction (R. Hay and R. Fleming, unpublished results). We therefore conclude that molecules of apolipoprotein can interact with lipid in a way at least superficially resembling a circulating lipoprotein particle (i.e., other than membrane associated in the organelle) as early as the endoplasmic reticulum.

It is likely that additional lipid can be added to a forming apolipoprotein-lipid particle as late as the Golgi apparatus. Using radiolabeling and kinetic analysis, Howell and Palade (85) and Janero and Lane (121) have provided evidence for at least an exchange, if not a net transfer, of lipid from the Golgi membranes into the Golgi VLDL. Even though a substantial proportion of apo A-I may be secreted in the absence of lipid, Nuñez and Swaney (122) have recently shown that purified apo A-I can under certain conditions extract lipid from isolated microsomes.

What, then, is the sequence of component acquisition by a forming lipoprotein particle? A consensus view of the observations discussed above would hold that for nVLDL, a primary core particle of apo B and associated lipid forms proximally in the secretory pathway, either within the rough ER or at the smooth ER-rough ER junction as proposed by Alexander et al. (112); that the VLDL-destined apo E and apo C components become coparticulate with the apo B during passage of the particle through the Golgi and from the Golgi to the plasma membrane; that the particle can continue to acquire lipid as it moves toward the plasma membrane; and that a certain proportion of apo E and apo C follows other routes, kinetically or spatially separate from the movement of the developing nVLDL particle (Fig. 5). Janero and Lane (121) have in fact obtained kinetic evidence that chicken liver apolipoprotein B acquires triglyceride early in nVLDL assembly, but that phospholipid is added at both early and late steps in the secretory process. Moreover, Miller and Lane (123) have recently suggested that different apolipoprotein species can compete for binding to the lipid surface of nVLDL, and that the spectrum of apolipoproteins associated with a particle can therefore be altered by changes in the levels of individual apolipoproteins within the lumen of secretory organelles. A corresponding model for intracellular HDL assembly is not easy to construct, because of the difficulty of identifying a fixed marker of the particle.

REGULATION OF LIPOPROTEIN AND APOPROTEIN BIOSYNTHESIS

Very little is known about molecular mechanisms whereby a cell increases or decreases the production rate for a particular plasma lipoprotein or apolipoprotein in response to a given metabolic stimulus. Since the time we previously reviewed this topic (124), however, there has been a dramatic increase in both the quantity and the sophistication of data regarding apolipoprotein and lipoprotein production in different metabolic settings. This section is meant both to summarize earlier observations in this field, and to incorporate more recent data and concepts.

First let us present some basic conclusions regarding the regulation of lipoprotein biogenesis:

1. One must distinguish the regulation of circulating lipoprotein levels from the regulation of lipoprotein production rates. The steady-state level of a circulating lipoprotein particle class may be affected by rates of production, rates of intravascular remodeling, rates of particle egress, or combinations of these. For example, the marked elevation of LDL in individuals with familial homozygous hypercholesterolemia is only partly attributable to an increase in LDL production rates. The defect in the structure or function of the (B,E) receptor accounts for most of the plasma LDL increment (28).
2. There is great variability in the response of different species, different organisms within a species, and different tissues within an organism to dietary and metabolic perturbation. Changes in the steady-state levels and production rates of lipoproteins vary in both direction and magnitude in response to a given metabolic stimulus. While it is relatively easy to raise plasma LDL levels in primates or rabbits by increasing their dietary cholesterol intake, species such as rats and dogs are highly resistant to cholesterol feeding in the absence of other manipulations. Different individuals within a primate species (human or nonhuman) show variable LDL levels at a given cholesterol load, a response which is at least in part genetically determined. Finally, in at least the mouse the intestinal output of apo A-I and the hepatic output of the same apolipoprotein change in opposite direction upon fat feeding.
3. Even though the circulating levels of VLDL and HDL are often related (11), their production rates are probably independently

regulated. Conditions have been found wherein the production of hepatic nascent HDL is enhanced far in excess of nascent VLDL (nephrosis); the production of nascent VLDL greatly exceeds that of nascent HDL (hypercholesterolemia); and nascent VLDL secretion can be completely arrested even though hepatic HDL secretion apparently continues (orotic acid fatty liver in rats). Humans with abetalipoproteinemia, genetically deficient in the expression of apolipoprotein B and therefore in the secretion of VLDL, nonetheless produce HDL.

4. The events that regulate apolipoprotein and lipid production rates are not tightly coupled. As we discussed earlier, the ability of enterocytes to vary their rates of production of lipoprotein surface components—apolipoproteins and phospholipids—is apparently more limited than their ability to absorb, resynthesize, and mobilize fat. The result of this limitation is that a range of particle sizes can be secreted, with a narrowly fixed surface stoichiometry but with a variable surface-to-core-mass ratio, reflecting the flux of triglyceride precursors through the enterocyte. A similar pattern holds for hepatic VLDL particles, although the excursion of surface-to-core ratio is not as great as for the intestinal particles.

With these general conclusions in mind, let us now examine in more detail a few of those factors found to be important in regulating plasma lipoprotein production. Factors affecting circulating plasma lipoprotein levels have been widely reviewed elsewhere.

Genetic Factors

Genetic variation has been shown to influence either the rate of expression or the structure of several apolipoproteins, with a wide spectrum of physiological consequences. These are discussed in depth by Breslow in Chapter 5.

Dietary Factors

Carbohydrate

Diets high in carbohydrate enhance VLDL production by the liver, probably both by direct stimulation of fatty acid synthesis (125) and by indirect hormonal effects. The influence of ethanol on VLDL production by the liver is probably due to increased availability of intracellular free fatty acids (126), resulting from the combination of reduced oxidation and increased synthesis. Virtually nothing is known about these regulatory phenomena at the molecular level.

Fatty Acid

The most obvious factor to influence plasma lipoprotein production is the supply of lipid and lipid substrates. Hepatic VLDL production rate increases in response to any of several factors that increase the delivery of fatty acids to the liver or that enhance hepatic fatty acid synthesis, e.g., ethanol, free fatty acid mobilization from adipocytes, and fatty acid absorption by the gut (presented to the liver later as chylomicron remnants). This enhanced VLDL production is attributable to increased triglyceride production and in some cases also to increased VLDL apoprotein production (127). All fatty acids are not equally effective at stimulating VLDL production. Larger VLDL particles are produced in response to unsaturated fatty acids than to saturated fatty acids; longer chain fatty acids are more stimulatory than are shorter chain fatty acids; and unsaturated fatty acids are more stimulatory than are saturated fatty acids of the same chain length (19,128).

Cholesterol

General effects: The effects of cholesterol feeding have been reviewed elsewhere (50,129). To summarize, cholesterol feeding alters both hepatic and intestinal lipoprotein production in a complex fashion, with very high species variability illustrated below. One common response is an increase in the plasma level, the size, and the cholesteryl ester content of plasma LDL, usually accompanied by a decrease in the circulating levels of plasma HDL. A more dramatic response is the appearance of two "abnormal" lipoprotein particles. These are designated beta-VLDL and HDL_c or HDL_1. The beta-VLDL particles observed in the plasma of cholesterol-fed dogs, rabbits, monkeys, rats, and humans (50) have a buoyant density characteristic of normal plasma VLDL, but they display beta rather than pre-beta electrophoretic mobility, an enrichment in cholesteryl ester relative to triglyceride, and an increased content of apolipoprotein E. The HDL_c or HDL_1 particles are "light" in the HDL density range, similar in size and cholesterol content to normal plasma LDL, and enriched relative to other HDL particles in apolipoprotein E. Some of these particles may contain apo E as their sole apolipoprotein constituent.

In the cholesterol-fed rabbit, the beta-VLDL particles predominantly represent remnants derived from the action upon chylomicrons of lipoprotein lipase (130). Kovanen et al. have shown that cholesterol feeding results in the saturation and suppression of the chylomicron remnant receptors in the rabbit, and hence in a delayed clearance of remnant particles from the circulation (131). Unlike the situation in rabbits, a high proportion of the beta-VLDL found in cholesterol-fed primates, dogs, and rats appears to be synthesized and secreted by the liver (21,22,132).

The HDL_c particles are thought to result from the acquisition of cholesterol and apolipoprotein E by "normal" circulating HDL, since a primary secretory product resembling HDL_c (i.e., an HDL rich in apo E and cholesteryl esters) has not yet been found (11). On the other hand, discoid HDL containing apo E and free cholesterol has been found in higher than normal amounts in perfusates from livers of cholesterol-fed African green monkeys (38) and of cholesterol-fed guinea pigs (133,134). Similar discoid HDL has been found in the peripheral lymph of cholesterol-fed dogs, perhaps reflecting peripheral synthesis (135). Potential pools of apo E upon which normal HDL could draw for this transformation include beta-VLDL, other HDL molecules, particle-free apo E if it exists, and certainly apo E secreted from extrasplanchnic tissues. To this point, Basu et al. have suggested that the apo E secreted by macrophages in vivo may participate in reverse cholesterol transport (37). Apo E and cholesterol, which are independently secreted from cholesterol-loaded macrophages, may bind to plasma HDL.

Responses in experimental animals

Rats and mice: Despite the appearance of beta-VLDL and HDL_c in their plasma, and an overall increase in the circulating level of apolipoprotein E, the levels of hepatic apo E mRNA in rats are not affected by cholesterol feeding alone. Levels of apo E mRNA as measured by translational activity in a heterologous system do, however, increase about twofold in livers of hypothyroid, cholesterol-fed rats (136). In mice fed a high-lipid diet, hepatic apo E mRNA levels show no significant change (106).

Although plasma apo A-I levels decline upon cholesterol feeding, there is some evidence that apo A-I mRNA levels are regulated differently in the liver and intestine. Mice fed a diet rich in cholesterol and saturated fat show a twofold increase in intestinal apo A-I mRNA, perhaps in order to package the increased load of dietary fat. Hepatic apo A-I mRNA decreases about twofold in these same animals, however. This finding suggests that apo A-I mRNA expression in the liver may be subject to negative feedback control by plasma cholesterol levels (137).

Guinea pigs: The guinea pig response to dietary lipid is very unusual. In normal guinea pigs the conversion rate of VLDL to LDL is high (27), and the bulk of plasma cholesterol is carried by LDL particles more dense (1.05 to 1.10 g/ml) than LDL of other species (138). Plasma HDL levels are very low in the guinea pig (12 mg protein/dl), with HDL transporting less than 5% of the total plasma cholesterol (139). Normal guinea pigs show the lowest reported plasma levels of apo A-I (6.2 mg/dl) and apo E (2.2 mg/dl) (133).

When guinea pigs are fed a 1% cholesterol diet supplemented with either cottonseed oil or corn oil (5%), their plasma cholesterol levels increase to about 300 mg/dl within 10 days (138,140). There is a three-to fourfold increase in particles of the IDL and LDL density range, but these particles are not HDL_C.

Plasma HDL levels increase 5- to 20-fold in guinea pigs with cholesterol feeding. These are isolated in the classical HDL density range and show alpha-1 mobility. However, they are discoidal particles of phospholipid, free cholesterol, and apo E, resembling the nascent HDL isolated before the action of LCAT (139,140), despite demonstrable LCAT activity in the plasma (141). Perhaps the high molar ratio of free cholesterol to phospholipid (2:1) interferes with LCAT activity (142).

Cholesterol feeding also alters the apolipoprotein profile of guinea pig lipoproteins. Plasma apo E levels increase more than 20-fold after 10 weeks on a 1% cholesterol/5% corn oil diet, with apo E appearing in all lipoprotein classes (133,143). The levels of apo E and free cholesterol are strongly correlated. Normal guinea pig apo E is more acidic than either human or rat apo E and three additional more acidic apo E isoforms are generated after cholesterol feeding. Using a nonrecirculating liver perfusion system, Guo et al. have shown both that hepatic apo E secretion increases twofold and that the apo E secreted from the cholesterol-fed guinea pig liver is more heavily sialylated than that secreted from normal liver (134).

Guo et al. have also compared the nascent lipoproteins secreted by livers of normal and cholesterol-fed guinea pigs (134). The normal liver secretes mainly triglyceride-rich VLDL and both spherical and discoidal HDL. Very little VLDL is secreted by the fatty liver, but it is similar to the beta-VLDL of the animals' plasma. The fatty liver perfusates contain a heterogeneous mixture of newly synthesized lipoproteins in the IDL and LDL density range that is rich in cholesteryl ester and in apo E, and a large amount of the free cholesterol-rich discoidal HDL. Apo E represents over 90% of the newly synthesized protein found in these discoidal HDL, which resemble those of the plasma.

The 7- to 10-fold increase in plasma apo E levels that follows a high cholesterol intake is associated with a doubling of the guinea pig hepatic levels of apo E mRNA (104). Cholesterol feeding also modulates apo E mRNA transcript levels in several extrahepatic guinea pig tissues. The spleen and adrenal respond to dietary lipid with increased tissue levels of both cholesterol ester and apo E mRNA transcripts after 4 weeks of diet. In the testis, however, the amount of translatable apo E mRNA declines to almost undetectable levels, and the tissue triglyceride content is decreased.

Nonhuman primates: In baboons and rhesus monkeys fed a mixture of polyunsaturated fatty acid (e.g., corn oil, 30%) and cholesterol (1%), the levels of plasma HDL decline. Hepatic apo A-I mRNA transcripts fall to about two-thirds of baseline levels after 6 weeks of diet, and to about half the baseline levels after 9 weeks of diet (J. C. Fox, et al., unpublished data). If a saturated fatty acid supplement is used (coconut oil), the apo A-I mRNA levels in the liver also fall to about two-thirds of baseline after 6 weeks, but do not fall further at later time points. In these same animals the intestinal apo A-I mRNA transcript levels are not significantly altered, nor are those of hepatic apo E mRNA or hepatic apo C-III mRNA under either dietary condition.

Hormones

Sex Hormones

Earlier studies found differences in lipoprotein metabolism between normal males and females of mammalian species, including a higher hepatic VLDL-triglyceride production rate in females. Several years ago we observed a fall in plasma LDL of male rats injected with high doses of estradiol (144), an effect now attributed to estrogen-induced expression of the hepatic LDL receptor (145). Estrogen administration to birds at more physiological doses had long been known to result in elevated plasma triglyceride and VLDL, an effect accompanied by a dramatic increase in hepatic VLDL protein synthesis (146,147).

The past few years have resulted in considerable progress in understanding regulation of apolipoprotein synthesis by hormones in two model systems:

Estrogen in birds: This topic has been reviewed extensively elsewhere (148) and is summarized only briefly here. Plasma VLDL of chickens contains predominantly two apoproteins (149). One resembles the apolipoprotein B_h of mammals. The other, designated apo VLDL-II, is found as a disulfide-linked dimer of two identical monomers of 9,444 Da (147,150). Expression of the apo VLDL-II gene begins in livers of chicks at the time of vitellogenesis. This apoprotein is not normally produced by livers of roosters; however, their apo VLDL-II genes can be activated by administration of estrogens. In the chick liver, this gene is initially unresponsive to estrogen during the early stages of embryogenesis, at a time when the cytosine residues in the 5'-flanking region of the gene are highly methylated. It has been shown that these residues undergo demethylation between days 7 and 9 of embryogenesis, so that the gene becomes estrogen-responsive and transcriptionally active by day 10 (151). Either in vivo or in tissue culture, chicken hepatocytes respond to estrogen administration with an elevated synthesis of apo B and with induction of apo VLDL-II (123,147). However, while the production of immunodetectable apo B increases from a basal level of about 1.5% to a stimulated level of about 4% of total protein secreted, immunoreactive apo VLDL-II secretion jumps from essentially nothing to about 3% of total secreted protein, calculated to be greater than a 200-fold increase (123). It is interesting to note that the induction of apo VLDL-II synthesis in vivo apparently involves not only an increase in the mRNA content per cell, but also a significant recruitment of hepatocytes into the production of apoprotein. Fewer than

5% of hepatocytes in cockerel livers are engaged in apo VLDL-II synthesis under basal conditions; however, upon estrogen stimulation this proportion increases to over 90% (152).

Follicle-stimulating hormone and cyclic AMP in ovary: Earlier experiments in our laboratory have established that steroidogenic organs actively synthesize apo E (104). The rat ovarian granulosa cell has been studied as a model of the steroid producing cell (153). Under some conditions, granulosa cells in culture retain their responsiveness to follicle-stimulating hormone (FSH) (154). It is well established that cyclic AMP (cAMP) functions as the second messenger for gonadotropin action (155,156).

Granulosa cells produce apo E that is identical to plasma apo E and is secreted in a form with a buoyant density of less than 1.21 g/ml, suggesting that it is lipidated. Although FSH does not stimulate total protein synthesis or total protein secretion in granulosa cells, the secretion of apo E by these cells is stimulated twofold in the presence of FSH (157). This stimulation also occurs in the presence of dibutyryl cyclic AMP (dbcAMP) even in the absence of FSH; moreover, the effect of FSH on both steroidogenesis and apo E secretion by these cells is potentiated by addition of a phosphodiesterase inhibitor. Cholera toxin, another agent that elevates intracellular cAMP levels, also stimulates granulosa cell apo E secretion. Approaches aimed at increasing the intracellular cAMP concentration can stimulate apo E production as much as 10- to 12-fold.

The effect of dbcAMP on apo E secretion is both dose and time dependent. The maximum stimulation is achieved by 48 hours. Although both apo E secretion and steroidogenesis are hormonally regulated in the granulosa cell, the production of apo E does not appear to be closely correlated with steroidogenesis or the production of a particular steroid.

Finally, synthesis of apo E may be developmentally regulated both in the granulosa cell and in bone marrow-derived macrophages (see Harmony, this volume) through the action of unknown mediators and mechanisms. FSH and cAMP both stimulate steroidogenesis and apo E secretion only in freshly isolated granulosa cells that have only cell-surface receptors for FSH. Addition of FSH or cAMP to granulosa cells for 48 hours induces the expression of receptors for LH and prolactin. Subsequent addition of gonadotropins or cAMP to these more mature cells still stimulates steroid production, but no longer influences the secretion of apo E.

CONCLUSION

It is clear that research in the next 5 to 10 years will reveal much about the molecular mechanisms involved in the synthesis of apolipoproteins and their incorporation into lipoprotein particles. Over the past 5 years the tools of cell and molecular biology have opened new vistas in this field.

The basis for the intracellular partitioning of apolipoproteins between the primary hepatic secretory lipoprotein particles, VLDL and HDL, remains a challenge for which no simple outcome can be predicted. Improved understanding of the mechanisms responsible for the intracellular assembly of nascent lipoprotein particles, and of the molecules involved in their passage through the secretory pathway, should provoke new experimental ideas and approaches for attacking this partitioning problem.

The elegance of genetic engineering technology offers exciting opportunities to ascertain the portions of each apoprotein necessary for the assembly and secretion of lipoproteins, for their functions as ligands in the metabolism and uptake of lipoproteins, and perhaps for other apolipoprotein functions we do not yet appreciate. The ubiquitous production of apoprotein E, for example, strongly suggests that it plays a role in overall cellular metabolism not commonly attributed to plasma apolipoproteins.

Finally, knowledge of mechanisms regulating apolipoprotein production by dietary lipids is bound to prove valuable in contemplating therapeutic approaches to hyperlipidemia, an obvious aggravating and almost certainly causative factor in atherogenesis.

One prediction we make with confidence is that the field of lipoprotein metabolism will benefit greatly from application of the techniques of cell and molecular biology, developed for studying other proteins of no particular direct interest to the lipoprotein physiologist and pathologist. Advancement in this field, as is the case now in so many others, will depend largely upon our ability to recruit to its ranks scientists broadly educated as cell and molecular biologists.

ACKNOWLEDGMENTS

We are very grateful to Ms. Linda McGuire and to Ms. Alice Snyder for help in preparing the manuscript. Experimental work in the authors' laboratories is supported by funding from the National Institutes of Health [HL 15062 (SCOR)] and from the Louis Block Fund. Donna Driscoll was a predoctoral trainee supported by NIH grants GM 07197 and HL 07237.

REFERENCES

1. Green, P. H. R., and Glickman, R. M., *J. Lipid Res.*, *22*: 1153–1173 (1981).

2. Eisenberg, S., and Rachmilewitz, D., *Biochim. Biophys. Acta*, *326*:391–405 (1973).

3. Brown, M. S., Kovanen, P. T., and Goldstein, J. L., *Science*, *212*:628–635 (1981).

4. Forester, G. P., Tall, A. R., Bisgaier, C. L., and Glickman, R. M., *J. Biol. Chem.*, *258*:5938–5943 (1983).

5. Bisgaier, C. L., and Glickman, A. M., *Ann. Rev. Physiol.*, *45*:625–636 (1983).

6. Imaizumi, K., Fainaru, M., and Havel, R. J., *J. Lipid Res.*, *19*:712–722 (1978).

7. Wu, A.-L., and Windmueller, H. G., *J. Biol. Chem.*, *254*: 7316–7322 (1979).

8. Imaizumi, K., Havel, R. J., Fainaru, M., and Vigne, J.-L., *J. Lipid Res.*, *19*:1038–1046 (1978).

9. Swift, L. L., Soulé, P. D., Gray, M. E., and LeQuire, V. S., *J. Lipid Res.*, *25*:1–13 (1984).

10. Ghiselli, G., Schaefer, E. J., Light, J. A., and Brewer, H. B., *J. Lipid Res.*, *24*:731–736 (1983).

11. Eisenberg, S., *J. Lipid Res.*, *25*:1017–1058 (1984).

12. Borensztajn, J., Getz, G. S., Padley, R. J., and Kotlar, T. J., *Biochem. J.*, *204*:609–612 (1982).

13. Hui, D. Y., Innerarity, T. L., Milne, R. W., Marcel, Y. L., and Mahley, R. W., *J. Biol. Chem.*, *259*:15060–15068 (1984).

14. Borensztajn, J., and Kotlar, T. J., *Proc. Natl. Acad. Sci. U.S.A.*, *81*:5863–5866 (1984).

15. Van't Hooft, F. M., Hardman, D. A., Kane, J. P., and Havel, R. J., *Proc. Natl. Acad. Sci. U.S.A.*, *79*:179–182 (1982).

16. Glickman, R. M., and Green, P. H. R., *Proc. Natl. Acad. Sci. U.S.A.*, *74*:2569–2573 (1977).

17. Green, P. H. R., Tall, A. R., and Glickman, R. M., *J. Clin. Invest.*, *61*:528–534 (1978).

18. Mougin–Schutz, A., Vache, D., and Girard–Globa, A., *Biochim. Biophys. Acta*, *754*:208–217 (1983).

19. Wilcox, H. G., Dunn, G. D., and Heimberg, M., *Biochim. Biophys. Acta*, *398*:39–54 (1975).

20. Noel, S.-P., Wong, L., Dolphin, P. J., Dory, L., and Rubinstein, D., *J. Clin. Invest.*, *64*:674–683 (1979).

21. Kris–Etherton, P. M., and Cooper, A. D., *J. Lipid Res.*, *21*:435–442 (1980).

22. Swift, L. L., Manowitz, N. R., Dunn, G. D., and LeQuire, V. S., *J. Clin. Invest.*, *66*:415–425 (1980).

23. Swift, L. L., Soulé, P. D., and LeQuire, V. S., *J. Lipid Res.*, *23*:962–971 (1982).

24. Faergeman, O., Sata, T., Kane, J. P., and Havel, R. J., *J. Clin. Invest.* *56*:1396–1403 (1975).

25. Kita, T., Brown, M. S., Bilheimer, D. W., and Goldstein, J. L., *Proc. Natl. Acad. Sci. U.S.A.*, *79*:5693–5697 (1982).

26. Ghiselli, G., *Biochim. Biophys. Acta*, *711*:311–315 (1982).

27. Barter, P., Faergeman, O., and Havel, R. J., *Metabolism*, *26*:615–622 (1977).

28. Goldstein, J. L., Kita, T., and Brown, M. S., *New Engl. J. Med.*, *309*:288–296 (1983).

29. Stalenhoef, A. F. H., Malloy, M. J., Kane, J. P., and Havel, R. J., *Proc. Natl. Acad. Sci. U.S.A.*, *81*:1839–1843 (1984).

30. Sparks, C. E., and Marsh, J. B., *J. Lipid Res.*, *22*:519–527 (1981).

31. Suissa, M., *Anal. Biochem.*, *115*:67–71 (1981).

32. Jones, L. A., Teramoto, T., Juhn, D. J., Goldberg, R. B., Rubenstein, A. H., and Getz, G. S., *J. Lipid Res.*, *25*:319–335 (1984).

33. Fless, G. M., Rolih, C. A., and Scanu, A. M., *J. Biol. Chem.*, *259*:11470–11478 (1984).

34. Mitchell, C. D., King, W. C., Applegate, K. R., Forte, T., Glomset, J. A., Norum, K. R., and Gjone, E., *J. Lipid Res.*, *21*:625–634 (1980).

35. Weidman, S. W., Ragland, J. B., and Sabesin, S. M., *J. Lipid Res.*, *23*:556–569 (1982).

36. Hamilton, R. L., Williams, M. C., Fielding, C. J., and Havel, R. J., *J. Clin. Invest.*, *58*:667–680 (1976).

37. Basu, S. K., Brown, M. S., Ho, Y. K., Havel, R. J., and Goldstein, J. L., *Proc. Natl. Acad. Sci. U.S.A.*, *78*:7545–7549 (1981).

38. Johnson, F. L., St. Clair, R. W., and Rudel, L. L., *J. Clin. Invest.*, *72*:221–236 (1983).

39. Johnson, F. L., St. Clair, R. W., and Rudel, L. L., *Circulation, 68*:III–118 (1983).

40. Zannis, V. I., Karathanasis, S. K., Keutmann, H. T., Goldberger, G., and Breslow, J. L., *Proc. Natl. Acad. Sci. U.S.A., 80*:2574–2578 (1983).

41. Sliwkowski, M. B., and Windmueller, H. G., *J. Biol. Chem., 259*:6459–6465 (1984).

42. Felker, T. E., Fainaru, M., Hamilton, R. L., and Havel, R. J., *J. Lipid Res., 18*:465–473 (1977).

43. Goldberg, R. B., Soltys, P. A., Cary, D., and Getz, G. S., *Circulation, 70*:II–119 (1984).

44. Glomset, J. A., Norum, K. R., Nichols, A. V., King, W. C., Mitchell, C. D., Applegate, K. R., Gong, E. L., and Gjone, E., *Scand. J. Clin. Lab. Invest., 35*(Suppl. 142):1–30 (1975).

45. Norum, K. R., Glomset, J. A., Nichols, A. V., Forte, T., Albers, J. J., King, W. C., Mitchell, C. D., Applegate, K. R., Gong, E. L., Cabana, V., and Gjone, E., *Scand. J. Clin. Lab. Invest., 35*(Suppl. 142):31–55 (1975).

46. Schmitz, G., Assmann, G., Rall, S. C., and Mahley, R. W., *Proc. Natl. Acad. Sci. U.S.A., 80*:6081–6085 (1983).

47. Gordon, J. I., Sims, H. F., Edelstein, C., Scanu, A. M., and Strauss, A. W., *J. Biol. Chem., 259*:15556–15563 (1984).

48. Hoffman, J. S., and Benditt, E. P., *J. Biol. Chem., 257*: 10510–10517; 10518–10522 (1982).

49. Glass, C. K., Pittman, R. C., Weinstein, D. B., and Steinberg, D., *Proc. Natl. Acad. Sci. U.S.A., 80*:5435–5439 (1983).

50. Mahley, R. W., in *Med. Clin. N. Am.: Lipid Disorders* (Havel, R. J., ed.), Saunders, Philadelphia, 1982, pp. 375–402.

51. Blum, C. B., Deckelbaum, R. J., Witte, L. D., Tall, A. R., and Cornicelli, J., *J. Clin. Invest., 70*:1157–1169 (1982).

52. Dory, L., Sloop, C. H., Boquet, L. M., Hamilton, R. L., and Roheim, P. S., *Proc. Natl. Acad. Sci. U.S.A. 80*:3489–3493 (1983).

53. Gordon, V., Innerarity, T. L., and Mahley, R. W., *J. Biol. Chem., 258*:6202–6212 (1983).

54. Shackelford, J. E., and Lebherz, H. G., *J. Biol. Chem., 258*: 7175–7180 (1983).

55. Kreil, G., *Ann. Rev. Biochem., 50*:317–348 (1981).

56. Driscoll, D. M., and Getz, G. S., *Methods Enzymol.*, in press.

57. Keller, W., *Cell, 39*:423–425 (1984).

58. Walter, P., Gilmore, R., and Blobel, G., *Cell, 38*:5–8 (1984).

59. Hay, R., Boehni, P., and Gasser, S., *Biochim. Biophys. Acta, 779*:65–87 (1984).

60. Kalderon, D., Roberts, B. L., Richardson, W. D., and Smith, A. E., *Cell, 39*:499–509 (1984).

61. Meyer, D. I., *Trends Biochem. Sci., 7*:320–321 (1982).

62. Sabatini, D. D., Kreibich, G., Morimoto, T., and Adesnik, M., *J. Cell Biol., 92*:1–22 (1982).

63. Gordon, J. I., Smith, D. P., Andy, R., Alpers, D. H., Schonfeld, G., and Strauss, A. W., *J. Biol. Chem., 257*: 971–978 (1982).

64. Gordon, J. I., Smith, D. P., Alpers, D. H., and Strauss, A. W., *J. Biol. Chem., 257*:8418–8423 (1982).

65. Gordon, J. I., Budelier, K. W., Sims, H. F., Edelstein, C., Scanu, A. M., and Strauss, A. W., *J. Biol. Chem., 258*: 14054–14059 (1983).

66. Reardon, C. A., Hay, R. V., Gordon, J. I., and Getz, G. S., *J. Lipid Res., 25*:348–360 (1984).

67. Blaufuss, M. C., Gordon, J. I., Schonfeld, G., Strauss, A. W., and Alpers, D. H., *J. Biol. Chem., 259*:2452–2456 (1984).

68. Sharpe, C. R., Sidoli, A., Shelley, C. S., Lucero, M. A., Shoulders, C. C., and Baralle, F. E., *Nucl. Acids Res., 12*: 3917--3932 (1984).

69. Jackson, C. L., Bruns, G. A. P., and Breslow, J. L., *Proc. Natl. Acad. Sci. U.S.A., 81*:2945–2949 (1984).

70. McLean, J. W., Elshourbagy, N. A., Chang, D. J., Mahley, R. W., and Taylor, J. M., *J. Biol. Chem., 259*:6498–6504 (1984).

71. Hubbard, S. C., and Ivatt, R. J., *Ann. Rev. Biochem., 50*: 555–583 (1981).

72. Lin-Lee, Y.-C., Bradley, W. A., and Chan, L., *Biochem. Biophys. Res. Commun., 99*:654–661 (1981).

73. Reardon, C. A., Ph.D. thesis, University of Chicago, Chicago, Ill., 1983.

74. Rall, S. C., Weisgraber, K. H., and Mahley, R. W., *J. Biol. Chem., 257*:4171–4178 (1982).

75. Zannis, V. I., and Breslow, J. L., *Biochemistry, 20*:1033–1041 (1981).

76. Pottenger, L. A., Frazier, L. E., DuBien, L. H., Getz, G. S., and Wissler, R. W., *Biochem. Biophys. Res. Commun., 54*: 770–776 (1973).

77. Siuta-Mangano, P., Howard, S. C., Lennarz, W. J., and Lane, M. D., *J. Biol. Chem., 257*:4292–4300 (1982).

78. Siuta-Mangano, P., Janero, D. R., and Lane, M. D., *J. Biol. Chem., 257*:11463–11467 (1982).

79. Davis, R. A., Clinton, G. M., Borchardt, R. A., Malone-McNeal, M., Tan, T., and Lattier, G. R., *J. Biol. Chem., 259*:3383–3386 (1984).

80. Lodish, H. F., Kong, N., Snider, N., and Strous, G. J. A. M., *Nature (London), 304*:80–83 (1983).

81. Balch, W. E., Glick, B. S., and Rothman, J. E., *Cell, 39*: 525–536 (1984).

82. Moore, H. P., Gumbiner, B., and Kelly, R. B., *Nature (London), 302*:434–436 (1983).

83. Schekman, R., and Novick, P., in *The Molecular Biology of the Yeast Saccharomyces: Metabolism and Gene Expression* (Strathern, J. N., Jones, E. W., and Broach, J. R., eds.) Cold Spring Harbor Laboratory, 1982, pp. 361–398.

84. Morré, D. J., and Ovtracht, L., *J. Ultrastruct. Res., 74*: 284–295 (1981).

85. Howell, K. E., and Palade, G. E., *J. Cell Biol., 92*:833–845 (1982).

86. Banerjee, D., and Redman, C. M., *J. Cell Biol., 96*:651–660 (1983).

87. Varki, A., and Kornfeld, S., *J. Biol. Chem., 258*:2808–2818 (1983).

88. Sly, W. S., and Fischer, H. D., *J. Cell. Biochem., 18*:67–85 (1982).

89. Krishnaiah, K. V., Walker, L. F., Borensztajn, J., Schonfeld, G., and Getz, G. S., *Proc. Natl. Acad. Sci. U.S.A., 77*: 3806–3810 (1980).

90. Kane, J. P., Hardman, D. A., and Paulus, H. E., *Proc. Natl. Acad. Sci. U.S.A., 77*:2465–2469 (1980).

91. Elovson, J., Huang, Y. O., Baker, N., and Kannan, R., *Proc. Natl. Acad. Sci. U.S.A., 78*:157–161 (1981).

92. Swift, L. L., Padley, R. J., LeQuire, V. S., and Getz, G. S., *Circulation*, *64*:IV–101 (1981).

93. Wu, A.-L., and Windmueller, H. G., *J. Biol. Chem.*, *256*: 3615–3618 (1981).

94. Soltys, P. A., Teramoto, T., Chang, L., and Getz, G. S., *Circulation*, *70*:II–270 (1984).

95. Curtiss, L. K., and Edgington, T. S., *J. Biol. Chem.*, *257*: 15213–15221 (1982).

96. Tikkanen, M. J., Cole, T. G., Hahm, K. S., Krul, E. S., and Schonfeld, G., *Arteriosclerosis*, *4*:138–146 (1984).

97. Marcel, Y. L., Hogue, M., Theolis, R., and Milne, R. W., *J. Biol. Chem.*, *257*:13165–13168 (1982).

98. Malloy, M. J., Kane, J. P., Hardman, A., Hamilton, R. L., and Dalal, K. B., *J. Clin. Invest.*, *67*:1441–1450 (1981).

99. Padley, R. J., Swift, L. L., and Getz, G. S., *Circulation*, *66*:II–101 (1982).

100. Cardin, A. D., Witt, K. R., Chao, J., Margolius, H. S., Donaldson, V. H., and Jackson, R. L., *J. Biol. Chem.*, *259*: 8522–8528 (1984).

101. Blue, M.-L., Protter, A. A., and Williams, D. L., *J. Biol. Chem.*, *255*:10048–10051 (1980).

102. Blue, M.-L., Ostapchuck, P., Gordon, J. S., and Williams, D. L., *J. Biol. Chem.*, *257*:11151–11159 (1982).

103. Elshourbagy, N. A., Liao, W. S., Mahley, R. W., and Taylor, J. M., *Proc. Natl. Acad. Sci. U.S.A.*, *82*:203–207 (1985).

104. Driscoll, D. M., and Getz, G. S., *J. Lipid Res.*, *25*:1368–1379 (1984).

105. Blue, M.-L., Williams, D. L., Zucker, S., Khan, S. A., and Blum, C. B., *Proc. Natl. Acad. Sci. U.S.A.*, *80*:283–287 (1983).

106. Reue, K. L., Quon, D. H., O'Donnell, K. A., Dizikes, G. J., Fareed, G. C., and Lusis, A. J., *J. Biol. Chem.*, *259*: 2100–2107 (1984).

107. Williams, D. L., Dawson, P. A., Newman, T. C., and Rudel, L. L., *J. Biol. Chem.*, *260*:2444–2451 (1985).

108. Boyles, J. K., Pitas, R. E., and Mahley, R. W., *Circulation*, *68*:III–17 (1984).

109. Newman, T. C., Dawson, P. A., Rudel, L. L., and Williams, D. L., *J. Biol. Chem.*, *260*:2452–2457 (1985).

110. Glaumann, H., Bergstrand, A., and Ericsson, J. L. E., *J. Cell Biol.*, *64*:356–377 (1975).

111. Claude, A. J., *J. Cell Biol.*, *47*:745–766 (1970).

112. Alexander, C. A., Hamilton, R. L., and Havel, R. J., *J. Cell Biol.*, *69*:241–263 (1976).

113. Christensen, N. J., Rubin, C. E., Cheung, M. C., and Albers, J. J., *J. Lipid Res.*, *24*:1229–1242 (1983).

114. Mahley, R. W., Bersot, T. P. LeQuire, V. S., Levy, R. I., Windmueller, H. G., and Brown, W. V., *Science*, *168*:380–382 (1970).

115. Pottenger, L. A., and Getz, G. S., *J. Lipid Res.*, *12*:450–459 (1971).

116. Nestruck, A. C., and Rubinstein, D., *Can. J. Biochem.*, *54*: 617–628 (1976).

117. Dolphin, P. J., *J. Lipid Res.*, *22*:971–989 (1981).

118. Gangl, A., and Ockner, R. K., *Gastroenterology*, *68*:167–186 (1975).

119. Marsh, J. B., *J. Biol. Chem.*, *238*:1752–1756 (1963).

120. Bungenberg de Jong, J. J., and Marsh, J. B., *J. Biol. Chem.*, *243*:192–199 (1968).

121. Janero, D. R., and Lane, M. D., *J. Biol. Chem.*, *258*: 14496–14504 (1983).

122. Nuñez, J. F., and Swaney, J. B., *J. Biol. Chem.*, *259*: 9141–9148 (1984).

123. Miller, K. W., and Lane, M. D., *J. Biol. Chem.*, *259*: 15277–15286 (1984).

124. Getz, G. S., and Hay, R. V., in *The Biochemistry of Atherosclerosis* (Scanu, A. M., Wissler, R. W., and Getz, G. S., eds.), Marcel Dekker, New York, 1978, pp. 151–188.

125. Heimberg, M., and Wilcox, H. G., *J. Biol. Chem.*, *247*:875–880 (1972).

126. Mistilis, S. P., and Ockner, R. K., *J. Lab. Clin. Med.*, *80*: 34–46 (1972).

127. Ruderman, N. B., Richards, K. C., de Bourges, V. V., and Jones, A. L., *J. Lipid Res.*, *9*:613–619 (1968).

128. Kohout, M., Kohoutova, B., and Heimberg, M., *J. Biol. Chem.*, *246*:5067–5074 (1971).

129. Mahley, R. W., and Innerarity, T. L., *Biochim. Biophys. Acta*, *737*:197–222 (1983).

130. Ross, A. C., and Zilversmit, D. B., *J. Lipid Res.*, *18*: 169–181 (1977).

131. Kovanen, P. T., Brown, M. S., Basu, S. K., Bilheimer, D. W., and Goldstein, J. L., *Proc. Natl. Acad. Sci. U.S.A.*, *78*:1396–1400 (1981).

132. Melchior, G. W., Mahley, R. W., and Buckhold, D. K., *J. Lipid Res.*, *22*:598–609 (1981).

133. Guo, L. S. S., Hamilton, R. L., Kane, J. P., Fielding, C. J., and Chen, G. C., *J. Lipid Res.*, *23*:531–542 (1982).

134. Guo, L. S. S., Hamilton, R. L., Ostwald, R., and Havel, R. J., *J. Lipid Res.*, *23*:543–555 (1982).

135. Sloop, C. H., Dory, L., Hamilton, R. L., Krause, B. R., and Roheim, P. S., *J. Lipid Res.*, *24*:1429–1440 (1983).

136. Lin-Lee, Y.-C., Tanaka, Y., Lin, C.-T., and Chan, L., *Biochemistry*, *20*:6474–6480 (1981).

137. Miller, J. C. E., Barth, R. K., Shaw, P. H., Elliott, R. W., and Hastie, N. D., *Proc. Natl. Acad. Sci. U.S.A.*, *80*:1511–1515 (1983).

138. Mills, G. L., Chapman, M. J., and McTaggart, F., *Biochim. Biophys. Acta*, *260*:401–412 (1972).

139. Puppione, D. L., Sardet, C., Yamanaka, W., Ostwald, R., and Nichols, A. V., *Biochim. Biophys. Acta*, *231*:295–301 (1971).

140. Sardet, C., Hansma, H., and Ostwald, R., *J. Lipid Res.*, *13*: 624–639 (1972).

141. Drevon, C. A., *Atherosclerosis*, *30*:123–136 (1978).

142. Fielding, C. J., Shore, V. G., and Fielding, P. E., *Biochim. Biophys. Acta*, *270*:513–518 (1972).

143. Guo, L. S., Meng, M., Hamilton, R. L., and Ostwald, R., *Biochemistry*, *16*:5807–5812 (1977).

144. Hay, R. V., Pottenger, L. A., Reingold, A. L., Getz, G. S., and Wissler, R. W., *Biochem. Biophys. Res. Commun.*, *44*: 1471–1477 (1971).

145. Kovanen, P. T., Brown, M. S., and Goldstein, J. L., *J. Biol. Chem.*, *254*:11367–11373 (1979).

146. Luskey, K. L., Brown, M. S., and Goldstein, J. L., *J. Biol. Chem.*, *249*:5939–5947 (1974).

147. Chan, L., Jackson, R. L., O'Malley, B. W., and Means, A. R., *J. Clin. Invest.*, *58*:368–379 (1976).

148. Chan, L., *Ann. Rev. Physiol.*, *45*:615–623 (1983).

149. Williams, D. L., *Biochemistry*, *18*:1056–1063 (1979).

150. Jackson, R. L., Lin, H.-Y., Chan, L., and Means, A. R., *J. Biol. Chem.*, *252*:250–253 (1977).

151. Colgan, V., Elbrecht, A., Goldman, P., Lazier, C. B., and Deeley, R., *J. Biol. Chem.*, *257*:14453–14460 (1982).

152. Lin, C.-T., and Chan, L., *Endocrinology*, *107*:70–75 (1980).

153. Hsueh, A. J. W., Adashi, E. Y., Jones, P. B. C., and Welsh, T. H., *Endocrinol. Rev.*, *5*:76–127 (1984).

154. Erickson, G. F., and Hsueh, A. J. W., *Endocrinology*, *102*: 1275–1282 (1978).

155. Richards, J. S., Jonassen, J. A., Rolfes, A. I., Kersey, K., and Reichert, L. E., *Endocrinology*, *104*:765–773 (1979).

156. Birnbaumer, L., and Kirchick, H. J., in *Factors Regulating Ovarian Function* (Greenwald, G. S., and Terranova, P. F., eds.), Raven Press, New York, 1983, pp. 287–310.

157. Driscoll, D. M., Schreiber, J., Schmit, V., and Getz, G. S., *Arteriosclerosis*, *4*:520a (1984).

3

Extracellular Posttranslational Proteolytic Processing of Apolipoproteins

CELINA EDELSTEIN and ANGELO M. SCANU The Pritzker School of Medicine, The University of Chicago, Chicago, Illinois

INTRODUCTION

The apolipoproteins, like most secretory proteins, are synthesized on the rough endoplasmic reticulum (RER) and translocated across the RER membrane during cotranslational cleavage of their signal peptides. The mechanisms by which these events occur have been reviewed recently (1,2) and the reader is referred to these accounts. The detailed secretory pathway that the apolipoproteins take and the steps involved in their assembly with lipids before they are exported from the cells are largely unknown. Information has been gathered on the NH_2-terminal sequences of the primary translation products of most of the apolipoprotein mRNAs: apo A-I, apo A-II, apo A-IV, apo C-I, apo C-II, apo C-III, and apo E (1). All of these apoproteins are secreted from the cells after they reach their mature form, with the exception of apo A-I and apo A-II, the major apoproteins of high-density lipoproteins (HDL), which are secreted as precursor proapoproteins. The processing of these two apoproteins to their mature forms is distinct from that of the other apoproteins in that maturation takes place extracellularly at unusual cleavage sites. Due to the intrinsic interest of these processes, aside from their physiological importance, these posttranslational events, which occur through the action of specific converting enzymes, will be discussed within the framework of our current general knowledge of the proteolytic processing occurring either intra- or extracellularly.

PROCESSING OF PROPROTEINS

General Mechanisms

Intracellular Processing

Ten to twenty minutes after synthesis and cotranslational removal of the signal peptide in the RER, general processing of propolypeptides begins during their transfer to the Golgi apparatus and subsequently in the secretory granules where they are concentrated. The cleavage of the prosegment occurs with half-lives ranging from 20 min to 1 hr or longer. As conversion nears completion, the secretory granules undergo morphological changes and may transform into storage granules. In the case of the peptide hormones and proalbumin, condensation of the products takes place before exocytosis. It has been postulated that the cleaving enzymes either interact directly with the precursor propeptides or become activated as they pass through the Golgi apparatus and then cosegregate into newly formed secretory granules (3,4).

Almost all prosegments of proproteins studied thus far contain cleavage sites at pairs of basic amino acids (Arg-Arg, Lys-Arg, Arg-Lys, or Lys-Lys, Fig. 1). Based on their frequency of distribution at peptide hormone converting sites, the basic amino acid pairs are cleaved in decreasing order Lys-Arg>Arg-Arg>Lys-Lys=Arg-Lys (5). This frequency suggests that the converting enzymes favor arginine in the second position of the dibasic pair. Except for the two basic amino acids, there is neither sequence homology surrounding these cleavage sites, nor defined secondary structural conformation. Moreover, not all basic pairs of amino acids in the protein are cleaved. These observations suggest that the specificity for cleavage may be related to the relative exposure of the cleavage site on the protein surface.

The presence of the paired basic amino acid residues in the prosegment appears essential for proper prohormone processing. Mutations in the dibasic pair, such as replacement of Arg-65 to His in the C chain at the C-A junction in abnormal proinsulin (6,7), or Arg-6 to Gln in the Christchurch proalbumin (8,9), or Arg-5 to His in proalbumin Lillie (10), or a dual alteration in catfish prosomatostatin peptide from Arg-Lys to Lys-Pro (11), have resulted in limited or no processing. Similarly, the replacement of Arg or Lys by canavanine or thialysine, respectively, during the biosynthesis of proproteins in vitro has also prevented cleavage of the prosegment (12,13). Although the presence of pairs of basic residues appears to be a general characteristic of propeptides, exceptions have been noted. In the following cases a single basic residue, usually arginine, is found in the COOH terminal of the propeptide and is cleaved to form the mature protein, e.g., chicken proalbumin (14), canine proinsulin (15), provasopressin/neurophysin II (4), cholecystokinin (16), canine pancreatic polypeptide (17), and vasoactive intestinal peptide (18). It remains to be established whether the protease(s) involved in the processing of these propeptides is the same as those cleaving after pairs of basic residues.

Based on evidence collected on the proteolytic processing of prohormones (4) such as proinsulin, proglucagon, progastrin, and proparathyroid, a common mechanism that has been invoked for the conversion of the proprotein into the mature form involves the combined action of an endopeptidase (trypsin or cathepsin B-like) and exopeptidase (carboxypeptidase B-like). The endoprotease that has been implicated in correctly cleaving after pairs of basic residues is a thiol protease whose properties resemble those of cathepsin B (19,20). However, Docherty et al. (21) have shown that purified cathepsin B derived from rat liver lysosomes does not accurately process proinsulin. It has also been found that cathepsin B is derived biosynthetically from a 44 kDa precursor that can be detected in islet secretion granule fractions using the site-specific probe ^{125}I-Tyr-Ala-Lys-Arg chloromethylketone (22). This evidence has led to the speculation that an active precursor, procathepsin B, may cosegregate along with proinsulin into the secretory granules and that both molecules may be intimately involved in their mutual processing.

Attending the endoproteolytic cleavage of the paired basic residues, there is an exoprotease resembling carboxypeptidase B activity, located in secretory granules. This enzyme removes the newly produced carboxyl-terminal basic residues from the partially processed fragments, is metal dependent, and has a molecular weight of 54 kDa. Unlike the pancreatic carboxypeptidase B, the exoprotease exhibits a pH optimum of 5.5. Moreover, its activity is inhibited by ethylendiamine tetraacetic acid (EDTA), β-mercaptoethanol, and o-phenanthroline, but not by diisopropylfluorophosphate (DFP) or iodoacetamide (4,22).

Extracellular Processing

Except for the activation of the classical zymogens (blood clotting factors, fibrinolysins, digestive enzymes), which are in a category of their own (for reviews see references 23 to 25), and the major HDL apoproteins (apo A-I and apo A-II), which will be considered in detail below, there are few examples of extracellular proprotein processing. These encompass procollagen, from which the NH_2- and COOH-terminal peptides are removed by specific proteases (26,27), and the protoxin, promelittin. The latter protein undergoes proteolytic processing by a dipeptidyl aminopeptidase that catalyzes the stepwise removal of dipeptides from the prosegment of promelittin. The melittin propeptide contains 11 sequential dipeptides of the structure X-Y, where X is either Ala, Glu, or Asp and Y is either Pro or Ala (28–30).

A dipeptidyl aminopeptidase also plays an essential role in the processing of the yeast alpha-mating factor. However, this polypeptide is processed intracellularly by the membrane-bound enzyme (31). Four

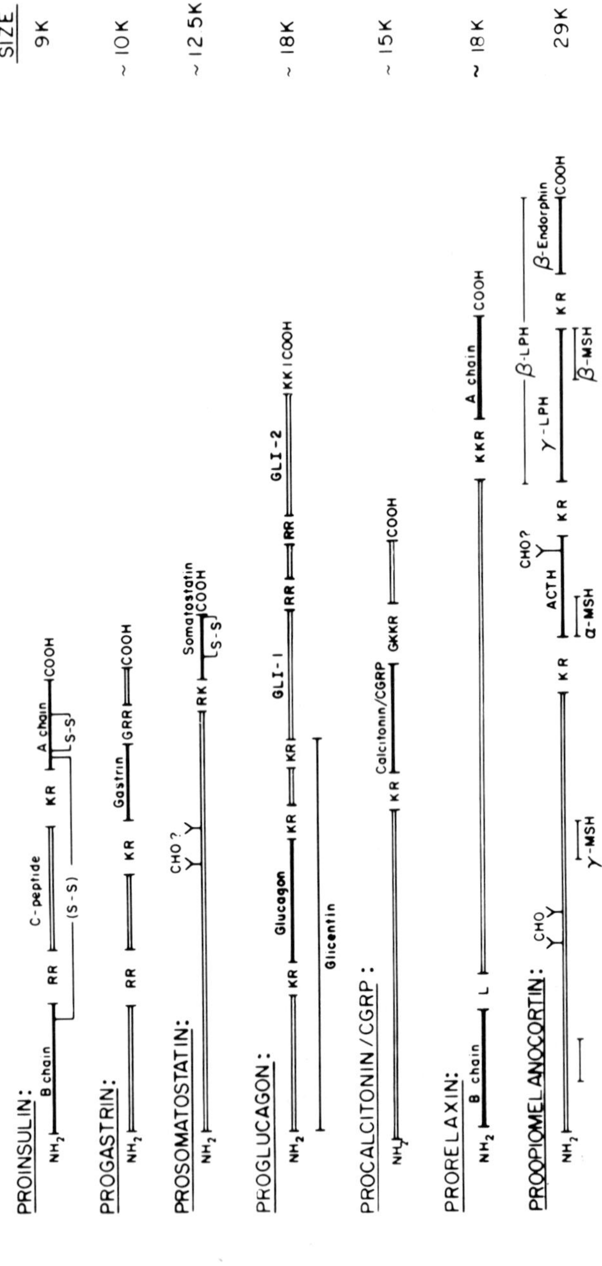
SIZE
PROINSULIN:
NH2
B chain
RR
C-peptide
(S-S)
KR
A chain
S-S
COOH
9K
PROGASTRIN:
NH2
RR
KR
Gastrin
GRR
COOH
~10K
PROSOMATOSTATIN:
NH2
CHO ?
RK
Somatostatin
S-S
COOH
~12.5K
PROGLUCAGON:
NH2
KR
Glucagon
KR
KR
GLI-1
RR
RR
GLI-2
KK I COOH
Glicentin
~18K
PROCALCITONIN/CGRP:
NH2
KR
Calcitonin/CGRP
GKKR
COOH
~15K
PRORELAXIN:
NH2
B chain
L
KKR
A chain
COOH
~18K
PROOPIOMELANOCORTIN:
NH2
CHO
γ-MSH
KR
ACTH
α-MSH
CHO?
KR
γ-LPH
β-LPH
β-MSH
KR
β-Endorphin
COOH
29K

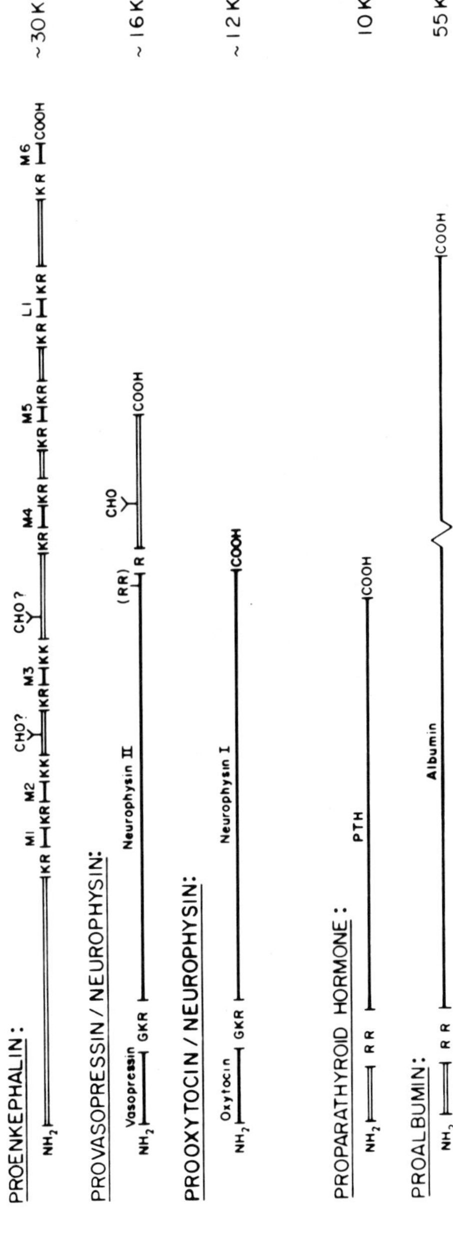

Fig. 1 Schematic representation of some polypeptide precursor forms showing residues at cleavage sites using the single letter amino acid notations. Heavy single lines indicate the biologically active products. Reproduced from reference 4 with permission from the publishers.

copies of proalpha factor are in tandem sequence, each consisting of a spacer peptide and the mature protein. Each spacer peptide contains paired basic amino termini followed by three repeats of a peptide with the sequence Glu-Ala-Asp-Ala-Glu-Ala (32). The paired basic amino termini are cleaved first, generating the repeat peptides that are further processed by the dipeptidyl aminopeptidase to produce the mature protein.

PROCESSING OF PROAPOLIPOPROTEINS A-I AND A-II

Intracellular Events

Upon cotranslational cleavage of the 18-amino-acid NH_2-terminal signal peptide extension in the RER (Fig. 2), both proapo A-I and proapo A-II move through the secretory pathway by means of an as yet undefined mechanism and are eventually secreted into the circulation. Gordon et al. (33) studied the relative rates of disappearance of proapo A-I and proapo A-II from Hep G2 cells. Near-confluent monolayers of these cells were pulse-labeled for 15 min with [^{3}H] valine and then chased with unlabeled amino acid. At various times of the chase, the apoproteins were immunoprecipitated from cell lysates and media, and the proteins were separated by gel electrophoresis in the presence of sodium dodecyl sulfate (SDS) and then fluorographed. The results showed that proapo A-II was no longer detectable within Hep G2 cells after 20 min, while proapo A-I was no longer detectable after a 2-hr chase (Fig. 3). The kinetic behavior of these two proapoproteins agrees in general with the kinetics of serum protein secretion by cultured hepatoma cells from the mouse (34), rat (35), and man (36). The evidence also supports multiple secretory pathways and is incompatible with bulk-phase movement, indicating that proapo A-I and proapo A-II are segregated into different vesicles at some time during cellular processing. This type of segregation would require signals that are intrinsic to the protein and recognized by a membrane-bound receptor that selectively mediates apoprotein transport. A distinguishing feature for these proapoproteins is the prosegment, a potential sorting signal that may permit it to function as a recognition marker. Lodish et al. (36) showed that human hepatoma secretory proteins move form the RER to the Golgi at characteristic limiting rates and that secretion of all the proteins from the Golgi requires 20 min. Clearly, in the case of proapo A-II, which contains paired basic residues at the COOH terminal of its prosegment and is processed extracellularly (see section on extracellular events), the relatively rapid secretion may point to a specific receptor-mediated transport vesicle protecting the protein from proteolysis by cathepsin B-like proteases. Alternatively, interaction of proapo A-II with lipids derived from the smooth ER membrane may aid in the transport of the proprotein. In the case of proapo A-I, the absence of

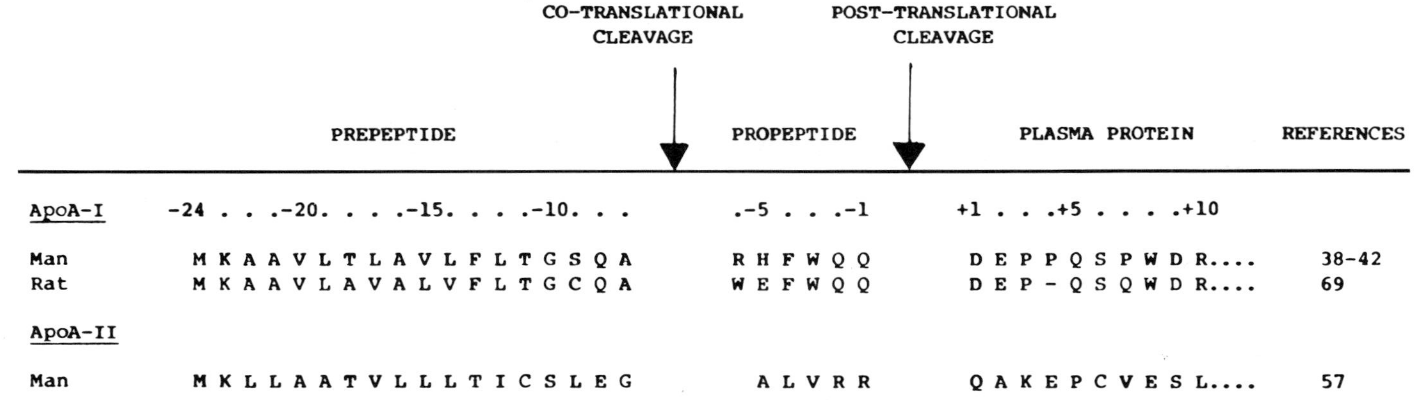

	PREPEPTIDE	PROPEPTIDE	PLASMA PROTEIN	REFERENCES
ApoA-I	-24 . . .-20. . . .-15. . . .-10. . .	.-5 . . .-1	+1 . . .+5 . . . .+10	
Man	M K A A V L T L A V L F L T G S Q A	R H F W Q Q	D E P P Q S P W D R....	38-42
Rat	M K A A V L A V A L V F L T G C Q A	W E F W Q Q	D E P - Q S Q W D R....	69
ApoA-II				
Man	M K L L A A T V L L L T I C S L E G	A L V R R	Q A K E P C V E S L....	57

Fig. 2 Amino acid sequences of the pre- and propeptides of plasma apoA-I and apo A-II. The arrows indicate the sites of co- and post-translational cleavage. Only the first 10 amino acids are presented for the mature plasma protein. (–), A deletion applied to obtain alignment of the sequences of man and rat. The single letter notation is used for the amino acids and is defined as: D, aspartic; N, asparagine; T, threonine; S, serine; P, proline; E, glutamic; Q, glutamine; G, glycine; A, alanine; V, valine; C, cysteine; M, methionine; I, isoleucine; L, leucine, Y, tyrosine; F, phenylalanine; K, lysine; H, histidine; R, arginine; W, tryptophan.

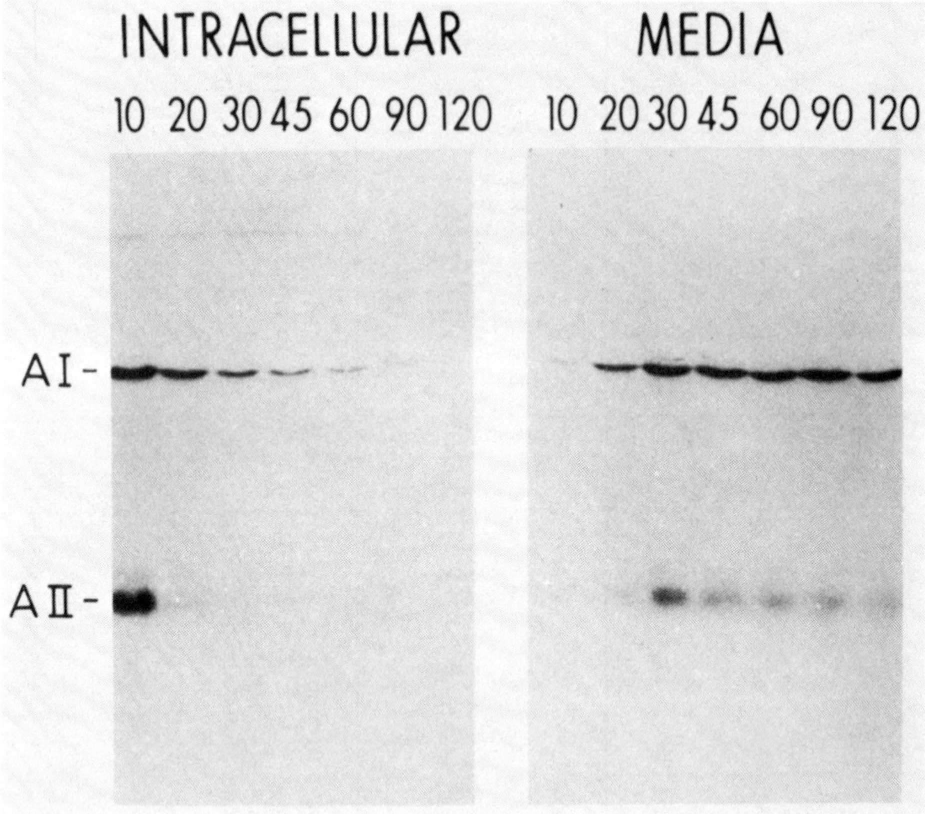

Fig. 3 Relative rates of secretion of apo A-I and apo A-II from HepG-2 cells. Near confluent monolayers were pulse-labeled for 15 min with [^{3}H]valine and then chased with unlabeled amino acid. Apolipoproteins were recovered from equal-sized aliquots of cell lysates or media obtained at various times during the chase using monospecific antibodies. Reproduced from reference 33 with permission from the publisher.

basic residues at the COOH terminal of the prosegment (see section on extracellular processing IIb and Fig. 2) may target the proprotein through different channels. Thus, the intracellular interaction of proapo A-I with lipids may not be a requirement. Accordingly, Alpers et al. (37) characterized intra- and extracellular apo A-I from the rat intestine and found that most of the apo A-I isolated from these compartments was not incorporated into lipid-rich particles.

Extracellular Events

Proapo A-I

Proapo A-I differs from its mature form by the presence of a hexapeptide amino-terminal extension with the sequence Arg-His-Phe-Trp-Gln-Gln- (38–42). The highly unusual COOH-terminal Gln-Gln sequence distinguishes it from other known vertebrate propeptide sequences that generally possess COOH-terminal paired basic amino acids (see section on general processing mechanisms). The proprotein is the stable intracellular form of apo A-I and is secreted as such, i.e., without proteolytic cleavage of its hexapeptide prosegment. The conversion of proapo A-I to apo A-I occurs extracellularly and has been studied in several laboratories, both in vitro (43,44) and in vivo (44,45).

Methods of analysis. In vitro the detection of the presence of proapo A-I and its conversion to the mature product have relied on three independent methods (46). Because of the small amounts of available proapo A-I, these methods utilize the radiolabeled proprotein, which is obtained from pulse-labeled cells.

1. Apo A-I isoform analysis. The technique of two-dimensional gel electrophoresis can resolve a total of six isoforms (pI 6.5 to 5.4) of plasma apo A-I (47). These are named according to their mobility in a pH gradient (from the most basic isoform 1 to the most acidic isoform 6). The origin of isoform 1 is unknown and may be artifactual. Isoforms 2 and 3 are attributed to the proapoprotein. Isoform 4 and isoforms 5 and 6 are the predominant species found in plasma and in HDL. At present, the structural basis for the differences in charge between isoforms 2 and 3 and between 4, 5, and 6 is not understood but may reflect deamidation of this glutamine-rich protein.
2. NH_2-terminal sequence analysis. Automated sequential Edman degradation of [^{3}H] proline-labeled proapo A-I can be used to determine the extent and accuracy of processing. Proapo A-I contains proline residues at positions 9 and 10, whereas mature apo A-I has proline residues at positions 3, 4, and 7 (38–42) (Fig. 2). From the distribution of the radioactive peaks it is possible to determine not only the occurrence of processing, but

also that it takes place at the correct cleavage site, i.e., at the Gln-Asp bond, the junction between the propeptide and the mature protein.

3. Trichloroacetic acid (TCA) assay. In this assay, developed in the authors' laboratory (46), [^{3}H]phenylalanine-labeled proapo A-I obtained from the Hep G2 cell medium is used as a substrate (38). Since the hexapeptide sequence contains phenylalanine, this amino acid is a convenient marker for detection of the cleaved prosegment. This assay is rapid and sensitive and is based on the different predicted solubilities of the hexapeptide prosegment and mature apo A-I molecule in 5% TCA.

Localization and properties of the enzyme that converts proapo A-I to apo A-I. The in vitro conversion of proapo A-I to apo A-I was initially studied by Edelstein et al. (43), who also partially characterized this extracellular activity. These authors found that human plasma, serum, or mesenteric lymph all induced proapo A-I to apo A-I conversion. The converting activity was associated with lymph chylomicrons as well as plasma very-low-density lipoprotein (VLDL) and HDL, the latter density class containing the highest specific activity of the converting enzyme. In addition, some activity was also found in the d>1.21 g/ml fraction. These results were supported by the in vitro studies with rat plasma using rat proapo A-I as a substrate (44). The proapo A-I cleavage site is identical in these two species with complete homology of the penultimate four COOH-terminal residues of both propeptides as well as of the first three NH_2-terminal residues of the mature proteins (Fig. 2). In fact, we have observed that human proapo A-I can be converted to its mature form using rat plasma as the source of the converting activity (unpublished observation). The kinetics of conversion of both human and rat proapo A-I to the mature form is on the order of hours and is in agreement with the slow conversion process reported for other proproteins such as proinsulin to insulin and G34 gastrin to gastrin (48). However, complete conversion of both human and rat proapo A-I to apo A-I is not achieved even after a 24-hr incubation.

Bojanovski et al. (45) provided proof in vivo that proapo A-I was converted to mature apo A-I. ^{125}I-Labeled normal human proapo A-I was infused into normolipidemic subjects and the conversion was followed by two-dimensional gel electrophoresis. The results showed that, contrary to the in vitro studies, proapo A-I was completely converted to mature apo A-I and that the average residence time of proapo A-I was almost 30-fold less than mature apo A-I (0.23 d compared to 6.5 d). In vivo pulse-chase studies in the rat (44a,b) are in accord with the results from human studies. In the rat the conversion proceeds to 80% completion compared to 20% in vitro. Thus, the partial conversion that is observed in vitro may be a result of the nonoptimal conditions of incubation or poor lability of the enzyme.

The converting activity in plasma is inhibited by 5 mM EDTA, 10 mM ethyleneglycol-bis-(β-amino ethylether)N,N-tetraacetic acid (EGTA),

1 mM dithiothreitol (DTT), and 10 mM 1,10 phenanthroline (43). The inhibition by EDTA is reversible upon dialysis into an EDTA-free buffer containing Ca^{++}. In addition, conversion is inhibited by high salt concentrations and is heat inactivated at 60°C. The serine protease inhibitors, diisopropylfluorophosphate (DFP) and phenylmethylsulfonylfluoride (PMSF), do not affect the activity; this is also true for the thiol-blocking agent, N-ethylenemaleimide (NEM). In partially purified preparations, Ca^{++} is essential for activity (unpublished observation). These properties permit the assignment of the enzyme to the class of metalloendopeptidases (49). At present, it is not clear whether one or more proteases are involved, as is the case for the prohormone intracellular processing.

Enzymes that exhibit properties similar to the converting enzyme have been reported in the literature. In these studies the enzyme preparations were tested for their ability to hydrolyze the artificial elastase substrate, succinyltrialanine nitroanilide. This enzyme activity has been detected in rheumatoid synovial fluid (50), human bile (51), human kidney (52), and human serum (53). Recent reports (54,55) have shown this enzyme activity to be associated with human serum lipoproteins. The enzyme activity derived from these sources was not due to leukocyte elastase, since cleavage of its naturally occurring substrate, elastin, was not demonstrated. In all cases, isolated fractions containing enzyme activity were lipophilic and were associated with either serum lipoproteins, lipids, or membrane fragments. It will be important to test these enzyme preparations for their ability to convert proapo A-I to mature apo A-I so that a clear assessment can be made on its identity with the converting enzyme.

The site of synthesis of the converting enzyme has been studied recently (56). Two types of cells have been examined, the hepatoma cell line Hep G2 and the myelocytic cell line ML-2, the latter both in the undifferentiated and differentiated macrophagic state. The cells were grown in heat-inactivated human serum, which consequently was devoid of converting activity. The cell medium was assessed for converting activity using radiolabeled proapo A-I as a substrate. Both Hep G2 and the differentiated ML-2 cells were found to secrete the converting activity that accumulated in the medium as a function of time. In contrast, the converting activity was absent in the undifferentiated ML-2 cell medium. Under the same culture conditions, both cell lines also secreted proapo A-I, which during the pulse chase studies was converted to mature apo A-I. The results thus far indicate that two cell lines grown in culture produce and secrete proapo A-I and converting activity that cleaves this precursor into the mature apoprotein; moreover, cell differentiation has an effect on this process. It is interesting to note that incubation of near-confluent Hep G2 cells for 16 hr in serum-free medium results in the secretion of proapo A-I but not of converting activity (38,43). This is suggestive of a role for a serum factor to stimulate either secretion and/or activation of the converting enzyme.

No information is available on the site of proapo A-I conversion, although since the enzyme is found associated with HDL, one may suspect the conversion to take place on a lipoprotein particle. In the in vitro systems studied, addition of a partially purified, delipidated, converting enzyme to a lipid-free proapo A-I substrate results in the formation of mature apo A-I (unpublished observation). This information does not rule out conversion at a lipoprotein surface, but indicates that such a surface, although sufficient, is not necessary. It is also conceivable that both proapo A-I and the converting enzyme are transported from the site of secretion to a region where conversion takes place. In this context it would be informative to identify a tissue that secretes either the enzyme or proapo A-I but not both.

Proapo A-II

Gordon et al. (57) studied the biosynthesis of human preproapo A-II in Hep G2 cells and found that the primary translation product of apo A-II contains a 23-amino-acid NH_2-terminal extension (Fig. 2). This extension consists of an 18-amino-acid-long signal peptide that is cleaved cotranslationally, and a 5-amino-acid-long propeptide, Ala-Leu-Val-Arg-Arg, which is cleaved extracellularly. The proteolytic processing of proapo A-II to its mature form represents a unique and novel pathway because cleavage occurs extracellularly after paired basic residues. The processing of precursors such as the zymogens takes place extracellularly but after a single basic residue, whereas processing after dibasic residues has been described for a variety of prohormones and proalbumin but takes place intracellularly.

The converting enzyme that cleaves proapo A-II to apo A-II. Proapo A-II is cleaved following secretion from Hep G2 cells. These cells secrete the protease responsible for prosegment removal (33). The converting activity present in media is not blocked by serine protease inhibitors such as PMSF, aprotinin, and furoyl saccharin or by a metalloprotease inhibitor 1,10 phenanthroline. The enzyme is, however, inhibited by the thiol protease reagents parachloromercuribenzoic acid (PCMB) and leupeptin. These properties are analogous to the cathepsin B-like enzyme implicated in the intracellular processing of prohormones. A thiol protease similar in enzymic and immunologic properties to lysosomal cathepsin B has been reported to be secreted from mouse mammary carcinomas (58), human breast tumors (59), and ascites fluid of patients with ovarian carcinoma (60). This proteinase has a larger molecular size (ca. 39000 daltons) than cathepsin B and has a striking size resemblance to the cathepsin-B-related protease in the insulin secretory granule (21). The secretion of this higher molecular weight enzyme may perhaps indicate an altered pathway of processing, at least in some tumor cells. The documentation of extracellular proapo A-II processing in the Hep G2 cell system may be yet another example of altered processing in a tumor cell line. Further evidence is needed using both in vivo (as demonstrated for proapo A-I) and in vitro systems, the latter in normal cell lines, to substantiate the site of proapo A-II processing.

At present, assessment of converting activity relies on the techniques of two-dimensional gel electrophoresis and sequence analysis of the products of proteolytic conversion of radiolabeled proapo A-II (33). Prosegment removal changes the pI from 6.61 (proapo A-II) to 4.95 (mature apo A-II). Extracellular proapo A-II processing, as studied in the Hep G2 cell line, is relatively slow ($t_{1/2}$ of 6 hr) and is comparable with the kinetics of both the in vivo and in vitro conversion of proapo A-I as well as with the kinetics of the intracellular conversion of prohormones. Lackner et al. (61) have recently identified proapo A-II in human plasma and thoracic duct lymph, albeit in very small quantities. This suggests that, unlike proapo A-I, proapo A-II is either not the predominant species secreted from normal organs such as the intestine or is very rapidly converted after secretion. It is clear that the processing of proapo A-II is not yet fully resolved.

SIGNIFICANCE OF THE PROPEPTIDES

The reason for the existence of the prosegment in proapo A-I and proapo A-II is largely unknown and this partially relates to the fact that neither of them has been isolated from the plasma and may in fact be subjected to extensive proteolysis. Both proapo A-I and proapo A-II have been shown to interact with lipoproteins in vitro (33,34). In addition, like mature apo A-I, proapo A-I is capable of activating LCAT (62). It is possible that the prosegment has some biological activity, but none has been determined so far even in the case of the propeptides of insulin or parathyroid hormone. The propeptide of apo A-II is not absolutely required for normal secretion since the replacement of arginines in the propeptide with canavanine does not alter the rate of secretion or the rate of dimer formation (57). Similarly, cleavage of proalbumin to albumin is not an absolute necessity for secretion since two reported variants of proalbumin, Christchurch and Lille proalbumin, have been found in circulation. In the case of the prohormones, they are inactive until cleaved, but secretion of proparathyroid hormone and of proinsulin can occur (63), so the attachment of the prosegment is not an obstacle to the act of secretion. In any case, other apoproteins such as apo A-IV, apo E, and the apo C peptides do not have prosegments and are secreted normally (1,2). Thus, the prosegment does not have to be a component in a general mechanism for secretion. On the other hand, the prosegment may facilitate transport through the cell, as discussed in the section on intracellular events. This may be particularly significant for the hexapeptide extension of proapo A-I since it has an exceptionally unusual sequence (Fig. 2).

The prosegment may have an important regulatory function in the synthesis of the apoproteins. In the case of the hexapeptide extension of proalbumin, studies in isolated hepatocytes and in a cell-free system (64) have shown that there is feedback inhibition of albumin synthesis by its propeptide. Also, the NH_2-terminal extension of the proalpha 1 chain of type I procollagen inhibits collagen synthesis in cell cultures and in the cell-free system (65). Studies such as these should also be performed for the proapoproteins.

A general function for the prosegment may be in the formation of the tertiary structure of the apoproteins. For example, the connecting segment in proinsulin appears to be required to facilitate the formation of the disulfide bridges of insulin and its proper folding (66,67). The hexapeptide of proapo A-I is predicted to be helical, but how that influences the secondary structure of the whole apoprotein molecule has not been investigated. Moreover, the mode of self-association may change due to the hexa- or pentapeptide extension in proapo A-I and proapo A-II, respectively, and requires further study.

From the evolutionary standpoint, except for the human and canine apo A-I amino acid sequence, complete sequence data for other species are not available even though this protein appears to be present in all higher animals (68). However, the hexapeptide extension of both human and rat can be compared (Fig. 2). It is interesting to note that the four penultimate COOH-terminal residues of the propeptide as well as the Gln-Asp cleavage site show complete homology. By comparison, the NH_2-terminal sequence of human plasma apo CII contains a region spanning residues 5 through 8 that mimics the processing site of proapo A-I (Gln-Gln-Asp-Glu) but does not contain the rest of the sequence that flanks the Gln-Gln-Asp site. As a result, apo C-II does not appear to be proteolytically cleaved. This information points to the importance of conserving the hexapeptide sequence. In the case of apo A-II, although the complete amino acid sequences of both the human and rhesus mature proteins are known and have been found to be highly homologous (68), the propeptide extension has been studied in humans only. It is obvious that amino acid and nucleotide sequence comparisons of these apoproteins among a large variety of species, both invertebrates and vertebrates, are needed to shed light on the importance and functionality, if any, of the propeptides.

CONCLUDING REMARKS

The extracellular processing of apo A-I and apo A-II is novel and brings into focus the first demonstration of an unusual posttranslational pathway. However, more work needs to be done with other cell lines, particularly in the case of proapo A-II. Similarly, isolation and characterization of the enzymes responsible for the proteolysis should help identify their localization and regulation. The role(s) that this novel processing mechanism plays in connection with lipoprotein biogenesis is at present undefined, although some work on the intra- and extracellular assembly of lipid-protein complexes has been already carried out (see Chapter 2). The potential functional properties of the propeptides are the least understood, and this applies not only to the apolipoproteins, but also to all of the proproteins studied thus far. Many questions remain to be answered. The present knowledge on posttranslational events should provide the groundwork for experimental studies directed at understanding proapolipoprotein processing mechanisms and their role in HDL biogenesis.

ACKNOWLEDGMENT

The work by the authors, cited in this review, was carried out by Program Project, Grant USPHS-HL 18577.

REFERENCES

1. Scanu, A. M., Byrne, R. E., and Edelstein, C., *J. Lipid Res.*, *25*:1593–1602 (1985).
2. Gordon, J. I., Sims, H. F., Strauss, A. W., Edelstein, C., Byrne, R. E., and Scanu, A. M., *CRC Crit. Rev. Biochem.*, in press.
3. Palade, G., *Science*, *189*:347–358 (1975).
4. Steiner, D. F., Docherty, K., and Carroll, B., *J. Cell Biochem.*, *24*:121–130 (1984).
5. Schwartz, T. W., Wittels, B., and Tager, H. S., in *Peptide: Structure and Function*, Proc. 8th Am. Peptide Symp., (Hruby, V. J. and Rich, D. L., eds.) Pierce Chemical Company, Rockford, Ill., 1984, pp. 229–238.
6. Robbins, D. C., Blix, P. M., Rubenstein, A. H., Karazawa, Y., Kosaka, K., and Tager, H. S., *Nature (London)*, *291*:679–681 (1981).
7. Shibaski, Y., Kanazawa, Y., Akanuma, Y., Kawakami, T., and Takaku, F., *Diabetes*, *33*(Suppl. 1):84A (1984).
8. Brennan, S. O., and Carrell, R. W., *Nature (London)*, *274*: 908–909 (1978).
9. Brennan, S. O., and Carrell, R. W., *Biochim. Biophys. Acta*, *621*:83–88 (1980).
10. Abdo, Y., Rousseaux, J., and Dautrevaux, M., *FEBS Lett.*, *131*:286–288 (1981).

11. Andrews, P. C., and Dixon, J. E., *J. Biol. Chem.*, *256*: 8267–8270 (1981).

12. Noe, B. D., *J. Biol. Chem.*, *256*:4940–4946 (1981).

13. Halban, P., *J. Biol. Chem.*, *257*:13,177–13,180 (1982).

14. Rosen, A. M., and Geller, D. M., *Biochem. Biophys. Res. Commun.*, *78*:1060 (1977).

15. Kwok, S. C. M., Chan, S. J., and Steiner, D. F., *J. Biol. Chem.*, *258*:2357 (1983).

16. Ryder, S. W., Straus, E., and Yalow, R. S., *Proc. Natl. Acad. Sci. U.S.A.*, *77*:3669 (1980).

17. Schwartz, T. W., and Tager, H. S., *Hoppe Seylers Z. Physiol. Chem.*, *363*:889 (1982).

18. Itoh, N., Obata, K., Yanaihara, N., and Okamoto, H., *Nature (London)*, *304*:547–549 (1983).

19. Docherty, K., Carroll, R. J., and Steiner, D. F., *Proc. Natl. Acad. Sci. U.S.A.*, *79*:4613–4617 (1982).

20. Docherty, K., Carroll, R. J., and Steiner, D. F., *Proc. Natl. Acad. Sci. U.S.A.*, *80*:3245–3249 (1983).

21. Docherty, K., Hutton, J. C., and Steiner, D. F., *J. Biol. Chem.*, *259*:6041–6044 (1984).

22. Docherty, K., and Hutton, J. C., *FEBS Lett.*, *162*:137–141 (1983).

23. Lorand, L., ed., *Methods in Enzymology*, Vol. XLV (Part B), Academic Press, New York, 1976.

24. Boyer, P. D., ed., *The Enzymes*, Vol. III, 3rd ed., Academic Press, New York, 1971.

25. Lorand, L., in *Proteases and Biological Control*, (Reich, E., Rifkin, D., and Shaw, E., eds.), Cold Spring Harbor, New York, 1975.

26. Halseth, D. L., Jr., and Veis, A., *Proc. Natl. Acad. Sci. U.S.A.*, *81*:3302–3306 (1984).

27. Gerstenfeld, L., Beldekes, J. C., Sonenshein, G. E., and Franzblau, C., *J. Biol. Chem.*, *259*:9158–9162 (1984).

28. Suchanek, G., Kreil, G., and Hermondson, M. A., *Proc. Natl. Acad. Sci. U.S.A.*, *75*:701–704 (1978).

29. Kreil, G., Mollay, C., Kaschnitz, R., Haiml, L., and Vilas, U., *Ann. N.Y. Acad. Sci.*, *343*:338–346 (1980).

30. Kreil, G., Haiml, L., and Suchanek, G., *Eur. J. Biochem.*, *111*:49–58 (1980).

31. Julius, D., Blair, L., Brake, A., Sprague, G., and Therner, J., *Cell*, *32*:839–852 (1983).

32. Kurjan, J., and Herskowitz, I., *Cell*, *30*:933–943 (1982).

33. Gordon, J. I., Sims, H. F., Edelstein, C., Scanu, A. M., and Strauss, A. W., *J. Biol. Chem.*, *259*:15,556–15,563 (1984).

34. Ledford, B. E., and Davis, D. F., *J. Biol. Chem.*, *258*: 3304–3308 (1983).

35. Strous, G. J. A. M., and Lodish, H. F., *Cell*, *22*:709–717 (1980).

36. Lodish, H. F., Kong, N., Snider, M., and Strous, G. J. A. M., *Nature (London)*, *304*:80–83 (1983).

37. Alpers, D. H., Lock, D. R., Lancaster, N., Poksay, K., and Schonfeld, G., *J. Lipid Res.*, *26*:1–10 (1985).

38. Gordon, J. I., Sims, H. F., Lentz, S. R., Edelstein, C., Scanu, A. M., and Strauss, A. W., *J. Biol. Chem.*, *258*: 4037–4044 (1983).

39. Law, S. W., Gray, G., and Brewer, H. B., Jr., *Biochem. Biophys. Res. Commun.*, *112*:257–264 (1983).

40. Law, S. W., and Brewer, H. B., Jr., *Proc. Natl. Acad. Sci. U.S.A.*, *81*:66–70 (1984).

41. Cheung, P., and Chan, L., *Nucleic Acids Res.*, *11*:3703–3715 (1983).

42. Zannis, V. I., Karathanasis, S. K., Keutmann, H. T., Goldberger, A., and Breslow, J. L., *Proc. Natl. Acad. Sci. U.S.A.*, *80*:2574–2578 (1983).

43. Edelstein, C., Gordon, J. I., Toscas, K., Sims, H. F., Strauss, A. W., and Scanu, A. M., *J. Biol. Chem.*, *258*: 11,430–11,433 (1983).

44a. Sliwkowski, M. B., and Windmueller, H. G., *J. Biol. Chem.*, *259*:6459–6465 (1984).

44b. Ghiselli, G., Gotto, A. M., Jr., Tanenbaum, S., and Sherrill, B. C., *Proc. Natl. Acad. Sci. U.S.A.*, *82*:874–878 (1985).

45. Bojanovski, D., Gregg, R. E., Ghiselli, G., Schaefer, E. J., Light, J. A., and Brewer, H. B., Jr., *J. Lipid Res.*, *26*: 185–193 (1985).

46. Edelstein, C., Gordon, J. I., Vergani, C. A., Catapano, A. L., Pietrini, V., and Scanu, A. M., *J. Clin. Invest.*, *74*: 1098–1103 (1984).

47. Zannis, V. I., Breslow, J. L., and Katz, A. J., *J. Biol. Chem.*, *255*:8612–8617 (1980).

48. Steiner, D. F., Quinn, P. S., Chen, S. J., Marsh, J., and Tager, H. S., *Ann. N.Y. Acad. Sci.*, *343*:1–16 (1980).

49. Barrett, A. J., in *Proteinases in Mammalian Cells and Tissues*, (Barrett, A. J., ed.), Vol. 2, North-Holland, New York, 1977, pp. 10–13.

50. Saklatvala, J., *J. Clin. Invest.*, *59*:794–801 (1977).

51. Ogawa, M., Kosaki, G., Tanaka, S., Iwaki, K., and Nomoto, M., *Clin. Chim. Acta*, *93*:235–238 (1979).

52. Ishida, M., Ogawa, M., Kosaki, G., Mega, T., and Ikenaka, T., *Biochem. Int.*, *3*:239–246 (1981).

53. Sasaki, M., Yoshikane, K., Nobata, E., Katagiri, K., and Takeuchi, T., *J. Biochem.*, *89*:609–614 (1981).

54. Jacob, M. P., Bellon, G., Robert, L., Hornebeck, W., Ayrault-Jarrier, M., Burdin, J., and Polonovski, J., *Biochem. Biophys. Res. Commun.*, *103*:311–318 (1981).

55. Maeda, H., Kobori, S., and Uzawa, H., *Arch. Biochem. Biophys.*, *226*:629–635 (1983).

56. Polacek, D., Edelstein, C., Ostrega, D., Gordon, J. I., Yachnin, S., and Scanu, A. M., *Fed. Proc.*, *44*:1453 (1985).

57. Gordon, J. I., Budelier, K. A., Sims, H. F., Edelstein, C., Scanu, A. M., and Strauss, A. W., *J. Biol. Chem.*, *258*: 14,054–14,059 (1983).

58. Recklies, A. D., Mort, J. S., and Poole, A. R., *Cancer Res.*, *42*:1026–1032 (1982).

59. Recklies, A. D., Poole, A. R., and Mort, J. S., *Biochem. J.*, *207*:633–636 (1982).

60. Mort, J. S., Leduc, M. S., and Recklies, A. D., *Biochim. Biophys. Acta*, *755*:369–375 (1983).

61. Lackner, K. J., Edge, S. B., Gregg, R. E., Hoeg, J. M., and Brewer, H. B., Jr., *J. Biol. Chem.*, *260*:703–706 (1985).

62. Menzel, H. J., Assmann, G., Rall, S. C., Weisgraber, K. H., and Mahley, R. W., *J. Biol. Chem.*, *259*:3070–3076 (1984).

63. Dean, R. T., and Judah, J. D., *Compr. Biochem.* (Florkin, M., and Stotz, E. J., eds.) Vol. 19B, Elsevier, New York, pp. 233–298 (1980).

64. Weigand, K., Schmid, M., Villringer, A., Birr, Ch., and Heinrich, P. C., *Biochemistry, 21*:6053–6059 (1982).

65. Horlein, D., McPherson, J., Goh, S. H., and Bornstein, P., *Proc. Natl. Acad. Sci. U.S.A., 78*:6163–6167 (1981).

66. Docherty, K., and Steiner, D. F., *Annu. Rev. Physiol., 44*: 625–638 (1982).

67. Tager, H. S., *Diabetes, 33*:693–699 (1984).

68. Scanu, A. M., Edelstein, C., and Keim, P., in *The Plasma Proteins*, (Putnam, F., ed.), 2nd ed., Academic Press, New York, 1974.

69. Gordon, J. I., Smith, D. P., Andy, R., Alpers, D. H., Schonfeld, G., and Strauss, A. W., *J. Biol. Chem., 257*: 971–978 (1982).

4

Lipoprotein(a): Biochemistry and Biology

GUNTHER M. FLESS and ANGELO M. SCANU The Pritzker School of Medicine, The University of Chicago, Chicago, Illinois

INTRODUCTION

Lipoprotein(a) is a variant of LDL in that it contains apo B, but differs from it because of the presence of an additional disulfide-linked apoprotein called apo(a) (1–3). Unlike the other lipoproteins, whose nomenclature is usually derived from their buoyant density, Lp(a) was named by the immunogeneticist K. Berg in 1963 to designate a factor or antigen present in the plasma of only a limited number of individuals (4). During a search for genetic variants of human lipoproteins, Berg discovered this antigen using antisera from rabbits hyperimmunized with LDL of different individuals. After absorbing out the antibodies to LDL with whole serum of different donors, he was left with antisera that reacted with sera of some but not other individuals. Those sera that formed precipitin lines upon double immunodiffusion he referred to as $Lp(a)^+$, and those that did not as $Lp(a)^-$. Subsequent studies showed that this antigen was associated with a lipoprotein having pre-β electrophoretic mobility on agarose gels and a hydrated density ranging from 1.05 to 1.12 g/ml.

ISOLATION AND HETEROGENEITY OF Lp(a)

When human plasma is placed on a density gradient that encompasses the density range between 1.0 and 1.25 g/ml and is subjected to ultracentrifugation, one can obtain an absorbance density profile of all the lipoproteins inclusive of Lp(a) (3,5). Fig. 1 shows lipoprotein profiles of individuals previously determined to be strongly Lp(a) positive by double immunodiffusion that demonstrates the density distribution of

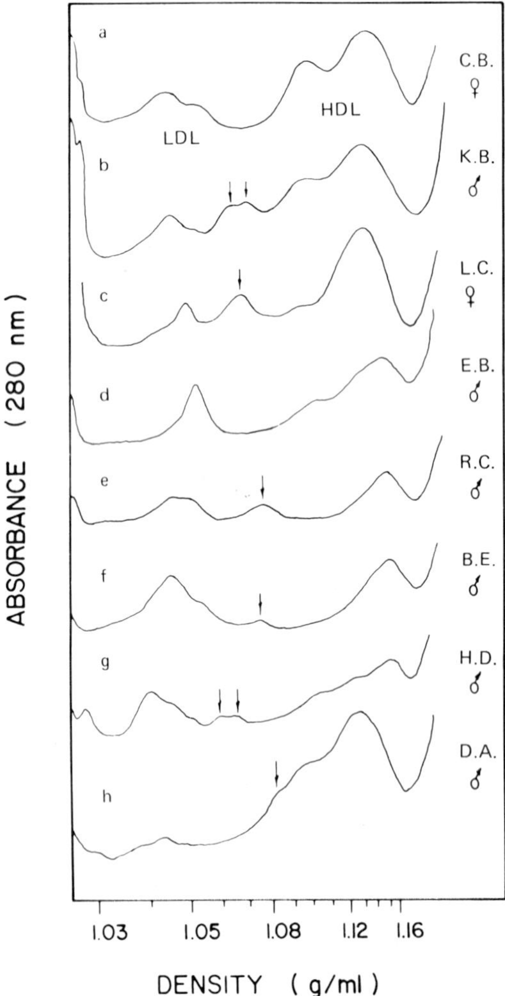

Fig. 1 "Single-spin" density gradient profiles of eight Lp(a)-positive individuals. The arrow identifies the position of Lp(a) on the gradient.

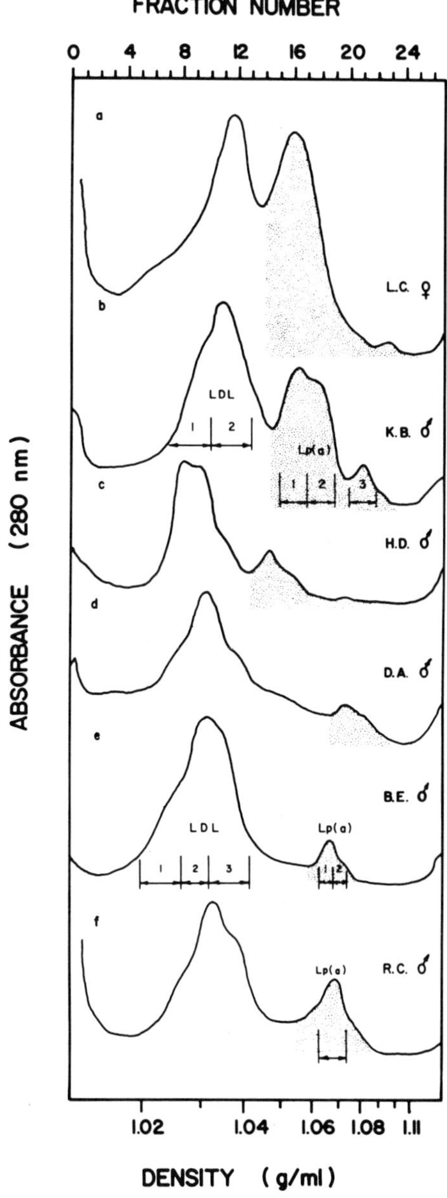

Fig. 2 Density gradient profiles of the apo-B-containing lipoproteins of six different individuals. The shaded portion of the gradients indicates the presence of Lp(a). Centrifugation was carried out in the SW-40 rotor, using a 0 to 12% NaBr gradient at 39,000 rpm for 48 hr at 20°C.

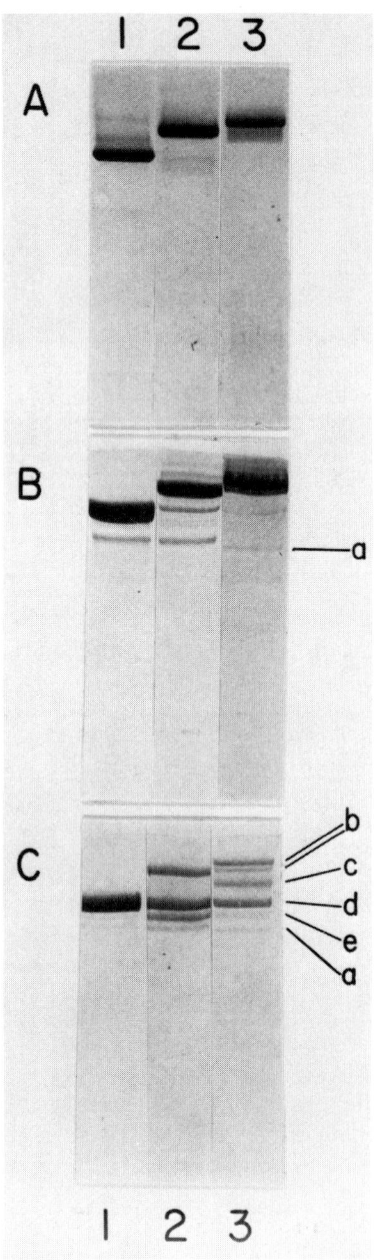

Fig. 3 Electrophoretic comparison of low- and high-density Lp(a). (A) Gradient gel electrophoresis (2.5 to 16%) of native lipoproteins runs

Lp(a) with respect to LDL and HDL, which are the major lipoproteins that have to be removed in order to obtain pure Lp(a). In technical terms, HDL can be separated from Lp(a) with relative ease either by gel filtration or rate zonal flotation on density gradients because Lp(a) is much larger than HDL. However, LDL is more difficult to separate from Lp(a) because of the smaller size difference between the two particles. Since a small fraction of LDL is isopycnic with Lp(a) and is therefore copurified during density gradient centrifugation, two methods were recently developed to ensure the isolation of Lp(a) free of LDL (3). One is heparin sepharose chromatography, which takes advantage of the differential affinity of these two lipoproteins for heparin; the other is chromatofocusing, which differentiates the particles according to charge or isoelectric point. Purified Lp(a) from different individuals was heterogeneous by density gradient centrifugation as shown by the great diversity in peak densities ranging from d 1.047 to 1.100 g/ml (Fig. 2). Moreover, most human subjects had more than one Lp(a) species that differed not only in their density but sometimes also in their electrophoretic behavior (Fig. 3a). Analytical ultracentrifugation confirmed the electrophoretic results, suggesting that the dense Lp(a) had a larger molecular weight than the low-density Lp(a). Part of this difference is caused by the fact that the apoprotein of high-density Lp(a) has a larger size than that of low-density Lp(a) (Fig. 3b). When the protein moiety of Lp(a) is analyzed by SDS gel electrophoresis in the presence of 2-mercaptoethanol, apo(a) dissociates from apo B. Under these conditions, the apo(a) of the lower-density Lp(a) is smaller and the apo(a) of the higher-density Lp(a) is larger than apo B-100 (Fig. 3c). Some individuals appear to have a third kind of Lp(a) with intermediate density that on reduction yields apo(a) and apo B-100 of equal mobility, which could only be differentiated using specific antibodies to the respective apoproteins by Western immunoblotting. Apo(a) stains poorly with Coomassie blue when compared to apo B-100; in fact, it has been reported that what may be a fourth form of apo(a) with a molecular weight higher than apo B-100 is not stained at all (1). The

---

Fig. 3 (continued)
in the absence of SDS. (B) Gradient gel electrophoresis (2.5 to 16%) of SDS-denatured lipoproteins. (C) SDS-gradient gel electrophoresis (2.5 to 16%) of lipoproteins run in the presence of 2-mercaptoethanol. Lane 1, LDL; lane 2, low-density Lp(a); lane 3, high-density Lp(a). The lipoproteins were taken from the density gradient shown in Fig. 2a. LDL, fractions 12+13; low density Lp(a), fractions 16+17; high density Lp(a), fraction 23. Identification of bands: (a) staining artifact caused by the presence of lipid, (b) unreduced apo Lp(a), (c) apo(a) from high-density Lp(a), (d) apoB, and (e) apo (a) from low-density Lp(a).

differential staining of the various forms of apo(a) with Coomassie blue is not understood, but may be due to variability in the extent of glycosylation. At this point, Lp(a) has been analyzed from only a limited number of human subjects; however, as this study is extended to a larger population, it is likely that the heterogeneity of Lp(a) and its apoproteins may become more complex than is currently thought.

COMPARATIVE PROPERTIES OF Lp(a) and OTHER LIPOPROTEINS

The chemical composition of Lp(a) has to be viewed from the context that Lp(a), as other lipoproteins, does not have a fixed molecular weight. This means that Lp(a) in the circulation consists of a set of particles of relatively similar molecular weight which differ in their lipid and in some cases their protein content. The mean number of lipid molecules associated with Lp(a) differs from individual to individual and is likely dependent on complex lipolytic and lipid transfer processes that these particles undergo during their residence time in the plasma. Therefore, the chemical composition of Lp(a) differs among and within individuals depending on the density interval from which it is isolated.

Compositional data of a typical Lp(a) species are shown in Table 1 and are compared to those of LDL, VLDL, and HDL. The values for molecular weight and density of Lp(a) species are generally larger than those of LDL. Yet, the molar content of the different lipid classes is almost the same, differing greatly from that of VLDL and HDL.

We can take advantage of the fact that the lipid compositions of LDL-1 and Lp(a)-2 of subject K.B. (see Table 1) are almost identical in order to make a general comparison of the structural differences between LDL and Lp(a). The similarity in lipid composition between the two lipoproteins in spite of their difference in size invites some consideration of the organization of the protein moiety of Lp(a) at the water-lipoprotein interface. Since their molar lipid volume is nearly the same, this suggests that apo B alone may be sufficient to stabilize the hydrophobic lipid constituents of the Lp(a) particle. This assumption is born out when the data are analyzed in terms of the packing of the protein and phospholipid at the water-lipoprotein interface (Fig. 4). Lp(a) is the only lipoprotein that is displaced from a common line formed by the other lipoproteins (chylomicrons, VLDL, LDL, HDL, and VHDL). This unusual behavior indicates that the protein moiety may be packed tighter in Lp(a) than in the other lipoproteins or that a significant portion is not amphiphilic in nature and is not tightly associated with the lipoprotein surface.

Table 1 Molar Composition of Lp(a) and Other Lipoproteins

	VLDL[a]	LDL[b]	Lp(a)[b]	HDL_2[a]
Molecular weight ($\times 10^{-6}$)	19.6	3.24	3.71	0.36
Density (g/ml)	0.97	1.030	1.062	1.09
Equivalent radius (A)	200	108	112	51
Protein $\times 10^{-5}$ (g/mol)	15.7	5.44	9.31	1.48
Phospholipid (mol/mol)	4,545	1,040	1,050	137
Free cholesterol (mol/mol)	3,539	829	786	50
Cholesteryl ester (mol/mol)	3,600	2,110	2,140	90
Triglycerides	11,500	229	278	19

[a] Data from Ref. 22.
[b] Compositional data of subfractions of LDL-1 and Lp(a)-2 of one individual (K.B.) from Ref. 3 (see Fig. 2b).

Several lines of evidence appear to support this hypothesis: (1) apo(a) is heavily glycosylated (27.9% carbohydrate), which favors its interaction with the aqueous medium (6); (2) Lp(a), in contrast to LDL, has a much higher viscosity; this would be in agreement with a spherical lipoprotein particle having part of its protein chains extending into the aqueous medium, thus increasing its effective radius of gyration (7); (3) limited trypsinization of Lp(a) causes the release of the antigenic determinants of apo (a) but not apo B (8); (4) electron spin resonance studies, with spin labels probing both the protein and lipid environments, indicated a constraining effect of apo(a) on the lipoprotein surface; this could be removed by trypsinization (8); and (5) Lp(a) has less α-helix and more random structure than LDL (1,3).

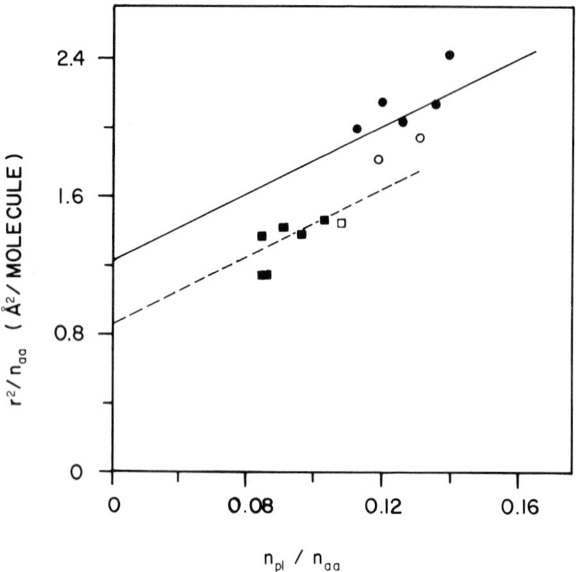

Fig. 4 Packing of phospholipids and protein at the lipoprotein-water interface. The solid line represents data for all lipoproteins (chylomicrons, VLDL, LDL, HDL, and VHDL) and is taken from Shen et al. (22). The parameters for LDL (●) and Lp(a) (■) were calculated from the data given in Ref. 3. Open circles and squares represent rhesus LDL and Lp(a), respectively, and were taken from Fless and Scanu (23) for comparison to the human data. The dotted line represents the data for Lp(a).

ISOLATION OF APO(a) FROM Lp(a)

The fact that apo(a) may be less amphiphilic in nature and has a relatively high content of random structure suggests that with the exception of its covalent attachment through disulfide bonds, apo(a) is loosely bound to Lp(a). This concept has served as the basis for devising a method for its isolation from the Lp(a) particle. Upon reduction of Lp(a) with 0.01 M DTT, apo(a) can be separated from Lp(a) under a high centrifugal field while apo B remains with the lipoprotein molecule (9). However, the fact that apo(a) cannot be removed from reduced Lp(a) by gel filtration in either low or high salt suggests that it must bind to the lipoprotein surface to some extent independent of its linkage to apo B through disulfide bonds, and that is overcome only after the application of a high centrifugal force. Apo(a) so prepared from low-density Lp(a) has an apparent molecular weight of 280,000 compared to 330,000 for apo B of Lp(a) as estimated by SDS gradient gel electrophoresis on 2.5 to 16% gels. This molecular weight is approximate because the carbohydrate of apo(a) may give it an anomalous mobility in SDS gel electrophoresis. The fact that apo(a) is a glycoprotein containing 27.9 weight percent carbohydrate is probably the reason why it is completely water soluble. Circular dichroism studies have indicated that the structure of apo(a) is mostly random, which is not surprising considering its carbohydrate and high proline content (6). Also, the high intrinsic viscosity of apo(a) suggests a more random structure rather than a globular configuration (6).

PHYSIOLOGICAL CONSIDERATIONS

Although from a structural viewpoint Lp(a) is becoming increasingly more understood, relatively little is known regarding its physiological role. Since the lipid content of Lp(a) is so much like that of LDL, it is tempting to speculate that the function of these two lipoproteins is analogous and is to serve as vehicles for cholesterol transport. However, apo(a) may confer some specificity to Lp(a) in targeting cholesterol entry into specialized tissues via a receptor (other than B,E)-mediated process. There is some controversy whether Lp(a) binds and competes with LDL via the apo B,E receptor and is similarly degraded, although a receptor-independent uptake for Lp(a) cannot be ruled out. However, from a quantitative viewpoint, this pathway may not be important since the concentration of Lp(a) in most human subjects is much lower than that of LDL. Metabolic studies have indicated that Lp(a) is removed from plasma by a mechanism similar to that of LDL (10). Their fractional catabolic rates are closely correlated, although that of Lp(a) was found to be about 30% lower. However, no relationship has been observed between serum levels of Lp(a) and LDL and their fractional catabolic rates. Instead it appears that the concentration of Lp(a) is regulated mainly by its synthetic rate.

The origin of Lp(a) in plasma has not been determined, although there is evidence indicating that it is not a metabolic product of other apo-B-containing lipoproteins such as VLDL or LDL (11). However, a recent preliminary report has shown that fat feeding results in the appearance of a component with immunological reactivity to anti-Lp(a) in lymph chylomicrons (12). Further studies are needed to show if the intestine may be capable of synthesizing and integrating apo(a) into triglyceride-rich particles and through their catabolism be ultimately responsible for the generation of plasma Lp(a). However, none of the observations reported thus far explains why Lp(a) retains relatively steady plasma levels even after severe dietary manipulations, which may indicate that the intestine does not play a major role in Lp(a) production (13,14). Unlike LDL, the levels of Lp(a) are also unaffected by pharmacological agents such as estrogen (13), clofibrate, and cholestyramine (15), except for the anabolic steroid, stanazolol, which has been shown to decrease dramatically the levels of plasma Lp(a) (16). Overall, these studies suggest that the metabolic control of Lp(a) is different from that of LDL and VLDL.

CLINICAL CONSIDERATIONS

Lp(a) is of clinical interest since several studies have shown a relationship between serum levels of Lp(a) and coronary heart disease (17,18). Indeed, high concentrations of Lp(a) have been considered to represent an independent risk factor for cardiovascular disease (19). In this context, it is important that Lp(a) has been demonstrated to be located in arterial atherosclerotic lesions (20). Since it has been demonstrated that Lp(a) interacts strongly with glycosaminoglycans present in the intima, and also with physiological concentrations of Ca^{++} (21), this may explain part of the atherogenicity of these particles. With more sensitive and specific probes for Lp(a), future studies should be able to clarify the physiological role of Lp(a), if any, and its significance in the process of atherosclerosis.

REFERENCES

1. Gaubatz, J. W., Heideman, C., Gotto, A. M., Jr., Morrisett, J. D., and Dahlen, G. H., *J. Biol. Chem.*, *258*:4582–4589 (1983).

2. Utermann, G., and Weber, W., *FEBS Lett.*, *154*:357–361 (1983).

3. Fless, G. M., Rolih, C. A., and Scanu, A. M., *J. Biol. Chem.*, *259*:11,470–11,478 (1984).

4. Berg, K., *Acta Pathol. Microbiol. Scand.*, *59*:369–382 (1963).

5. Foreman, J. R., Karlin, J. B., Edelstein, C., Juhn, D. J., Rubenstein, A. H., and Scanu, A. M., *J. Lipid Res.*, *18*: 759–767 (1977).

6. Fless, G. M., ZumMallen, M. E., Scanu, A. M., and Aggerbeck, L., submitted.

7. Schurz, J., Niedermayer, H., Jurgens, G., Kostner, G. M., and Holasek, A., *Colloid Polym. Sci.*, *257*:1068–1072 (1979).

8. Nothig-Laslo, V., and Jurgens, G., *Arch. Biochem. Biophys.*, *215*:329–338 (1982).

9. Fless, G. M., ZumMallen, M. E., and Scanu, A. M., *J. Lipid Res.*, *26*:1224–1229 (1985).

10. Krempler, F., Kostner, G. M., Roscher, A., Haslauer, F., Bolzano, K., and Sandhofer, F., *J. Clin. Invest.*, *71*:1431–1441 (1983).

11. Krempler, F., Kostner, G. M., Bolzano, K., and Sandhofer, F., *Biochim. Biophys. Acta*, *575*:63–70 (1979).

12. Bersot, T. P., Innerarity, T. L., and Mahley, R. W., *Arteriosclerosis*, *4*:536a (1984).

13. Albers, J. J., Cabana, V. G., Warnick, G. R., and Hazzard, W. R., *Metabolism*, *24*:1047–1054 (1975).

14. Fless, G. M., Fischer-Dzoga, K., Juhn, D. J., Bates, S. R., and Scanu, A. M., *Arteriosclerosis*, *2*:475–486 (1982).

15. Vessby, B., Kostner, G., Lithell, H., and Thomis, J., *Atherosclerosis*, *44*:61–71 (1982).

16. Albers, J. J., Taggart, H. McA., Applebaum-Bowden, D., Haffner, S., Chestnut, C. H., III, and Hazzard, W. R., *Biochim. Biophys. Acta*, *795*:293–296 (1984).

17. Dahlen, G., Ericson, C., Furberg, C., Lundqvist, L., and Svardsudd, K., *Acta Med. Scand. Suppl.*, *531*:1–29 (1972).

18. Berg, K., in *The Biochemistry of Atherosclerosis* (Scanu, A. M., ed.), Marcel Dekker, New York, 1979, pp. 419–490.

19. Kostner, G. M., Avogaro, P., Cazzolato, G., Marth, E., Bittolo-Bon, G., and Qunici, G. B., *Atherosclerosis*, *38*:51–61 (1981).

20. Walton, K. W., Hitchens, J., Magnani, H. N., and Khan, M., *Atherosclerosis*, *20*:323–346 (1974).

21. Ericson, C., Dahlen, G., and Berg, K., *Clin. Genet.*, *11*:433–440 (1977).

22. Shen, B. W., Scanu, A. M., and Kezdy, F. J., *Proc. Natl. Acad. Sci. U.S.A.*, *74*:837–841 (1977).

23. Fless, G. M., and Scanu, A. M., *J. Biol. Chem.*, *254*:8653–8661 (1979).

5

Genetics of the Human Apolipoproteins

JAN L. BRESLOW The Rockefeller University, New York, New York

PERSPECTIVES AND SUMMARY

Apolipoproteins are important structural constituents of lipoprotein particles and have been shown to participate in lipoprotein synthesis, secretion, processing, and catabolism. These subjects have been reviewed recently (1,2). In the last 15 years, advances in protein chemistry techniques have allowed the identification, isolation, and characterization of at least eight apolipoproteins (Table 1). Protein sequencing techniques have allowed the derivation of the primary amino acid sequence of the plasma form of six of these polypeptides. In the last 2 years, cDNA and in some cases genomic clones have been derived for seven of the apolipoproteins. The DNA sequences combined with cell-free synthesis and tissue and organ culture studies have revealed the presence of apolipoprotein precursors containing NH_2-terminal extensions, including prepeptides and in some cases propeptides. In addition, most of the apolipoprotein genes have been mapped in the human genome (Table 2). Finally, human mutations in the apolipoprotein genes have been identified at both the amino acid and DNA level. Some of these have profound effects on lipoprotein metabolism and are associated with premature atherosclerosis. This chapter will review current knowledge of apolipoprotein gene structure, function, and genetic variation.

APO A-I

Apo A-I is the major protein constituent of high-density lipoproteins (HDL). HDL particles are about 50% protein and 50% lipid, and apo

Table 1 Apoproteins and Their Association with Human Diseases

Apoprotein	Plasma concentration (mg/dl)	Isoelectric point (PI)	MW	Function	Association with clinical disorders
A-I	1.0 –1.2	5.85–5.40[a]	28K	Activates LCAT	Tangier disease Apo A-I, apo CIII deficiency Atherosclerosis
A-II	0.3 –0.5	5.0	8.5K	–	–
A-IV	0.16	5.5	46K	–	–
B-100	0.7 –1.0	–	400K	Receptor mediated catabolism of LDL	Abetalipoproteinemia Normotriglyceridemic abetalipoproteinemia (B-100 deficiency) Atherosclerosis
B-48	–	–	200K	Chylomicron production	–

CI	0.04–0.06	7.5	6.5K	Activates (moderately) LCAT	–
CII	0.03–0.05	4.9	9K	Activates lipoprotein lipase	Familial type I hyperlipoproteinemia
CIII	0.12–0.14	4.7 –5.0[b]	9K	Inhibits catabolism of triglyceride-rich lipoproteins	Apo A-I, apo CIII deficiency
E	0.025–0.050	6.0 –5.7[c]	34.2K	Receptor mediated catabolism of apo E-containing lipoproteins	Familial type III hyperlipoproteinemia

[a]The isoelectric points of apo A-I isoproteins are apo $A\text{-}I_2$ = 5.85; apo $A\text{-}I_3$ = 5.74; apo $A\text{-}I_4$ = 5.65; apo $A\text{-}I_5$ = 5.52; apo $A\text{-}I_6$ = 5.40. The major plasma isoprotein is apo $A\text{-}I_4$.
[b]The isoelectric points of individual apo CIII isoproteins are apo CIII-0 = 5.0; apo CIII-1 = 4.85; apo CIII-2 = 4.65.
[c]The isoelectric points of individual apo E3 isoproteins are apo E3 = 6.02; apo $E3_{s-1}$ = 5.89, apo $E3_{s-2}$ = 5.78; apo $E3_{s-3}$ = 5.68. The isoelectric points of the common apo E variants are apo E2 = 5.89; apo E4 = 6.18.

A-I constitutes 70% of HDL protein (2). HDL levels are inversely related to susceptibility to coronary artery disease, and recently the same association has been demonstrated for apo A-I (3). Apo A-I is abundant in plasma with a concentration of 1.0 to 1.2 mg/ml. Apo A-I is thought to participate via two mechanisms in the reverse transport of cholesterol from tissues to the liver for excretion. Apo A-I can promote cholesterol efflux from tissues (4), perhaps through a recently described receptor that is up-regulated by cholesterol loading (5). Apo A-I also displays cofactor activity for the lecithin cholesterol acyltransferase (LCAT) enzyme, which is responsible for almost all plasma cholesterol esterification (6). This reaction is thought to play a role in transforming nascent HDL to mature HDL particles. In mammals, apo A-I synthesis is approximately equally divided between liver and small intesting; in avians, other major sites of synthesis have been identified (see Ref. 1).

Apo A-I cDNA

Apo A-I cDNA clones have been obtained by several laboratories, and their DNA sequences have been derived (7–13) (Fig. 1). From this information, apo A-I mRNA is thought to be 893 bp in length and includes a 5' untranslated region of 35 bp, a region coding for 267 amino acids of 801 bp, a termination codon, TGA, and a 3' untranslated region of 54 bp followed by a poly A tail. This is compatible with an apo A-I mRNA size of 950 bp determined by Northern blotting analysis of human liver RNA.

The cDNA sequence and NH_2-terminal microsequencing of the primary translation product of apo A-I mRNA in cell-free synthesis experiments indicate translation initiation at the methionine 24 amino acids upstream of the NH_2 terminus of the mature protein. The 18

Table 2 Human Apolipoproteins

	Amino acid sequence[a]	cDNA clone[b]	Genomic clone[c]	Chromosome mapping[d]
Apo A-I[e]	243	267	R(3IVS)	11q13
Apo A-II[f]	77	100	NR	1
Apo A-IV[g]	—	391	NR	11
Apo B[h]	—	—	NR	—
Apo CI[i]	57	83	NR	19
Apo CII[i]	79	101	R	19pter → q13

Table 2 (continued)

	Amino acid sequence[a]	cDNA clone[b]	Genomic clone[c]	Chromosome mapping[d]
Apo CIII[i]	79	99	R(3IVS)	11q13
Apo E[i]	299	317	R(3IVS)	19pter → q13

[a]Amino acid sequence derived by protein sequencing techniques from the plasma form of the protein. Number of amino acids specified.
[b]cDNA clones isolated, sequenced, and length of primary translation product deduced. Number of amino acids specified.
[c]Genomic clones have been reported (R) and not reported (NR) as indicated. Apo A-I, apo CIII, and apo E each have 3 introns in similar locations. The apo CII introns are currently being characterized.
[d]Six apolipoprotein genes have been localized through the use of somatic cell hybrids and DNA probes. Apo A-I and apo CIII are within 2.5 kb of each other and linkage studies have tentatively placed apo A-IV in this region.
[e]The 24-amino-acid NH_2-terminal extension of the primary translation product includes an 18-amino-acid prepeptide and a 6-amino-acid propeptide. The latter has an unusual amino acid configuration of R-H-F-W-Q-Q. Apo A-I is secreted in its pro form, which is cleaved extracellularly.
[f]In human plasma, apo A-II exists as a dimer of two 77-amino-acid monomers connected by a disulfide bridge at amino acid 6. The 23-amino-acid NH_2-terminal extension of the primary translation product includes an 18-amino-acid prepeptide and a 5-amino-acid propeptide.
[g]The amino acid sequence of apo A-IV has not been reported, but partial sequence of a prepeptide 20 amino acids long has been determined. The information given for the length of the primary translation product is for rat preapo A-IV, which is 391 amino acids long and also contains a 20-amino-acid prepeptide and a 371-amino-acid-long coding segment for the mature protein.
[h]There is very little structural information about apo B due to its size and great insolubility after delipidation. Physicochemical measurements indicate it has MW 400,000 and, therefore, may have a primary amino acid sequence approximately 4,000 amino acids long. Apo B is made in two forms: the long form (apo B-100) mainly from liver, and an antigenically similar molecular of approximately half that length (apo B-48) mainly from intestine.
[i]The cDNA sequences for apo CI, apo CII, apo CIII, and apo E suggest they are synthesized with 26-, 22-, 20-, and 18-amino-acid NH_2-terminal extensions. These sequences are compatible with prepeptide sequence. The primary translation product of rat apo CIII has been shown to have a 20-amino-acid NH_2-terminal extension.

HUMAN APO A-I cDNA

```
        10         20         30         40         50         60         70         80         90        100        110        120
GACTGCGAGA AGGAGGTCCC CCACGGCCCT TCAGGATGAA AGCTGCGGTG CTGACCTTGG CCGTGCTCTT CCTGACGGGG AGCCAGGCTC GGCATTTCTG GCAGCAAGAT GAACCCCCCC
                                        M K  A  A  V  L  T  L  A  V  L  F  L  T  G  S  Q  A  R  H  F  W  Q  Q  D  E  P  P
                                       -24                                                                   -1 +1

       130        140        150        160        170        180        190        200        210        220        230        240
AGAGCCCCTG GGATCGAGTG AAGGACCTGG CCACTGTGTA CGTGGATGTG CTCAAAGACA GCGGCAGAGA CTATGTGTCC CAGTTTGAAG GCTCCGCCTT GGGAAAACAG CTAAACCTAA
Q  S  P  W  D  R  V  K  D  L  A  T  V  Y  V  D  V  L  K  D  S  G  R  D  Y  V  S  Q  F  E  G  S  A  L  G  K  Q  L  N  L

       250        260        270        280        290        300        310        320        330        340        350        360
AGCTCCTTGA CAACTGGGAC AGCGTGACCT CCACCTTCAG CAAGCTGCGC GAACAGCTCG GCCCTGTGAC CCAGGAGTTC TGGGATAACC TGGAAAAGGA GACAGAGGGC CTGAGGCAGG
K  L  L  D  N  W  D  S  V  T  S  T  F  S  K  L  R  E  Q  L  G  P  V  T  Q  E  F  W  D  N  L  E  K  E  T  E  G  L  R  Q▲

       370        380        390        400        410        420        430        440        450        460        470        480
AGATGAGCAA GGATCTGGAG GAGGTGAAGG CCAAGGTGCA GCCCTACCTG GACGACTTCC AGAAGAAGTG GCAGGAGGAG ATGGAGCTCT ACCGCCAGAA GGTGGAGCCG CTGCGCGCAG
E  M  S  K  D  L  E  E  V  K  A  K  V  Q  P  Y  L  D  D  F  Q  K  K  W  Q  E  E  M  E  L  Y  R  Q  K  V  E  P  L  R  A

       490        500        510        520        530        540        550        560        570        580        590        600
AGCTCCAAGA GGGCGCGCGC CAGAAGCTGC ACGAGCTGCA AGAGAAGCTG AGCCCACTGG GCGAGGAGAT GCGCGACCGC GCGCGCGCCC ATGTGGACGC GCTGCGCACG CATCTGGCCC
E  L  Q  E  G  A  R  Q  K  L  H  E  L  Q  E  K  L  S  P  L  G  E  E  M  R  D  R  A  R  A  H  V  D  A  L  R  T  H  L  A

       610        620        630        640        650        660        670        680        690        700        710        720
CCTACAGCGA CGAGCTGCGC CAGCGCTTGG CCGCGCGCCT TGAGGCTCTC AAGGAGAACG GCGGCGCCAG ACTGGCCGAG TACCACGCCA AGGCCACCGA GCATCTGAGC ACGCTCAGCG
P  Y  S  D  E  L  R  Q  R  L  A  A  R  L  E  A  L  K  E  N  G  G  A  R  L  A  E  Y  H  A  K  A  T  E  H  L  S  T  L  S

       730        740        750        760        770        780        790        800        810        820        830        840
AGAAGGCCAA GCCCGCGCTC GAGGACCTCC GCCAAGGCCT GCTGCCCGTG CTGGAGAGCT TCAAGGTCAG CTTCCTGAGC GCTCTCGAGG AGTACACTAA GAAGCTCAAC ACCCAGTGAG
E  K  A  K  P  A  L  E  D  L  R  Q  G  L  L  P  V  L  E  S  F  K  V  S  F  L  S  A  L  E  E  Y  T  K  K  L  N  T  Q
                                                                                                                        243

       850        860        870        880        890
GCGCCCGCCG CCGCCCCCCT TCCCGGTGCT CAGAATAAAC GTTTCCAAAG TGGA(n)
```

Fig. 1 Apo A-I cDNA is 893 bp in length plus a poly A tail. The coding regions for the prepeptide, propeptide, and mature protein are bp's 36 to 89, 90 to 107, and 108 to 836. The six 66-bp tandem repeats are in the region of bp's 402 to 797. The polyadenylation signal AATAAA occurs in the 3' untranslated region from bp's 874 to 879. The arrow at bp 359 indicates a probable site of true variation with some alleles having a G, as shown, and other alleles having an A. In either case, the codon specifies Glu.

NH_2-terminal amino acids, which can be cotranslationally cleaved by microsomal membranes, represent the apo A-I prepeptide. The six amino acids adjacent to the NH_2 terminus of the mature apo A-I is the propeptide and has the rather unusual sequence Arg-His-Phe-Trp-Gln-Gln (14–16). The propeptide is not cleaved intracellularly, but rather is present in secreted apo A-I (15–19). Thus it is necessary to postulate the existence of a previously unsuspected protease activity in lymph or plasma required to cleave this hexapeptide and generate mature apo A-I. This converting protease presumably plays a role in apo A-I processing and may be an important determinant of apo A-I and, thereby, HDL metabolism. Recently, protease activity, which is inhibited by EDTA, has been demonstrated in human serum and on the surface of human endothelial cells and hepatoma cells (20,21). The reported cDNA sequences specify an amino acid sequence for mature apo A-I of 243 amino acids, which is very similar to that derived previously by protein sequencing methods (22). The only difference is at residue 34, where the protein sequence is specified Gln and the cDNA sequence indicates Glu.

It has been noted previously that the apo A-I amino acid sequence from residues 99 to 230 is composed of 6 tandem 22 amino acid repeats, 5 of the 6 repeats beginning with proline (23,24). Examination of the DNA sequence in this region confirms this and shows a tandemly repeated DNA structure 66 bp in length (11). This finding suggests that this portion of the apo A-I gene arose by intragenic duplications. When the six 66-bp repeats are aligned and a consensus nucleotide at each position of the repeat is derived, the consensus sequence is 64 to 80% homologous with each of the repeats (11) (Fig. 2a). Translation of the consensus sequence reveals an interesting underlying protein structure for this region of apo A-I (Fig. 2a). As noted from the protein structure, proline, an alpha-helix breaker, occurs every 22 amino acids. The intervening amino acids, when placed in an Edmundson wheel diagram (25), specify an alpha-helix with a nonpolar and a polar face (Fig. 2b). This is the general character of the amphipathic alpha-helical configuration, which is a common feature of the apolipoproteins (26). It is thought that the nonpolar face interacts with the hydrophobic lipid core of the lipoprotein particle, whereas the polar face interacts with the aqueous plasma environment. In addition, the positively charged residues tend to cluster between the nonpolar and polar faces. The latter has been shown to be important in stabilizing the lipid protein association (27). A recent, more sophisticated computer analysis derived to specifically look for DNA repeats in apo A-I reveals that the basic structure is a 33-bp (11-codon) repeat—a model based on gene duplication and unequal crossing-over events has been derived (28).

APO A-I 66bp DNA REPEATS

```
Repeat Amino Acid                                                                          % Homology

#1 (099-120)    CCCTACCTGGACGACTTCCAGAAGAAGTGGCAGGAGGAGATGGAGCTCTACCGCCAGAAGGTGGAG     69
#2 (121-142)    CCGCTGCGCGCAGAGCTCCAAGAGGGCGCGCGCCAGAAGCTGCACGAGCTGCAAGAGAAGCTGAGC     80
#3 (143-164)    CCACTGGGCCAGGAGATGCGCGACCGCGCGCGCGCCCATGTGGACGCGCTGCGCACGCATCTGGCC     74
#4 (165-186)    CCCTACAGCGACGAGCTGCGCCAGCGCTTGGCCGCGCGCCTTGAGGCTCTCAAGGAGAACGGCGGC     74
#5 (187-208)    GCCAGACTGGCCGAGTATCACGCCAAGGCCACCGAGCATCTGAGCACGCTCAGCGAGAAGGCCAAG     69
#6 (209-230)    CCCGCGCTCGAGGACCTCCGCCAAGGCCTGCTGCCCGTGCTGGAGAGCTTCAAGGTCAGCTTCCTG     64
-----------------------------------------------------------------------------------------------------

Consensus       CCCXXGCGCGACGAGCTCCGCGAGXGCGCGCXCGCGCAGCTGGAGGCGCTCCGCGAGAAGGTGGXG
Sequence               T           A              A         C       AA         C  C

-----------------------------------------------------------------------------------------------------

Translated      Pro---ArgAspGluLeuArgGlu---Ala---AlaGlnLeuGluAlaLeuArgGluLysVal---
Amino Acid            Leu         His            Glu      Asp      Ser
Sequence                                                           His
                                                                   Asn
-----------------------------------------------------------------------------------------------------

Amino Acid
Charges          0  ? +½ -1 -1  0 +1 -1  ?  0  ? -½  0  0 -1  0  0 +½ -1 +1  0  ?

-----------------------------------------------------------------------------------------------------
```

(a)

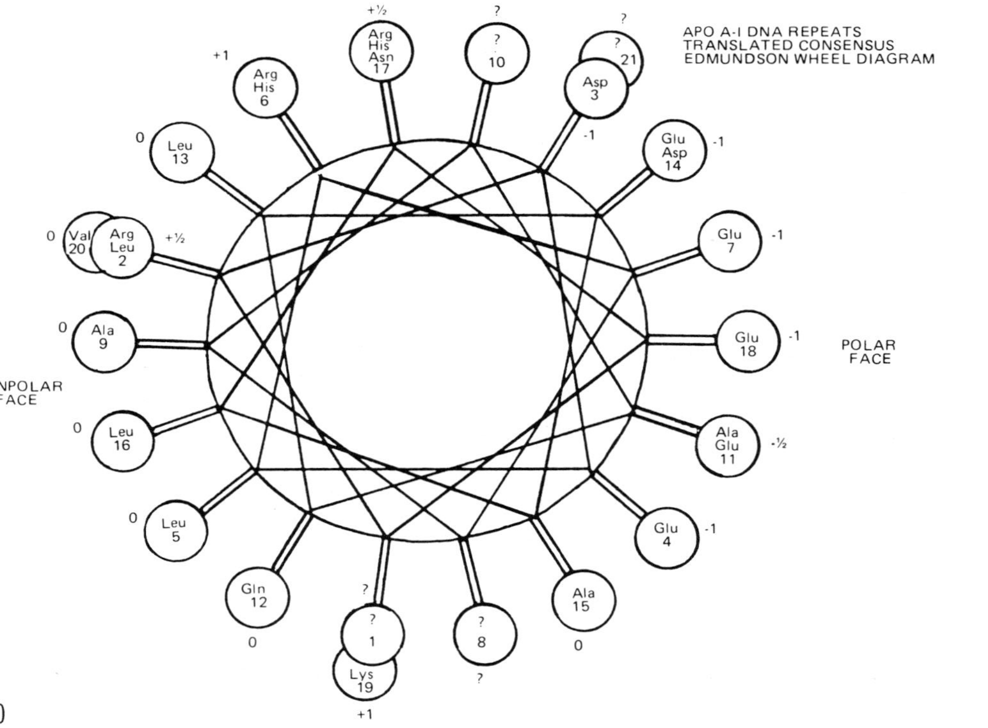

Fig. 2 (a) The apo A-I 66-bp DNA repeats were aligned and a consensus sequence generated. The homology of each of the repeats with the consensus is shown. Charges of the amino acids are specified. (b) As shown in the diagram the helix clearly contains a nonpolar and a polar face. The positively charged residues tend to cluster between nonpolar and polar faces.

HUMAN APO A-I GENE

```
        10         20         30         40         50         60         70         80         90        100        110        120
AAAGAAGAGC ACTGGTGGGA GGACAGGGCG GGGGAAGGGG GAGGGGAGTG AAGTAGTCTC CCTGGAATGC TGGTGGTGGG GGAGGCAGTC TCCTTGGTGG AGGAGTCCCA GCGTCCCTCC
---------- ---------- ---------- ---------- ---------- ---------- ---------- ---------- ---------- ---------- ---------- ----------

       130        140        150        160        170        180        190        200        210        220        230        240
CCTCCCCTCC TCTGCCAACA CAATGGACAA TGGCAACTGC CCACACACTC CCATGGAGGG GAAGGGGATG AGTGCAGGGA ACCCCGACCC CACCCGGGAG ACCTGCAAGC CTGCAGACAC
---------- ---------- ---------- ---------- ---------- ---------- ---------- ---------- ---------- ---------- ---------- ----------

       250        260        270        280        290        300        310        320        330        340        350        360
TCCCCTCCCG CCCCCACTGA ACCCTTGACC CCTGCCCTGC ACGCCCCGCA GCTTGCTGTT TGCCCACTCC TATTTGCCCA GTCCCAGGGA CAGAGCTGAT CCTTGAACTC TTAAGTTCCA
---------- ---------- ---------- ---------- ---------- ---------- ---------- ---------- ---------- ---------- ---------- ----------

                                                                              "TATA" Box
       370        380        390        400        410        420        430        440        450        460        470        480
CATTGCCAGG ACCAGTGAGC AGCAACAGGG CCAGGGCTGG GCTTATCAGC CTCCCAGCCC AGACCCTGGC TGCAGACATA AATAGGCCCT GCAAGAGCTG GCTGCTTAGA GACTGCGAGA
---------- ---------- ---------- ---------- ---------- ---------- ---------- ---------- ---------- ---------- ----------

       490        500        510        520        530        540        550        560        570        580        590        600
AGGAGGTGCG TCCTGCTGCC TGCCCCGGTC ACTCTGGCTC CCCAGCTCAA GGTTCAGGCC TTGCCCCAGG CCGGGCCTCT GGGTACCTGA GGTCTTCTCC CGCTCTGTGC CCTTCTCCTC
     [---- ---------- ---------- ---------- ---------- ---------- ---------- ---------- ---------- ---IVS-1-- ---------- ----------

       610        620        630        640        650        660        670        680        690        700        710        720
ACCTGGCTGC AATGAGTGGG GGAGCACGGG GCTTCTGCAT GCTGAAGGCA CCCCACTCAG CCAGGCCCTT CTTCTCCTCC AGGTCCCCCA CGGCCCTTCA GGATGAAAGC TGCGGTGCTG
---------- ---------- ---------- ---------- ---------- ---------- ---------- ---------- -]                       M  K  A   A  V  L

       730        740        750        760        770        780        790        800        810        820        830        840
ACCTTGGCCG TGCTCTTCCT GACGGGTAGG TGTCCCCTAA CCTAGGGAGC CAACCATCGG GGGGCTTTCT CCCTAAATCC CCGTGGCCCA CCCTCCTGGG CAGAGGCAGC AGGTTTCTCA
 T  L  A   V  L  F  L   T [---- ---------- ---------- ---------- -----▲---- ---------- ---------- ---------- ---------- ----------

       850        860        870        880        890        900        910        920        930        940        950        960
CTGGCCCCCT CTCCCCCACC TCCAAGCTTG GCCTTTCGGC TCAGATCTCA GCCCACAGCT GGCCTGATCT GGGTCTCCCC TCCCACCCTC AGGGAGCCAG GCTCGGCATT TCTGGCAGCA
---------- ---------- --IVS-2--- ---------- ---------- ---------- ---------- ---------- ---------- -]G  S  Q   A  R  H   F  W  Q  Q
                                                                                                                                -1

       970        980        990       1000       1010       1020       1030       1040       1050       1060       1070       1080
AGATGAACCC CCCCAGAGCC CCTGGGATCG AGTGAAGGAC CTGGCCACTG TGTACGTGGA TGTGCTCAAA GACAGCGGCA GAGACTATGT GTCCCAGTTT GAAGGCTCCG CCTTGGGAAA
  D  E  P   F  Q  S   P  W  D  R   V  K  D   L  A  T   V  Y  V  D   V  L  K   D  S  G   R  D  Y  V   S  Q  F   E  G  S   A  L  G  K
 +1
```

```
      1090       1100       1110       1120       1130       1140       1150       1160       1170       1180       1190       1200
ACAGCTAAAG TAAGGACCCA GCCTGGGGTT GAGGGCAGGG GCAGGGGGCA GAGGCCTGTG GGATGATGTT GAAGCCAGAC TGGCCGAGTC CTCACCTAAT ATCTGATGAG CTGGGCCCCA
  Q  L  N[ ---------- ---------- ---------- ---------- ---------- ---------- ---------- ---------- ---------- ---------- ----------

      1210       1220       1230       1240       1250       1260       1270       1280       1290       1300       1310       1320
CAGATGGTCT GGATGGAGAA ACCGGAATGG ATCTCCAGGC AGGGTCACAG CCCATGTCCC CTGCAAAGGA CAGACCAGGG CTGCCCGATG CGTGATCACA GAGCCACATT GTGCCTGCAA
---------- ---------- ---------- ---------- ---------- ---------- ---------- ---------- ---------- ---------- ---------- ----------

      1330       1340       1350       1360       1370       1380       1390       1400       1410       1420       1430       1440
GTGTAGCAAG CCCCTTTCCC TTCTTCACCA CCTCCTCTGC TCCTGCCCAG CAAGACTGTG GGCTGTCTTC GGAGAGGAGA ATGCGCTGGA GGCATAGAAG CGAGGTCCTT CAAGGGCCCA
---------- ---------- ---------- ---------- ---------- ---------- --IVS-3--- ---------- ---------- ---------- ---------- ----------
```

(continued on p. 96)

Fig. 3 From the proposed transcription initiation site (bp 472) to the polyadenylation site (bp 2334), the apo A-I gene is 1863 bp in length. Three introns (IVS-1, IVS-2, and IVS-3) are indicated by brackets and underlining, and are located from bp 486 to 682, 746 to 932, and 1090 to 1677. A 7-bp "AT" containing region "TATA Box" begins 33 bp 5' to the proposed transcription initiation site and is indicated. Sequences 5' and 3' to the gene are underlined but not bracketed. The apo A-I gene sequence was originally reported from two laboratories (11,12). A comparison of the sequences showed 16 sites of difference. Barralle and colleagues have reported a second sequence (13) in which they changed the sequence at four sites of difference (236, 508, 766, and 1801) to correspond with the sequence reported by Breslow and colleagues. The latter group is currently resequencing the apo A-I gene, and unpublished data indicate agreement with the British group at five sites (562, 612, 618, 653, and 808), but persisting disagreement at site 786 (Breslow and colleagues, C; Barralle and colleagues, T), with the situation at sites 281, 287, 309, 322, 393, and 400 as yet unresolved. Thus, site 786 may represent true genetic variation (thick arrow). The DNA sequence shown in the figure resolves previous differences and where uncertainty still exists is compatible with the second sequence reported by Barralle and colleagues.

```
      1450       1460       1470       1480       1490       1500       1510       1520       1530       1540       1550       1560
CTTTGGAGAC CAACGTAACT GGGCACCAGT CCCAGCTCTG TCTCCTTTTT AGCTCCTCTC TGTGCCTCGG TCCAGCTGCA CAACGGGGCA TGGCCTGGCG GGGCAGGGGT GTTGGTTGAG
---------- ---------- ---------- ---------- ---------- ---------- ---------- ---------- ---------- ---------- ---------- ----------

      1570       1580       1590       1600       1610       1620       1630       1640       1650       1660       1670       1680
AGTGTACTGG AAATGCTAGG CCACTGCACC TCCGCGGACA GGTGTCACCC AGGGCTCACC CCTGATAGGC TGGGGCGCTG GGAGGCCAGC CCTCAACCCT TCTGTCTCAC CCTCCAGCCT
---------- ---------- ---------- ---------- ---------- ---------- ---------- ---------- ---------- ---------- ---------- ------]  L

      1690       1700       1710       1720       1730       1740       1750       1760       1770       1780       1790       1800
AAAGCTCCTT GACAACTGGG ACAGCGTGAC CTCCACCTTC AGCAAGCTGC GCGAACAGCT CGGCCCTGTG ACCCAGGAGT TCTGGGATAA CCTGGAAAAG GAGACAGAGG GCCTGAGGCA
 K  L  L    D  N  W    D  S  V  T   S  T  F    S  K  L    R  E  Q  L   G  P  V    T  Q  E    F  W  D  N   L  E  K    E  T  E    G  L  R  Q

      1810       1820       1830       1840       1850       1860       1870       1880       1890       1900       1910       1920
GGAGATGAGC AAGGATCTGG AGGAGGTGAA GGCCAAGGTG CAGCCCTACC TGGACGACTT CCAGAAGAAG TGGCAGGAGG AGATGGAGCT CTACCGCCAG AAGGTGGAGC CGCTGCGCGC
 E  M  S    K  D  L    E  E  V  K   A  K  V    Q  P  Y    L  D  D  F   Q  K  K    W  Q  E    E  M  E  L   Y  R  Q    K  V  E    P  L  R  A

      1930       1940       1950       1960       1970       1980       1990       2000       2010       2020       2030       2040
AGAGCTCCAA GAGGGCGCGC GCCAGAAGCT GCACGAGCTG CAAGAGAAGC TGAGCCCACT GGGCGAGGAG ATGCGCGACC GCGCGCGCGC CCATGTGGAC GCGCTGCGCA CGCATCTGGC
 E  L  Q    E  G  A    R  Q  K  L   H  E  L    Q  E  K    L  S  P  L   G  E  E    M  R  D    R  A  R  A   H  V  D    A  L  R    T  H  L  A

      2050       2060       2070       2080       2090       2100       2110       2120       2130       2140       2150       2160
CCCCTACAGC GACGAGCTGC GCCAGCGCTT GGCCGCGCGC CTTGAGGCTC TCAAGGAGAA CGGCGGCGCC AGACTGGCCG AGTACCACGC CAAGGCCACC GAGCATCTGA GCACGCTCAG
 P  Y  S    D  E  L    R  Q  R  L   A  A  R    L  E  A    L  K  E  N   G  G  A    R  L  A    E  Y  H  A   K  A  T    E  H  L    S  T  L  S

      2170       2180       2190       2200       2210       2220       2230       2240       2250       2260       2270       2280
CGAGAAGGCC AAGCCCGCGC TCGAGGACCT CCGCCAAGGC CTGCTGCCCG TGCTGGAGAG CTTCAAGGTC AGCTTCCTGA GCGCTCTCGA GGAGTACACT AAGAAGCTCA ACACCCAGTG
 E  K  A    K  P  A    L  E  D  L   R  Q  G    L  L  P    V  L  E  S   F  K  V    S  F  L    S  A  L  E   E  Y  T    K  K  L    N  T  Q

      2290       2300       2310       2320       2330       2340       2350       2360       2370       2380       2390
AGGCGCCCGC CGCCGCCCCC CTTCCCGGTG CTCAGAATAA ACGTTTCCAA AGTGGGAAGC AGCTTCTTTC TTTTGGGAGA ATAGAGGGGG GTGCGGGGAC ATCCGGGGGA GCCCGGC
                                                            ----- ---------- ---------- ---------- ---------- ---------- -------
```

Fig. 3 (continued)

Apo A-I Gene

The apo A-I gene has been isolated and its DNA sequence derived (11–13) (Fig. 3). The gene is 1863 bp in length. A comparison of the sequence of the apo A-I gene with the cDNA reveals 3 introns (IVS) in the apo A-I gene. IVS-1 is 197 bp long and occurs in the 5' untranslated region between bases 20 and 21 upstream of the codon for Met that initiates translation. IVS-2 is 186 bp long and interrupts the codon specifying amino acid 10, which is in the apo A-I prepeptide. IVS-3 is 588 bp long and interrupts the codon-specifying amino acid 43 of the mature protein. The intron locations indicate that apo A-I exons may code for functionally distinct regions of apo A-I. For instance, exon 2 contains most of the apo A-I prepeptide and exon 3 contains the propeptide and the NH_2-terminal sequences, whereas exon 4 contains codons for the 200 amino acids that comprise the COOH-terminal portion of the molecule. The latter includes the 66-bp tandem DNA repeats.

The apo A-I gene transcription initiation site has been designated (Fig. 4) based on the length of several apo A-I cDNA clones (13). Further experiments have failed to find sequences upstream of this

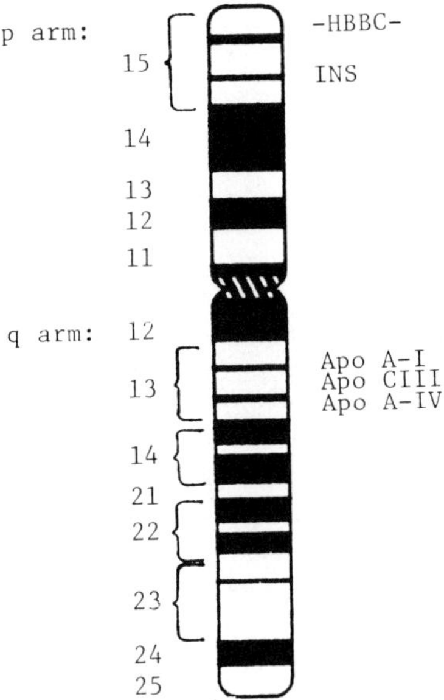

Fig. 4 A map of human chromosome 11 has been assembled at the Seventh International Workshop on Human Gene Mapping and many loci regionalized to either short (p) arm or long (q) arm or specific bands (35). The apo A-I, apo A-IV, and apo CIII loci have been mapped to the vicinity of 11q13. The polymorphic nonalpha-globin (-HBBC-), and insulin (INS) loci, have been mapped to p15.

site occurring commonly in liver-derived apo A-I mRNA. Upstream of the proposed apo A-I transcription initiation site is a 7-bp-long AT-rich region that may be the apo A-I promoter, "TATA box" (11–13). It is of interest that an apo A-I cDNA clone pAI-121 has been reported which includes 96 bp 5' to the translation initiation codon (11). This cDNA clone contains the "TATA box" sequences, which implies that transcription can begin 5' to this sequence, even though this may be an uncommon event. Examination of the DNA sequence several hundred bases 5' to the sequences in the pAI-121 clone does not reveal another suitable AT-rich promoter region.

Apo A-I Gene Location

Somatic cell hybrids and DNA probes have been used to map the gene for human apo A-I (29–31). In all studies, the apo A-I gene appears to be at a single locus and cosegregates with human chromosome 11. Some of the hybrids examined contained only a portion of chromosome 11, and apo A-I cosegregated with p11→qter (29), p11→q13 (30), and q13→qter (31) in three different studies. In the mouse, apo A-I has been mapped to chromosome 9 (32) and shown to be 1.3 ± 0.7 centimorgans from uroporphyrinogen I synthase (33). The latter has been mapped in humans to chromosome region 11q13→qter (34). These data strongly suggest that the human apo A-I gene is located on the long arm of chromosome 11 in the vicinity of q13 (35) (Fig. 4).

Apo A-I Mutations

Apo A-I is the principal structural protein in HDL. Because of the importance of HDL levels in predicting atherosclerosis susceptibility, attention has been paid to apo A-I by screening for variants in populations, principally by isoelectric focusing, as well as by studying apo A-I in individuals with altered HDL levels. Thus far, these studies have resulted in the discovery of eight proven apo A-I genetic variants (Table 3). Seven of these variants have been shown in people who appear to be heterozygotes for one normal apo A-I structural allele and another allele that specifies a gene product that is either one charge unit more acidic or one charge unit more basic than wild type. The acidic alleles have been designated $A\text{-}I_{Milano}$ (36,37), $A\text{-}I_{Marburg}$ (38,39), and $A\text{-}I_{Munster2}$ (40). The former mutation results from a substitution of Cys for Arg at residue 173 (37), whereas both of the latter two mutations appear to be due to a deletion of Lys at residue 107 (41). The basic alleles have been designated $A\text{-}I_{Giessen}$ (38), $A\text{-}I_{Munster3A}$, $A\text{-}I_{Munster3B}$, and $A\text{-}I_{Munster3C}$ (40). These mutations result from substitutions of Arg for Pro at residue 143 (41), Asn for Asp at residue 103, Arg for Pro at residue 4, and His for Pro at residue 3 (42), respectively. $A\text{-}I_{Milano}$ and

Table 3 Apo A-I Genetics Variants

Name[a]	Charge difference[b]	Defect[c]	HDL level[d]
A-I$_{Milano}$	−1	$Arg_{173} \rightarrow Cys$	↓
A-I$_{Marburg}$	−1	$Lys_{107} \rightarrow 0$	↓
A-I$_{Munster2}$	−1	$Lys_{107} \rightarrow 0$	NL NL
A-I$_{Giessen}$	+1	$Pro_{143} \rightarrow Arg$	NL
A-I$_{Munster3A}$	+1	$Asp_{103} \rightarrow Asn$	NL
A-I$_{Munster3B}$	+1	$Pro_{4} \rightarrow Arg$	NL
A-I$_{Munster3C}$	+1	$Pro_{3} \rightarrow His$	NL
A-I-CIII Deficiency	NA	A-I gene insert	↓↓

[a]The apo A-I genetic variants, except for A-I-CIII deficiency, have been named for the cities in which they were discovered. A-I-CIII deficiency was discovered in Detroit by Norum et al. and designates a clinical syndrome of severe premature atherosclerosis associated with low HDL levels and plasma deficiency of two apolipoproteins, apo A-I and apo CIII.

[b]The major normal human apo A-I isoprotein has an isoelectric point of pH 5.64. Individuals with apo A-I charge variants are heterozygotes with one normal major apo A-I isoprotein and one major apo A-I isoprotein with an isoelectric point of either pH 5.52 (−1) or pH 5.74 (+1).

[c]For each of the charge variants, the altered protein has been isolated, protein sequence determined, and the altered amino acid residue identified. For two of the variants, it appears that Lys_{107} has been deleted. In apo A-I-CIII deficiency, a DNA insert in the apo A-I gene has rendered it dysfunctional.

[d]HDL levels in probands have been determined and found to be either normal (NL), mildly reduced(↓), or severely reduced (↓↓) as indicated.

A-I$_{Marburg}$, but not the other structural variants, have been associated with reduced HDL levels (36,39). Normal apo A-I activates lecithin cholesterol acyl transferase, and A-I$_{Giessen}$ has been reported to be defective in this regard (41). The apo A-I genetic variant designated apo A-I, apo C-III deficiency appears to be due to a DNA insertion in the coding region of the apo A-I gene and will be discussed in a subsequent section (43–46).

Another disorder, called Tangier disease, characterized by an autosomal recessive form of inheritance, very low HDL levels, and cholesteryl ester accumulation in reticuloendothelial cells (2), may be associated with an apo A-I abnormality (47). Normal apo A-I is synthesized as a prepropeptide. After cleavage of the 18-amino-acid presegment, apo A-I is secreted as the propeptide with a 6-amino-acid NH_2-terminal extension. The propeptide is cleaved, presumably by a lymph or plasma protease, to achieve the mature form of the plasma protein (15–19). Normal plasma apo A-I has a ratio of propeptide to mature peptide of 0.01 to 0.02, whereas in Tangier disease this ratio is 1 to 1.5 (47). It was hypothesized that this observation could be due to a lack of Tangier-converting protease activity, a defective substrate precluding normal conversion, or a very unstable conversion product (47). Each of these possibilities has been studied. Conversion of proapo A-I to apo A-I appears to be normal (48), and NH_2-terminal sequencing of Tangier proapo A-I reveals a normal amino acid sequence around the cleavage point, suggesting a normal substrate for conversion (49). There is some suggestion of instability of mature Tangier apo A-I. Altered lipid binding (50) as well as enhanced in vivo catabolism (51) have been demonstrated for the isolated material. However, the Tangier apo A-I gene has recently been cloned (V. I. Zannis and J. L. Breslow, unpublished observations). Thus far, the DNA sequence of one allele from one patient analyzed has shown that the coding region appears to specify a normal amino acid sequence. If this is replicated in studies of other alleles from other patients, it would indicate that a structural apo A-I abnormality does not underlie Tangier disease. Other explanations would have to be found for the altered lipid binding, accelerated in vivo catabolism, and increased ratio of proapo A-I to apo A-I. Apo A-I is not a glycoprotein; therefore, altered posttranslational modification with sugars cannot be involved as a mechanism.

APO A-II

Apo A-II is the second most abundant protein in HDL, comprising approximately 20% of its protein (2). Plasma apo A-II concentrations are 0.3 to 0.5 mg/ml. In vitro apo A-II has been shown to displace apo A-I from HDL particles (52) as well as to activate hepatic lipase

HUMAN APO A-II cDNA

```
        10         20         30         40         50         60         70         80         90        100        110        120
CGCCCTCCCC ACTGTTACCA ACATGAAGCT GCTCGCAGCA ACTGTGCTAC TCCTCACCAT CTGCAGCCTT GAAGGAGCTT TGGTTCGGAG ACAGGCAAAG GAGCCATGTG TGGAGAGCCT
                        M  K  L   L  A  A   T  V  L   L  L  T  I   C  S  L   E  G  A   L  V  R  R   Q  A  K   E  P  C   V  E  S  L
                      -23                                                                    -1   +1

       130        140        150        160        170        180        190        200        210        220        230        240
GGTTTCTCAG TACTTCCAGA CCGTGACTGA CTATGGCAAG GACCTGATGG AGAAGGTCAA GAGCCCAGAG CTTCAGGCCG AGGCCAAGTC TTACTTTGAA AAGTCAAAGG AGCAGCTGAC
  V  S  Q   Y  F  Q  T   V  T  D   Y  G  K   D  L  M   E  K  V  K   S  P  E   L  Q  A   E  A  K  S   Y  F  E   K  S  K  E   Q  L  T

       250        260        270        280        290        300        310        320        330        340        350        360
ACCCCTGATC AAGAAGGCTG GAACGGAACT GGTTAACTTC TTGAGCTATT TCGTGGAACT TGGAACACAG CCTGCCACCC AGTGAAGTGT CCAGACCATT GTCTTCCAAC CCCAGCTGGC
  P  L  I   K  K  A   G  T  E  L   V  N  F   L  S  Y   F  V  E  L . G  T  Q   P  A  T  Q
                                                                                         77

       370        380        390        400        410        420        430        440
CTCTAGAACA CCCACTGGCC AGTCCTAGAG CTCCTGTCCC TACCCACTCT TTGCTACAAT AAATGCTGAA TGAATCCA(n)
```

Fig. 5 Apo A-II cDNA is at least 437 bp in length plus a poly A tail. The coding regions for the prepeptide, and mature protein are bp's 23 to 76, 77 to 91, and 92 to 322. The polyadenylation signal AATAAA occurs in the 3' untranslated region from bp's 418 to 423.

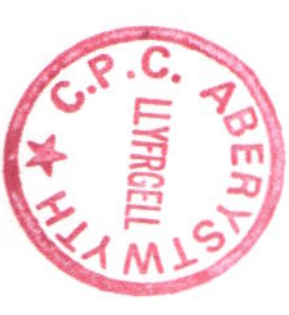

(53) and to inhibit LCAT (6). However, the physiological role of apo A-II has not been determined, and primary qualitative or quantitative abnormalities of human apo A-II have not been reported. Apo A-II is made in the liver and intestine (54).

Apo A-II cDNA

Apo A-II cDNA clones have been isolated and the longest sequence reported is 437 bp (13) (Fig. 5). The transcription initiation site has not been identified but 22 bp of 5' untranslated sequence has been reported. The rest of the DNA sequence specifies a region coding for 100 amino acids of 300 bp, a termination codon TGA, and a 3' untranslated region of 112 bp.

The cDNA sequence (13) and NH_2-terminal microsequencing of the primary translation product of apo A-II mRNA in cell-free synthesis experiments (55) indicate translation initiation at the methionine 23 amino acids upstream of the NH_2 terminus of the mature protein. Cotranslational cleavage of the primary translation product by microsomal membranes removes the 18 NH_2-terminal amino acids, which presumably represent the apo A-II prepeptide. The remaining five amino acids adjacent to the NH_2 terminus of mature apo A-II is a propeptide with the sequence Ala-Leu-Val-Arg-Arg. The occurrence of two basic amino acids in the propeptide adjacent to the NH_2 terminus of the mature protein is rather typical of propeptides and quite different from the apo A-I propeptide (14–16). Therefore, apo A-II should be cleaved intracellularly, in contrast to apo A-I. Studies with the human hepatoma cell line, Hep G2 (55), indicate that proapo A-II can be cleaved intracellularly but only approximately half is cleaved before export. The explanation for this may be of interest physiologically, or may be a function of this particular in vitro system.

The cDNA sequence specifies an amino acid sequence for mature apo A-II of 77 amino acids, very similar to the previously reported amino acid sequence determined by protein sequencing methods (56). The difference was at residue 35, where the DNA sequence predicts Glu, and the protein-derived sequence specified Gln. In human plasma, apo A-II exists as a dimer; the monomers are connected by a disulfide bridge between the only cysteine in the mature protein which resides at amino acid residue 6 (56). At this time, apo A-II gene structure has not been reported. Recently, apo A-II has been mapped to human chromosome 1 using a cDNA probe and a panel of somatic cell hybrids (57).

APO A-IV

Apo A-IV was originally discovered as a major constituent of rat HDL (58). In humans, it is a relatively minor HDL protein with most apo

A-IV in the nonlipoprotein plasma fraction (59). Human plasma apo A-IV concentrations are approximately 0.16 mg/ml. In rats, apo A-IV synthesis occurs equally in intestine and liver (54) and in this animal fat feeding doubles intestinal apo A-IV synthesis (60). On this basis, it is hypothesized that apo A-IV plays a role in the biogenesis and secretion of intestinal triglyceride-rich lipoproteins, but direct proof of this or any other functional role for apo A-IV is lacking.

Apo A-IV cDNA

Human apo A-IV cDNA clones have not yet been reported; however, some relevant information is available. RNA from human intestinal mucosa has been isolated and translated in wheat germ lysates (61). The NH_2-terminal sequence of the primary translation product has been analyzed by microsequencing techniques and compared to the NH_2-terminal sequence of the mature protein. in this manner, it was determined that human apo A-IV contains a prepeptide sequence 20 amino acids in length. Unlike apo A-I and apo A-II, apo A-IV does not contain a propeptide. The apo A-IV prepeptide is conserved between rats (62) and humans with at least a 55% sequence homology at the amino acid level. The rat apo A-IV prepeptide is very similar to the rat apo A-I prepeptide (14), with 67% homology at the amino acid level.

The rat apo A-IV cDNA sequence has recently been reported (63) (Fig. 6). From this information, rat apo A-IV mRNA is thought to be 1422 bp in length and includes a 5' untranslated region of 90 bp, a region coding for 391 amino acids of 1173 bp, a termination codon, TGA, and a 3' untranslated region of 156 bp followed by a poly A tail. The deduced protein sequence was analyzed and 13 repetitions of segments approximately 22 amino acids in length with amphipathic alpha-helical character were identified. In analogy with the previous findings for human apo A-I (11), eight of the apo A-IV repeats, from amino acids 95 through 270, occur as tandem repetitions of exactly 22 amino acids. Seven of these eight repeats begin with proline. When the DNA segments coding for these repeats are aligned and a consensus nucleotide at each position of the repeat derived, the consensus sequence is 64 to 83% homologous with each of the rat apo A-IV repeats (Fig. 7a) and 49% homologous with a similarly derived consensus sequence for the six human apo A-I DNA repeats that code for apo A-I residues 99 to 230 (11). In an Edmundson wheel diagram, the consensus codes for an alpha-helix with a polar and nonpolar face (Fig. 7b) as shown for apo A-I (Fig. 2b). In the cases of rat apo A-IV and human apo A-I, repetitive amino acid and DNA sequences may exist outside of the region of amino acids 95 to 270 and 99 to 230, respectively, but the requirement for exact tandem repetition of 22

```
        10         20         30         40         50         60         70         80         90        100        110        120
ATCCTCACAG CGACACAGTG AACCATTTCT TCTGACGCTA CGAAACATCC AGTGTAGCTG AGGCTGTCCC AACCCAGTGA GGAGCCCAGG ATGTTCCTGA AGGCTGTGGT GCTGACCGTG
                                                                                                  M  F  L    K  A  V  V  L  T  V
                                                                                                 -20

       130        140        150        160        170        180        190        200        210        220        230        240
GCCCTGGTGG CCATCACCGG GACCCAGGCT GAGGTCACTT CCGACCAGGT GGCCAATGTG ATGTGGGACT ACTTCACCCA GCTAAGCAAC AATGCCAAGG AGGCTGTGGA ACAACTGCAG
 A  L  V   A  I  T  G  T  Q  A   E  V  T   S  D  Q  V  A  N  V   M  W  D   Y  F  T  Q  L  S  N   N  A  K   E  A  V  E  Q  L  Q
                             -1  +1

       250        260        270        280        290        300        310        320        330        340        350        360
AAGACAGATG TCACTCAACA GCTCAATACC CTCTTCCAGG ACAAACTTGG GAACATTAAC ACCTATGCCG ATGACCTGCA GAACAAGCTG GTGCCCTTCG CCGTTCAACT GAGTGGACAT
 K  T  D   V  T  Q  Q  L  N  T   L  F  Q   D  K  L  G  N  I  N   T  Y  A   D  D  L  Q  N  K  L   V  P  F   A  V  Q  L  S  G  H

       370        380        390        400        410        420        430        440        450        460        470        480
CTAACCAAGG AAACAGAGAG GGTGAGGGAA GAGATCCAGA AGGAGCTCGA GGACCTACGG GCCAACATGA TGCCCCATGC CAACAAAGTG AGCCAGATGT TCGGGGACAA CGTGCAGAAG
 L  T  K   E  T  E  R  V  R  E   E  I  Q   K  E  L  E  D  L  R   A  N  M   M  P  H  A  N  K  V   S  Q  M   F  G  D  N  V  Q  K

       490        500        510        520        530        540        550        560        570        580        590        600
TTGCAGGAAC ACCTGAGGCC CTATGCCACG GACCTGCAAG CTCAGATCAA CGCACAGACC CAGGATATGA AACGCCAGCT GACCCCCTAC ATCCAGCGCA TGCAGACCAC AATACAAGAC
 L  Q  E   H  L  R  P  Y  A  T   D  L  Q   A  Q  I  N  A  Q  T   Q  D  M   K  R  Q  L  T  P  Y   I  Q  R   M  Q  T  T  I  Q  D

       610        620        630        640        650        660        670        680        690        700        710        720
AATGTGGAAA ACCTGCAGTC CTCCATGGTG CCCTTTGCCA ACGAGCTAAA GGAAAAGTTT AACCAGAATA TGGAAGGGCT CAAGGGGCAA CTAACCCCCC GTGCCAACGA GCTGAAGGCC
 N  V  E   N  L  Q  S  S  M  V   P  F  A   N  E  L  K  E  K  F   N  Q  N   M  E  G  L  K  G  Q   L  T  P   R  A  N  E  L  K  A
```

```
       730        740        750        760        770        780        790        800        810        820        830        840
ACGATCGACC AGAACCTGGA AGACCTGCGC AGCAGACTGG CCCCTCTCGC GGAGGGTGTG CAGGAAAAAC TCAACCATCA GATGGAAGCC TTGGCCTTCC AGATGAAGAA GAACGCTGAG
 T  I  D   Q  N  L  E   D  L  R   S  R  L   A  P  L  A   E  G  V   Q  E  K   L  N  H  Q   M  E  G   L  A  F   Q  M  K  K   N  A  E

       850        860        870        880        890        900        910        920        930        940        950        960
GAGCTCCATA CCAAAGTCTC CACAAATATC GACCAGCTGC AGAAGAATCT GGCCCCGCTG GTGGAAGATG TGCAAAGCAA GCTGAAAGGC AACACGGAAG GACTGCAGAA GTCTCTGGAA
 E  L  H   T  K  V  S   T  N  I   D  Q  L   Q  K  N  L   A  P  L   V  E  D   V  Q  S  K   L  K  G   N  T  E   G  L  Q  K   S  L  E

       970        980        990       1000       1010       1020       1030       1040       1050       1060       1070       1080
GACCTGAACA AGCAGCTGGA CCAGCAGGTG GAGGTGTTCC GGCGTGCTGT GGAGCCCCTG GGGGATAAGT TCAACATGGC TCTGGTGCAG CAGATGGAGA AGTTCAGGCA GCAGCTGGGC
 D  L  N   K  Q  L  D   Q  Q  V   E  V  F   R  R  A  V   E  P  L   G  D  K   F  N  M  A   L  V  Q   Q  M  E   K  F  R  Q   Q  L  G

      1090       1100       1110       1120       1130       1140       1150       1160       1170       1180       1190       1200
TCCGATTCGG GGGACGTGGA AAGCCACTTG AGCTTCCTGG AGAAGAACCT GAGGGAAAAG GTCAGCTCCT TTATGAGCAC CCTGCAAAAA AAGGGGAGCC CAGACCAGCC CCTAGCCCTC
 S  D  S   G  D  V  E   S  H  L   S  F  L   E  K  N  L   R  E  K   V  S  S   F  M  S  T   L  Q  K   K  G  S   P  D  Q  P   L  A  L

      1210       1220       1230       1240       1250       1260       1270       1280       1290       1300       1310       1320
CCCCTCCCGG AGCAGGTTCA GGAACAGGTC CAGGAGCAGG TGCAGCCCAA ACCTCTGGAG AGCTGAGCTG TCCCTGTGTC CTCGGCCCAT CACAGCAGCA GACACCTGCC CTGCCCCACC
 P  L  P   E  Q  V  Q   E  Q  V   Q  E  Q   V  Q  P  K   P  L  E   S
                                                                    371

      1330       1340       1350       1360       1370       1380       1390       1400       1410       1420
ACCTGTCTGT CACTCTGTTC CCAAGCACTT CTCGTACCAG CTTGAGGACA CATGTCCTGT GGGTGACGAT ACCTCCTCTC GTTACTCAAT AAAGCATCTG AGA(n)
```

Fig. 6 Rat apo A-IV cDNA is 1422 bp in length plus a poly A tail. The coding regions for the prepeptide and mature protein are bp's 91 to 150 and 151 to 1236, respectively. The eight 66-bp tandem repeats are in the region of bp's 433 to 960. The polyadenylation signal AATAAA occurs in the 3' untranslated region from bp's 1408 to 1413.

APO A-IV 66bp DNA REPEATS

Repeat	Amino Acid	Sequence	% Homology
#1	(095-116)	CCCCATCCCAACAAAGTGAGCCAGATGTTCGGGGACAACGTGCAGAAGTTGCAGGAACACCTGAGG	64
#2	(117-138)	CCCTATGCCACGGACCTGCAAGCTCAGATCAACGCACAGACCCAGGATATGAAACGCCAGCTGACC	76
#3	(139-160)	CCCTACATCCAGCGCATGCAGACCACAATACAAGACAATGTGGAAAACCTGCAGTCCTCCATGGTG	64
#4	(161-182)	CCCTTTGCCAACGAGCTAAAGGAAAAGTTTAACCAGAATATGGAAGGGCTCAAGGGGCAACTAACC	76
#5	(183-204)	CCCCGTGCCAACGAGCTGAAGGCCACGATCGACCAGAACCTGGAAGACCTGCGCAGCAGACTGGCC	83
#6	(205-226)	CCTCTCGCGGAGGGTGTGCAGGAAAAACTCAACCATCAGATGGAAGGCTTGGCCTTCCAGATGAAG	66
#7	(227-248)	AAGAACGCTGAGGAGCTCCATACCAAAGTCTCCACAAATATCGACCAGCTGCAGAAGAATCTGGCC	66
#8	(249-270)	CCGCTGGTGGAAGATGTGCAAAGCAAGCTGAAAGGCAACACGGAAGGACTGCAGAAGTCTCTGGAA	64

```
Consensus     CCCCATGCCAAGGAXCTGCAGGCCAAGXTCAACGAXAAXATGGAAGAXCTGCAGXXCCAXCTGACC
Sequence                                                                     G

Translated    ProHisAlaLysAspLeuGlnAlaLysPheAsnAspAsnMetGluAspLeuGln---HisLeuThr
Amino Acid                Glu               Leu   GluLys      Glu         Gln   Ala
Sequence                                    Ile
                                            Val

Amino Acid
Charges        0 +1  0 +1 -1  0  0  0 +1  0  0 -1 +½  0 -1 -1  0  0  ? +½  0  0
```

(a)

Fig. 7 (a) The apo A-IV 66-bp DNA repeats were aligned and a consensus sequence generated. The homology of each of the repeats with the consensus is shown. The translated amino acid sequence derived from the consensus is shown, as are the charges of the amino acids specified. 9b) The Edmundson wheel diagram showing the positions of the consensus-derived amino acids and their charges in an alpha-helical configuration. The helix clearly contains a nonpolar and a polar face. The positively charged residues tend to cluster between the nonpolar and polar faces.

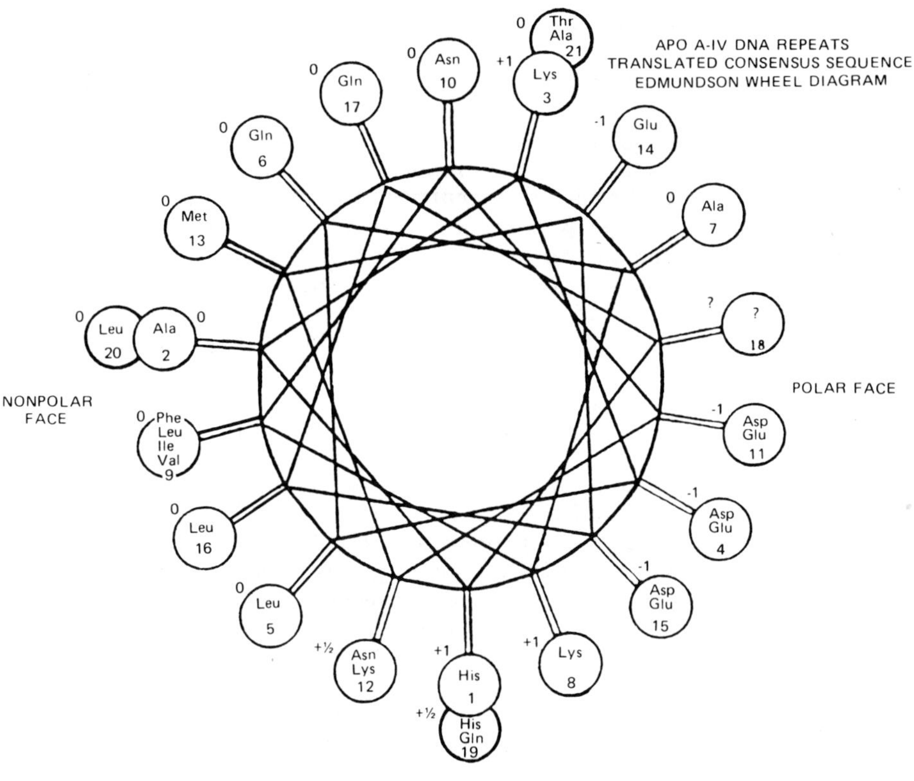

(b)

Fig. 7 (continued)

amino acid segments has been lost. This presumably represents relaxation of a biological requirement outside of these regions, but future work will be necessary to validate this hypothesis.

Apo A-IV Gene and Genetic Variation

The genomic structure has not been reported for either the human or rat apo A-IV genes. However, genetic variation in human apo A-IV has been demonstrated (38,40). In most people, isoelectric focusing of plasma apo A-IV results in a single major isoprotein of pH 5.50, whereas other people have this isoprotein plus another one charge unit more basic, and a few people have just the more basic isoprotein. In a large German study, the frequencies of these patterns in a normal population were 85.6, 13.8, and 0.6%, respectively (40). Genetic studies were consistent with a single genetic locus, two-allele model (64). From these data, the major allele frequency, specifying the more acidic gene product, was 92.5%, and the minor allele frequency, specifying the more basic gene product, was 7.5%. Neither hetero- nor homozygosity for the minor allele has been associated with plasma lipoprotein abnormalities or atherosclerosis susceptibility. The apo A-IV protein polymorphism is potentially useful in studying linkage relationships of the apo A-IV gene to other genes. In family studies, a preliminary result showing cosegregation of the apo A-IV protein variant with an apo A-I protein variant has been reported (Lod = 2.7 at 0 = 0.0) (35). If this is confirmed, it would mean that the apo A-IV gene resides on human chromosome 11 in the region of q13.

APO B

Apo B is the major protein constituent of low-density lipoproteins (LDL), but is also found in chylomicrons and VLDL (2). LDL particles are approximately 25% protein and 75% lipid and virtually all of the protein is apo B. LDL levels are directly correlated with coronary artery disease susceptibility and recently the same association has been demonstrated for apo B levels (3). Apo B is abundant in plasma with a concentration of 0.7 to 1.0 mg/ml. Apo B is thought to be required for the secretion into plasma of intestinal and hepatic triglyceride-rich lipoproteins (2). Apo B is also recognized by specific high affinity receptors that mediate clearance of LDL particles from plasma (65).

Human apo B is a glycoprotein that occurs in two forms, designated B-100 and B-48 (66). B-100 is thought to be a single polypeptide of molecular weight (MW) approximately 400,000 daltons and produced primarily in liver; B-48 is approximately half that MW and is produced primarily in the small intestine (66). Very little information about the primary structure of apo B is available. Two problems have been encountered. The protein becomes quite insoluble after delipidation, and standard methods of proteolytic digestion have not resulted in a high enough yield of unique peptides for structural studies (66). It has been suggested that the insolubility problem is due to an abnormal sensitivity of the protein to oxidation after delipidation, and recently, with proper precautions, soluble preparations of delipidated apo B have been obtained (67). In addition, the use of bacterial proteases has improved the yield of unique apo B peptides (68). A recent report provides the partial amino acid sequence of two peptides and more structural data should be forthcoming in the near future (68).

The paucity of data on apo B structure, using standard protein chemistry techniques, has led to immunochemical studies to gain relevant information about this protein. In this regard, several groups have developed monoclonal antibodies to human apo B that recognize distinct epitopes and some interesting information has been derived. In one study, the immunoreactivity of apo B in VLDL changed significantly after in vitro lipolysis, suggesting that apo B conformation might change at different stages of lipoprotein metabolism (69). In another study, epitopes of apo B-100 have been mapped in a linear nonrepetitive array. For one subset of these epitopes, the monoclonal antibodies disrupt apo B binding to the LDL receptor but do not bind to B-48. For another subset of epitopes, the monoclonal antibodies bind B-48 but do not disrupt receptor binding (70). Thus B-48 and B-100 are antigenically related, and it has been suggested that B-48 represents approximately one half of the B-100 protein and that this part of apo B is not involved in receptor binding (66,70).

Apo B Genetic Variation

Genetically determined variation in both the quality and quantity of apo B has been demonstrated. Antisera from multiply transfused patients have been used to define two series of allelic variants called Lp and Ag. Both systems appear to have marginal effects on plasma cholesterol levels and risk of atherosclerosis (see Ref. 71 for a recent review). Recently, in some individuals reduced binding to each of three anti-apo B monoclonal antibodies has been demonstrated (72). Three phenotypes of strong, weak, and intermediate binding have been identified, and family studies suggest a genetic basis for this consistent with a single genetic locus with two alleles specifying strong and weak binding forms of apo B. Thus, the intermediate binding pattern is the result of heterozygosity for the strong and weak binding alleles, whereas the other two patterns represent homozygosity for their respective alleles. In a study of the phenotype frequencies in a small number of unrelated individuals, the major allele frequency was found to be 70% (72). It was suggested that this apo B antigenic variation resulted from an alteration in the amino acid sequence of the apo B polypeptide affecting the configuration of a single domain in which the epitopes recognized by the three monclonal antibodies reside. The effect of this recently described genetic variation in apo B on plasma lipoprotein levels has yet to be determined.

Inherited disorders of lipoprotein metabolism associated with diminished plasma levels of apo B have been described. The most striking of these is abetalipoproteinemia (2). In this disorder, individuals suffer from fat malabsorption and lack apo-B-containing lipoproteins in their plasma, including chylomicrons, VLDL, and LDL. Parents of affected individuals have normal lipoprotein and apo B levels; however, siblings with this disorder have been described and inheritance is assumed to be autosomal recessive. Immunologically detectable apo B is absent from both the plasma and tissues of these individuals and the disorder is thought to be a genetic defect in apo B synthesis. A phenotypically similar disorder has been described and termed homozygous hypobetalipoproteinemia, in which parents of affected individuals have half-normal levels of LDL cholesterol and apo B (2). This condition may also involve a genetic defect in apo B synthesis, but by a different mechanism. Finally, individuals have been described with normal fat absorption and the ability to produce chylomicrons but low to absent levels of LDL cholesterol (73,74). Apparently these individuals can produce the intestinal form of apo B, B-48, but not the hepatic form, B-100. The existence of this disorder suggests separate genetic control of B-48 and B-100 synthesis. However, at this time it cannot be determined whether these two gene products are the result of distinct genetic loci or represent differential splicing of the transcript produced from a single genetic locus.

Increased apo B levels are associated with atherosclerosis susceptibility (3). In familial hypercholesterolemia (FH), an autosomal dominant disorder is characterized by premature atherosclerosis; apo B and cholesterol in LDL are elevated; and the genetic lesion is a defect in the apo B/E receptor (65). A substantial fraction of non-FH individuals with coronary disease has been shown to have increased apo B, but normal cholesterol in LDL. This phenotype has been called hyperapobetalipoproteinemia (75). A subset of these individuals may have the autosomal dominant disorder associated with premature atherosclerosis, familial combined hyperlipidemia (FCHL) (76). Plasma from these individuals consistently contains elevated plasma apo B levels, but only occasionally is the LDL cholesterol elevated (77). One possible genetic explanation for the hyperapobetalipoproteinemia phenotype could be a primary overproduction of apo B (78,79). Further efforts aimed at studying the regulation of apo B synthesis are hampered by the absence of cDNA and genomic clones for apo B.

APO CI

Apo CI is a constituent of VLDL and HDL (2). VLDL particles are approximately 10% protein and 90% lipid, and apo CI constitutes 10% of VLDL protein. As previously noted, HDL particles are approximately 50% protein and 50% lipid, and apo CI constitutes 2% of HDL protein. Human plasma apo CI concentrations are in the range of 0.04 to 0.06 mg/ml. In vitro apo CI has been shown to activate LCAT but not as efficiently as apo A-I (80). The physiological role(s) of apo CI has not been defined. Synthesis occurs mainly in the liver and to a minor degree in the intestine but has not been evaluated in other organs (2). Primary qualitative or quantitative abnormalities of human apo CI have not been reported.

HUMAN APO C-I cDNA

```
        10         20         30         40         50         60         70         80         90        100        110        120
CCCGCAGCTC AGCCACGGCA CAGATCAGCA CCACGACCCC TCCCTCGGGC CTCGCCATGA GGCTCTTCCT GTCGCTCCCG GTCCTGGTGG TGGTTCTGTC GATCGTCTTG GAAGGCCCAG
                                                           M   R  L  F  L   S  L  P   V  L  V   V  V  L  S   I  V  L   E  G  P
                                                          -26

       130        140        150        160        170        180        190        200        210        220        230        240
CCCCAGCCCA GGGGACCCCA GACGTCTCCA GTGCCTTGGA TAAGCTGAAG GAGTTTGGAA ACACACTGGA GGACAAGGCT CGGGAACTCA TCAGCCGCAT CAAACAGAGT GAACTTTCTG
A  P  A  Q   G  T  P   D  V  S   S  A  L  D   K  L  K   E  F  G   N  T  L  E   D  K  A   R  E  L   I  S  R  I   K  Q  S   E  L  S
           -1 +1

       250        260        270        280        290        300        310        320        330        340        350        360
CCAAGATGCG GGAGTGGTTT TCAGAGACAT TTCAGAAAGT GAAGGAGAAA CTCAAGATTG ACTCATGAGG ACCTGAAGGG TGACATCCAG GAGGGGCCTC TGAAATTTCC CACACCCCAG
A  K  M  R   E  W  F   S  E  T   F  Q  K  V   K  E  K   L  K  I   D  S
                                                                    57

       370        380        390        400        410        420
CGCCTGTGCT GAGGACTCCC GCCATGTGGC CCCAGGTGCC ACCAATAAAA ATCCTACCGA(n)
```

Fig. 8 The reported sequence of human apo CI cDNA is 419 bp in length plus a poly A tail. The coding regions for the prepeptide and mature protein are bp's 57 to 134 and 135 to 305, respectively. The polyadenylation signal AATAAA occurs in the 3' untranslated region from bp's 404 to 409.

Apo CI cDNA

Apo CI cDNA clones between 400 and 480 bp in length have recently been isolated (81). Northern blotting of adult human liver RNA with a probe made from apo CI cDNA indicated two species of apo CI mRNA approximately 530 and 580 bp in length. This meant both that there could be heterogeneity in the transcription initiation of apo CI mRNA and that the inserts in the cDNA clones were not full length. The inserts appeared to lack sequences corresponding to the 5' end of apo CI mRNA. Primer extension on a template of human liver mRNA indicated that apo CI mRNAs have 63 and 40 bp 5' untranslated regions. The DNA sequence provided includes 56 bp in the 5' untranslated region. The rest of the DNA sequence specifies a region coding for 83 amino acids of 249 bp, a termination codon, TGA, and a 3' untranslated region of 111 bp (Fig. 8).

The DNA-derived amino acid sequence contains the 57 residues of mature apo CI and agrees entirely with the results derived by protein sequencing techniques (82,83). The DNA sequence also specifies a 26-amino-acid NH_2-terminal extension (81). This amino acid sequence is compatible with the entire 26 amino acids, being the apo CI prepeptide. However, the possible existence of an apo CI propeptide with an unusual sequence and two-step processing of the apo CI primary translation product must be formally excluded.

Apo CI gene structure has not yet been reported. Recently, utilizing somatic cell hybrids and a cDNA probe, the apo CI gene has been mapped to human chromosome 19 (84).

APO CII

Apo CII is a constituent of VLDL and HDL and comprises 10% of VLDL protein and approximately 1% of HDL protein (2). Human plasma apo CII concentrations are in the range of 0.03 to 0.05 mg/ml. Purified apo CII has cofactor activity for the enzyme lipoprotein lipase, which catalyzes the hydrolysis of triglycerides in chylomicrons and VLDL. The physiological importance of apo CII in activating lipoprotein lipase has been established by the discovery of patients with inherited apo CII deficiency, who are severely hypertriglyceridemic and have functional lipoprotein lipase deficiency (see Ref. 85 for review). In such cases, both the hypertriglyceridemia and the lipase deficiency can be relieved by an exogenous source of apo CII (86). Studies using tryptic fragments of apo CII have shown that the COOH-terminal amino acids 55 to 79 are necessary for maximal lipoprotein lipase activation (87,88). Synthesis of apo CII takes place mainly in the liver and to a minor degree in the intestine.

Apo CII cDNA

Apo CII cDNA clones have been obtained by several laboratories (13, 89,90). DNA sequence information is not yet available on the 5' untranslated region; however, beginning with the codon that initiates translation, 450 bp of sequence has been specified. Northern blotting analysis of liver and intestine RNA indicates that apo CII mRNA is approximately 500 bp in length (90). This suggests a short 5' untranslated region of, at most, 50 bp. The cDNA sequence indicates a coding region for 101 amino acids of 303 bp, a termination codon, TAA, and a 3' untranslated region of 144 bp followed by a poly A tail (Fig. 9).

The DNA-derived amino acid sequence contains the 79 residues of mature apo CII. This is in agreement with a recent result derived by protein sequencing techniques (91), but differs somewhat from the previously derived amino acid sequence (92). In the latter case, a polypeptide of 78 amino acids was reported. In addition, the DNA sequence indicates that residues 2 and 17 are glutamine, not glutamic acid; amino acid 27 is glutamic acid, not glutamine; and amino acids 20 through 26 are Glu-Ser-Leu-Ser-Ser-Tyr-Trp, not the reported Glu-Trp-Leu-Ser-Ser-Tyr. The DNA sequence also specifies a 22-amino-acid NH_2-terminal extension compatible with the existence of an apo CII prepeptide (13,89,90).

There is a striking homology between the NH_2-terminal regions of both apo A-I and apo CII at the amino acid level. Apo A-I amino acids −2, −1, +1, +2 are identical to apo CII amino acids 5, 6, 7, and 8, and, in each case, specify Gln-Gln-Asp-Glu. This region spans the site of cleavage of the protease that converts proapo A-I to mature apo A-I. This suggests that apo CII should be a substrate for the apo-A-I-converting protease. However, in plasma, mature apo CII is found to be the full 79 amino acids in length and is fully active as a lipoportein lipase activator in this form. Thus, for reasons that remain to be elucidated, apo CII is not a physiological substrate for the apo-A-I-converting protease. Preliminary analysis of the apo A-I and apo CII cDNA sequences reveals extensive homology at the DNA level extending between apo A-I bp 102 to 285 (amino acids −2 to 59) (Fig. 1) and apo CII bp 79 to 261 (amino acids 5 to 65) (Fig. 9). Alignment of the DNA sequences in these regions by metric analysis indicates 56% overall matching with runs of matches 11, 8, and 10 bp in length (B. Erickson and J. L. Breslow, unpublished observations). These observations suggest a close phylogenetic relationship between apo A-I and apo CII.

Apo CII Gene Structure, Mapping, and Genetic Variation

The apo CII gene has been isolated and a restriction map reported (89,93) (Fig. 10). Preliminary sequencing information reveals introns

HUMAN APO C-II cDNA

```
                                                         ↓
        10         20         30         40         50         60         70         80         90        100        110        120
ATGGGCACAC GACTCCTCCC AGCTCTGTTT CTTGTCCTCC TGGTATTGGG ATTTGAGGTC CAGGGGACCC AACAGCCCCA GCAAGATGAG ATGCCTAGCC CGACCTTCCT CACCCAGGTG
 M  G  T    R  L  L  P   A  L  F    L  V  L   L  V  L  G   F  E  V    Q  G  T   Q  Q  P  Q   Q  D  E   M  P  S    P  T  F  L   T  Q  V
-22                                                                   -1 +1

       130        140        150        160        170        180        190        200        210      ↓ 220        230        240
AAGGAATCTC TCTCCAGTTA CTGGGAGTCA GCAAAGACAG CCGCCCAGAA CCTGTACGAG AAGACATACC TGCCCGCTGT AGATGAGAAA CTCAGGGACT TGTACAGCAA AAGCACAGCA
 K  E  S    L  S  S  Y   W  E  S    A  K  T   A  A  Q  N   L  Y  E   K  T  Y    L  P  A  V   D  E  K    L  R  D   L  Y  S  K   S  T  A

       250        260        270        280        290        300        310        320        330        340        350        360
GCCATGAGCA CTTACACAGG CATTTTTACT GACCAAGTTC TTTCTGTGCT GAAGGGAGAG GAGTAACAGC CAGACCCCCC ATCAGTGGAC AAGGGGAGAG TCCCCTACTC CCCTGATCCC
 A  M  S    T  Y  T  G   I  F  T    D  Q  V   L  S  V  L   K  G  E   E
                                                                   79

       370        380        390        400        410        420        430        440        450
CCAGGTTCAG ACTGAGCTCC CCCTTCCCAG TAGCTCTTGC ATCCTCCTCC CAACTCTAGC CTGAATTCTT TTCAATAAAA AATACAATTCA(n)
```

Fig. 9 The longest human apo CII cDNA sequence reported is 450 bp plus a poly A tail. The coding regions for the prepeptide and mature protein are bp's 1 to 66 and 67 to 303, respectively. Sequence information in the 5' untranslated region has not been reported. The polyadenylation signal AATAAA occurs in the 3' untranslated region from bp's 434 to 439. Partial sequence determination of an apo CII genomic clone has revealed introns after bp's 58 and 215 (arrows).

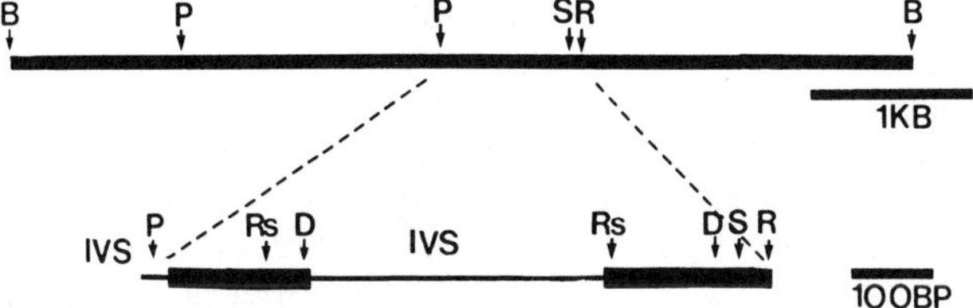

Fig. 10 Restriction map of the human genome in the vicinity of the apo CII gene. The approximately 1.0-kb PstI to EcoRI restriction fragment has been subjected to partial DNA sequence analysis and two intronic regions (IVS) are shown. Restriction sites are indicated as follows: B, BamHI; P, PstI; S, SacI; R, EcoRI; Rs, RsaI; D, DdeI.

interrupting the codons specifying amino acids −3 and 50. There are introns in similar locations in the other apolipoprotein genes where this has been studied. This is discussed in the sections on the apo A-I, apo CIII, and apo E genes. In addition, these other genes all have introns interrupting the 5' noncoding region of their cDNAs. Therefore, it is expected that apo CII will also have an intron in this location, but this information is not yet available. The two known apo CII introns divide the DNA sequence coding for the signal peptide from that coding for the mature protein, and the DNA sequence coding for the NH_2 from that coding for the COOH-terminal portions of the mature protein, respectively.

Somatic cell hybrids and a probe made from an apo CII cDNA clone have been used to map the gene for human apo CII to chromosome 19 (89,93). A discordancy was noted with a somatic cell hybrid that contained a rearranged chromosome 19 and that lacked two markers for the distal end of the long arm of the chromosome. Apo CII can therefore be localized to 19pter—q13 (89,93).

Southern blotting analysis of human DNA after digestion with the restriction endonuclease TaqI reveals a common polymorphism in the vicinity of the apo CII gene (94,95). The major allele frequency in normal individuals is 0.60 (95). As will be discussed in the section on apo E, the human apo E gene also resides on chromosome 19 and a common polymorphism has been demonstrated. The exact relationship between the apo CII and apo E genes has not been defined. However, family studies done by two different groups show cosegregation of the apo CII TaqI polymorphism and the apo E protein polymorphism (in each case, Lod = >4.0 at $\theta - 0.0$) (94,95). In addition, linkage disequilibrium has been demonstrated between the alleles of both genes (95). The combined data from the two studies indicate that no recombinations have occurred in 53 observed meioses. Therefore, these two genes appear to be less than 2 centimorgans apart.

The genomic clone for apo CII does not hybridize strongly with the cDNA clone for apo E and vice versa. From the location of these genes on their respective genomic clones, one can conclude that they are no closer than 5 to 7 kb (J. L. Breslow, unpublished data).

Several patients have been described who lack apo CII in their plasma. They are functionally lipoprotein lipase deficient and are severely hypertriglyceridemic. Apo CII deficiency appears to be a recessive genetic disorder with obligate heterozygotes having half-normal apo CII levels but normal triglyceride concentrations (85). Southern blotting analysis with a probe made from an apo CII cDNA clone reveals that at least a subset of these patients possesses the apo CII gene and that it is grossly intact (96). Two independent families of probands with this disorder have been studied using the TaqI polymorphism to assess disease linkage with the apo CII gene locus. In each family, cosegregation was observed, which is consistent with the defect in this condition being within or near the apo CII gene (96).

A protein polymorphism of apo CII has also been described (97). In most individuals, plasma apo CII is a single spot on two-dimensional gels and a single band on one-dimensional size or charge separation gels. Recently, three hypertriglyceridemic individuals have been described who have a normal apo CII component and an apo CII isoprotein one charge unit more acidic than normal (97). It has been determined that this is due to a substitution of glutamine for lysine at residue 55. The apo CII DNA sequence at this residue determined for cDNA clone pCII-711 is AAA, which specifies lysine. It is possible to explain the occurrence of glutamine at this residue by a single base substitution in the first base of this codon, substituting C for A. Although this mutant form of apo CII was isolated from hypertriglyceridemic patients, it appears to activate lipoprotein lipase normally. Thus the relationship between the amino acid substitution and the hypertriglyceridemia probably is not cause and effect.

APO CIII

Apo CIII is a constituent of VLDL and HDL and comprises about 50% of VLDL protein and 2% of HDL protein (2). Human plasma apo CIII concentrations are in the range of 0.12 to 0.14 mg/ml. Apo CIII is a glycoprotein containing 1 mol each of galactose and galactosamine, and either 0, 1, or 2 mol of sialic acid (98). The three resultant isoproteins recognizable by isoelectric focusing are designated CIII-0, CIII-1, and CIII-2 and comprise 14, 59, and 27% of plasma apo CIII, respectively (99). In vitro, apo CIII has been shown to inhibit the activities of both lipoprotein lipase (100,101) and hepatic lipase (102). Apo CIII has also been shown to decrease the uptake of lymph chylomicrons by the perfused rat liver (103–106). These in vitro studies suggest that apo CIII might delay catabolism of triglyceride-rich particles. Recently, patients with combined apo A-I, apo CIII deficiency were shown to have low plasma triglyceride levels (43), and in vivo studies showed that they rapidly convert VLDL to LDL (107). In vitro lipolysis of their VLDL was inhibited by added apo CIII (107). Thus it appears that primary abnormalities in the quantity or quality of apo CIII may affect plasma triglyceride levels and the physiological role of apo CIII may be in the regulation of the catabolism of triglyceride-rich lipoproteins. Functional domains of apo CIII have been demonstrated. The 40 NH_2-terminal amino acids do not bind phospholipid, whereas the 39 COOH-terminal amino acids do (108). Synthesis of apo CIII is mainly in liver and to a lesser degree in intesting (2).

Apo CIII cDNA

Apo CIII cDNA sequence has been reported (13,45,109) (Fig. 11). The complete sequence of the apo CIII 5' untranslated region is not currently known, but 20 bp of sequence information is available. These data indicate that apo CIII mRNA is at least 507 bp in length and includes a coding region for 99 amino acids of 297 bp, a termination codon, TGA, and a 3' untranslated region of 187 bp followed by a poly A tail. This is compatible with the size of an apo CIII mRNA of about 550 bp determined by Northern blotting analysis of human liver mRNA (13).

The DNA-derived apo CIII amino acid sequence (13,109) differs from the previously reported protein-derived apo CIII amino acid sequence (98) at residues 32, 33, 37, and 39. At these locations, the DNA sequence predicts Glu, Ser, Gln, Ala, respectively, whereas the previously reported protein-derived sequence specified Ser, Gln, Ala, Gln, respectively. Three cDNA clones from two separate cDNA libraries (13,109) all have shown the same DNA-derived amino acid sequence. In addition, the DNA sequence coding for residues 32 and 33, GAGTCC, includes a recognition site for the restriction endonuclease HinfI (GANTC), whereas the DNA sequence required to code for the corresponding residues in the protein-derived sequence could not possibly contain a HinfI recognition site (109). Southern blotting analysis of genomic DNA from four normal and two hypertriglyceridemic individuals identifies a HinfI site in this region, which is also compatible with the DNA-derived amino acid sequence (109). Thus the protein sequence, unless it was derived from a person homozygous for a rare apo CIII allele, is probably in error and should be revised.

The DNA-derived amino acid sequence indicates a 20-amino-acid NH_2-terminal extension for the primary translation product of apo CIII (13,109). The sequence is compatible with previously reported prepeptide sequences. Cell-free synthesis experiments using mRNA from rat liver and intestine indicate that rat apo CIII is made with a

HUMAN APO C-III cDNA

```
  ↓10         20         30         40         50         60         70     ↓  80         90        100        110        120
GCTCCAGGAA CAGAGGTGCC ATGCAGCCCC GGGTACTCCT TGTTGTTGCC CTCCTGGCGC TCCTGGCCTC TGCCCGAGCT TCAGAGGCCG AGGATGCCTC CCTTCTCAGC TTCATGCAGG
                      M  Q  P    R  V  L  L   V  V  A    L  L  A    L  L  A  S   A  R  A    S  E  A    E  D  A  S   L  L  S    F  M  Q
                     -20                                                                -1    +1

                                                                                  ↓
       130        140        150        160        170        180        190        200        210        220        230        240
GTTACATGAA GCACGCCACC AAGACCGCCA AGGATGCACT GAGCAGCGTG CAGGAGTCCC AGGTGGCCCA GCAGGCCAGG GGCTGGGTGA CCGATGGCTT CAGTTCCCTG AAAGACTACT
G ▲Y M K    H  A  T    K  T  A    K  D  A  L   S  S  V    Q  E  S    Q  V  A  Q   Q  A  R    G  W  V    T  D  G  F   S  S  L    K  D  Y

       250        260        270        280        290        300        310        320        330        340        350        360
GGAGCACCGT TAAGGACAAG TTCTCTGAGT TCTGGGATTT GGACCCTGAG GTCAGACCAA CTTCAGCCGT GGCTGCCTGA GACCTCAATA CCCCAAGTCC ACCTGCCTAT CCATCCTGCG
W  S  T  V   K  D  K    F  S  E    F  W  D  L   D  P  E    V  R  P    T  S  A  V   A  A                                              ▲
                                                                           79

       370        380        390        400        410        420        430        440        450        460        470        480
AGCTCCTTGG GTCCTGCAAT CTCCAGGGCT GCCCCTGTAG GTTGCTTAAA AGGGACAGTA TTCTCAGTGC TCTCCTACCC CACCTCATGC CTGGCCCCCC TCCAGGCATG CTGGCCTCCC
------                           ▲

       490        500        510
AATAAAGCTG GACAAGAAGC TGCTATGA(n)
```

Fig. 11 Sequence information of 507 bp is available for human apo CIII cDNA. The coding regions for the prepeptide and the mature protein are bp's 21 to 80 and 81 to 317, respectively. The sequence information in the 5' untranslated region is incomplete. The polyadenylation signal AATAAA occurs in the 3' untranslated region from bp's 481 to 486. Partial sequence determination of an apo CIII genomic clone has revealed introns after bp's 7, 75, and 199 (thin arrows). The thick arrows at bp's 123, 360, and 391 indicate probable sites of true variation (see text). The sequence shown is the allele containing restriction endonuclease site SacI in the 3' untranslated region from bp's 360 to 365 (underlined).

20-amino-acid NH_2-terminal extension (110). This can be cotranslationally cleaved by signal peptidase to yield a product with the same NH_2 terminus as the mature protein (110). Therefore, apo CIII is made as a preprotein and does not contain a propeptide sequence.

Apo CIII Gene Structure, Mapping, and Genetic Variation

Apo CIII cDNA clones were used to identify the apo CIII gene on human genomic DNA cloned in lambda phage that contained the apo A-I gene (45). Mapping of the apo CIII gene reveals that it is about 2500 bp from the 3' end of the apo A-I gene (45). Further mapping and DNA sequence analysis reveals that these genes are coded for by opposite DNA strands (45,109). The 3' end of the apo CIII gene is located closest to the 3' end of the apo A-I gene, and the 5' end of the apo CIII gene, containing the apo CIII promoter, is farthest away from the apo A-I gene. Thus, these two genes are convergently transcribed. It is not known where their primary transcripts end, or whether there is any functional significance to this unusual configuration.

The apo CIII gene is approximately 3000 bp in length and contains 3 introns (109) (Fig. 12). IVS-1 is approximately 600 bp long and occurs in the 5' untranslated region between bases 13 and 14 upstream of the codon for Met that initiates translation. IVS-2 is approximately 125 bp long and interrupts the codon specifying amino acid −2, which is in the apo CIII prepeptide. IVS-3 is about 1800 bp long and interrupts the codon specifying amino acid 40 of the mature protein. Thus, as for apo A-I and apo CII, the intron locations indicate that apo CIII exons may code for functionally important domains of the protein. For instance, intron 2 separates the prepeptide from the mature protein, and intron 3 seems to separate the phospholipid-binding domain from the nonbinding domain.

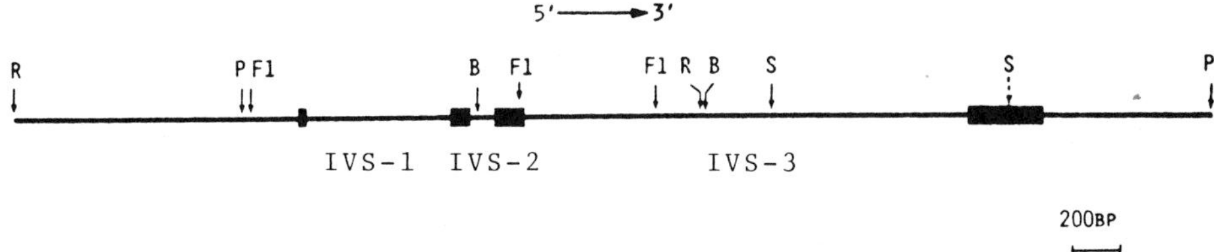

Fig. 12 Restriction map of the human genome in the vicinity of the apo CIII gene. Four exons (thick lines) and three introns (IVS) have been defined. Restriction sites are indicated as follows: R, EcoRI; B, BamHI; P, PstI; S, SacI; F1, HinfI. The polymorphic (see text) SacI restriction site is shown by a dotted-line arrow.

Apo CIII cDNA clones and somatic cell hybrids have been used to map the apo CIII gene to a single locus on human chromosome 11 (29). This is compatible with the close linkage demonstrated by finding both genes on a single cloned genomic fragment of DNA (45). Thus the human apo A-I, apo CIII, and probably apo A-IV (35) genes all reside in the same region of the genome in the vicinity of 11q13.

Human genetic variation in apo CIII has been documented. Southern blotting analysis of human DNA after digestion with SstI or its isoschizomer, SacI, along with an apo A-I probe revealed a DNA polymorphism flanking the apo A-I gene (111). This was subsequently shown to be due to a single base substitution in the 3' untranslated region of the neighboring apo CIII gene (45). A clinical study of 28 hypertriglyceridemic subjects found 10 heterozygotes and 2 homozygotes for this polymorphism, whereas in 70 controls only 3 were found to be heterozygotes (111). Thus an association was suggested between hypertriglyceridemia and genetic variation in the apo CIII gene (111). This is compatible with the proposed physiological role of apo CIII in regulating the metabolism of triglyceride-rich lipoproteins. However, it will be necessary to confirm this association by studying other hypertriglyceridemic as well as control populations. It also remains to be determined how a DNA base substitution in the 3' untranslated region could affect the quantity or quality of the apo CIII protein in a person's plasma. To this end, three apo CIII cDNA clones containing the entire coding region, one with and two without the SacI site, have been sequenced (13,109). Three sites of variation, including the polymorphic SacI site, have been identified (Table 4). One site of variation is in the coding region affecting the third

Table 4 Human Apo CIII Genetic Variation

	Base pair[b]			
Clone[a]	123	360	391	SacI site[c]
1	T	G	G	+
2	C	C	T	–
3	T	C	G	–

[a]cDNA clones were sequenced in two different laboratories. Clones 1 and 2 were from the same laboratory constructed from liver mRNA of a donor who was heterozygous for the SacI site. Clone 3 was from a different library.
[b]Refers to bp location in Fig. 11.
[c]SacI site GAGCTC refers to bp 360–365 in Fig. 11.

base of a codon specifying amino acid residue 14, but in each case, the codon specifies glycine. The other two sites of variation are 31 bp apart in the 3' untranslated region. Thus far, the SacI polymorphism cannot be associated with another DNA variation affecting the primary amino acid sequence and thereby the quality of apo CIII. Whether the bp variations identified in the 3' untranslated region can affect the quantity of apo CIII remains to be determined.

Apo A-I, Apo CIII Gene Rearrangement

A family has been described in which two sisters had very low HDL but normal LDL levels, xanthomas, severe premature atherosclerosis, and absent plasma apo A-I and apo CIII (43). First-degree relatives of these individuals had half-normal plasma levels of HDL, apo A-I, and apo CIII. Southern blotting analysis of genomic DNA from the probands, after digestion with EcoRI, along with an apo A-I cDNA probe revealed a single band of 6.5 kb, whereas normals showed a single 13-kb band (44). First-degree relatives, including the mother and father, of the probands showed one normal band and one abnormal band (44). Therefore, they appeared to be carriers of a mutant allele associated with the apo A-I gene, and the probands appeared to be homozygous for this mutant allele (Fig. 13). Southern blotting analysis of probands' DNA, after digestion with other restriction endonucleases, along with an apo A-I cDNA probe consistently revealed differences from wild type (46). This suggested that the genetic lesion was not a single bp substitution, but rather a more major DNA alteration. Southern blotting analysis with other probes derived from the region of the apo A-I gene indicated the lesion was an insertion of at least 7.5 kb in length into the fourth exon of the apo A-I gene (46). This interrupts the normal coding region of the apo A-I gene at approximately the codon specifying residue 80 of the mature protein, and may explain the lack of apo A-I in the plasma of these patients. To define the nature of the DNA insertion, a genomic library was made from the DNA of one of the probands, and clones containing the apo A-I gene and the contigous up- and downstream portions of the insertion were isolated (S. K. Karathanasis, V. I. Zannis, and J. L. Breslow, unpublished data). Southern blotting analysis of genomic DNA from normal individuals, after digestion with EcoRI, and with a probe that included apo A-I sequences and insertion sequences, revealed the normal 13-kb apo A-I genomic fragment, as expected, plus another unique band. In the probands the same probe revealed only the 6.5-kb band. This suggested that in the probands a unique piece of DNA, normally present in the genome, had been deleted and was inserted into the apo A-I gene. Further experiments with a probe made to just the insert showed that it hybridized to a region approximately 5 kb to

APO A-I APO CIII DEFICIENCY
PROBANDS AND FIRST-DEGREE RELATIVES
SOUTHERN BLOT ANALYSIS
APO A-I GENE

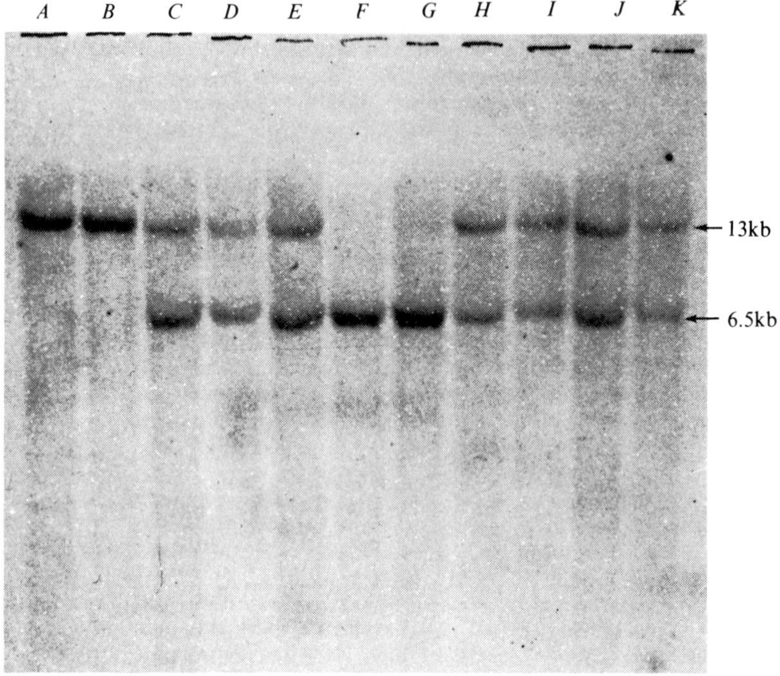

Fig. 13 Southern blotting analysis of EcoRI-digested DNA from a normal individual (A) and from the apo A-I-deficient probands (F) and (G). Blots are also shown for the maternal grandfather (B), father (C), mother (D), and brother (E) of the probands. In addition, the son (H) and daughter (I) of proband (G), and the son (J) and daughter (K) of proband (F) are also shown.

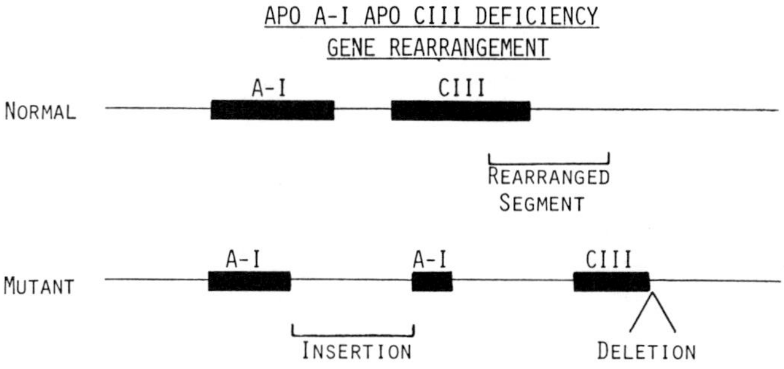

Fig. 14 A schematic diagram showing the normal and mutant genomes in the region of the apo A-I and apo CIII genes.

the 3' direction of the apo A-I gene in normal individuals. Since the apo CIII gene is in the opposite orientation to the apo A-I gene, this corresponds to the promoter region of the apo CIII gene. Thus it appears that the promoter region of the apo CIII gene was eliminated in the probands and that this is the underlying molecular basis of their apo CIII deficiency (Fig. 14).

APO E

Apo E in normal plasma is equally divided between VLDL and HDL. It comprises about 10 to 20% of VLDL protein and 1 to 2% of HDL protein. Apo E occurs in a metabolically distinct subfraction of HDL particles where it is a larger fraction of the protein (2). Human plasma apo E concentrations are in the range of 0.025 to 0.050 mg/ml. Two-dimensional gel electrophoresis of human plasma apo E has shown it to consist of several isoproteins that differ in size and charge (112,113). This is the result of both common genetic variation of apo E in the population and posttranslational modification of apo E with carbohydrate chains containing sialic acid (112–116). Apo E is synthesized and secreted as sialo apo E and subsequently desialated in plasma (18,19,117), but the physiological significance of this process is unknown. Apo E can be recognized by high-affinity receptors and mediate the binding, internalization, and catabolism of lipoprotein particles. Apo E can serve as a ligand for the LDL (apo B/E) receptor present on hepatic as well as extrahepatic tissues (118–120). Hepatic tissues also possess a high-affinity receptor that recognizes particles that contain apo E, but not apo B (121–123). This receptor is genetically distinct from the LDL receptor and has been called the chylomicron remnant or apo E receptor. Mature apo E is a 299-amino-acid polypeptide (124), and the receptor binding region has been

HUMAN APO E cDNA

```
        10         20         30         40    ↓    50         60         70         80         90        100        110↓       120
ACTCAGCCCC AGCGGAGGTG AAGGACGTCC TTCCCCAGGA GCCGACTGGC CAATCACAGG CAGGAAGATG AAGGTTCTGT GGGCTGCGTT GCTGGTCACA TTCCTGGCAG GATGCCAGGC
    ▲                                                                   M   K  V  L  W  A  A  L  L  V  T  F  L  A  G  C  Q  A
                                                                      -18                                                      -1

       130        140        150        160        170        180        190        200        210        220        230        240
CAAGGTGGAG CAAGCGGTGG AGACAGAGCC GGAGCCCGAG CTGCGCCAGC AGACCGAGTG GCAGAGCGGC CAGCGCTGGG AACTGGCACT GGGTCGCTTT TGGGATTACC TGCGCTGGGT
 K  V  E   Q  A  V  E  T  E  P  E  P  E  L  R  Q  Q  T  E  W  Q  S  G  Q  R  W  E  L  A  L  G  R  F  W  D  Y  L  R  W  V
+1

       250        260        270        280        290        300   ↓    310        320        330        340        350        360
GCAGACACTG TCTGAGCAGG TGCAGGAGGA GCTGCTCAGC TCCCAGGTCA CCCAGGAACT GAGGGCGCTG ATGGACGAGA CCATGAAGGA GTTGAAGGCC TACAAATCGG AACTGGAGGA
 Q  T  L   S  E  Q  V  Q  E  E  L  L  S  S  Q  V  T  Q  E  L  R  A  L  M  D  E  T  M  K  E  L  K  A  Y  K  S  E  L  E  E
                       50

       370        380        390        400        410        420        430        440        450        460        470        480
ACAACTGACC CCGGTGGCGG AGGAGACGCG GGCACGGCTG TCCAAGGAGC TGCAGGCGGC GCAGGCCCGG CTGGGCGCGG ACATGGAGGA CGTGTGCGGC CGCCTGGTGC AGTACCGCGG
 Q  L  T   P  V▲ A  E  E  T  R  A  R  L  S  K  E  L  Q ▲A  A  Q  A  R  L  G  A  D  M  E  D  V ▲C  G  R  L  V  Q  Y  R  G
                                                         100

       490        500        510        520        530        540        550        560        570        580        590        600
CGAGGTGCAG GCCATGCTCG GCCAGAGCAC CGAGGAGCTG CGGGTGCGCC TCGCCTCCCA CCTGCGCAAG CTGCGTAAGC GGCTCCTCCG CGATGCCGAT GACCTGCAGA AGCGCCTGGC
 E  V  Q   A  M  L  G  Q  S  T  E  E  L  R  V  R  L  A  S  H  L  R  K  L  R  K  R  L  L  R  D ▲A  D  D  L  Q  K  R  L  A
                                                                                            150

       610        620        630        640        650        660        670        680        690        700        710        720
AGTGTACCAG GCCGGGGCCC GCGAGGGCGC CGAGCGCGGC CTCAGCGCCA TCCGCGAGCG CCTGGGGCCC CTGGTGGAAC AGGGCCGCGT GCGGGCCGCC ACTGTGGGCT CCCTGGCCGC
 V  Y  Q   A  G  A  R  E  G  A  E  R  G  L  S  A  I  R  E  R  L  G  P  L  V  E  Q  G  R  V  R  A  A  T  V  G  S  L  A  G
                                                                                                                              200

       730        740        750        760        770        780        790        800        810        820        830        840
CCAGCCGCTA CAGGAGCGGG CCCAGGCCTG GGGCGAGCGG CTGCGCGCGC GGATGGAGGA GATGGGCAGC CGGACCCGCG ACCGCCTGGA CGAGGTGAAG GAGCAGGTGG CGGAGGTGCG
 Q  P  L   Q  E  R  A  Q  A  W  G  E  R  L  R  A  R  M  E  E  M  G  S▲ R  T  R  D  R  L  D  E  V  K  E  Q  V  A  E  V  R

       850        860        870        880        890        900        910        920        930        940        950        960
CGCCAAGCTG GAGGAGCAGG CCCAGCAGAT ACGCCTGCAG GCCGAGGCCT TCCAGGCCCG CCTCAAGAGC TGGTTCGAGC CCCTGGTGGA AGACATGCAG CGCCAGTGGG CCGGGCTGGT
 A  K  L   E  E  Q  A  Q▲ Q  I  R  L  Q  A  E  A  F  Q  A  R  L  K  S  W  F  E  P  L  V  E  D  M  Q  R  Q  W  A  G  L  V
                             250

       970        980        990       1000       1010       1020       1030       1040       1050       1060       1070       1080
GGAGAAGGTG CAGGCTGCCG TGGGCACCAG CGCCGCCCCT GTGCCCAGCG ACAATCACTG AACGCCGAAG CCTGCAGCCA TGCGACCCCA CGCCACCCCG TGCCTCCTGC CTCCGCGCAG
 E  K  V   Q  A  A  V  G  T  S  A  A  P  V  P  S  D  N  H
                                                       299

      1090       1100       1110       1120       1130       1140       1150       1160
CCTGCAGCGG GAGACCCTGT CCCCGCCCCA GCCGTCCTCC TGGGGTGGAC CCTAGTTTAA TAAAGATTCA CCAAGTTTCA CGCA(n)
```

localized to the middle portion of the polypeptide chain between residues 140 and 150, with residue 158 being important for the conformation of the binding domain (125–127). Structural mutations in apo E affect receptor recognition and are believed to underlie type-III hyperlipoproteinemia (HLP), a condition associated with increased plasma levels of cholesterol and triglycerides, xanthomas, and premature atherosclerosis (for reviews, see Refs. 128,129).

Apo E synthesis occurs in liver and to a minor extent in intestine. However, in contrast to the other apolipoproteins, synthesis has been documented in a wide variety of other tissues, including kidney, adrenal gland, and reticuloendothelial cells (130,131).

Apo E cDNA

Apo E cDNA sequences have been reported (117,132–135) (Fig. 15). From the proposed transcription initiation point (136), these data indicate that apo E mRNA is 1163 bp in length and includes a 5' untranslated region of 67 bp, a region coding for 317 amino acids of 951 bp, a termination codon, TGA, and a 3' untranslated region of 142 bp. This is compatible with an apo E mRNA size of 1150 bp determined by Northern blotting analysis of human liver mRNA (134).

The cDNA sequence and NH_2-terminal microsequencing of the primary translation product of apo E mRNA in cell-free synthesis experiments indicate translation initiation at the methionine 18 amino acids upstream of the mature protein (117). The NH_2-terminal 18 amino acids can be cotranslationally cleaved by microsomal membranes and represents the apo E signal peptide (117). There is no propeptide.

In analogy with both apo A-I and apo A-IV, human apo E contains 8 tandem repetitions of exactly 22 amino acids from residues 62 to 237 (136). Only one of these repeats actually begins with proline. However, the sequence of charges of the amino acids in each repeat is strikingly similar. For example, two consecutive acidic amino acids occur in the same position in six of the eight repeats. When the DNA

Fig. 15 Apo E cDNA is 1163 bp in length plus a poly A tail. The coding regions for the prepeptide and mature protein are bp's 68 to 121 and 122 to 1018, respectively. The eight 66-bp tandem repeats are in the region of bp's 305 to 832. The polyadenylation signal AATAAA occurs in the 3' untranslated region from bp's 1139 to 1144. Partial sequence determination of an apo E genomic clone has revealed introns after bp's 44, 110, and 303 (thin arrows). The thick arrows at bp's 9, 376, 416, 455, 575, 790, and 865 indicate probable sites of true variation determined by DNA sequencing of different apo E clones (see text).

APO E 66bp DNA REPEATS

```
Repeat Amino Acid                                                                                % Homology

#1  (062-083)   GCGCTGATGGACGAGACCATGAAGGAGTTGAAGGCCTACAAATCGGAACTGGAGGAACAACTGACC    56
#2  (084-105)   CCGGTGGCGGAGGAGACGCGGGCACGGCTGTCCAAGGAGCTGCAGGCGGCGCAGGCCCGGCTGGGC    75
#3  (106-127)   GCGGACATGGAGGACGTGTGCGGCCGCCTGGTGCAGTACCGCGGCGAGGTGCAGGCCATGCTCGGC    75
#4  (128-149)   CAGAGCACCGAGGAGCTGCGGGTGCGCCTCGCCTCCCACCTGCGCAAGCTGCGTAAGCGGCTCCTC    71
#5  (150-171)   CGCGATGCCGATGACCTGCAGAAGCGCCTGGCAGTGTACCAGGCCGGGGCCCGCGAGGGCGCCGAG    60
#6  (172-193)   CGCGGCCTCAGCGCCATCCGCGAGCGCCTGGGGCCCCTGGTGGAACAGGGCCGCGTGCGGGCCGCC    62
#7  (194-215)   ACTGTGGGCTCCCTGGCCGGCCAGCCGCTACAGGAGCGGGCCCAGGCCTGGGGCGAGCGGCTGCGC    51
#8  (216-237)   GCGCGGATGGAGGAGATGGGCAGCCGGACCCGCGACCGCCTGGACGAGGTGAAGGAGCAGGTGGCG    73
------------------------------------------------------------------------------------------------
Consensus       CCGGXGATGGAGGAGATGCGGGAGCGGCTGGXGGAGCACCTGGACGAGGTGCGGGAGCGGCTGGXC
Sequence                C           C     C                         A         C
------------------------------------------------------------------------------------------------
Translated      ProValMetGluGluMetArgGluArgLeuValGluHisLeuAspGluValArgGluArgLeuVal
Amino Acid         AlaIle                      Ala                                Ala
Sequence           Glu                         Glu                                Asp
                   Gly                         Gly                                Gly
------------------------------------------------------------------------------------------------
Amino Acid
Charges          0 -¼  0 -1 -1  0 +1 -1 +1  0 -¼ -1 +1  0 -1 -1  0 +1 -1 +1  0 -¼
------------------------------------------------------------------------------------------------
```

(a)

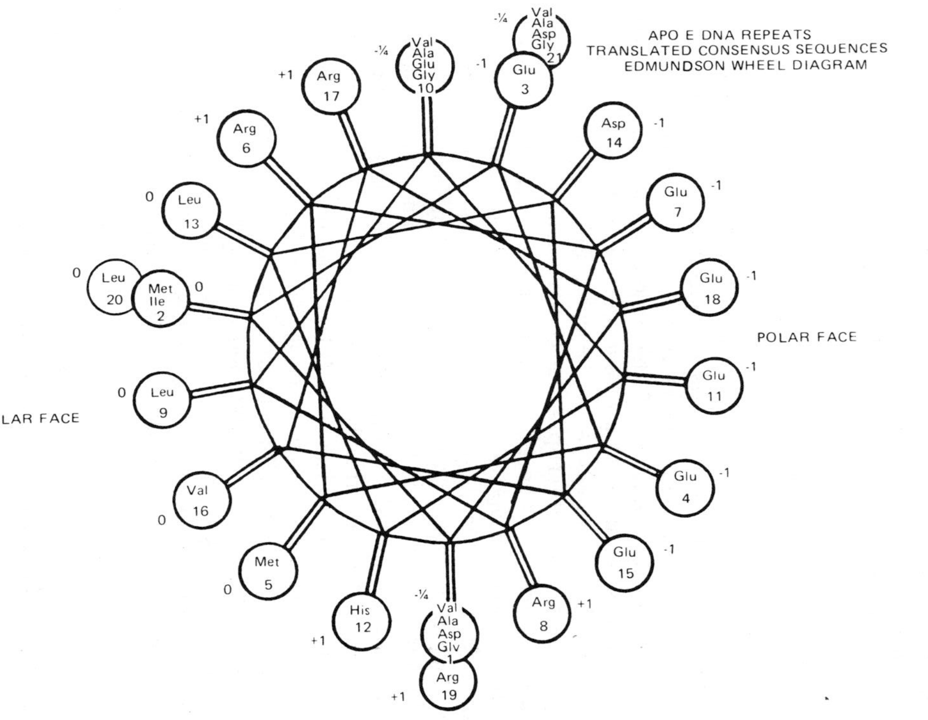

(b)

Fig. 16 (a) The apo E 66-bp DNA repeats were aligned and a consensus sequence generated. Homology of each of repeats with the consensus is shown. The charges of the amino acids are specified. (b) As shown in the wheel diagram the positively charged residues tend to cluster between the nonpolar and polar faces.

segments coding for these repeats are aligned and a consensus nucleotide at each position of the repeat derived, the consensus sequence is 51 to 75% homologous with each of the apo E repeats (Fig. 16a) and 72% homologous to a similarly derived consensus sequence for the six human apo A-I DNA repeats that code for apo A-I residues 99 to 230. Thus, extreme similarity exists with respect to the 66-bp repeats in apo E, apo A-I, and apo A-IV, suggestive of a common ancestral origin of this portion of these three apolipoprotein genes. The consensus amino acid sequence, when placed in an Edmundson wheel diagram, specifies an amphipathic alpha-helix (Fig. 16b).

Apo E Gene Structure and Mapping

The apo E gene has been isolated, a restriction map determined (Fig. 17), and its DNA sequence almost completed (136). The gene is about 3.7 kb in length and contains 4 exons and 3 introns (IVS). IVS-1 is about 700 bp long and occurs in the 5' untranslated region between bases 23 and 24 upstream of the codon for Met that initiates translation. IVS-2 is about 1100 bp long and interrupts the codon specifying amino acid −4, which is in the apo E prepeptide. IVS-3 is about 600 bp long and interrupts the codon specifying amino acid 61 of the mature protein. The intron locations are strikingly similar to those identified for the apo A-I, apo CII, and apo CIII genes and, as previously suggested, may indicate that each exon codes for a functionally distinct region of apo E. Similar intron locations of the apolipoprotein genes may be in favor of a common ancestral origin of this gene family as previously suggested (23). The apo E transcription initiation site has been tentatively assigned to the A 44 bp upstream of the GT that begins the first intron based on Sl nuclease protection experiments with human liver mRNA (136). The sequence TATAATT occurs beginning 33 bp upstream of the proposed transcription initiation site and is the putative apo E promoter.

Family studies were used to show that the inheritance of the apo E protein polymorphism cosegregated with the protein polymorphism for the third component of complement (137). Since the latter has

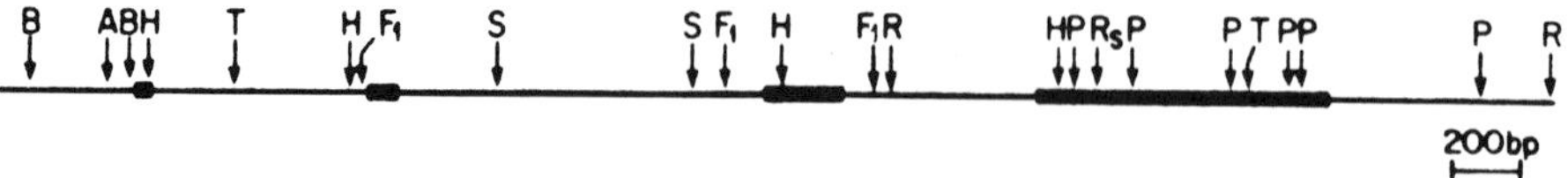

Fig. 17 Restriction map of the human genome in the vicinity of the apo E gene. Four exons (thick lines) and three introns (IVS) have been defined. Restriction sites are indicated as follows: B, BamHI; A, HaeIII; H, HpaII; T, TaqI; Fl, Hinfl; S, Sau3AI, R, EcoRI, P, PstI; R, RsaI.

been mapped using a DNA probe and somatic cell hybrids to human chromosome 19 (138), the apo E gene was also assigned to this chromosome (137). Apo E cDNA probes and somatic cell hybrids have now been used to confirm this assignment (136). As previously noted, the apo CI (84) and apo CII (89) genes have also been mapped to chromosome 19. The apo E and apo CII genes are within 2 centimorgans (94,95), but their exact relationship, or the relationship of either gene to apo CI, has not been defined. The disorder familial hypercholesterolemia involves a defect in the LDL (apo B/E) receptor where the receptor gene has been assigned to chromosome 19 (139). It is of interest that the gene for a receptor and one of its ligands both reside on the same chromosome. However, preliminary data suggest that they are not closely linked (140).

Apo E Mutations

One-dimensional isoelectric focusing of human plasma apo E reveals several bands whose relative concentrations vary between different individuals (114,116). Utilizing two-dimensional gel electrophoresis, it was possible to determine that some of these bands were due to sialo apo E isoproteins, and others due to variations in the isoelectric point of the major asialo apo E isoprotein(s) (112,113). Studies of large numbers of individuals revealed six common apo E phenotypes in the population (112,113). Family studies showed that these phenotypes were the result of a single apo E gene locus with three common alleles (112,113). The alleles have been designated $\varepsilon 4$, $\varepsilon 3$, and $\varepsilon 2$, and their gene products from basic to acidic are E4, E3, and E2, respectively. There are three homozygous phenotypes, E4/4, E3/3, and E2/2, and three heterozygous phenotypes, E4/3, E3/2, and E4/2 (141) (Fig. 18). Five relatively large studies of apo E phenotype prevalence have been reported (129,142–145) (Table 5). These have been done in diverse geographical areas but primarily in Caucasians. The range of allele frequencies were $\varepsilon 4$ 11 to 15%, $\varepsilon 3$ 74 to 78%, and $\varepsilon 2$ 8 to 13%. Large studies assessing the frequencies of the apo E alleles in other racial groups have not been reported. In Caucasians, it appears that apo E allele frequencies are similar worldwide.

This common apo E polymorphism has been found to play a role in type III HLP (112–114, 146). This disorder is characterized by elevated cholesterol and triglyceride levels as a result of delayed chylomicron remnant clearance, xanthomas, and premature coronary, as well as peripheral vascular disease (128,129). Over 90% of individuals with type III HLP have the E2/2 phenotype (129,147), whereas this occurs in only 0.5 to 1.4% (Table 5) of normal individuals (129,142–145). In addition, when E2 is isolated and studied in vitro, it does not bind as well as E3 or E4 to high affinity lipoprotein receptors (148–150). It has been suggested that chylomicron remnants with E2 on their surface are poorly recognized by receptors, clear slowly from

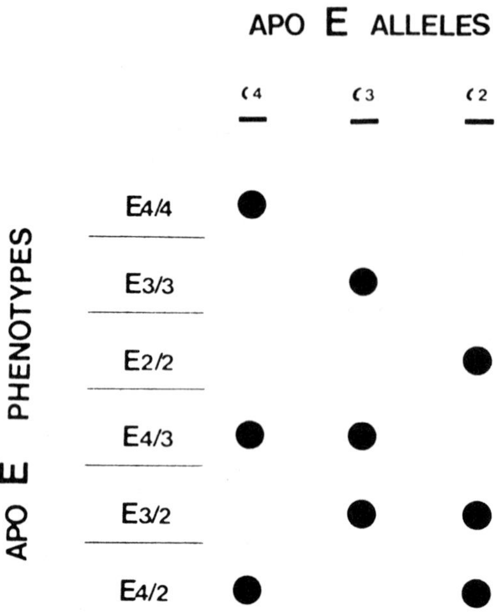

Fig. 18 Schematic presentation of the three-allele model of apo E inheritance and nomenclature of the apo E alleles and phenotypes. The closed circles represent the major asialo apo E isoproteins.

plasma, and accumulate in plasma. Chylomicron remnants are quite potent stimulators of macrophage cholesteryl ester accumulation in vitro, and high plasma concentrations of these particles may be involved in the atherogenic process in vivo (reviewed in Refs. 128 and 129). These data all suggest that homozygosity for the ε2 allele may be the underlying cause of type III HLP. However, the disease frequency is such that only 1 to 2% of people with the E2/2 phenotype actually express the disease. It is known that other hormonal and environmental factors are necessary for disease expression. However, the current belief is that type III HLP is the result of two gene defects. One of these is in the apo E structural gene and the other in a gene that influences chylomicron remnant synthesis or catabolism in a synergistic fashion. The second gene product has yet to be defined (128,129).

In addition to the striking involvement of the E2/2 phenotype in type III HLP, it appears that the apo E gene locus may be one of the factors influencing lipid levels in the general population. A recent review of five studies in the literature suggests that the ε2 allele exerts a stepwise gene dosage effect on lowering LDL cholesterol

Table 5 Apo E Phenotype Prevalence in Population Studies: Derived Apo E Allele Frequencies[a]

Phenotype	Utermann	Assmann	Breslow	Wardell	Cumming
E4/4	2.8	2.2	3.0	1.0	1.0
E3/3	59.8	62.2	58.0	51.4	58.3
E2/2	1.0	0.9	1.3	1.4	0.5
E4/3	22.9	19.9	14.0	25.0	24.8
E4/2	1.5	2.9	2.0	1.2	2.8
E3/2	12.0	11.7	22.0	20.0	12.8
No. of subjects	1031	1557	152	426	400
Allele					
ε4	15	14	11	14	15
ε3	77	78	76	74	77
ε2	8	8	13	12	8

[a]Relatively large studies of apo E phenotype prevalence reported in primarily Caucasian populations. The studies were done in Germany (142), Germany (143), United States (Boston) (129), New Zealand (144), and Scotland (145), respectively. The apo E phenotype frequencies are given as percent of that phenotype occurring in the population under study. Allele frequencies were calculated and given as percent of total.

levels (129). The ε2 allele also appears to influence the VLDL fraction and results in an increase in VLDL cholesterol and triglyceride levels in a similar stepwise manner (129). Recent studies have found E2 more frequent in patients with hypertriglyceridemia, E4 more frequent in hypercholesterolemia, and E2 and E4 more frequent in mixed hyperlipidemia, and suggested a specific effect of E4 on blood lipid values (142,143). Future studies will have to determine the exact nature of the effect of the apo E phenotype on plasma lipid levels in the general population.

Amino acid sequence analysis established that the two common variants of apo E, E4 and E2, differ from E3 by single amino acid substitutions (124). E4 differs from E3, at residue 112, because of an arginine for cysteine substitution; E2 differs from E3, at residue 158, because of a cysteine for arginine substitution. Isoelectric focusing and amino acid and DNA sequencing have identified other rare apo E

Table 6 Human Apo E Protein Polymorphism

Name[a]	Charge difference[a]	Defect[b]
E5	+2	?
E4	+1	$Cys_{112} \rightarrow Arg$
E3	0	—
E3*	0	$Ala_{99} \rightarrow Thr$, $Ala_{152} \rightarrow Pro$
E3**	0	$Cys_{112} \rightarrow Arg$, $Arg_{142} \rightarrow Cys$
E2	−1	$Arg_{158} \rightarrow Cys$
E2*	−1	$Arg_{145} \rightarrow Cys$
E2**	−1	$Lys_{146} \rightarrow Gln$
El	−2	$Gly_{127} \rightarrow Asp$, $Arg_{158} \rightarrow Cys$

[a]Nomenclature for the apo E allele gene products recognized by the isoelectric focusing position of their major asialo apo E isoprotein as specified by Zannis et al. (141). The most common allele gene product, E3, has an isoelectric point of pH 6.02. Alleles specifying gene products E4 and E5 are 1 and 2 charge units, respectively, more basic, and E2 and E1 are 1 and 2 charge units, respectively, more acidic than wild type. *, ** Indicate rare apo E variants recently discovered with the same isoelectric focusing pattern as E3 and E2.
[b]The amino acid sequence of the most common allele gene product, E3, has been specified by protein and DNA sequencing (Fig. 15). Further protein sequencing studies of apo E derived from different individuals has revealed amino acid substitutions as indicated. The nature of the protein defect responsible for E5 has yet to be determined.

alleles. In all, nine alleles are known and these are listed in Table 6. In all but one of these alleles, E5 (151), the amino acid substitution underlying the variation has been identified. Alleles E3** (127), E2 (124), E2* (150), E2** (152), and E1 (153) all involve amino acid substitutions replacing positively charged amino acids with neutral ones in the apo E receptor binding region. Where information is available, these gene products have been shown to be defective in receptor binding and/or isolated from individuals with the type III HLP phenotype. This emphasizes the importance of the positively charged amino acid residues in the receptor binding region. Allele E3* was determined from the DNA sequence (135), but the substitution of proline for alanine at residue 152 might have a significant effect on the conformation of the receptor binding region. Functional studies of this gene product have not yet been reported. Finally, the alteration responsible for the E4 allele is not in the receptor binding region, and this gene product is fully functional in receptor binding studies (148–150).

Further information about apo E genetic variation has been forthcoming from DNA sequencing. Four cDNA clones and one genomic clone have been sequenced and seven sites of variation identified (117,132,133,135). A consensus DNA sequence for allele ε3 has been

Table 7 Human Apo E Genetic Variation

	Base pair[b]							
Clone[a]	9	376	416	455	575	790	865	Gene product[c]
pE-368	G	G	G	T	G	C	G	E3
λapo E #1	C	G	G	C	G	C	G	E4
pHAE-112	C	G	G	T	G	C	A	E3
pHAE-178	C	G	G	T	G	C	A	E3
pHAE-813	C	A	A	T	C	T	G	E3*

[a]cDNA and genomic clones were sequenced in two different laboratories. pE-368, pHAE-112, pHAE-178, and pHAE-813 are cDNA clones. λapo E #1 is a genomic clone.
[b]Refers to bp location in Fig. 15.
[c]Gene product specified by that allele. E3* refers to a new allele identified by DNA sequencing. This allele has the same isoelectric focusing pattern as the E3 allele but differs in 2 uncharged amino acids and 4 bp.

presented in Fig. 14. cDNA clone pE-368 varies at bp 9 (117); cDNA clones pHAE-112 and pHAE-178 vary at bp 865 (135). cDNA clone pHAE-813 differs at 4 bp: 376, 416, 575, and 790 (135). Two of the bp substitutions actually change the coding sequence and result in the gene product E3* discussed above and presented in Table 6. The lambda apo E #1 clone of genomic DNA differs at bp 455 and appears to specify the E4 gene product (136). Thus, in addition to the nine apo E alleles specified in Table 7, DNA sequence analysis reveals the presence of at least two more alleles. In addition to the large number of mutations in the apo E exonic regions, other significant variations may exist in the apo E gene, as suggested by the recent report of an individual with absence of plasma apo E and type III HLP phenotype (154).

ACKNOWLEDGMENTS

This work was supported by grants from the National Institutes of Health (HL32354, HL32435, AG04727). Dr. Jan L. Breslow is an Established Investigator of the American Heart Association. I would like to express my sincere appreciation to Miss Lorraine Duda, Mr. Jeffrey Levine, and Mr. Alexander Pertsemlidis for their extraordinary and expert assistance in preparing this review.

REFERENCES

1. Zannis, V. I., and Breslow, J. L., *Adv. Hum. Genet.*, in press.
2. Herbert, P. N., Assmann, G., Gotto, A. M., Jr., and Frederickson, D. S., in *The Metabolic Basis of Inherited Disease* (Stanbury, J. B., Wyngaarden, J. B., Fredrickson, D. S., Goldstein, J. L., and Brown, M. D., eds.), McGraw-Hill, New York, 1982, pp. 589–651.
3. Heiss, G., and Tyroler, H. A., in *Proceedings of the Workshop on Apolipoprotein Quantification* (Lippel, K., ed.), U.S. Department of Health and Human Services, National Institutes of Health (NIH Pub. No. 83-1266), Bethesda, Md., 1982, pp. 7–42.
4. Stein, O., and Stein, Y., *Biochim. Biophys. Acta, 326*:232 (1973).
5. Brinton, E. A., and Bierman, E. L., *J. Clin. Invest., 72*:1611 (1983).
6. Fielding, C. J., Shore, V. G., and Fielding, P. E., *Biochim. Biophys. Acta, 270*:513 (1973).

7. Breslow, J. L., Ross, D., McPherson, J., Williams, H., Kurnit, D., Nussbaum, A., Karathanasis, S. K., and Zannis, V. I., *Proc. Natl. Acad. Sci. U.S.A.*, *79*:6861 (1982).

8. Shoulders, C. C., and Baralle, F. E., *Nucl. Acids Res.*, *10*: 4873 (1982).

9. Cheung, P., and Chan, L., *Nucl. Acids Res.*, *11*:3703 (1983).

10. Law, S. W., and Brewer, H. B., Jr., *Proc. Natl. Acad. Sci. U.S.A.*, *81*:66 (1984).

11. Karathanasis, S. K., Zannis, V. I., and Breslow, J. L., *Proc. Natl. Acad. Sci. U.S.A.*, *80*:6147 (1983).

12. Shoulders, C. C., Kornblihtt, A. R., Munro, B. S., and Baralle, F. E., *Nucl. Acids Res.*, *11*:2827 (1983).

13. Sharpe, C. R., Sidoli, A., Shelley, C. S., Lucero, M. A., Shoulders, C. C., and Baralle, F. E., *Nucl. Acids Res.*, *12*: 3917 (1984).

14. Gordon, J. I., Smith, D. P., Andy, R., Alpers, D. H., Schonfeld, G., and Strauss, A. W., *J. Biol. Chem.*, *257*:971 (1982).

15. Zannis, V. I., Karathanasis, S. K., Keutmann, H., Goldberger, G., and Breslow, J. L., *Proc. Natl. Acad. Sci. U.S.A.*, *80*: 2574 (1983).

16. Gordon, J. I., Sims, H. F., Lentz, S. R., Edelstein, C., Scanu, A. M., and Strauss, A. W., *J. Biol. Chem.*, *258*:4037 (1983).

17. Zannis, V. I., Breslow, J. L., and Katz, A. J., *J. Biol. Chem.*, *255*:8612 (1980).

18. Zannis, V. I., Breslow, J. L., SanGiacomo, T. R., Aden, D. P., and Knowles, B. B., *Biochemistry*, *20*:7089 (1981).

19. Zannis, V. I., Kurnit, D. M., and Breslow, J. L., *J. Biol. Chem.*, *257*:536 (1982).

20. Edelstein, C., Gordon, J. I., Toscas, K., Sims, H. F., Strauss, A. W., and Scanu, A. M., *J. Biol. Chem.*, *258*:11,430 (1983).

21. Kooistra, T., VanHinsbergh, V., Havekas, L., and Kempen, H. J., *FEBS Lett.*, *170*:109 (1984).

22. Brewer, H. B., Jr., Fairwell, T., LaRue, A., Ronan, R., Houser, A., and Brouzert, T. J., *Biochem. Biophys. Res. Commun.*, *80*:623 (1978).

23. Barker, W. C., and Dayhoff, M. O., *Comp. Biochem. Physiol.*, *57B*:309 (1977).

24. Fitch, W. M., *Genetics*, *86*:623 (1977).

25. Schiffer, M., and Edmundson, A. B., *Biophys. J.*, *7*:121 (1967).

26. Segrest, J. P., Jackson, R. L., Morrisett, J. D., and Gotto, A. M., *FEBS Lett.*, *38*:247 (1974).

27. Segrest, J. P., Chung, B. H., Brouillette, C. G., Kanellis, P., and McGahan, R., *J. Biol. Chem.*, *258*:2290 (1983).

28. Fitch, W. M., Smith, T., and Breslow, J. L., in *Methods in Enzymology* (Segrest, J. P., and Albers, J. J., eds.), Academic Press, New York, 1984, Chap. 99.

29. Bruns, G. A. P., Karathanasis, S. K., and Breslow, J. L., *Arteriosclerosis*, *4*:97 (1984).

30. Law, S. W., Gray, G., Brewer, H. B., Jr., Sakaguchi, A. Y., and Naylor, S. L., *Biochem. Biophys. Res. Commun.*, *118*:934 (1984).

31. Cheung, P., Kao, F. T., Law, M. L., Jones, C., Puck, T. T., and Chan, L., *Proc. Natl. Acad. Sci. U.S.A.*, *81*:508 (1984).

32. Lusis, A. J., Taylor, B. A., Wangenstein, R. W., and LeBoeuf, R. L., *J. Biol. Chem.*, *258*:5071 (1983).

33. Antonucci, T. K., VonDeimling, O. H., Rosenblum, B. B., Skow, L. C., and Meisler, M. H., *Genetics*, *107*:463 (1984).

34. Meisler, M. H., Wanner, L., Kao, F. T., and Jones, C., *Cytogenet. Cell Genet.*, *31*:124 (1981).

35. Gerald, P. S., and Grzeschik, K. H., *Cytogenet. Cell Genet.*, *37*:103 (1984).

36. Franceschini, G., Sirtori, C. R., Capurso, A., Weisgraber, K. H., and Mahley, R. W., *J. Clin. Invest.*, *66*:892 (1980).

37. Weisgraber, K. H., Rall, S. C., Bersot, T. P., Mahley, R. W., Franceschini, G., and Sirtori, C. R., *J. Biol. Chem.*, *258*:2508 (1983).

38. Utermann, G., Geussner, G., Franceschini, G., Haas, J., and Steinmetz, A., *J. Biol. Chem.*, *257*:501 (1982).

39. Utermann, G., Steinmetz, A., Paetzold, R., Wilk, J., Fuessner, G., Kaffarnik, H., Mueller–Eckhardt, C., Seidel, D., Vogelbert, K. H., and Zimmer, F., *Hum. Genet.*, *61*:329 (1982).

40. Menzel, H. J., Kladetzky, L., and Assmann, G., *J. Lipid Res.*, *23*:915 (1982).

41. Rall, S. C., Menzel, H. J., Assmann, G., Utermann, G., Haas, J., Harris, R. J., Weisgraber, K. H., Bersot, T. P., and Mahley, R. W., *Arteriosclerosis*, *3*:515a (1983).

42. Menzel, H. J., Assman, G., Rall, S. C., Weisgraber, K. H., and Mahley, R. W., *J. Biol. Chem.*, *259*:3070 (1984).

43. Norum, R. A., Laker, J. B., Goldstein, S., Angel, A., Goldberg, R. B., Block, W. D., Noffze, D. K., Dolphin, P. J., Edelglass, J., Bogorad, D. D., and Alaupovic, P., *New Engl. J. Med.*, *306*:1513 (1982).

44. Karathanasis, S. K., Norum, R. A., Zannis, V. I., and Breslow, J. L., *Nature (London)*, *301*:718 (1983).

45. Karathanasis, S. K., McPherson, J., Zannis, V. I., and Breslow, J. L., *Nature (London)*, *304*:371 (1983).

46. Karathanasis, S. K., Zannis, V. I., and Breslow, J. L., *Nature (London)*, *305*:823 (1983).

47. Zannis, V. I., Lees, A. M., Lees, R. S., and Breslow, J. L., *J. Biol. Chem.*, *257*:4978 (1982).

48. Bojanovski, D., Gregg, R. E., Zech, L. A., Meng, M. S., Ronan, R., and Brewer, H. B., *Clin. Res.*, *32*:390a (1984).

49. Brewer, H. B., Jr., Fairwell, T., Meng, M., Kay, L., and Ronan, R., *Biochem. Biophys. Res. Commun.*, *113*:934 (1983).

50. Rosseneu, M., Assmann, G., Taveirne, M. J., and Schmitz, G., *J. Lipid Res.*, *25*:111 (1984).

51. Schaefer, E. J., Kay, L. L., Zech, L. A., Brewer, H. B., Jr., *J. Clin. Invest.*, *70*:934 (1982).

52. Logocki, P. A., and Scanu, A. M., *J. Biol. Chem.*, *255*:3701 (1980).

53. Schinomiya, M., Sasaki, N., Barnhart, R. L., Shirai, K., and Jackson, R. L., *Biochim. Biophys. Acta*, *713*:292 (1982).

54. Wu, A. L., and Windmueller, H. G., *J. Biol. Chem.*, *254*:7316 (1979).

55. Gordon, J. I., Budelier, K. A., Sims, H. E., Edelstein, C., Scanu, A. M., and Strauss, A. W., *J. Biol. Chem.*, *258*: 14,054 (1983).

56. Brewer, H. B., Jr., Lux, S. E., Ronan, R., and John, K. M., *Proc. Natl. Acad. Sci. U.S.A.*, *69*:1304 (1972).

57. Moore, M. N., Kao, F. T., Tsao, Y. K., and Chan, L., *Biochem. Biophys. Res. Commun.*, *123*:1 (1984).

58. Swaney, J. B., Reese, H., and Eder, H. A., *Biochem. Biophys. Res. Commun.*, *59*:513 (1974).

59. Weisgraber, K. H., Bersot, T. P., and Mahley, R. W., *Biochem. Biophys. Res. Commun.*, *85*:287 (1978).

60. Gordon, J. I., Smit, D. P., Alpers, D. H., and Strauss, A. W., *Biochemistry*, *21*:5424 (1982).

61. Gordon, J. I., Disgaier, C. L., Sims, H. F., Sachdev, O. P., Glickman, R. M., and Strauss, A. W., *J. Biol. Chem.*, *259*: 468 (1984).

62. Gordon, J. I., Smith, D. P., Alpers, D. H., and Strauss, A. W., *J. Biol. Chem.*, *257*:8418 (1982).

63. Boguski, M. S., Elshourbagy, N., Taylor, J. M., and Gordon, J. I., *Proc. Natl. Acad. Sci. U.S.A.*, *81*:5021 (1984).

64. Menzel, H. J., Kovary, P. M., and Assmann, G., *Hum. Genet.*, *62*:349 (1982).

65. Goldstein, J. L., and Brown, M. S., in *Metabolic Basis of Inherited Disease* (Stanbury, J. B., Wyngaarden, J. B., Fredrickson, D. S., Goldstein, J. L., and Brown, M. D., eds.), McGraw-Hill, New York, 1982, pp. 672–712.

66. Kane, J. P., *Ann. Rev. Physiol.*, *45*:637 (1983).

67. Lee, D. M., Valente, A. J., Kuo, W. H., and Maeda, H., *Biochim. Biophys. Acta*, *666*:133 (1981).

68. LeBoeuf, R. C., Miller, C., Shiverly, J. E., Schumaker, V. N., Balla, M. A., and Lusis, A. J., *FEBS Lett.*, *170*:105 (1984).

69. Schonfeld, G., Patsch, W., Pfleger, B., Witztum, J. L., and Weidman, S. W., *J. Clin. Invest.*, *64*:1288 (1979).

70. Marcel, Y. L., Hogue, M., Theolis, R., and Milne, R. W., *J. Biol. Chem.*, *257*:13,165 (1982).

71. Berg, K., in *Progress in Medical Genetics* (Steinberg, A. G., Bearn, A. G., Motulsky, A. R., and Childs, B., eds.), Saunders, Philadelphia, 1983, pp. 35–90.

72. Schumaker, V. N., Robinson, M. T., Curtiss, L. K., Butler, R., and Sparkes, R. S., *J. Biol. Chem.*, *259*:6423 (1984).

73. Malloy, M. J., Kane, J. P., Hardman, D. A., Hamilton, R. L., and Dolal, K. B., *J. Clin. Invest.*, *67*:1441 (1981).

74. Hyams, J., Herbert, P., Benner, D., Saribelli, A., Lynch, K., and Berman, M., *Clin. Res.*, *32*:399a (1984).

75. Sniderman, A. D., Shapiro, S., Marpole, D., Skinner, B., Teng, B., and Kwiterovich, P. O., *Proc. Natl. Acad. Sci. U.S.A.*, *77*:604 (1980).

76. Goldstein, J. L., Schrott, H. G., Hazzard, W. R., Bierman, E. L., and Motolsky, A. R., *J. Clin. Invest.*, *52*:1544 (1973).

77. Brunzell, J. D., Albers, J. J., Chait, A., Grundy, S. M., Groszek, E., and McDonald, G. B., *J. Lipid Res.*, *24*:147 (1983).

78. Chait, A., Albers, J. J., and Brunzell, J. D., *Eur. J. Clin. Invest.*, *10*:17 (1980).

79. Janus, E. D., Nicoll, A. M., Turner, P. R., Magill, P., and Lewis, B., *Eur. J. Clin. Invest.*, *10*:161 (1980).

80. Soutar, A. K., Garner, C. W., Baker, H. N., Sparrow, J. J., and Jackson, R. L., *Biochemistry*, *14*:3057 (1975).

81. Knott, T. J., Robertson, M. E., Priestley, L. M., Urdea, M., Wallis, S., and Scott, J., *Nucl. Acids Res.*, *12*:3909 (1984).

82. Jackson, R. L., Sparrow, J. T., Baker, H. N., Morrisett, J., Taunton, O. D., and Gotto, A. M., Jr., *J. Biol. Chem.*, *249*: 5308 (1974).

83. Shulman, R. S., Herbert, P. N., Wehrly, K., and Fredrickson, D. S., *J. Biol. Chem.*, *280*:182 (1975).

84. Tata, F., Henri, I., Markham, A., Weil, D., Williamson, R., Humphries, S., and Junien, C., *Hum. Genet.*, *69*:345 (1985).

85. Nikkila, E. A., in *The Metabolic Basis of Inherited Disease* (Stanbury, J. B., Wyngaarden, J. B., Fredrickson, D. S., Goldstein, J. L., and Brown, M. D., eds.), McGraw-Hill, New York, 1983, pp. 622–642.

86. Breckenridge, W. C., Little, J. A., Steiner, G., Chow, A., and Poapst, M., *New Engl. J. Med.*, *298*:1265 (1978).

87. Musliner, T. A., Church, E. C., Herbert, P. N., Kingston, M. J., and Shulman, R. S., *Proc. Natl. Acad. Sci. U.S.A.*, *74*:5358 (1977).

88. Kinnunen, P. K. J., Jackson, R. L., Smith, L. C., Gotto, A. M., and Sparrow, J. T., *Proc. Natl. Acad. Sci. U.S.A.*, *74*:4848 (1977).

89. Jackson, C. L., Bruns, G. A. P., and Breslow, J. L., *Proc. Natl. Acad. Sci. U.S.A.*, *81*:2945 (1984).

90. Myklebost, O., Williamson, B., Markham, A. F., Myklebost, S. R., Rogers, J., Woods, D. E., and Humphries, S. E., *J. Biol. Chem.*, *259*:4401 (1984).

91. Hoispattankar, A. V., Fairwell, T., Ronan, R., and Brewer, H. B., Jr., *J. Biol. Chem.*, *259*:318 (1984).

92. Jackson, R. L., Baker, H. N., Gilliam, E. B., and Gotto, A. M., *Proc. Natl. Acad. Sci. U.S.A.*, *74*:1942 (1977).

93. Jackson, C. J., Bruns, G. A. P., and Breslow, J. L., in *Methods in Enzymology* (Segrest, J. P., and Albers, J. J., eds.), Academic Press, New York, 1984, Chap. 89.

94. Myklebost, O., Rogne, S., Olaisen, B., Gedde-Dahl, T., Jr., and Prydz, H., *Hum. Genet.*, *67*:309 (1984).

95. Humphries, S. E., Berg, K., Gill, L., Cumming, A. M., Robertson, F. W., Stalenhort, A. F. H., Williamson, R., and Borresen, A. L., *Clin. Genet.*, *26*:389 (1984),

96. Humphries, S. E., Williams, L. Myklebost, O., Stalenhoef, A. F. H., Demacker, P. N. M., Baggio, G., Crepaldi, G., Galton, D. J., and Williamson, R., *Hum. Genet.*, *67*:151 (1984).

97. Havel, R. J., Kotite, L., and Kane, J. P., *Biochem. Med.*, *21*:121 (1979).

98. Brewer, H. B., Shulman, R., Herbert, P., and Ronan, R., *J. Biol. Chem.*, *249*:4975 (1974).

99. Kashyap, M. L., Srivastava, L. S., Hynd, B. A., Gartside, P. S., and Perisutti, G., *J. Lipid Res.*, *22*:800 (1981).

100. Brown, W. V., and Baginsky, M. L., *Biochem. Biophys. Res. Commun.*, *46*:375 (1972).

101. Krauss, R. M., Herbert, P. N., Levy, R. I., and Fredrickson, D. S., *Circ. Res.*, *33*:403 (1973).

102. Kinnunen, P. K. J., and Ehnholm, C., *FEBS Lett.*, *65*:354 (1976).

103. Windler, E., Chao, Y., and Havel, R. J., *J. Biol. Chem.*, *255*:5475 (1980).

104. Shelburne, F., Hanks, J., Meyers, W., and Quarfordt, S., *J. Clin. Invest.*, *65*:652 (1980).

105. Windler, E., Chao, Y., and Havel, R. J., *J. Biol. Chem.*, *255*:8303 (1980).

106. Quarfordt, S. H., Michalopoulos, G., and Shirmer, B., *J. Biol. Chem.*, *257*:14,642 (1982).

107. Ginsberg, H., Le, N. A., Norum, R. A., Bigson, J., and Brown, W. V., *Clin. Res.*, *32*:396a (1984).

108. Sparrow, J. T., Pownall, H. J., Hsu, F. J., Blumenthal, L. E., Culwell, A. R., and Gotto, A. M., *Biochemistry*, *16*: 5427 (1977).

109. Karathanasis, S. K., Zannis, V. I., and Breslow, J. L., *J. Lipid Res.*, *26*:451 (1985).

110. Blaufuss, M. C., Gordon, J. I., Schonfeld, G., Strauss, A. W., and Alpers, D. H., *J. Biol. Chem.*, *259*:2452 (1984).

111. Rees, A., Shoulders, C. C., Stocks, J., Galton, D. J., and Baralle, F. E., *Lancet*, *1(8322)*:444 (1983).

112. Zannis, V. I., Just, P. W., and Breslow, J. L., *Am. J. Hum. Genet.*, *33*:11 (1981).

113. Zannis, V. I., and Breslow, J. L., *Biochemistry*, *21*:1033 (1981).

114. Utermann, G., Jaeschke, M., and Mangel, J., *FEBS Lett.*, *56*:352 (1975).

115. Jain, R. S., and Quarfordt, S. H., *Life Sci.*, *25*:1315 (1979).

116. Utermann, G., Langenback, U., Beisiegel, U., and Weber, W., *Am. J. Hum. Genet.*, *32*:3398 (1980).

117. Zannis, V. I., McPherson, J., Goldberger, G., Karathanasis, S. K., and Breslow, J. L., *J. Biol. Chem.*, *259*:5495 (1984).

118. Pitas, E., Innerarity, T. L., Arnold, K. S., and Mahley, R. W., *Proc. Natl. Acad. Sci. U.S.A.*, *76*:2311 (1981).

119. Bersot, T. P., Mahley, R. W., Brown, M. S., and Goldstein, J. L., *J. Biol. Chem.*, *251*:2395 (1976).

120. Innerarity, T. L., and Mahley, R. W., *Biochemistry*, *17*:1440 (1978).

121. Hui, D. Y., Innerarity, T. L., and Mahley, R. W., *J. Biol. Chem.*, *256*:5646 (1981).

122. Carrela, M., and Cooper, A. D., *Proc. Natl. Acad. Sci. U.S.A.*, *76*:338 (1979).

123. Sherrill, B. C., Innerarity, T. L., and Mahley, R. W., *J. Biol. Chem.*, *255*:1804 (1980).

124. Rall, S. C., Weisgraber, K. H., and Mahley, R. W., *J. Biol. Chem.*, *257*:4171–4178 (1981).

125. Innerarity, T. L., Friedlander, E. J., Rall, S. C., Jr., Weisgraber, K. H., and Mahley, R. W., *J. Biol. Chem.*, *258*: 12,341 (1983).

126. Weisgraber, K. H., Innerarity, T. L., Harder, K. J., Mahley, R. W., Milne, R. W., Marcel, Y. L., and Sparrow, J. T., *J. Biol. Chem.*, *258*:12,348 (1983).

127. Innerarity, T. L., Weisgraber, K. H., Arnold, K. S., Rall, S. C., Jr., and Mahley, R. W., *J. Biol. Chem.*, *259*:7261 (1984).

128. Mahley, R. W., and Angelin, B., *Adv. intern. Med.*, *29*:385 (1984).

129. Breslow, J. L., and Zannis, V. I., in *Arteriosclerosis Reviews*, Raven Press, New York, in press.

130. Blue, M. L., Williams, D. L., Zucker, S., Khan, S. A., and Blum, C. B., *Proc. Natl. Acad. Sci. U.S.A.*, *80*:283 (1983).

131. Basu, S. K., Brown, M. S., Ho, Y. K., Havel, R. J., and Goldstein, J. L., *Proc. Natl. Acad. Sci. U.S.A.*, *78*:7545 (1981).

132. Breslow, J. L., McPherson, J., Nussbaum, A. L., Williams, H. W., Lofquist-Kahl, F., Karathanasis, S. K., and Zannis, V. I., *J. Biol. Cehm.*, *257*:14,639 (1982).

133. Breslow, J. L., McPherson, J., Nussbaum, A. L., Williams, H. W., Lofquist-Kahl, F., Karathanasis, S. K., and Zannis, V. I., *J. Biol. Chem.*, *258*:11,422 (1983).

134. Wallis, S. C., Rogne, S., Gill, L., Markham, A., Edge, M., Woods, D., Williamson, R., and Humphries, S., *EMBO J.*, *2*:2369 (1983).

135. McLean, J. W., Elshourbagy, N. A., Chang, D. J., Mahley, R. W., and Taylor, J. M., *J. Biol. Chem.*, *259*:6498 (1984).

136. Das, H. K., McPherson, J., Bruns, G. A. P., Karathanasis, S. K., and Breslow, J. L., *J. Biol. Chem.*, *260*:6240 (1985).

137. Olaisen, B., Teisberg, P., and Gedde-Dahl, T., *Hum. Genet.*, *62*:233 (1982).

138. Whitehead, A. S., Bruns, G. A. P., Markham, A. P., Colten, H. R., and Woods, D. E., *Science*, *221*:69 (1983).

139. Francke, U., Brown, M. S., and Goldstein, J. L., *Proc. Natl. Acad. Sci. U.S.A.*, *81*:2826 (1984).

140. Berg, K., Borresen, A. L. Heiberg, A., and Maartmann-Moe, K., *Cytogenet. Cell Genet.*, *37*:418a (1984).

141. Zannis, V. I., Breslow, J. L., Utermann, G., Mahley, R. W., Weisgraber, K. H., Havel, R. J., Goldstein, J. L., Brown, M. S., Schonfeld, G., Hazzard, W. R., and Blum, C. B., *J. Lipid Res.*, *23*:911 (1982).

142. Utermann, G., Kindermann, I., Kaffarnik, H., and Steinmetz, A., *Hum. Genet.*, *65*:232 (1984).

143. Assmann, G., Schmitz, G., Menzel, H. J., and Schulte, H., *Clin. Chem.*, *30/5*:641 (1984).

144. Wardell, M. R., Suckling, P. A., and Janus, E. D., *J. Lipid Res.*, *23*:1174 (1982).

145. Cumming, A. M., and Robertson, F. W., *Clin. Genet.*, *25*:310 (1984).

146. Zannis, V. I., Breslow, J. L., *J. Biol. Chem.*, *255*:1759 (1980).

147. Breslow, J. L., Zannis, V. I., SanGiacomo, T. R., Third, J. L. H. C., Tracy, T., and Glueck, C. J., *J. Lipid Res.*, *23*:1224 (1982).

148. Schneider, W. J., Kovanen, P. T., Brown, M. S., Goldstein, J. L., Utermann, G., Weber, W., Havel, R. J., Kotite, L., Kane, J. P., Innerarity, T. L., and Mahley, R. W., *J. Clin. Invest.*, *68*:1075 (1981).

149. Weisgraber, K. H., Innerarity, T. L., and Mahley, R. W., *J. Biol. Chem.*, *257*:2518 (1982).

150. Rall, S. C., Jr., Weisgraber, K. H., Innerarity, T. L., and Mahley, R. W., *Proc. Natl. Acad. Sci. U.S.A.*, *79*:4696 (1982).

151. Yamamura, T., Yamamoto, A., Hiramori, K., and S. Nambu, *Atherosclerosis*, *50*:159 (1984).

152. Rall, S. C., Jr., Weisgraber, K. H., Innerarity, T. L., Bersot, T. P., Mahley, R. W., and Blum, C. B., *J. Clin. Invest.*, *72*:1288 (1983).

153. Weisgraber, K. H., Rall, S. C., Jr., Innerarity, T. L., Mahley, R. W., Kuusi, W., and Ehnholm, C., *J. Clin. Invest.*, *73*:1024 (1984).

154. Ghiselli, G., Schaefer, E. J., Gascon, P., and Brewer, H. B., Jr., *Science*, *214*:1239 (1981).

6

Biological Membranes

THEODORE L. STECK The Pritzker School of Medicine, The University of Chicago, Chicago, Illinois

INTRODUCTION

Biological membranes are the structures that delimit cells and organelles to create their functional compartments. Their relationship to plasma lipoproteins has at least two facets: (1) universal constituents of biological membranes—amphipathic lipids—are conveyed to and from cells in higher organisms by these lipoproteins, and (2) the synthesis, assembly, and secretion of lipoproteins and their assimilation and disposal in target cells are mediated by membrane processes. This chapter briefly describes and illustrates membrane structure and function in order to explain the related processes that are the subjects of other chapters in this volume. (Some recent monographs providing an overview of this topic are cited in Refs. 1–4.)

MEMBRANE LIPIDS

Biological membranes are composed of lipids, proteins, and carbohydrates, the latter taking the form of glycolipids and glycoproteins. The lipids provide the basis for membrane structure. Moreover, the information required for membrane assembly is implicit in the structure of the lipid molecules themselves. This is readily demonstrated in the laboratory by the creation of artificial lipid membranes, which resemble their biological counterparts to a surprising degree, simply by dispersing purified lipids in water. Membrane assembly is thus driven by a thermodynamic mechanism: the minimization of free energy. The structure of membrane lipid molecules tells the story.

Lipid Classes (1–3)

There are three major types of membrane lipids: glycerolipids, sphingolipids, and sterols. Glycerolipids, the most universal of membrane constituents, form a class of enormous diversity in molecular detail but striking uniformity in overall design. Coupled to the first and second carbon atoms of the glycerol backbone are long-chain fatty acids, most often in ester linkage. The fatty acids have chain lengths in the range of 14 to 24 methylene groups, the most common being 16 to 18 in length. They may have zero to three or more unsaturations, most often double bonds in the cis configuration. The fatty acid linked to the first carbon atom of the glycerol is usually saturated and the second fatty acid is usually unsaturated. Other modifications of the alkyl chains include branching, hydroxylation, and propanyl or epoxy rings.

The third carbon atom on the glycerol backbone bears a polar group, typically an oligosaccharide or a phosphate ester. The phosphate group is usually also esterified to a polar alcohol such as choline, ethanolamine, serine, inositol, or a second glycerol (itself sometimes further modified).

Sphingolipids are built upon the aliphatic amine-alcohol, sphingosine. Sphingosine serves both as a backbone and as the bearer of one of the two long alkyl chains of these lipids. The other alkyl chain derives from a fatty acid linked as an amide to the primary amino group. As with the glycerolipids, the polar head groups of sphingolipids are either oligosaccharides or phosphodiesters (e.g., phosphorylcholine in sphingomyelin).

Sterols such as cholesterol are polycyclic hydrocarbons, devoid of polar centers except for the single oxygen atom in the hydroxyl group at carbon three.

There are also other, less common membrane lipids and special lipids devoted to specific functions (e.g., quinones and dolichols). It is worth noting that many types of cellular lipids are not present in biological membranes in more than trace amounts; among these are mono-, di-, and triglycerides, fatty acids, lysophosphatides, and sterol esters.

Membrane lipid profiles vary characteristically throughout phylogeny for reasons we do not understand. Prokaryotes generally utilize glycerolipids containing fatty acids with no more than one unsaturation. Gram-positive bacteria and plants are rich in glycoglycerolipids, while animals utilize glycosphingolipids. Sterols are ubiquitous in eukaryotes and rare in prokaryotes; they, like sphingolipids, are enriched in plasma membranes. A complex membrane lipid, diphosphatidylglycerol or cardiolipin, is a specific component of gram-negative bacteria, mitochondrial inner membranes, and the thylakoid membranes of chloroplasts. The most common polar head group in animals, phosphorylcholine, is absent from prokaryotes.

Amphipathy (5)

Membrane lipids share a special feature: they are all amphipaths or amphiphiles, i.e., built into each molecule are substantial polar and nonpolar centers. The polar moieties naturally seek association with water and dissolved ions. This chemical affinity is manifested in a substantial negative enthalpy change for thier dissolution. The nonpolar portions of the amphipaths do not associate with the solvent; thus, the enthalpy change for their interaction with water is nearly zero. However, hydrocarbons reduce the freedom of motion of water molecules around them. The consequent increase in the ordering of the solvent lowers the entropy of the system. The unfavorable entropy change, uncompensated by a favorable enthalpy of bonding to water, drives hydrocarbons and other nonpolar solutes from water. This thermodynamic mechanism is called the *hydrophobic effect*. Each methylene group in an alkyl chain adds approximately 0.8 kcal/mol to the energy expelling it from water.

Since membrane lipids typically have both a large polar head group and two fatty acyl chains of 16 or more methylene units, the asymmetric forces driving their orientation in water are enormous. The thermodynamic mandate for such lipids is to find a disposition compatible with their amphipathy (Fig. 1). One solution is for these amphipaths to accumulate at air-water interfaces as monomolecular

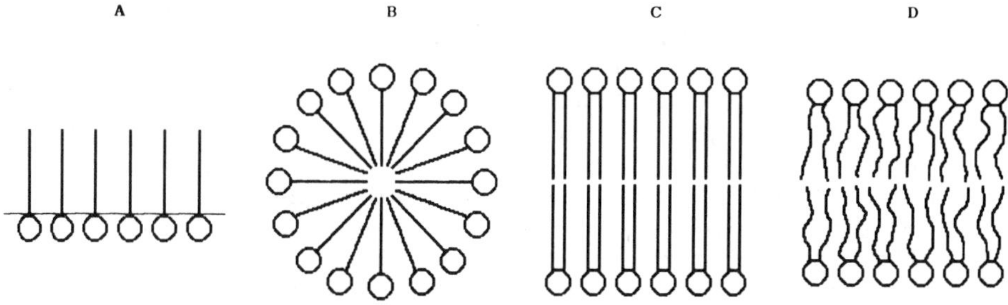

Fig. 1 Hydrophobic aggregation of amphipaths in water can create ordered arrays. (A) A monomolecular film or monolayer at an air-water interface. (B) A micelle. (C) A bimolecular leaflet or bilayer in a crystalline or solid state. (D) The same bilayer following a thermal transition to a liquid crystalline or fluid state. These figures are cross-sections through arrays; in A, C and D the arrays are indefinite in extent, while in micelles (B), the arrays are usually finite (spheres, ellipsoids, or cylinders). Note that micelles could not form if the head group of the amphipath were not larger in cross-section than the apolar tails, and that bilayers require that head and tail be of similar cross-section.

films; however, except for surfactant in the lung, this option is not generally available in the body. Instead, amphipaths usually create their own nonpolar compartments by hydrophobic associations that remove their nonpolar groups, but not their polar groups, from water.

Some lipids, such as lysophosphatides, in which the polar head group is large in size relative to the nonpolar moiety, associate to form water-soluble micelles, i.e., discrete, cooperatively assembled aggregates. Micelles may contain hundreds of molecules and may be spheres, ellipsoids, or cylinders of indefinite length. If the polar and nonpolar portions of the amphipath are approximately equal in cross-section, the ensemble will tend to be planar, two molecules thick, and of unlimited extent, rather than small, curved, and closed.

The Bilayer (1–5)

The universal configuration of membrane lipids and the fundamental unit of membrane organization is, in fact, such a bimolecular leaflet of polar lipids, commonly called a bilayer. In this structure, two monomolecular layers are joined through the hydrophobic apposition of the ends of their apolar chains to create a membrane approximately 50 Å thick. Phospholipids and glycolipids must have evolved expressly to create such structures. These lipids have long hydrocarbon tails to confer insolubility, hence a stable membrane phase; they also have a balance between the cross-section of their head and tail groups, which confers a planar configuration and assures that the molecules do not slip past one another across the central plane of the bilayer. Is it not now evident why most nonmembrane lipids do not form bilayers? Consider this laboratory exercise: Neither cholesterol nor lysolecithin forms bilayers by itself; the former lacks a sufficient head group and forms instead water-insoluble droplets, while the latter, with too large a head for its tail, forms spherical micelles. Mixed one-to-one, however, their complementary contours create planar bilayers in the absence of other membrane lipids.

The hydrophobic edges of planar bilayers are not stable and will take up more lipid indefinitely. This restlessness is resolved if the bilayer closes into a spherical shell; generically, a vesicle. This process occurs spontaneously when membrane lipids are simply dispersed vigorously in water. It is this configuration—the closed sac—in which all biological membranes are found and which confers their primary function—creating impermeable boundaries for cellular compartments of any size and shape.

Phase Behavior and Lipid Motion in Bilayers (3,5,6)

To a first approximation, lipid bilayers may be regarded as microphases that can pass from the solid (gel or crystalline) to the fluid (liquid crystalline) state at a critical temperature. Such melting behavior reflects the cooperative disordering of their fatty acyl chains from a relatively close-packed, linear configuration to a more expanded array of kinked chains. The heat taken up drives the creation of a few gauche isomers (i.e., 120° rotations around carbon-carbon bonds) in otherwise all-trans alkyl chains (with only 180° rotations). The gauche conformers appear and disappear up and down the chain approximately 10^9 times per second, but only a few exist in a molecule in the liquid state at any instant.

The gel or crystalline state is characterized by a high degree of order; there is close molecular packing, slow intra- and intermolecular thermal motion, and a low capacity to dissolve exogenous amphipaths in the bilayer. The liquid crystalline state exhibits disordered packing, increased molecular motion, increased mean molecular volume despite a shortening of net chain length, and increased solvent properties. An analogy is soldiers on parade versus soldiers on the dance floor.

Molecular motion in the fluid membrane has been well characterized by a variety of physical techniques in terms of rotations about individual carbon-carbon bonds, wagging motion of segments of the molecules, rotation of lipid molecules about their long axis, and lateral diffusion of molecules in the plane of the membrane. Viscosity (the inverse of fluidity) is commonly 1 to 5 poise in fully disordered bilayers, 100 to 500 times that of water (0.01 poise). The simple bilayer thus has a resistance to flow comparable to that of a light oil. In such medium, a phospholipid molecule diffuses at the rate of 1 μm/sec or more and can migrate around an organelle or bacterial cell membrane in just a few seconds.

Cells adjust the fluidity of their membranes biosynthetically. The most important determinant of the melting temperature of a bilayer is the structure of its fatty acyl substituents (Table 1). The melting temperature rises with alkyl chain length because of increased van der Waals attractions. Conversely, covalent modifications that thwart close packing reduce the melting temperature. The most important of these are unsaturations, cis double bonds being far more potent than trans. Branching, hydroxylation, etc., serve a similar function. The alkyl chain at C-2 dominates over that at C-1 in determining the melting temperature. Furthermore, phospholipids with bulky head groups, such as phosphatidylcholine, melt more readily than those with smaller head groups, such as phosphatidylethanolamine, because the close packing of their acyl chains is compromised. Bilayers composed of a single lipid species have a sharp melting curve, while even the simplest of naturally occurring membranes contain mixtures of diverse lipids and have correspondingly broad thermal transition profiles.

In the mid-range of the thermal transition, the bilyaer is a mosaic of gel-like patches, each containing hundreds of lipid molecules in

Table 1 Melting Temperatures of Selected Phospholipids

Variable	Phospholipid (acyl chains)	T (°C)
Chain length	Dimyristoyl phosphatidylcholine (1,2 di 14:0)	24
	Dipalmitoyl phosphatidylcholine (1,2 di 16:0)	42
	Distearoyl phosphatidylcholine (1,2 di 18:0)	55
Chain position	1-Myristoyl, 2-palmitoyl phosphatidylcholine	35
	1-Palmitoyl, 2-myristoyl phosphatidylcholine	27
	1-Stearoyl, 2-palmitoyl phosphatidylcholine	47
	1-Palmitoyl, 2-stearoyl phosphatidylcholine	44
Chain saturation	Dipalmitoyl phosphatidylcholine (1,2 di 16:0)	42
	Dielaidoyl phosphatidylcholine (1,2 di 18:1, 9 trans)	5
	Dioleoyl phosphatidylcholine (1,2 di 18:1, 9 cis)	−22
Head group	Dipalmitoyl phosphatidylcholine	42
	Dipalmitoyl phosphatidylglycerol	41
	Dipalmitoyl phosphatidylethanolamine	63
	Dipalmitoyl phosphatidic acid	67

Source: Ref. 3.

physical continuity and diffusional equilibrium with the surrounding fluid phase (Fig. 2). In a bilayer composed of a mixture of lipids, the gel and fluid phases will contain the different lipid species in different proportions, and the solid patches need not be identical to one another in composition.

It is characteristic of biological membranes that their lipids melt at a temperature near the growth temperature of the organism. When poikilothermic microbes are grown at a new temperature, their synthesis of lipids changes, and the melting temperature of the membrane shifts accordingly. The goal cannot simply be to maintain the membrane in a melted state, for the organism could assure complete fluidity at all times by synthesizing lipids with short-chain, polyunsaturated tails and bulky head groups. Instead, the organism seeks to

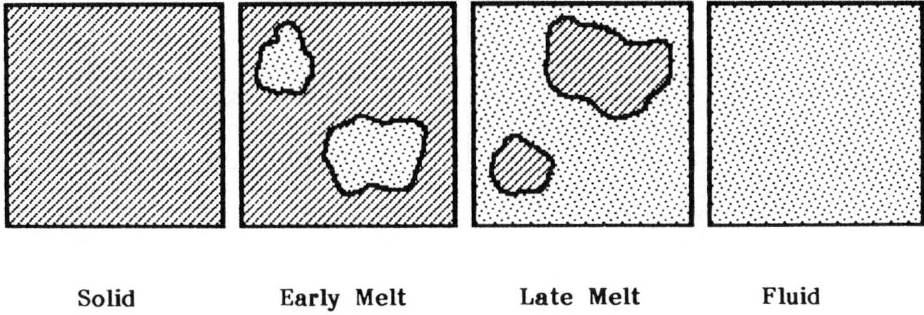

Fig. 2 Thermal phase transition of a bilayer (viewed from its surface). As the crystalline array is warmed, discontinuous islands of liquid crystalline phase emerge, surrounded by a continuous crystalline phase. As the temperature is raised, the liquid phase becomes confluent and surrounds patches of the solid, which disappear on further warming.

center the growth temperature near the middle of a broad membrane melting curve. For what purpose? Consider that in this mid-range, the bilayer is a multiphasic system, containing solid and liquid domains. Just as the lipid composition of the microphases is not the same, their physical properties, affinity for specific membrane proteins, passive permeability, and mechanical properties also can differ. Furthermore, the half-melted bilayer has special structures, namely boundaries between solid and fluid phases which may have unique properties. It may be that the compositionally heterogeneous bilayer is tailored to carry out a more complex and subtle repertoire of functions than we now recognize.

Transverse Asymmetry (3,7)

While lateral motion is unrestricted, diffusion of membrane lipids across the plane of the bilayer is, in general, exceedingly slow. The energy of hydration of the polar head groups of phospholipids presumably prevents them from entering the core of the bilayer. Phospholipids thus "flip" across bilayers with half-times measured in hours, days, or longer. Sterols are different: they are the only membrane constituents known to diffuse across the membrane on a physiological time-scale—seconds or less.

Given the low rate of transverse diffusion in bilayers, it is not surprising that naturally occurring membranes maintain a high degree of lipid asymmetry. In the best-studied system, the human erythrocyte, the outer leaflet is rich in phosphatidylcholine and sphingomyelin and contains all of the glycolipids; the inner leaflet is rich in phosphatidylethanolamine and the minor anionic phospholipids bearing serine, glycerol, and inositol. The mechanisms creating lipid asymmetry and its purposes are obscure. Transverse asymmetry could be generated during the synthesis of the bilayer, following which the lipids might not redistribute. Alternatively, since the environments of the two membrane surfaces are different, they could create and sustain an asymmetrical distribution of lipids even if the lipids diffused across the bilayer. Recently, evidence was presented for an ATP-dependent process catalyzing the trans-bilayer movement of phospholipids in the red blood cell membrane (8).

Membrane Fusion and Fission (9,10)

Lipid bilayers not only demarcate sealed aqueous compartments but can also unite existing compartments and segregate new ones without loss of membrane integrity (Fig. 3). Both in the laboratory and in the cell, two membrane-bound vesicles can coalesce at a point of contact to form one; this is fusion. By a process which, in our ignorance of mechanism, we can call the reverse, a single vesicle can be drawn into two; this is fission. The former process allows secretory vesicles in the cytoplasm to expel their contents (e.g., peptide hormones, neurotransmitters, serum lipoproteins, and antibodies) through the plasma membrane. The latter process creates such intracellular

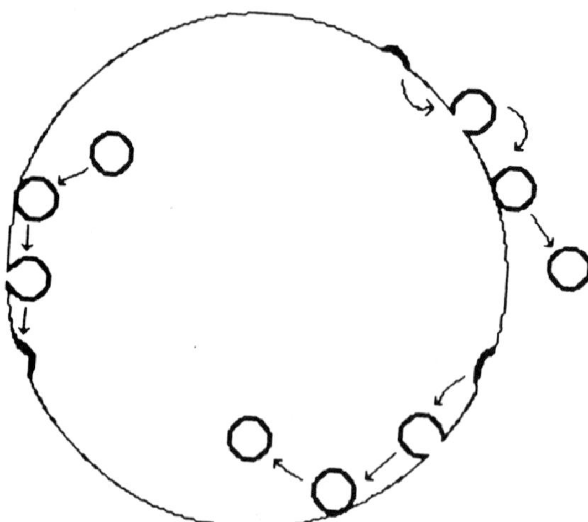

Fig. 3 One example of membrane fusion (left) and two examples of membrane fission (right).

vesicles in the first place and underlies phagocytosis, pinocytosis, the budding of enveloped viruses, and cell division.

MEMBRANE PROTEINS

Membrane function is carried out by and large by proteins. Among these functions are solute transport, information transduction, energy conversion, and other metabolic processes. The proteins involved are specific, as is their prevalence in the membrane, their localization, and their association with lipids and with one another. Each membrane and each function has its own proteins; none is universal. Some membranes of limited function contain less than 25% protein by mass; myelin, the membranous insulator wrapped around nerve axons, is an example. Busy membranes, such as the mitochondrial inner membrane, are comprised of 75% protein or more by weight. Similarly, myelin and viral envelopes have only a few types of proteins, while the inner mitochondrial membrane and *Escherichia coli* membranes have dozens. (See Ref. 1 to 4 and 11 to 13 for an overview.)

Association of Proteins with Membranes (Fig. 4)

There are two ways in which proteins are associated with membranes. Integral or intrinsic proteins are anchored by being dissolved in the core of the bilayer. As might be expected, these proteins have hydrophobic contact surfaces for this purpose. There are instances of proteins covalently bound to membrane lipids; in most cases, these proteins are also integrated into the bilayer, but a few are attached to the membrane through this lipid link only.

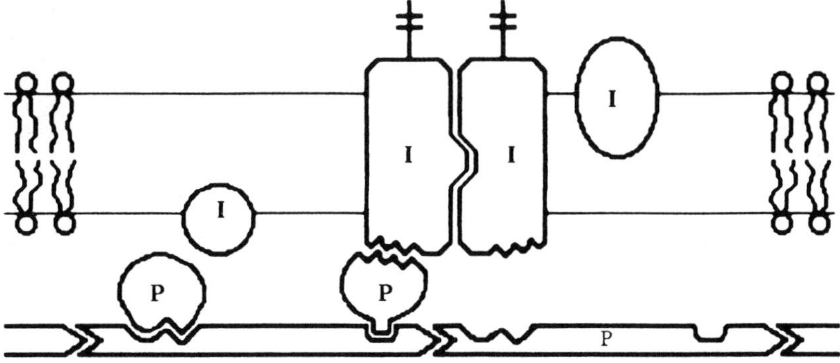

Fig. 4 Integral (I) and peripheral (P) membrane proteins.

The second class of membrane proteins is termed peripheral or extrinsic. These are associated through stereochemical, lock-and-key binding to specific membrane sites. In general, each peripheral protein binds to its membrane site with a defined stoichiometry and affinity. It is difficult to document instances of peripheral proteins whose physiological site of membrane association is the polar head groups of lipids. Thus, membrane proteins generally seem to be either integral or bound to integral proteins (or to peripheral proteins bound to integral proteins, etc.).

Solubilization and Purification of Membrane Proteins

There is a simple functional test for the mode of association of a protein with a membrane. A protein solubilized from the membrane without dissolving or disrupting the bilayer is most likely peripheral in its disposition. This is because agents that solubilize peripheral proteins do so by reversing their specific linkages. For example, high ionic strength buffers weaken electrostatic contacts. Low ionic strength buffers promote dissociation by increasing charge repulsions between like-charged (generally, polyanionic) proteins. Chaotropic agents such as urea or guanidine-HCl or covalent modifying agents such as succinic anhydride denature proteins and thus unfold their binding sites. While integral proteins are also denatured by these treatments, they remain dissolved in the lipid bilayer, which itself is resistant to all but the strongest chaotropic agents.

A major goal in this work is to dissolve the lipid without denaturing the proteins or allowing them to aggregate into insoluble precipitates. Organic solvents generally denature globular proteins, as do ionic detergents such as sodium dodecylsulfate. Nonionic detergents and bile salts, however, have found great utility in forming water-soluble complexes with integral proteins; these detergents merely dissolve the lipid and replace it at the hydrophobic contact surface of the protein with a unimolecular detergent coat without altering protein conformation.

Purification of solubilized membrane proteins is open to all the major tools of conventional protein isolation. The task is made complex, however, by the propensity of some of these proteins to aggregate irreversibly, even when dissolved in detergent. Furthermore, some membrane proteins may be weakly complexed with each other in the membrane, reversibly associated by virtue of their high local concentration; these associations may be undone by mass action when the membranes are dissolved and diluted in detergent solutions.

Composition of Membrane Proteins

Membrane proteins contain the same amino acids as water-soluble proteins; membrane glycoproteins are conjugated with the same oligosaccharides as are soluble glycoproteins. Most membrane proteins tend to be acidic in charge. Peripheral proteins usually resemble water-soluble proteins in amino acid composition. Integral proteins may be enriched in hydrophobic residues if their contact surface with the core of the bilayer is extensive. Membrane proteins may be covalently conjugated to fatty acids or other lipids and may bear chromophores or other cofactors.

Disposition of Membrane Proteins

Peripheral proteins are found at both surfaces of the membrane; however, in many cells such as the erythrocyte, they preponderate at the cytoplasmic surface. Peripheral proteins may be globular or filamentous, monomeric or polymeric, just like their nonmembrane counterparts. Integral proteins are more distinctive. They are amphipathic, making contact with water and lipid polar head groups as well as apolar fatty acyl chains. Some are confined to one membrane surface while others span the membrane, thereby communicating with three compartments. If glycosylated, the oligosaccharides invariably lie in the space opposite the cytoplasm; if phosphorylated, the phosphate groups are confined to the cytoplasmic aspect of the protein. Integral proteins may be anchored in the bilayer by a single strand of amino acids spanning the membrane, a patch of hydrophobic residues, or an extensive hydrophobic domain. In some cases, the bulk of the protein is submerged in lipid. Figure 5 provides an illustration.

The amino acid sequence of integral proteins may provide major insights into their spatial organization (14–16). Water-soluble and membrane-intercalated domains may lie in separate segments of the primary structure of the protein. These domains may fold independently and may be cleaved apart experimentally by limited proteolysis if they are joined by an exposed hinge region. A common feature of the primary structure of integral proteins are segments approximately 25 residues in length composed almost entirely of nonpolar residues (14,15). These hydrophobic sequences are usually compatible with an α-helical secondary structure. In fact, α-helixes are particularly stable in the lipid environment, since water competes for and hence weakens intrapeptide hydrogen bonds. At 1.5 Å per residue, the length of such helical segments is just that required to span the apolar core of the bilayer, approximately 40 Å. The rarity of hydrophobic stretches longer than 30 residues suggests that these helical segments are essentially linear and perpendicular to the plane of the membrane; more complex transmembrane dispositions are as yet unknown. Several such hydrophobic segments may occur in sequence, typically separated by 2 to 10 polar residues. These helixes thus lace back and forth across the bilayer in an antiparallel array (Fig. 5). A bundle of such helixes itself may have a twist, creating a coiled-coil structure (15).

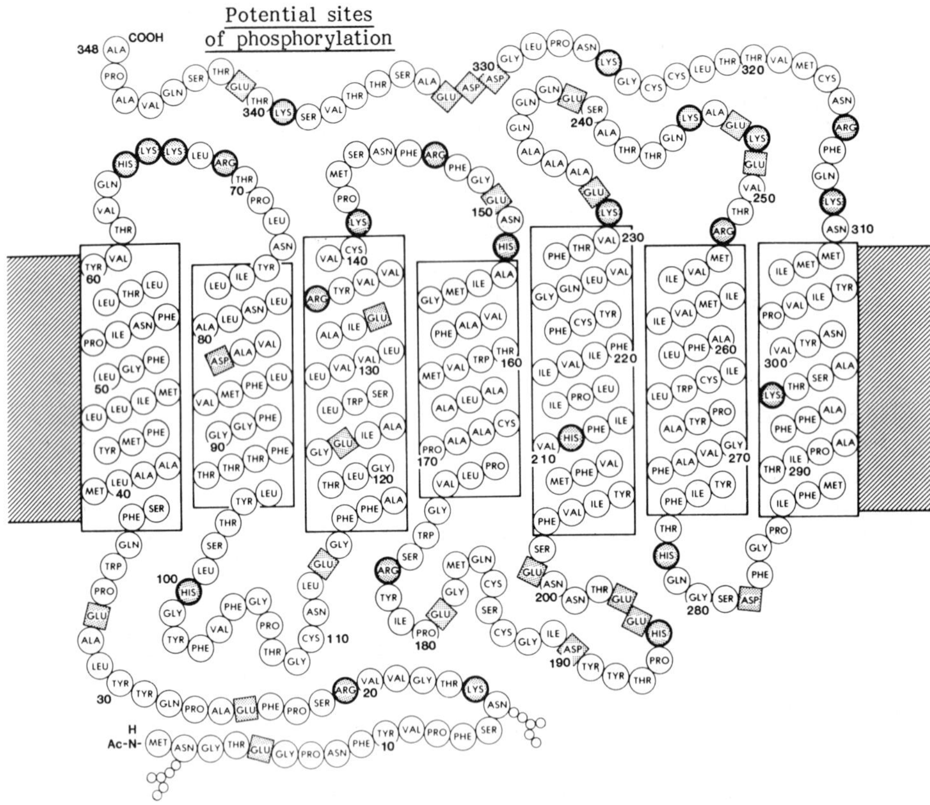

Fig. 5 A model for the organization of rhodopsin in the membrane of the rod outer segment disk. The carboxyl terminus of the protein as well as multiple sites of phosphorylation are in the cytoplasmic space, while the acetylated amino terminus and the oligosaccharides linked to asparagine residues 2 and 15 lie within the disk space. Note that the seven peptide segments placed within the bilayer are composed primarily of nonpolar residues with only rare polar or charged groups, while the reverse is true of the extramembrane segments linking them. (Modified from Ref. 14. With permission.)

Integral membrane proteins are frequently found to be oligomeric (12,13). Dimers and tetramers are common, compounded of either identical, similar (isomeric), or dissimilar subunits. Channel-forming proteins are typically polymeric. Where an axis of symmetry exists, it lies normal to the plane of the membrane. Certain integral membrane proteins congregate into patches containing dozens of hundreds of units, often in a hexagonal array, which reflects maximum packing density. (An example is the gap junction.) Some integral proteins also form heterocomplexes with peripheral proteins on the two membrane surfaces.

Integral membrane proteins interact somewhat specifically with their lipid environment (3,17,18). They may selectively bind or shun certain lipids. Their hydrophobic contact surfaces may perturb bilayer organization and lipid motion. The activity of transport systems and enzymes embedded in the membrane often responds profoundly to the lipid head groups and/or fatty acyl chains in their vicinity. The activity of some integral proteins also may be too sensitive to the state of fluidity of the bilayer and even to bilayer thickness, which presumably should just match the span of the hydrophobic contact surface of the protein (19).

Some integral proteins display a diffusional mobility commensurate with the fluidity of the lipids in which they are dissolved (3). In many cases, however, lateral motion is constrained by protein-protein association, e.g., the formation of large patches or the tethering of integral proteins to peripheral filaments. Integral proteins may also be sequestered within the interstices of submembrane protein networks or may be kept in one portion of a cell surface by proteinaceous barriers, such as the tight junctions found in epithelial sheets. The latter devices allow cells to have long-range topographical variation in their surfaces without impeding the local mobility of the proteins.

Finally, membrane proteins face an overwhelming energy barrier to translocation across the plane of the bilayer, even when the protein spans the membrane. This thermodynamic mechanism maintains the absolute asymmetry or "sidedness" characteristic of the two faces of each biological membrane (11,12).

MEMBRANE RECONSTITUTION (3)

One of the ways biochemists ascertain the validity of their hypotheses about membrane structure and function is to take apart these complex ensembles and reconstitute them from their purified components. The issue for many peripheral proteins is straightforward; they will often reassociate with their physiological binding site whether it is in the membrane, solubilized in detergent, or liberated as a water-soluble fragment by limited proteolysis. Of course, it is best that neither the peripheral protein nor its binding site be denatured during isolation if reassociation is desired.

The reassociation of integral proteins with phospholipids to form functional membranes is directed by the information implicit in their structure and is driven primarily by the minimization of hydrophobic free energy. Several simple strategies have been devised, principally by Racker and associates. In the first, phospholipids and proteins were purified in cholate and then mixed; when the detergent was dialyzed away, the lipids and proteins condensed into small membranous vesicles. A similar result was obtained when such mixtures were merely diluted so as to lower the detergent concentration below its critical micellar concentration (at which point the detergent cannot maintain the membrane constituents in solution). A comparable outcome can be achieved by removing the detergent by gel filtration chromatography. Racker's group later found that when certain integral proteins were freed of most of their detergent and sonicated in the presence of phospholipids, functional lipid-protein vesicles were generated. Recently it was discovered that when detergent-depleted proteins such as cytochrome c oxidase were simply added to preformed lipid vesicles in buffer, they rapidly entered the membranes in a uniform, rather asymmetrical orientation. These vesicles were well sealed and the proteins were active (20).

Such reconstitution systems have revealed that certain integral proteins often have preferences for specific phospholipid partners for both their integration and their function. The presence of other proteins can also influence the uptake of an integral protein into preformed vesicles.

MEMBRANE TRANSPORT (1,2)

While cell membranes create barriers between aqueous compartments, these barriers must be breached to allow the movement of specific solutes. The various modes of transport can be grouped into two classes according to the source of energy driving solute movement: (1) Solutes may move by diffusion from a distribution of high potential energy to one of lower potential energy. The transmembrane potential energy difference for a solute derives from the difference in its concentration and if charged, its response to the electrical field across the membrane. For example, in the case of K^+, a concentration difference of 10-fold or a membrane potential of 59 mV imposes a driving force of approximately 1.4 kcal/mol. (2) Some solutes are moved by the dissipation of a source of energy external to the membrane, e.g., "active transport" fueled by ATP, respiration, or light. In these cases, the dissipation of energy is coupled to solute movement by obliging a single protein to catalyze both processes in a single conformational cycle. Some common mechanisms of solute transport are outlined below and illustrated in Fig. 6.

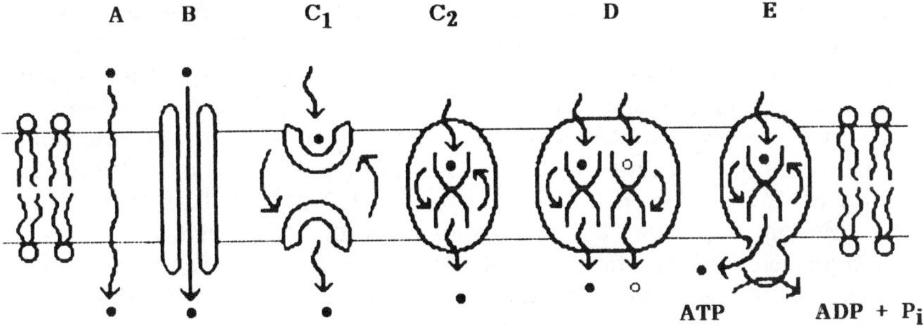

Fig. 6 Rudimentary sketches of some common mechanisms of membrane transport. Each solute molecule (•) is shown twice, at the beginning and at the end of its translocation. Class A: simple diffusion. The solute dissolves in and diffuses through the lipid bilayer. Class B: channels. The solute diffuses through a water-filled pore. Class C: reciprocating transporters. The solute binds to a transporter that either itself diffuses through the bilayer (C_1), or undergoes a conformational change to effect such translocation (C_2). In both cases, a reciprocal movement is required to complete the cycle. Depending on the system, this second step can occur with the transporter occupied or unoccupied by solute. Class D: coupled transport. Two solutes must bind simultaneously to the transporter before a conformational change translocates them both. The binding sites for the solutes may be on the same (as shown) or opposite sides of the membrane at any given time. Class E: ATP-driven transport. The solute translocation cycle (conformational change upon solute binding) proceeds only if ATP is cleaved. Coupling translocation to ATP hydrolysis drives solutes against their electrochemical gradient.

Simple Diffusion in Bilayers

A primordial form of transport is the unaided diffusion of lipid-soluble molecules through the lipid bilayer. This is the mechanism by which we get our oxygen and our alcohol. Some complex bimolecules, such as steroid hormones, presumably also take this direct route. The more hydrophobic the molecule, the greater its partition into the lipid phase and the faster its diffusion across the bilayer.

Membrane Channels

Some membranes possess pores that create aqueous continuity between the two water compartments adjoining the membrane and permit the transmembrane diffusion of polar solutes. Since no barrier is crossed, this mode of transport is the most rapid known: some channels conduct more than 10^7 ions per second even though they are only a few angstroms wide. These systems are constructed of specific proteins, and each exhibits a characteristic selectivity, reflecting the size of the aqueous pore and the energy barriers imposed by the chemical structure of the pathway. Solute selectivity implies a transient association of the solute with the channel, although the flux is so fast that this binding must be quite short-lived, hence weak.

Simple models for this class of transporters are found in channel-forming antibiotics such as the gramicidins and amphotericins (21). Pairs of these molecules associate end-to-end to create transmembrane "tubes." The water-filled interior is approximately 4 to 8 Å in diameter and is lined by polar groups; the exterior surface of the cylinder is quite hydrophobic.

The outer envelopes of gram-negative bacteria are fenestrated by multiple channels permeable to polar solutes of less than 1000 daltons. These channels are created by the aggregation of six 58-residue amphipathic helical peptides (see Chapter 1) to form a coiled coil with a central pore 13 Å in diameter. (The peptides, called porins, are also notable for their covalently bound fatty acids.) The outer membranes of mitochondria have comparable structures performing a similar function: the rapid movement of microsolutes, nutrients, and wastes.

Higher organisms have more complex channels (22). In many tissues, cells are coupled by gap junctions: tightly packed assemblies of repeating units called connexons that span the plasma membranes of closely apposed cells to create aqueous paths between their cytoplasmic compartments. Metabolites of up to approximately 1000 daltons can thus flow freely between neighboring cells through these 12-Å-diameter pores. However, if a cell is injured, the increase in its cytoplasmic Ca^{++} and/or the drop in its cytoplasmic pH closes its channels, isolating the damaged cell from its neighbors.

The most interesting channels are excitable, e.g., those of nerve and muscle. Neurotransmitters such as acetylcholine bind to receptor proteins that are built into the complex channels of synaptic membranes. The binding event triggers the rapid opening of a small (approximately 5 Å in diameter) cation-selective pore, presumably by imposing a conformational change. Sodium ions immediately flow into the cell and potassium ions flow out, both down their concentration gradients. Within a few milliseconds, another, slower conformational change, triggered by the same acetylcholine binding event, closes the pore. In this way, the conductance of the channel is terminated long before the acetylcholine departs from its receptor, sparing the cell the deleterious effects of prolonged stimulation. Much later, the acetylcholine dissociates from its receptor and the channel regains its original closed conformation (23).

Scattered along the length of the plasma membrane of these excitable cells are other channels, selective for either Na^+ or K^+ (24).

They are opened by the drop in membrane potential triggered by the flow of cations through the chemically gated channels at the synapse. These channel proteins presumably undergo conformational changes in response to changes in the surrounding electrical field when the membrane is depolarized. Since the flow of Na^+ through the open Na^+ channels causes further depolarization in its vicinity, these voltage-gated channels propagate an action potential along the length of the cell. At the next synapse, there are electrically sensitive calcium channels that translate the action potential into a rise in cytoplasmic Ca^{++}. This stimulates the secretion of neurotransmitter and thus communicates excitation to the next cell. It will be interesting to learn whether the several chemically and electrically gated membrane channels share similar mechanisms of transient conformation-dependent porosity (22,23).

Reciprocating Transporters

Several kinds of transporters bind solutes and move them across the membrane; they must then complete the cycle by returning through a reciprocal step. Inorganic ions do not generally permeate membranes by themselves, but there are hydrophobic antibiotics that form complexes with them and diffuse through the bilayer. The best known of these ionophores is valinomycin, which forms a rather specific 1:1 association with K^+. Because it can cross the membrane loaded and return empty, valinomycin can mediate the net transfer of charge and thus create or dissipate a K^+ gradient. This ionophore is therefore said to be electrogenic. Another antibiotic, nigericin, only enters the membrane when carrying a cation; its transport is obliged to be one-for-one exchange, hence electrically neutral. These antibiotics have no physiological counterpart; cells do not employ transporters as mobile (diffusible) carriers.

Nevertheless, the kinetics of transport of glucose, amino acids, and anions in erythrocytes and certain other cells resemble the transport kinetics of the ionophores. The similarity reflects a formal (but not mechanistic) correspondence in their multistep transport pathways. In both cases (1) the solute first binds to the transport molecule; (2) the solute is moved across the membrane; (3) the solute is discharged; and (4) the transporter returns to its original disposition. The transporter may return empty; however, in some systems, it can only return when loaded.

Since physiological transport proteins are not free to diffuse across the membrane, the part of them to which the solute is bound must undergo a conformational change which transfers the solute from facing one compartment to the other; the reciprocal change completes the conformational cycle. As with the ionophores, if the transporter is unable to cycle without bearing a solute, transport will be strictly one-for-one, and the transporter is often called an exchanger. This is essentially the case for the anion transporter in the erythrocyte, which rapidly and randomly swaps bicarbonate and chloride ions to facilitate the movement of carbon dioxide from the tissues to the lungs. A second example are sodium/proton exchangers. In contrast to these one-for-one systems, transporters such as those for glucose in erythrocytes can cycle empty, hence mediate the net transfer of solutes down their concentration gradients. The rate of transport in these systems is a function of the local solute concentration and the affinity for the solute (hence, the fractional saturation of the binding sites at each side of the membrane), as well as the velocity of transit of the transporter, whether loaded or empty, in each direction (25).

Coupled Transport (26)

Imagine a reciprocating transporter with separate binding sites for two different solutes, e.g., Na^+ and glucose. If this device cannot cycle without both solute species being bound simultaneously, the transport of the two solutes will be coupled. Furthermore, the steeper of the two concentration gradients (that having higher potential energy) will drive the other until the two gradient energies balance. In our example, the movement of Na^+ down its gradient can drive glucose up its gradient and vice versa. In actuality, the large gradient of Na^+, which exists across intestinal and other epithelial plasma membranes, is exploited to drive the absorption of glucose and certain other solutes into these cells. Microbes use proton gradients in a similar way to drive the uptake of many nutrients.

Depending on the system, the coupled solutes may be required to bind on the same or on opposite sides of the membrane for their transporter to cycle. In the case of the Na^+/glucose pair mentioned above, the solutes must come from the same side. However, in other systems, Na^+ gradients can drive the movement of Ca^{++} from the opposite side of the membrane (and vice versa). When the driving and the driven solutes move in the same direction, the process is called cotransport; when they move in opposite directions, the process is called countertransport. Such co- and countertransport systems probably do not differ fundamentally in molecular mechanism but only in the coupling of binding sites to the conformational cycle. This type of transport is "active" only in the sense that accumulation of a solute can be driven by a source of energy other than its own concentration gradient, namely the gradient of its partner solute.

Transport ATPases (27)

Cation pumps, powered by the hydrolysis of ATP, are ubiquitous throughout phylogeny. They may transport Na^+, K^+, H^+, or Ca^{++}.

Some of these pumps trade one cation for another and therefore do not change the electrical potential of the membrane; the H^+/K^+ ATPase of the stomach is an example. The familiar Na^+/K^+ ATPase, on the other hand, expels 3 Na^+ from the cell for every 2 K^+ taken up and is therefore electrogenic.

The mechanism by which these transporters function also appears to involve a reciprocating conformational cycle. In this case, the cycle is tightly coupled to the hydrolysis of ATP. That is, hydrolysis occurs only as the appropriate cations, bound to their specific sites, cross the membrane in the mandated direction, converting the energy of hydrolysis into concentration gradients. The process is entirely reversible; in the laboratory properly arranged cation gradients can drive the synthesis of ATP. As with other enzymes, partial reactions—segments of the cycle—can still be observed when the complete pathway is blocked. For example, 1:1 exchange of isotopes of Na^+ ions across the plasma membranes is catalyzed by the Na^+/K^+ pump in the absence of K^+. While the presence of ATP is required for 1:1 exchange, it is not hydrolyzed nor is there a net movement of Na^+.

Redox-Driven Transport (28)

The change in free energy of many chemical reactions can be coupled to the movement of solutes across membranes against their electrochemical gradient by an appropriately disposed membrane protein. An ancient and ubiquitous illustration is the tapping of the free energy of redox reactions in the form of proton gradients. The transmembrane proton gradient is as universal an energy currency as ATP and can be tapped to drive many other processes, including the synthesis of ATP (oxidative phosphorylation). Similarly, a primary consequence of the absorption of light by photosynthetic organisms is the generation of a proton gradient that is subsequently harvested in the form of "high-energy" chemical compounds.

MEMBRANE TRANSDUCTION

Just as the plasma membrane mediates the selective passage of solutes, so must it also transmit information from outside the cell to the cytoplasm. The term transduction implies that the signals are transformed as they are relayed across the membrane. Let us consider a few examples of the coupling of stimulus to response.

Stimuli (29)

Other than steroid hormones, which are designed to dissolve in and diffuse through membranes on their way to intracellular receptors, hormones and neurotransmitters generally act at the cell surface. This group includes, e.g., insulin, glucagon, prostaglandins, catecholamines, and acetylcholine. Chemoattractants, antigens, and growth factors also have their primary effect at the outer surface of the plasma membrane. The consequences of the interaction of these agents with plasma membranes are manifold and include changes in the concentration of cytoplasmic second messengers (e.g., cyclic nucleotides, Ca^{++}, and other inorganic cations) and the covalent modifications of proteins and phospholipids.

Membrane Receptors (30–33)

Specific to each stimulus is a receptor, an integral (glyco) protein that asymmetrically spans the plasma membrane. Receptor proteins tend to be large (60,000 daltons or more); some are monomeric, others are oligomeric. Transduction occurs when the receptor binds its ligand at the outer surface, undergoes a change (discussed below), and manifests that change at the cytoplasmic surface. Receptors are often trace components of the plasma membrane and therefore difficult to identify. Their isolation is often aided, however, by their exceptional affinity for their signal molecules.

The activity of membrane receptors is physiologically regulated in at least two ways. Some are automatically shut off soon after activation even though the stimulus is still bound (e.g., the acetylcholine receptor, discussed above and in Ref. 23). Since the debinding of a highly avid ligand may be very slow, such "desensitization" spares the cell from enduring prolonged responses to transient stimuli. Activity is ultimately regained as the ligand departs. A second, slower mode of regulation is through the control of receptor concentration, i.e., the rate of receptor introduction into and removal from the cell surface (30–33). Receptors (whether liganded or not) are commonly internalized by endocytosis, the pinching off of vesicles from the plasma membrane into the cytoplasm (34). These vesicles usually bear a high concentration of clustered receptors; their cytoplasmic surfaces are coated with a scaffold of the protein clathrin. Internalized receptors soon return to the cell surface by exocytosis, the fusion of their carrier vesicles with the plasma membrane. Two functions for this vesicle traffic are apparent. First, the fraction of the total receptor pool at the cell surface (hence, available for stimulation) can be adjusted by changing the kinetic constants for internalization and return.* Second, the internalized receptor quickly sheds

---

*A striking illustration of this type of process is the mechanism by which insulin stimulates glucose transport levels in target cells: insulin binding promotes fusion with the plasma membrane of cytoplasmic vesicles rich in glucose transporters. Removing the insulin leads to reinternalization of these transporters.

the tightly bound ligand inside the cell, thereby terminating the response. This happens because the internalized vesicles fuse with intracellular vesicles (endosomes). These endosomes maintain an acidic internal pH through the action of an ATP-driven proton pump. Because the affinity of the receptor for its ligand drastically falls with decreasing pH, the bound hormone is released. The discarded hormone is disposed of by transfer to lysosomes, while the free receptor is returned to the cell surface. Receptors enjoy dozens of circuits before they too are degraded in the lysosomes (34,35).

Signal Transmission Mechanisms (Table 2)

How is the binding of a stimulus at the cell surface communicated to the cytoplasm? Four mechanisms can be described in detail; many others presumably await elucidation. First, there is direct alteration of membrane permeability by receptors that also are transporters. The classical example are chemically gated channels such as that for acetylcholine (23,24). The flow of cations can have the effect of altering membrane potential or changing the level of an intracellular messenger such as Ca^{++}.

A second mechanism involves the lateral aggregation of receptors in the membrane (36,37). Recall that many integral membrane proteins can diffuse rapidly and randomly in the plane of the membrane and therefore collide frequently. Certain stimuli appear to induce their receptors to cluster. The multimeric resulting receptor-ligand complex triggers a cytoplasmic response, perhaps through a change in membrane cation permeability or by affecting the activity of an enzyme at the cytoplasmic membrane surface. A well-studied example of this class involves the allergic response. Immunoglobulin E (IgE) antibodies bind to specific receptors on the surface of mast cells and other granulated leukocytes. When multivalent allergens such as pollen become covered with IgE molecules, this can induce the close association of IgE receptors on mast cells. The plasma membrane then becomes selectively permeable to Ca^{++}, presumably reflecting channels activated by the aggregates of IgE receptors (36,38). A cascade of intracellular responses leads to the secretion of vasoactive compounds such as histamine and serotonin through the fusion of their storage granules with the plasma membrane: an allergic response. There is evidence that insulin and epidermal growth factor may also act by inducing lateral aggregation of their receptors (37). This would explain why antibodies to these receptors and even plant agglutinins, which bind to the oligosaccharides on the receptors, can mimic or potentiate the action of these hormones.

In a third mechanism, the binding of an extracellular stimulus activates an enzyme that is built into the cytoplasmic domain of the receptor. The receptors for epidermal growth factor and insulin contain tyrosine kinases in their cytoplasmic domains, which phosphorylate

Table 2 Receptor-Mediated Membrane Transduction

Effector	Target cells	Receptor protein	Receptor response	Cellular response	Effect
Acetylcholine	Skeletal muscle	Pentamer of 40–64-kDA subunits	Conformational change opens cation channels	Membrane depolarization opens Ca^{++} channels	Muscle contraction
Allergen-IgE complex	Mast cells Basophils	Dimer of 33- and 50-kDA subunits	Clustering opens Ca^{++} channels	Secretory vesicles fuse with plasma membrane	Secretion of of vasoactive agents (e.g., histamine)
Epidermal growth factor	Epithelial cells	160-kDA glycoprotein	Protein tyrosine phosphorylation	Poorly defined	Mitosis and differentiation
Insulin	Hepatocytes Adipocytes Muscle cells	Tetramer of pairs of 125- and 90-kDa subunits	Clustering and protein tyrosine phosphorylation	Fusion of special intracellular vesicles with plasma membrane	Glucose transporters inserted into plasma membrane
Epinephrine	Hepatocytes Muscle cells	60-kDa glycoprotein	Conformational change activates G protein	Activation of adenylate cyclase	Altered cell metabolism
Light	Retinal rod and cone cells	Rhodopsin (41-kDa glycoprotein)	Conformational change activates G protein (transducin)	Activation of a phosphodiesterase closes plasma membrane Na^+ channels	Nerve impulse

tyrosine residues both in the receptor and on other proteins. The physiological consequences of this tyrosine phosphorylation are under investigation (33).

In a fourth mechanism, the resting receptor binds and holds inactive a separate signal protein on its cytoplasmic domain. Ligand binding to the receptor presumably imposes a transmembrane conformational change that cause the release of the signal protein and its consequent activation. The signal protein triggers a cascade of consequences in the cytoplasm, which effect the response. The classic example of this mechanism is the β-adrenergic receptor (32). The binding of catecholamines such as epinephrine to their receptors causes the release of a signal protein, variously referred to as the N, G, or G/F protein. The G protein migrates to and activates adenylate cyclase, which is also located on the cytoplasmic surface of the plasma membrane. The period of 3',5'-cyclic AMP synthesis is limited by a special clock. When the G protein is released from the receptor by epinephrine, it binds a molecule of GTP at a GTPase site within it. This GTP enables the G protein to activate adenylate cyclase. The GTPase site soon catalyzes the hydrolysis of GTP, causing the G protein to become inactive and to return to the β-adrenergic receptor, completing the response.

There is an illuminating parallel between the β-adrenergic receptor transduction system and the first steps in visual excitation. The absorption of light by the visual pigment, rhodopsin, drives it into a new conformation. As a result, rhodopsin releases a signal protein, transducin, from its cytoplasmic surface (39). Transducin then binds GTP and becomes an activator of a phosphodiesterase for 3',5'-cyclic GMP. The consequent decrease in cyclic GMP levels leads to a reduction in the cation permeability of the retinal cell plasma membrane (40). This change in permeability is read as a signal by the visual pathway. Transducin bears a GTPase activity and soon becomes inactive as it hydrolyzes its bound GTP. The spontaneous GTPase activity apparently serves to keep photoresponses short. Recent studies have shown several striking resemblances between retinal transducin and the G protein of the β-adrenergic system.

MEMBRANE CONNECTIONS

Cells and their organelles are not afloat; rather, their membranes are coupled to filamentous matrixes both within the cell and without. The function of these supramolecular arrays is generally mechanical: to strengthen the fluid membranes and their liquid contents (i.e., to bear and distribute tension), to determine membrane contour, and to direct cell and organelle movement and positioning.

The Cytoskeleton (41,42)

When eukaryotic cells are treated with a nondenaturing detergent such as Triton X-100, their bilayers are dissolved and their water-soluble contents are dispersed. What remains is a water-insoluble, filamentous matrix (12,43). (An analogous matrix fills the nucleoplasm.) The filaments are polymers of actin (in the form of microfilaments), tubulin (in the form of microtubules), and a diverse family of keratins and related structural proteins (in the form of intermediate filaments). These three classes of filaments are coupled to a variety of accessory proteins to create a complex and dynamic skeletal meshwork that traverses the space between the cell surface and the cytoplasmic organelles. All three types of filaments confer mechanical strength; the first two also mediate motility.

Each type of cytoskeletal filament system makes specific contacts with cellular membranes. Intermediate filaments anchored to the plasma membrane gird the cell like heavy cables. Microtubules determine the position of structures like the Golgi apparatus and small transport vesicles. Bundles of microfilaments mediate ameboid motion and define complex cell contour, e.g., the microvilli in the brush border of epithelial cells. The human red blood cell membrane is stabilized by a "two-dimensional" network, composed of actin and other filamentous proteins, which is linked to the bilayer through several hundred thousand copies of peripheral anchor proteins bound to specific integral membrane proteins, as illustrated in Fig. 4 (12, 44,45). It is this skeleton that gives the erythrocyte its durability and flexibility (Fig. 7).

The Extracellular Matrix (2,46,47)

The outer surface of most cells enjoys a sugar-coated environment. In higher animals, the extracellular face of the plasma membrane itself is studded with glycolipids and glycoproteins. Many of the soluble extracellular proteins in the vicinity (e.g., serum proteins and peptide hormones) are also glycoproteins. The insoluble filamentous matrix in which tissue cells are imbedded is compounded of glycosylated macromolecules: glycoproteins such as collagen and glycosaminoglycans such as hyaluronic acid and chondroitin sulfate. In bacteria, we find cell envelopes containing lipopolysaccharides and proteoglycans; in plants and primitive eukaryotes, we find cell walls of polysaccharides and cell coats of mucopolysaccharides. These supramolecular structures, referred to as the glycocalyx, protect, confer tensile strength against shear stress, and align cells into tissues. For example, consider the basement membrane or basal lamina of epithelia and the giant glycoprotein assemblies that link sponge cells together (2).

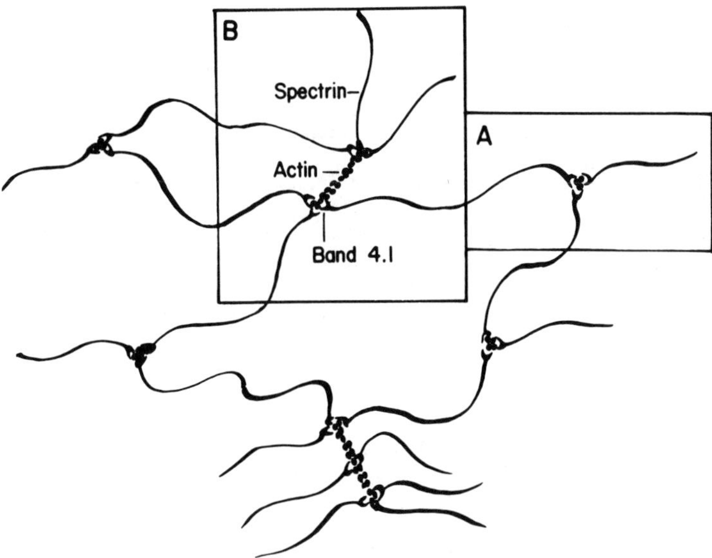

Fig. 7 The human erythrocyte membrane skeleton. Short filaments of actin are the attachment sites for multiple long, thin, and supple filaments of spectrin. Oligomers of band 4.1 stabilize the junctions of spectrin and actin and gather the spectrin ends into clusters that are particularly prevalent at the ends of the actin filaments. Not shown are multiple linkages to the overlying membrane through the binding of peripheral accessory proteins to integral, transmembrane glycoproteins (as in Fig. 4). (From Ref. 45. With permission.)

Fibronectin (48) is a large filamentous glycoprotein that binds to both tissue cell surfaces and to intercellular matrix molecules such as collagen, fibrin, and glycosaminoglycans. These multiple associations help to link the cell to its periphery. Fibronectin filaments are often gathered into focal arrays or patches on the cell surface. In parallel array on the opposite (cytoplasmic) side of the plasma membrane are filaments of actin in association with several actin-binding proteins (Fig. 8). It appears that the intra- and extracellular matrixes are linked and coordinated at such junctions, which are called fibronexuses (49). We can infer that tension imposed on the extracellular matrix does not come to bear on the plasma membrane, but is transmitted through it and through the cytoplasm by this grid of structural proteins (see Fig. 8).

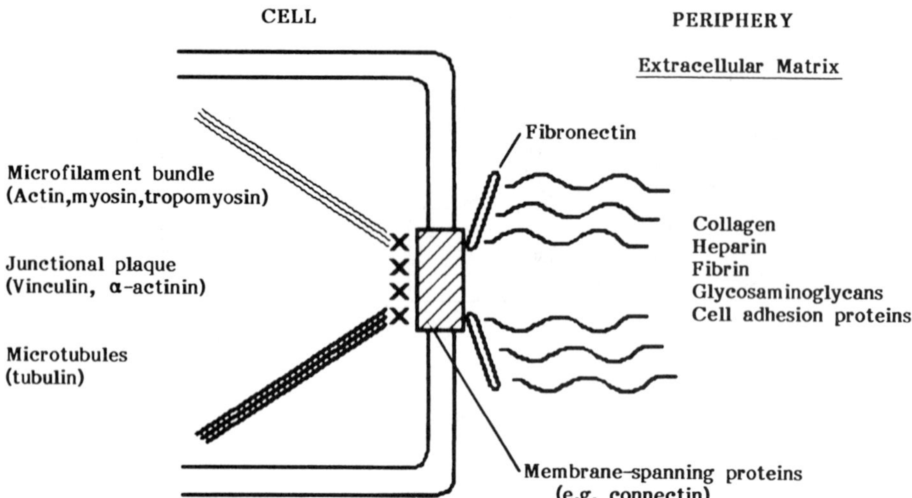

Fig. 8 Communication of the cytoskeleton with the extracellular matrix. A highly idealized scheme combining features of several different systems. Various cytoplasmic filament systems make contact with the plasma membrane through peripheral accessory proteins at specialized regions. These junctions may be organized by transmembrane proteins, such as connectin. At the extracellular surface, fibronectin and other peripheral proteins link binding proteins in the plasma membrane to a variety of intercellular matrix glycoproteins, some of which may guide specific cell-cell adhesion.

THE BIOGENESIS OF MEMBRANES AND ORGANELLES (1,3)

Lipids

Generally speaking, membranes are built by the assimilation of new molecular components into preexisting membranes that act not only as templates for their assembly but as participants. Most of those phospholipids, glycosphingolipids, and sterols not imported via plasma lipoproteins are synthesized or at least initiated in the endoplasmic reticulum and are then delivered to outlying membranes. The pathway of transport of membrane lipids to their site of destination is largely uncharted but could entail, as in the case of proteins, diffusion along the endoplasmic reticulum, packaging in small transport vesicles, and delivery through fusion of these vesicles with target membranes. In addition, mitochondria and chloroplasts have the capacity to synthesize some of their own phospholipids, cardiolipin (diphosphatidylglycerol) in particular.

Complex Carbohydrates

Complex carbohydrates are added to glycoproteins and glycolipids in two ways. In the first, monosaccharide residues are transferred stepwise from sugar nucleotides to growing oligosaccharide chains by specific glycosyl transferases in the endoplasmic reticulum and Golgi apparatus. In the second, oligosaccharide cores are presynthesized on dolichol phosphate carriers and then transferred to asparagine residues on nascent proteins soon after they emerge into the lumen of the rough endoplasmic reticulum. The trimming and extension of these oligosaccharides accompany, and perhaps guide, the transit of these glycoproteins through the endoplasmic reticulum, Golgi apparatus, and transport vesicles to their sites of destination (50).

Proteins

Proteins take diverse routes from the cytoplasmic ribosomes on which they are initiated to their destinations in membranes, organelles, and extracellular space (51). Consider first a scenario for integral proteins destined for the plasma membrane. A newly synthesized polypeptide chain extends from a cytoplasmic ribosome until a sequence of 20 or more nonpolar residues emerges. This hydrophobic signal becomes bound to a cytoplasmic ribonucleoprotein complex called the signal recognition particle (SRP) (52). Further elongation of the polypeptide by the ribosome is temporarily halted by the SRP; this effect prevents polypeptides destined to be integral proteins from being adventitiously completed in the cytoplasm. When the SRP binds to a receptor on the rough endoplasmic reticulum, the hydrophobic segment of the nascent protein is inserted across the bilayer. The mechanism of this crucial event is unknown. The SRP is soon discharged, and protein synthesis resumes on what are now membrane-bound ribosomes. A pair of polypeptides, called ribophorins, anchor the ribosomes to the membrane during this time (53). As translation of the chain proceeds to completion, the polypeptide is folded into its mature structure in the membrane. Protein folding often involves the integration of several strands of hydrophobic sequence into the bilayer.

Many integral membrane proteins are synthesized as precursors with temporary hydrophobic signal sequences extending from their aminoterminal ends. These sequences promote the prompt insertion of the nascent polypeptide in the membranes and are then cleaved from the protein by a signal peptidase at the lumenal surface of the rough endoplasmic reticulum. The newly completed integral protein is thought to diffuse along the endoplasmic reticulum membrane until it enters and is discharged with the membrane of a small transport vesicle that carries it to the Golgi apparatus. A similar process conveys the appropriate proteins from the Golgi stack to the plasma membrane (54).

A second class of proteins resembles that described above except that the entire polypeptide chain is threaded through the membrane of the rough endoplasmic reticulum and deposited, in a water-soluble form, in its lumen (51). In the process, the amino-terminal signal sequences usually found on these nascent proteins are removed by the signal peptidase so as to release them from the membrane. Once mature, these proteins are delivered to the interior of an organelle or, in the case of secretory proteins such as peptide hormones, immunoglobulins, and lipoproteins, are released from the cell by fusion of their transport vesicles with the plasma membrane. The information directing the routing of newly synthesized proteins to their destination is now understood in the case of lysosomal hydrolases (Fig. 9). These enzymes carry a temporary signal—one or more phosphate groups esterified to terminal mannose residues on their oligosaccharides (55). Receptors for this signal are scattered on various membranes of the cell, presumably to assist in the movement of the hydrolases to the lysosomes (56). Once the newly made enzymes reach a lysosome, the signal phosphate moieties are excised, and the enzymes assume their final disposition (55).

A third class of membrane proteins is synthesized entirely on ribosomes free in the cytoplasm rather than bound to the endoplasmic reticulum (51). Some of these products bind as peripheral proteins to specific sites on the cytoplasmic surface of various cellular membranes. Others integrate into the bilayer of organelle membranes; a classic example is cytochrome b_5 of the endoplasmic reticulum. Still others are taken up into the interior of organelles such as peroxisomes, chloroplasts, and mitochondria. Indeed, even though the latter two organelles have fully functioning ribosomes, the bulk of their membrane and soluble proteins is coded for by nuclear genes and synthesized on soluble cytoplasmic ribosomes (57). These findings show that integral membrane proteins can exist as water-soluble precursors, presumably utilizing special mechanisms to sequester their hydrophobic contact surfaces prior to insertion.

The incorporation of various proteins from the cytoplasm into mitochondria has recently been studied in detail (58). Porin (the channel-forming protein mentioned earlier) simply partitions from the cytoplasm into the outer membrane of the mitochondrion, coincident with a conformational change to its mature form. However, most imported proteins must pass completely through the outer mitochondrial membrane. They appear to do so in a precursor form, often bearing a hydrophilic, amino-terminal extension of varied length. Their transit is dependent on specific receptors at the outer surface of the mitochondrion. Cytochrome c, however, lacks an amino-terminal extension. It is transported through the outer membrane as the apoprotein and is then deposited in the space between the outer and inner mitochondrial membranes where it receives its heme, assumes its native conformation, and becomes reversibly associated with the inner mitochondrial

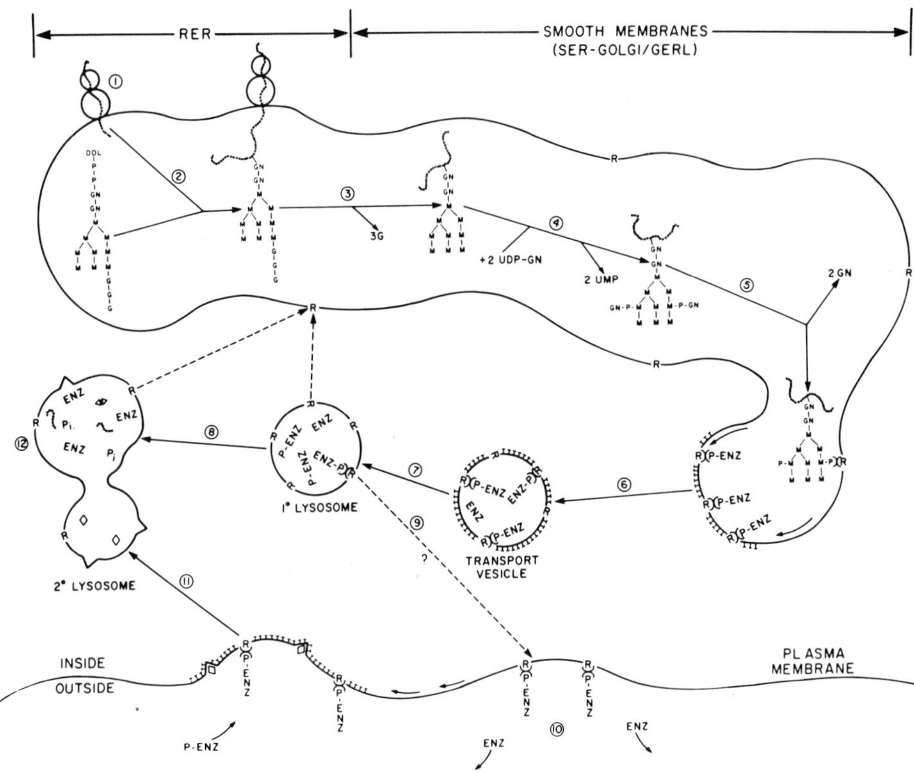

Fig. 9 The routing of lysosomal enzymes. Newly synthesized lysosomal hydrolases (step 1) are glycosylated from dolichol donors in the rough endoplasmic reticulum (step 2). As these glycoproteins travel to the Golgi apparatus, glucose residues are trimmed away (step 3), and N-acetylglucosamine phosphate is added to the oligosaccharides (step 4). Removal of the N-acetylglucosamine groups exposes mannose-6-phosphate residues (step 5), which are recognized by and bound to specific receptors in the smooth membranes. The complexes of hydrolases and mannose-6-phosphate receptors leave the Golgi apparatus in small vesicles (step 6) that fuse with lysosomes (step 7). There the mannose phosphate ester link is cleaved by an acid phosphatase. This reduces the affinity of the receptor for the oligosaccharide, releasing the newly arrived enzyme to the interior of the lysosome and freeing the receptor for another delivery cycle (step 8). Steps 9 to 12 show a side path whereby receptors can deliver and retrieve lysosomal enzymes to and from the plasma membrane and hence the extracellular space. (From Ref. 55. With permission.)

membrane as a peripheral protein. Those precursors destined to be integral inner mitochondrial membrane proteins or matrix proteins enclosed within the inner membrane utilize not only specific outer surface receptors and amino-terminal extensions, but the electrochemical potential maintained across the inner membrane by respiration. These precursors are matured by proteolytic cleavage as they reach their destination within the organelle. Presumably, these posttranslational modifications trigger the conformational changes requisite to the proper placement of the proteins.

Finally, the polypeptides synthesized within the mitochondria and those imported from the cytoplasm must collaborate in the assembly of hybrid oligomeric enzymes such as cytochrome c oxidase and the F_1ATP synthetase. There is even coordination in the expression of the cognate genes within the nucleus and the organelle (58).

Wondrous things, these biological membranes.

REFERENCES

1. Jain, M. K., and Wagner, R. C., *Introduction to Biological Membranes*, John Wiley & Sons, New York, 1980.
2. Harrison, R., and Lunt, G. G., *Biological Membranes*, 2nd ed., John Wiley & Sons, New York, 1980.
3. Houslay, M. D., and Stanley, K. K., *Dynamics of Biological Membranes*, John Wiley & Sons, New York, 1982.
4. Sim, E., *Membrane Biochemistry*, Chapman & Hall, New York, 1982.
5. Tanford, C., *The Hydrophobic Effect*, 2nd ed., John Wiley & Sons, New York, 1980.
6. Thompson, T. E., and Huang, C., in *Physiology of Membrane Disorders* (Andreoli, T. E., Hoffman, J. F., and Fanestill, D. D., eds.), Plenum Press, New York, 1978, pp. 27–48.
7. Op den Kamp, J. A. F., *Annu. Rev. Biochem.*, *48*:47 (1979).
8. Seigneuret, M., and Devaux, P. F., *Proc. Natl. Acad. Sci. U.S.A.*, *81*:3751 (1984).
9. Poste, G., and Nicolson, G. L., *Membrane Fusion*, North-Holland, New York, 1978.
10. Wilschut, J., and Haekstra, D., *Trends Biochem. Sci.*, *9*:479 (1984).
11. Steck, T. L., and Fox, C. F., in *Membrane Molecular Biology* (Fox, C. F., and Keith, A., eds.), Sinauer Associates, Stamford, Conn., 1972, pp. 27–75.

12. Steck, T. L., *J. Cell Biol.*, *62*:1 (1974).

13. Guidotti, G., *Physiology of Membrane Disorders* (Andreoli, T. E., Hoffman, J. F., and Fanestil, D. D., eds.), Plenum Press, New York, 1978, pp. 49–60.

14. Dratz, E. A., and Hargrave, P. A., *Trends Biochem. Sci.*, *8*:131 (1983).

15. Engelman, D. M., Henderson, R., McLachlan, A. D., and Wallace, B. A., *Proc. Natl. Acad. Sci. U.S.A.*, *77*:2023 (1980).

16. Eisenberg, D., *Annu. Rev. Biochem.*, *53*:595 (1984).

17. Grover, A. K., Slotboom, A. J., de Haas, G. H., and Hammes, G. G., *J. Biol. Chem.*, *250*:31 (1975).

18. Gennis, R. B., and Jonas, A., *Annu. Rev. Biophys. Bioeng.*, *6*:195 (1977).

19. Johannsson, A., Keightley, C. A., Smith, G. A., Richards, C. D., Hesketh, T. R., and Metcalfe, J. C., *J. Biol. Chem.*, *256*:1643 (1981).

20. Eytan, G. D., Matheson, M. J., and Racker, E., *J. Biol. Chem.*, *251*:6831 (1976).

21. Finkelstein, A., and Anderson, O. S., *J. Membr. Biol.*, *59*:155 (1981).

22. Miller, C., *Physiol. Rev.*, *63*:1209 (1983).

23. Maelicke, A., and Prinz, H., *Modern Cell Biol.*, *1*:171 (1983).

24. Reichardt, L. F., and Kelley, R. B., *Annu. Rev. Biochem.*, *52*:871 (1983).

25. Knauf, P. A., *Curr. Topics Membr. Transport*, *12*:249 (1979).

26. Overath, P., and Wright, J. K., *Trends Biochem. Sci.*, *8*:404 (1983).

27. Carafoli, E., and Scarpa, A., eds., *Ann. New York Acad. Sci.*, *402* (1982).

28. Nicholls, D. G., *Bioenergetics*, Academic Press, New York, 1982.

29. Bitensky, M., Collier, R. J., Steiner, D. F., and Fox, C. F., *Transmembrane Signalling*, Alan R. Liss, New York, 1979.

30. Carpenter, G., and Cohen, S., *Annu. Rev. Biochem.*, *48*:193 (1979).

31. Czech, M. P., Massague, J., and Pilch, P. F., *Trends Biochem. Sci.*, *6*:222 (1981).

32. Lefkowitz, R. J., Stadel, J. M., and Caron, M. G., *Annu. Rev. Biochem.*, *52*:159 (1983).

33. Carpenter, G., *Cell*, *37*:357 (1984).

34. Anderson, R. G. W., and Kaplan, J., *Modern Cell Biol.*, *1*:1 (1983).

35. Brown, M. S., Anderson, R. G. W., and Goldstein, J. L., *Cell*, *32*:663 (1983).

36. Kagey-Sobotka, A., MacGlashan, D. W., and Lichtenstein, L. M., *Fed. Proc.*, *41*:12 (1982).

37. Schreiber, A. B., Libermann, T. A., Lax, I., Yarden, Y., and Schlessinger, J., *J. Biol. Chem.*, *258*:846 (1983).

38. Kanner, B. I., and Metzger, H., *Proc. Natl. Acad. Sci. U.S.A.*, *80*:5744 (1983).

39. Stryer, L., Hurley, J. B., and Fung, B. K.-K., *Trends Biochem. Sci.*, *6*:245 (1981).

40. Bownds, M. D., *Curr. Topics Membr. Transport*, *15*:203 (1981).

41. The Cytoplasmic Matrix and the Integration of Cellular Function, *J. Cell Biol.*, *99*:1x–248s (1984).

42. Fulton, A. B., *The Cytoskeleton*, Chapman & Hall, New York, 1984.

43. Fey, E. G., Capco, D. G., Krochmalnic, G., and Penman, S., *J. Cell Biol.*, *99*:2035 (1984).

44. Cohen, C., *Semin. Hematol.*, *20*:141 (1983).

45. Shen, B. W., Josephs, R., and Steck, T. L., *J. Cell Biol.*, *99*:810 (1984).

46. Hughes, R. C., *Essays Biochem.*, *11*:1 (1975).

47. Höök, M., Kjellen, L., Johansson, S., and Robinson, J., *Annu. Rev. Biochem.*, *53*:847 (1984).

48. Yamada, K. M., *Annu. Rev. Biochem.*, *52*:761 (1983).

49. Singer, I. I., Kawka, D. W., Kazazis, D. M., and Clark, R. A. F., *J. Cell Biol.*, *98*:2091 (1984).

50. Hubbard, S. C., and Ivatt, R. J., *Annu. Rev. Biochem.*, *50*:555 (1981).

51. Sabatini, D. D., Kreibich, G., Morimoto, T., and Adesnik, M., *J. Cell Biol.*, *92*:1 (1982).

52. Walter, P., Gilmore, R., and Blobel, G., *Cell*, *38*:5 (1984).

53. Marcantonio, E. E., Amar-Costesec, A., and Kreibich, G., *J. Cell Biol.*, *99*:2254 (1984).

54. Green, J., Griffiths, G., Louvard, D., Quinn, P., and Warren, G., *J. Mol. Biol.*, *152*:663 (1981).

55. Sly, W. S., and Fischer, H. D., *J. Cell Biochem.*, *18*:67 (1982).

56. Brown, W. J., and Farquhar, M. G., *Cell*, *36*:295 (1984).

57. Schatz, G., and Butow, R. A., *Cell*, *32*:316 (1983).

58. Hay, R., Bohni, P., and Gasser, S., *Biochim. Biophys. Acta*, *779*:65 (1984).

7

Membrane Cholesterol

YVONNE LANGE Rush-Presbyterian-St. Luke's Medical Center, Chicago, Illinois

INTRODUCTION

Cholesterol plays a major role in the pathophysiology of atherosclerotic cardiovascular disease and is a major component of our diet and a principal constituent of plasma lipoproteins. In addition to their role as precursors of steroid hormones and bile acids, sterols are universal constituents of the plasma membranes of all eukaryotes. However, neither the physiological function nor the precise disposition of these compounds within the cell is well understood.

In this chapter the distribution and movement of cholesterol molecules between membranes and across membranes within animal cells will be discussed. While cholesterol has been the most studied, there is no reason to assume that other membrane sterols in organisms less familiar than man will behave differently.

CHOLESTEROL STRUCTURE

The cholesterol molecule (Fig. 1) measures 7.2 × 5 × 20 Å (1) and can be characterized as having three regions: (1) an alcoholic hydroxyl group covalently attached at carbon 3 of the steroid nucleus; (2) a fixed tetracyclic ring system 9 Å in length that is stereochemically rigid (the CPK space-filling molecular model shows that the α-surface of the fused ring system is planar, but the β-surface is puckered due to the presence of two angular methyl groups at C_{10} and C_{13}); and (3) a branched, extended hydrocarbon side chain attached to carbon 17 of the ring system. Cholesterol is a weak amphiphile.

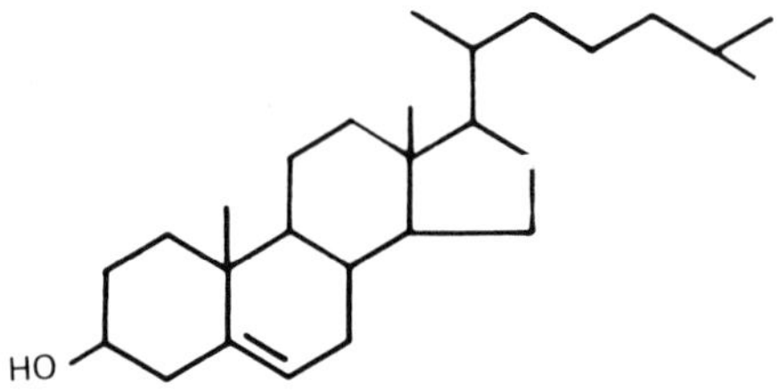

Fig. 1 The structure of cholesterol.

CHOLESTEROL FUNCTION

Most of our information on the position of the cholesterol molecule in membranes and its effect on membrane properties has been obtained in model system studies. The molecule is believed to take up a position with its paraffin side chain extended towards the center of the bimolecular lipid leaflet with the steroid nucleus interdigitated between the fatty acyl chains of the phospholipid molecules. The sole hydrophilic hydroxyl group of the molecule is weakly exposed to water. This model was proposed on the basis of x-ray diffraction studies of lecithin-cholesterol-water lamellar phases (2) and confirmed using total erythrocyte lipids (3). Further support came from studies of hydrated egg lecithin-cholesterol bilayers using NMR (4), circular dichroism (5), x-ray diffraction (6), and neutron diffraction (7).

The effect of cholesterol on the physical state of model phospholipid membranes has been investigated by various techniques. It has been shown that the interaction between cholesterol and the phospholipid hydrocarbon chains gives rise to restricted motion of the portion of the hydrocarbon chain nearest to the bilayer surface, but an increased motion of the terminal methyl groups in the hydrophobic core of the membrane bilayer (4,8). In this way, cholesterol maintains the membrane in a state of "intermediate fluidity," permitting motion of hydrocarbon chains in the gel phase while restricting motion in the liquid crystalline phase (for a review, see Ref. 9).

A comprehensive model for the structure of the phospholipid-cholesterol complex in bilayers has been proposed based on the considerable body of experimental data available (10). According to this model, the 3β-hydroxyl group of cholesterol is hydrogen bonded to the ester carbonyl oxygens of phospholipid molecules in bilayers. In addition, the model proposes that the saturated chains of phosphatidylcholine molecules are in all trans conformation and appose the planar α-face of the steroid nucleus, whereas the puckered β-face of the steroid nucleus is in contact with the unsaturated fatty acyl chains. In this manner, van der Waals interactions between the steroid nucleus and the fatty acyl chains provide a stabilizing force for the cholesterol-phospholipid complex in membranes and account for the observed decrease in the mean molecular surface area of phospholipid molecules on addition of cholesterol.

It is well established that the permeability of artificial phospholipid membranes to a large number of solutes decreases considerably upon incorporation of cholesterol in the membrane. An illustration of this effect is given in Fig. 2. In this study, the permeability of liposomes to glycerol and erythritol was assessed by measuring the swelling of the structure in isotonic solutions of these compounds. The addition of cholesterol to the membrane caused a marked reduction in permeability. This observation can be understood in terms of the influence of cholesterol on the fluidity of the hydrocarbon region of the membrane (12) as described below.

In the case of biological membranes, much less is known about the role of cholesterol and its position in the membrane. There is some direct evidence that cholesterol is important in controlling the fluidity

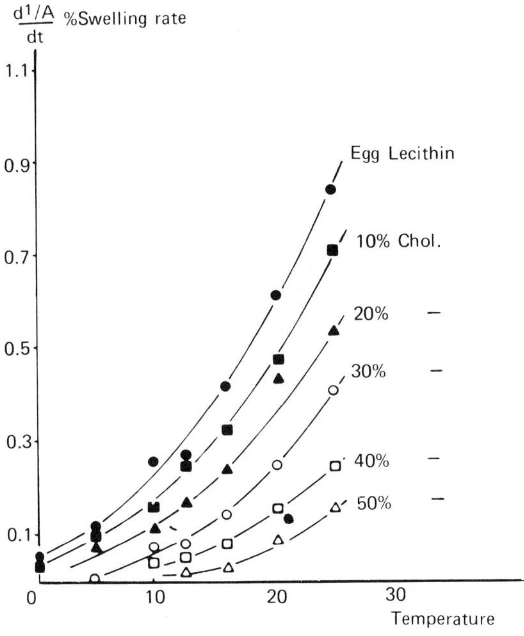

Fig. 2 The effect of cholesterol on bilayer permeability. The initial swelling rate in isotonic glycerol of liposomes prepared from phosphatidylcholine with varied amounts of cholesterol. (From Ref. 11.)

of biological membrane phospholipids as it is in artificial membranes. Such evidence has been limited by the difficulties inherent in altering the cholesterol content of biological membranes. However, some information has been obtained through studies of certain microorganisms and erythrocytes, systems in which it is possible to alter the amount of membrane cholesterol.

In one such study, the microorganism *Mycoplasma mycoides* (var. *capri*), which requires sterol for growth, was maintained in serum-free medium supplemented with decreasing amounts of cholesterol (13,14). These conditions resulted in the adaptation of the organism to growth without added cholesterol. Adapted cell membranes contained about 10% of the cholesterol in native membranes, a change that was accompanied by an increase in the saturation of the polar lipids. Thus, the lack of cholesterol was offset by the preferential incorporation into membrane phospholipids of saturated fatty acids from the growth medium. In this organism cholesterol functions as a regulator of membrane fluidity, and cells deprived of sterol compensate by altering their fatty acid composition so as to increase the rigidity of the acyl chains in the interior of the bilayer.

The effect of cholesterol on the fluidity of guinea pig erythrocyte membranes was studied by electron spin resonance using spin-labeled fatty acids as probes (15). This approach showed that cholesterol enrichment resulted in an increase in the local viscosity of the membrane compared to the controls. Similarly, in human erythrocyte membranes, cholesterol enrichment led to a decrease in the molecular motion in the hydrophobic portion of the membrane as reported by the fluorescent anisotropy of a stearic acid analog (16).

Cholesterol also appears to affect the permeability of biological membranes. Incorporation of cholesterol into the membrane decreased the permeability of *Acholeplasma laidlawii* to glycerol and erythritol (17). The partial removal of human erythrocyte membrane cholesterol was found to lead to an increase in the permeability of the membrane to glycerol (18), although the permeability to water was unaltered (19). Nonelectrolyte and Na^+ transfer were decreased in guinea pig erythrocytes after dietary elevation of membrane cholesterol (20).

It has long been known that red cell cholesterol is in dynamic equilibrium with the unesterified cholesterol in plasma lipoproteins (21). Indeed, it appears that red cell cholesterol content is set by the cholesterol to phospholipid mole ratio (C/P) of plasma lipoproteins (22,23), although the physiological significance of this finding is obscure. The high cholesterol content of red cells from patients with spur cell anemia is secondary to the elevated unesterified cholesterol levels in the plasma lipoproteins of these individuals, since the abnormality was shown to develop in normal transfused erythrocytes (24). Similarly, if red cells are incubated with cholesterol-depleted serum, the membrane loses cholesterol until a new equilibrium is established (23). Red cells enriched in cholesterol are less deformable than normal or cholesterol-depleted cells and have an increased surface area and broad, flattened contour (22).

Recent studies of the effect of cholesterol content on membrane contour suggested a novel role for cholesterol. Whereas normal ghosts as well as ghosts depleted of cholesterol underwent invagination at low ionic strength to form inside-out vesicles, enrichment to $C/P \geqslant 0.95$ promoted right-side-out vesicle formation instead (25). By analogy with other intercalating amphipaths, these data were interpreted as indicating a slight excess of cholesterol in the outer leaflet of the bilayer relative to the inner. Other studies have also suggested that the external surface of the red cell membrane is enriched in cholesterol, although there is disagreement as to the extent of the differential (see section on the plasma membrane). In the study cited (25), it also was shown that the breakdown of ghosts into endocytic vesicles in dilute alkaline media and the concomitant release and dissolution of the submembrane protein reticulum were retarded by excess cholesterol and promoted by cholesterol removal. Thus, cholesterol may act physiologically both to stabilize the membrane and to constrain its contour against invagination.

CHOLESTEROL TRANSFER BETWEEN MEMBRANES AND LIPOPROTEINS

Red cell membrane cholesterol exchanges readily with the unesterified cholesterol of plasma lipoproteins both in vivo (21) and in vitro (26) (Fig. 3). Studies of cholesterol exchange have shown that the process is nonenzymatic and does not require energy (27). Cholesterol exchange also occurs between erythrocyte membranes and sonicated liposomes of phospholipid and cholesterol (28). Although the mechanism of cholesterol exchange is not known, three hypotheses have been advanced: (1) cholesterol may be transferred by diffusion through the aqueous medium (26); (2) cholesterol may exchange via hydrophobic collision complexes formed during contact among red cell membranes or between the cells and lipoproteins or vesicles (29); and (3) there may be saturable binding sites on the red cell membrane which mediate cholesterol transfer, as suggested for serum lipoproteins (30). The dependence of transfer rate on the concentration of donor and acceptor can, in principle, distinguish among these mechanisms. Thus, transfer by simple collision depends on the product of donor and acceptor concentrations; transfer by diffusion becomes independent of acceptor concentration when it is sufficiently high; and specific sites show saturation kinetics and fixed stoichiometry.

Several studies have led to diverse conclusions regarding the mechanism of cholesterol transfer between a variety of donor and

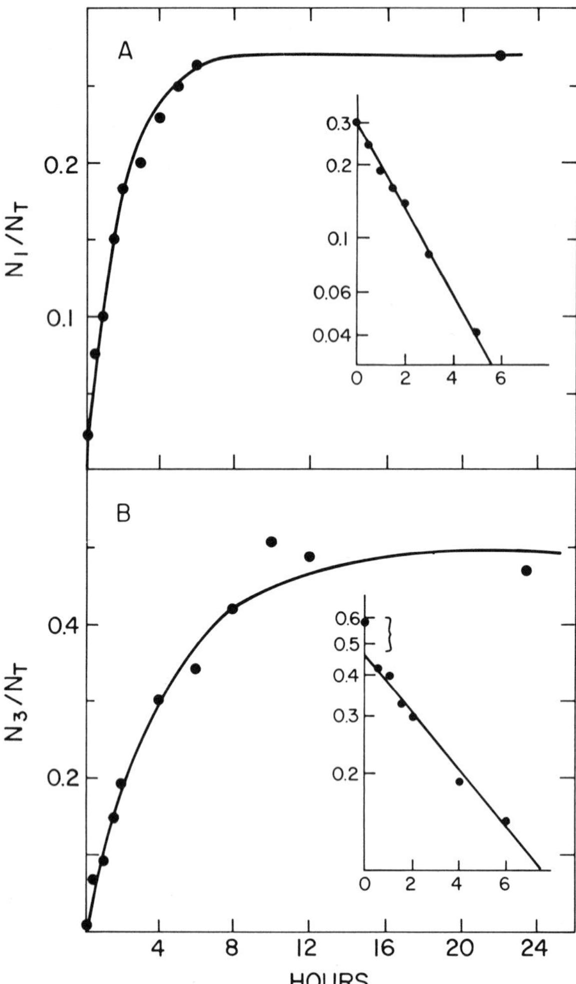

Fig. 3 The exchange of [^{3}H] cholesterol between human red cells and plasma at 37°C. (A) The transfer of [^{3}H] cholesterol from labeled plasma to red cells. N_1/N_T is the fractional label recovered in the red cells as a function of incubation time. (B) The transfer of [^{3}H] cholesterol from labeled red cells to plasma. N_3/N_T is the fractional label recovered in the plasma. Insets show semilog plots of the approach to equilibrium. (From Ref. 34.)

acceptor particles. On the basis of weak concentration dependence of transfer rate, a diffusion mechanism was invoked in studies of cholesterol transfer between liposomes (31,32), between red cells and plasma (33,34), and between different classes of lipoproteins (35). However, stable complexes were inferred in one study of cholesterol transfer between red cells and purified plasma lipoproteins (30). Similarly, a transient collision mechanism was proposed for transfer between red cells and liposomes (36). In the latter two studies, transfer rate was found to saturate at high concentrations. The transfer of cholesterol between the membrane of vesicular stomatitis virus and sonicated liposomes was found to be dependent on liposome concentration, suggestive of a collision-mediated mechanism (37).

The differences in these findings notwithstanding, all of the transfer rates measured exhibited similar half-times of 1 to 2 hours at 37°C. At the present time, the concensus of opinion favors the aqueous diffusion model of cholesterol transfer. Nonetheless, there is some evidence that this is incorrect. Cholesterol was found to transfer extremely slowly with a half-time in excess of 50 hr between different populations of red cells and between red cells and ghosts (38). Transfer was greatly accelerated by the addition of plasma to the system. These observations are incompatible with a diffusion mechanism. If transfer of cholesterol between membranes occurred by diffusion through the aqueous phase, the rate-limiting step would most likely be its desorption from the membrane, as has been proposed for the transfer of cholesterol between different populations of liposomes (35). Addition of plasma to the system should not affect this step. It follows that the plasma-induced acceleration of transfer between red cells must involve collisions between lipoproteins and membranes. Unfortunately, due to its very slow time course, a kinetic analysis of the mechanism of transfer of cholesterol between red cells is difficult.

Further evidence against a simple diffusion mechanism for cholesterol transfer between membranes comes from recent studies in nucleated cells. (See section on intracellular movement of cholesterol.) It has been shown that the major fraction of cell cholesterol resides in the plasma membrane (39). The cell thus maintains a considerable gradient in cholesterol concentration between surface and internal membranes. This gradient appears to be established by a unidirectional transfer of cholesterol from its site of synthesis (the endoplasmic reticulum) to the plasma membrane (40). Furthermore it has been demonstrated directly that cholesterol in the plasma membrane does not enter internal pools as would be the case if cholesterol diffused spontaneously between membranes (40).

TRANSMEMBRANE MOVEMENT OF CHOLESTEROL

In order for cholesterol exchanged into the plasma membrane to enter the cell interior it first must cross the membrane. The first measurement of the rate at which sterol molecules translocate between the two leaflets of a lipid bilayer ("flip-flop") was made by Smith and Green (41). In this study, the fluorescent sterol analog, sterophenol (1-methyl-19-nor-cholesta-1,3,5(10)tiren-3-ol) was incorporated into sonicated phosphatidylcholine liposomes at the time of preparation so that it was present in both bilayer leaflets. The liposomes were incubated with plasma low-density lipoproteins to deplete the outer surface of sterophenol molecules. Iodide ions that quenched the fluorescence of sterophenol were added to the system and the fluorescence measured. In this way, the appearance of sterophenol at the outer surface, a measure of flip rate, was monitored. A half-time of 70 min at 37°C was calculated from these data.

Subsequently, the transmembrane movement of cholesterol in sonicated liposomes and red cell membranes was studied by several workers using a nonperturbative approach based on the measurement of the exchangeability of membrane cholesterol. All the cholesterol in intact erythrocytes or erythrocyte ghosts was found to exchange with the unesterified cholesterol of plasma lipoproteins or sonicated liposomes (23,28). These observations indicated that transmembrane movement of cholesterol occurred but did not provide information on the rate of the process. Later, careful kinetic studies of the exchange of radiocholesterol between erythrocytes and plasma or sonicated liposomes placed an upper bound of 50 min (42) or a value of 2.3 hr (43) on the half-time of cholesterol flip across the cell membrane. A similar approach applied to the measurement of cholesterol flip in sonicated liposomes led to conflicting results. Some authors (44) concluded that cholesterol flip was immeasurably slow, whereas others (45) reported half-times on the order of hours. A study of the kinetics of transfer of radioactive cholesterol from influenza virus to sonicated liposomes prepared from phosphatidylcholine and cholesterol showed that all of the cholesterol in the virus membrane was not available for exchange (46). If the nonexchangeable cholesterol was located at the inner bilayer leaflet, these data indicated that cholesterol does not flip in this membrane. However, similar studies of vesicular stomatitis virus (37) and Sindbis virus (47) indicated that cholesterol in both membrane leaflets was available for transfer to phospholipid vesicles.

More recently, a different approach to the study of cholesterol flip has demonstrated that the process is very fast. The method makes use of the enzyme cholesterol oxidase, which interacts with cholesterol in phospholipid bilayers of the appropriate composition, converting it to cholestenone (48). Using this method, it was found that all the cholesterol in sonicated egg phosphatidylcholine-cholesterol liposomes was oxidized rapidly (49). Since the enzyme had access only to the outer bilayer leaflet, these data demonstrated that cholesterol flip occurred. From the time course of oxidation, the authors estimated an upper bound of 1 min at 37°C for the half-time of cholesterol flip. A similar approach showed that cholesterol in the erythrocyte membrane undergoes rapid flip (50). In these experiments, red cells were enriched in cholesterol, a treatment that renders membrane cholesterol susceptible to oxidation by cholesterol oxidase. The time course of oxidation was determined at 37°C (Fig. 4). Since no lysis of the cells occurred during the time of the experiment, the finding that the entire pool of membrane cholesterol was oxidized indicates that cholesterol at the inner membrane leaflet must have flipped rapidly across the bilayer. From these studies it was estimated that the transmembrane movement of cholesterol in the erythrocyte membrane occurs with a half-time of less than 3 sec at 37°C (Fig. 4B).

The transmembrane movement of phospholipids in various membrane systems generally occurs with a half-time on the order of hours to days (51). Thus, cholesterol flips much more rapidly than do phospholipids, a result in keeping with the magnitude of their respective

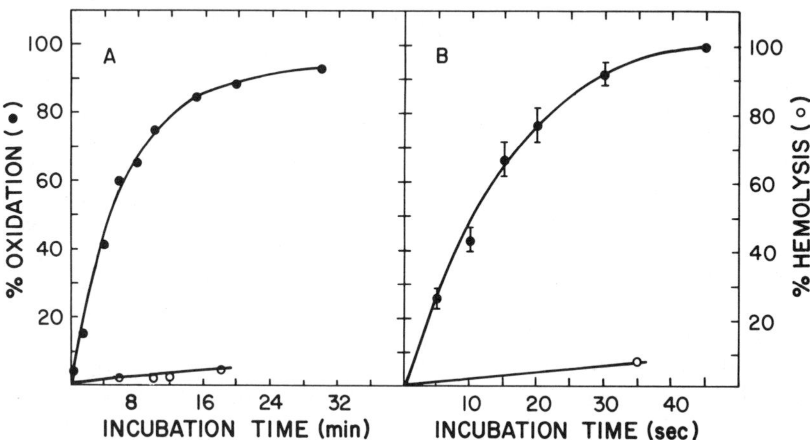

Fig. 4 Time course of cholesterol oxidation in erythrocytes. Cholesterol-enriched red cells were incubated at 37°C in 0.15 M NaCl, 5 mM NaP_i (pH 7.5) containing cholesterol oxidase. The appearance of cholestenone (•) and hemolysis (○) was determined. (A) Low enzyme. The red cell cholesterol/phospholipid mole ratio was 1.4; the cholesterol concentration was 86 μg/ml; and the cholesterol oxidase concentration was 1.25 IU/ml. (B) High enzyme. The red cell cholesterol/phospholipid mole ratio was 1.2; the cholesterol concentration was 52 μg/ml; and the cholesterol oxidase concentration was 20 IU/ml. (From Ref. 50.)

polar head groups. Indeed, sterols appear to be the only major component of plasma membranes that can cross the membrane on the physiological time scale of less than 1 sec.

The rapid transmembrane movement of cholesterol suggests a novel function for sterols. As a membrane is constrained to change shape by mechanical or physiological forces, the coupled compression and expansion of the two lipid leaflets will offer resistance to bending. A rapid redistribution of membrane sterol could relieve this resistance and thus facilitate and stabilize changes in shape. A role for sterols as a surface area buffer in bilayers undergoing deformation is consistent with the universally observed enrichment of these lipids in plasma membranes of eukaryotes, since the cell surface is particularly subject to frequent and rapid changes in contour.

DISTRIBUTION OF CHOLESTEROL WITHIN THE CELL

The broad diversity of membrane lipid molecules within even the simplest of cells has been well documented but poorly rationalized. Likewise, it is well established that the distribution of lipids between different membranes in animal cells is nonuniform, although the significance of this finding is obscure. Plasma membranes have a much higher concentration of sphingolipids, glycolipids, and cholesterol than intracellular membranes (52). Conversely, internal membranes are enriched in phosphatidylethanolamine compared to surface membranes (52), and mitochondria contain cardiolipin. Furthermore, within a single membrane, there is a difference in the lipid composition of the two halves of the bilayer (51). The mechanisms by which the specific lipid compositions are established and maintained in cell membranes are not understood. Since most of the lipids are synthesized in the endoplasmic reticulum, some sorting and targeting must occur intracellularly. In addition, it is possible that the lipid composition of plasma membranes is strongly influenced by equilibration with plasma lipoproteins, as has been shown in the red cell. In this section, the distribution of cholesterol between the two halves of the plasma membrane and among the different cell membranes is discussed.

The Plasma Membrane

It is well established that the red cell membrane has a compositional asymmetry in its phospholipid components: choline-containing phospholipids (sphingomyelin and phosphatidylcholine) are located predominantly in the outer half of the membrane and anionic phospholipids, e.g., phosphatidylserine, phosphatidylethanolamine, phosphatidylinositol, phosphatidylglycerol, and phosphatidic acid at the inner half (51). Cholesterol is a relatively unreactive molecule; therefore, information on its localization within the membrane has been less readily attainable. Nonetheless, several studies have addressed the transmembrane distribution of cholesterol.

The first report on the transbilayer distribution of cholesterol came from an x-ray diffraction study of nerve myelin (53). In this work, the authors suggested that the asymmetric electron density profile they observed was a manifestation of differences in cholesterol composition of the two bilayer leaflets with a slight enrichment of the outer surface. A similar study of gap junction membranes led to comparable conclusions (54). However, in neither of these studies was it demonstrated directly that the asymmetry in electron density was due to cholesterol as opposed to some other membrane constituent such as protein. A more direct approach was taken in studies in which an attempt was made to determine the chemical composition of the two halves of the erythrocyte membrane using a freeze-fracture procedure (55). This study suggested that the external surface of the membrane was significantly richer in cholesterol than the cytoplasmic surface; however, the uncertainties in these experiments are considerable.

More recently, a study of the effect of cholesterol on membrane contour in ghosts led to the suggestion that there is a very slight enrichment of cholesterol in the outer membrane leaflet (25) When ghosts are incubated in low ionic strength alkaline buffers they break down and vesiculate by endocytosis, forming sealed vesicles of the opposite orientation from the parent membrane (inside-out) (56). Ghosts from erythrocytes slightly enriched in cholesterol formed right-side-out vesicles under conditions that generated inside-out vesicles in control membranes (25). A simple explanation for the effect of cholesterol on vesicle sidedness is that it, like other uncharged amphipaths (57), partitions in favor of, and thus differentially expands, the outer leaflet of the membrane. The requisite asymmetry is minimal, since the maximal difference in the surface area of the two leaflets of a red cell membrane (in the extreme of a sphere) is only 0.3%.

A study of the effect of lysophosphatidylcholine on the shape of erythrocytes of modified cholesterol content also led to the conclusion that there was a small excess (∿1%) of cholesterol in the outer membrane leaflet (58). It is possible that this unequal distribution of cholesterol results from the difference in phospholipid composition between the two halves of the erythrocyte membrane (51). There have been reports based on differential scanning calorimetry studies that cholesterol has different affinity for different phospholipids (59,60). These studies demonstrated that in mixtures of phosphatidylcholine and phosphatidylethanolamine showing phase separation, cholesterol had preferential affinity for phosphatidylcholine. In mixtures of sphingomyelin and phosphatidylcholine or phosphatidylethanolamine, cholesterol had a greater affinity for the sphingolipid. Thus, in the erythrocyte membrane, the phospholipids having the higher affinity for cholesterol are concentrated at the outer membrane leaflet. It is tempting to conclude that this side of the membrane should contain more cholesterol than the cytoplasmic leaflet (60). However, the interpretation of the differential scanning calorimetry studies cited above in terms of cholesterol affinity for phospholipids has been questioned. In particular, the report that cholesterol has higher affinity for sphingomyelin than for phosphatidylcholine was not confirmed in two independent studies (61,62). Furthermore, the finding that cholesterol distributes nearly equally between the two leaflets of the erythrocyte membrane (58), the dramatic differential in sphingomyelin content notwithstanding, argues against a preferential affinity of cholesterol for this phospholipid.

There have been suggestions that cholesterol is not uniformly distributed in the plane of the plasma membrane. For example, in rat intestinal mucosa, the basolateral membranes are more enriched in cholesterol than the brush border membranes (63). This observation is intriguing in view of the rapid lateral diffusion of cholesterol in membranes (64). The explanation may lie in the exclusion of cholesterol from tight junctions and gap junctions (65). It was originally believed that cholesterol is absent in those regions of the plasma membrane which invaginate to form coated pits during endocytosis (66). However, recent reports suggested that the vesicles that form by invagination and budding off of these regions of the membrane contain the same amount of cholesterol as the parent membrane (67). Retinal rod outer segments provide a striking example of nonuniformity in membrane cholesterol distribution. In these structures, the free-floating stacked discs that form by invagination of the plasma membrane contain very little cholesterol (68), suggesting that in this system there is a mechanism for extruding cholesterol from the plasma membrane.

Cellular Cholesterol

A striking feature of the distribution of cholesterol in eukaryotes is the very large differential in cholesterol content among the various membranes of the cell (Table 1). Early studies based on subcellular fractionation of cells by density gradient centrifugation showed that the plasma membrane fraction contained a high concentration of cholesterol, whereas preparations of mitochondria and rough endoplasmic reticulum had little sterol. Golgi membranes and smooth endoplasmic reticulum (ER) were reported to have more cholesterol than mitochondria. The relatively high values reported for the cholesterol content of Golgi and endoplasmic reticulum membranes (Table 1) may well reflect contamination of these preparations with plasma membrane. Recent studies have shown that greater than 90% of total cell cholesterol is in the plasma

Table 1 Cholesterol Content of Various Cell Membranes

	Mole sterol/mole phospholipid	
Membrane	Liver	LM cells[a]
Outer mitochondria	0.065	
Mitochondria	0.034	0.02
Rough ER	0.070	0.19
Smooth ER	0.237	
Golgi	0.215	
Plasma membrane	0.50	0.65
Whole cells	0.19	0.21

[a]The sterol in these cells is desmosterol. Values taken from Ref. 69. Liver values given are averages obtained from Refs. 52, 70, and 71.

membrane in fibroblasts and Chinese hamster ovary cells (39). Hepatocytes have 80% of total cellular cholesterol in the plasma membrane (39). The larger internal pool of unesterified cholesterol in hepatocytes probably reflects the involvement of these cells in lipoprotein synthesis. These measurements were made using the enzyme cholesterol oxidase, which catalyzes the oxidation of plasma membrane cholesterol to cholestenone in intact cells, while leaving cholesterol in internal pools untouched. Because of the rapid transmembrane movement of cholesterol, the entire plasma membrane pool was oxidized. Thus, cholesterol in the plasma membrane could be separated and distinguished from intracellular cholesterol. Based on the value of 80% for the proportion of phospholipid that is located intracellularly in hepatocytes (39), this means that, on average, internal membranes have only 6% of the cholesterol concentration (per unit phospholipid) found in the cell surface.

The mechanism by which cells maintain this large differential in cholesterol content between internal membranes and the plasma membrane is not known, although various possibilities have been raised. The data certainly appear to preclude the possibility that cholesterol is free to move around the cell by diffusion since, as discussed below, newly synthesized cholesterol is transferred in a unidirectional manner from its site of synthesis, the endoplasmic recticulum, to the plasma membrane. However, it is possible that cholesterol in the various membranes is in diffusional equilibrium and the unequal distribution is a manifestation of a relatively high affinity of plasma membrane phospholipids for cholesterol. In the case of hepatocytes, using the values given above, the overall partition coefficient for surface versus internal cholesterol would be (cholesterol/phospholipid)$_{surface}$ divided by (cholesterol/phospholipid)$_{internal}$ or approximately 80/20 divided by 20/80 = 16. Recent studies have shown that various subcellular organelles will take up cholesterol in vitro when presented in mixed lipid vesicles (72). There was a nonuniformity in the equilibrium distribution of cholesterol among subcellular fractions; however, it was insufficient to account for the observed inhomogeneity in whole cells (39). Further evidence that the low cholesterol content of internal membranes is not due to their phospholipid composition or architecture came from a study using the membrane discs of bovine retinal rod outer segments (73). These membranes provide a favorable system for examination of these questions, since they are formed by invagination of the plasma membrane and yet contain only a trace of cholesterol (68). Moreover, since the bulk of the cell membrane is internal, plasma membrane contamination of isolated discs is minimal. Discs were incubated with an excess of human plasma labeled with [^{3}H]cholesterol. The membranes readily took up cholesterol, increasing their sterol content from 0.09 to 0.28 mol/mol phospholipid in 24 hours at 37°C (73). The amount taken up reflected equilibration with the plasma unesterified cholesterol pool. These data support the hypothesis that the low cholesterol content of these membranes is not due to a low affinity for cholesterol. Rather, it must be that in vivo internal membranes are not presented with a source of cholesterol.

INTRACELLULAR MOVEMENT OF CHOLESTEROL

Over the past few years, considerable insight has been obtained into mechanisms by which newly synthesized proteins are inserted into the plasma membrane (74,75). In contrast, very little is known about the biogenesis of the lipid component of cell surface membranes. Phospholipid and cholesterol are synthesized in the endoplasmic reticulum in most eukaryotes and subsequently inserted into the various membranes of the cell. (Endogenous mitochondrial lipid synthesis is an exception.) Specific targeting must occur since the lipid composition of the various cell membranes varies widely. Several mechanisms by which lipid can be moved around the cell can be visualized: (1) diffusion through the cytoplasm, (2) protein-mediated transport, and (3) vesicular transport.

The small amount of data currently available regarding the transfer of phospholipid from its site of synthesis to the plasma membrane does not suggest a single mechanism. Thus, there is evidence that in *Dictyostelium discoideum*, newly synthesized phospholipids are transferred to the plasma membrane by a special class of phospholipid-rich vesicle (76). However, in Chinese hamster fibroblasts it seems that newly synthesized phosphatidylethanolamine is transferred to the plasma membrane by one of the other two mechanisms mentioned above (77).

The bulk of cellular cholesterol is associated with the plasma membrane and only a few percent with internal membranes (39). There are two obvious sources for plasma membrane cholesterol: plasma lipoproteins and cellular biosynthesis. Low-density lipoproteins enter cells both by receptor- (78) and non-receptor-mediated (79) pathways. The subsequent release of the cholesterol in the particle and its effect on cellular processes have been described in detail (78). However, the extent to which this internalized low-density lipoprotein cholesterol subsequently contributes to the plasma membrane cholesterol pool has not been addressed. Nor is it known to what degree the cell plasma membrane cholesterol level is regulated by a passive transfer of unesterified cholesterol from the plasma lipoprotein pool at the cell surface. Cholesterol equilibrates between red cell membranes and plasma lipoproteins (21), and a similar process may well be important in establishing surface membrane cholesterol content in all cells that are exposed to lipoproteins. Indeed, there is evidence that purified high-density lipoproteins can remove cholesterol from cells (80), although the contribution of the plasma membrane pool to this efflux from the cell is not known.

Studies of the rate of transfer of cholesterol from its site of synthesis to the plasma membrane have given conflicting results. In a study of radiocholesterol movement between human skin fibroblasts and sonicated liposomes, no movement of endogenously synthesized cholesterol to the cell surface was detected in the course of several hours (81). However, data obtained using a plasma membrane isolation procedure showed that the movement of newly synthesized cholesterol to the plasma membrane in Chinese hamster ovary cells occurred with a half-time of 10 min at 37°C (82). Subsequent studies using cholesterol oxidase to distinguish between plasma membrane cholesterol and internal cholesterol reported a transfer half-time of about 1 hr in human skin fibroblasts and Chinese hamster ovary cells (40). The mechanism of transfer was not elucidated in any of these studies; however, there is evidence that it is unidirectional (40). Thus, radiocholesterol introduced into the plasma membrane did not subsequently move to the cell interior. It is unlikely, therefore, that cholesterol transfer occurs by simple diffusion within the cell. Furthermore, an active transport mechanism in which newly synthesized cholesterol is transported against its concentration gradient to the plasma membrane and then diffuses back down the gradient to the cell interior is excluded by experiments showing that exogenous [^{14}C]-cholesterol inserted into the plasma membrane did not mingle with newly synthesized [^{3}H]cholesterol over a time period of many hours at 37°C (40).

It is likely that the transfer of newly synthesized cholesterol to the plasma membrane in fibroblasts is mediated by a membrane vesicle since no evidence for involvement of a carrier protein was obtained in at least one study (40; see below). The composition of such a vesicle and whether it carries newly synthesized phospholipid and protein as well as cholesterol are issues of great interest which await resolution.

Several soluble cytoplasmic proteins that play a role in sterol biosynthesis have been identified in tissues in which cholesterol turnover is high, including liver, adrenal, and ovaries (83). Proteins that specifically stimulate the metabolism of cholesterol precursors by microsomal enzymes have been purified and characterized. Supernatant protein factor (SPF) (84) and sterol carrier protein (SCP) (85), soluble cytoplasmic proteins isolated from rat liver, stimulate squalene epoxidase and squalene-2,3-oxide-lanosterol cyclase. There is some question as to whether these proteins function by binding sterols. There have been reports that SCP binds various cholesterol precursors (86); however, SPF binds neither squalene nor squalene-2,3-oxide, although it does interact strongly with anionic phospholipids (87). Thus, the original proposal that these proteins exert their effect on microsomal conversions by actually carrying insoluble substrate to the microsome is in doubt. It now seems likely that they act at the microsomal membrane by facilitating the access of substrate to specific membrane sites (88). It has been shown that SPF can promote the transfer of squalene from one microsomal vesicle population to another (88). Subsequent studies showed that these proteins also promote the transfer of later intermediates in sterol biosynthesis between microsomes (89).

A suggestion that the sterol carrier proteins are involved directly in cholesterol movement comes from studies using adrenal tissue. A major function of adrenal cortical cells is the synthesis of steroid hormones from cholesterol. The rate-limiting step in steroidogenesis, conversion of cholesterol to pregnenolone, is catalyzed by a cytochrome P-450 located at the matrix side of the inner mitochondrial membrane (90). Several studies have indicated that the increase in steroid hormone synthesis that occurs in response to corticotropin probably reflects an increased availability of cholesterol to the cytochrome P-450 (91). Since the cholesterol used for steroid hormone synthesis comes from the hydrolysis of cholesterol esters stored in cytoplasmic lipid droplets, a mechanism for the transport of this cholesterol to the inner mitochondrial membrane is required. Several studies suggest that sterol carrier protein may be involved in the movement of cholesterol both from lipid droplets to mitochondria and from the outer to the inner mitochondrial membrane (92–94).

These findings raise interesting questions regarding the mechanism of cholesterol transfer between membranes and lipoproteins (discussed above). If cholesterol transfer occurred by simple diffusion through the cytoplasm, there would be no need for a specific carrier protein to bring cholesterol to mitochondria. Furthermore, in view of the rapid transmembrane movement of cholesterol, cholesterol, once at the outer mitochondrial membrane, could readily reach the inner membrane matrix without assistance from a carrier protein. The demonstrated role of sterol carrier proteins in steroidogenesis therefore argues against cholesterol diffusion through the aqueous phase.

REFERENCES

1. Crowfoot, D., *Vitam. Horm.*, *2*:409 (1944).
2. Small, D. M., and Bourges, M., *Mol. Cryst.*, *1*:541 (1966).
3. Rand, R. P., and Luzatti, V., *Biophys. J.*, *8*:125 (1968).
4. Darke, A., Finer, E. G., Flook, A. G., and Phillips, M. C., *J. Mol. Biol.*, *63*:265 (1972).
5. Green, J. R., Edwards, P. A., and Green, C., *Biochem. J.*, *135*:63 (1973).
6. Franks, N. P., *J. Mol. Biol.*, *100*:345 (1976).
7. Worcester, D. L., and Franks, N. P., *J. Mol. Biol.*, *100*:359 (1976).
8. Verma, S. P., and Wallach, D. F. H., *Biochim. Biophys. Acta*, *330*:122 (1973).
9. Chapman, D., in *Biological Membranes*, Vol. 2, Academic Press, New York, 1973.
10. Huang, C. H., *Lipids*, *12*:348 (1977).
11. de Gier, J., Mandersloot, J. G., and van Deenen, L. L. M., *Biochim. Biophys. Acta*, *150*:666 (1968).
12. Oldfield, E., and Chapman, D., *Biochem. Biophys. Res. Commun.*, *43*:610 (1971).
13. Rottem, S., Yashouv, Z., Ne'eman, Z., and Razin, S., *Biochim. Biophys. Acta*, *323*:495 (1973).
14. Rottem, S., Cirillo, V. P., DeKruyff, B., Shinitzky, M., and Razin, S., *Biochim. Biophys. Acta*, *323*:509 (1973).
15. Kroes, J., Ostwald, M., and Keith, A., *Biochim. Biophys. Acta*, *274*:71 (1972).
16. Vanderkooi, J., Fischkoff, S., Chance, B., and Cooper, R. A., *Biochemistry*, *13*:1589 (1974).

17. DeKruyff, B., Demel, R. A., and Van Deenen, L. L. M., *Biochim. Biophys. Acta, 255*:331 (1972).

18. Bruckdorfer, K. R., Demel, R. A., de Gier, J., and van Deenen, L. L. M., *Biochim. Biophys. Acta, 183*:334 (1969).

19. Shaafi, R. I., Gary Bobo, C. M., and Solomon, A. K., *Biochim. Biophys. Acta, 173*:141 (1969).

20. Kroes, J., and Ostwald, R., *Biochim. Biophys. Acta, 249*:647 (1971).

21. Taylor, C. B., and Gould, R. G., *Circulation, 2*:467 (1950).

22. Cooper, R. A., Arner, E. C., Wiley, J. S., and Shattil, S. J., *J. Clin. Invest., 55*:115 (1975).

23. Lange, Y., and d'Alessandro, J. S., *Biochemistry, 16*:4339 (1977).

24. Cooper, R. A., *J. Clin. Invest., 48*:1820 (1969).

25. Lange, Y., Cutler, H. B., and Steck, T. L., *J. Biol. Chem., 255*:9331 (1980).

26. Hagerman, J. S., and Gould, R. G., *Proc. Soc. Exp. Biol. Med., 78*:329 (1951).

27. Murphy, J. R., *J. Lab. Clin. Med., 60*:571 (1962).

28. Bruckdorfer, K. R., Edwards, P. A., and Green, C., *Eur. J. Biochem., 4*:506 (1968).

29. Gurd, F. R. N., in *Lipid Chemistry* (Hanahan, D. J., ed.), John Wiley & Sons, New York, 1960, pp. 208–259.

30. Gottlieb, M. H., *Biochim. Biophys. Acta, 600*:530 (1980).

31. McLean, L. R., and Phillips, M. C., *Biochemistry, 20*:2893 (1981).

32. Backer, J. M., and Dawidowicz, E. A., *Biochemistry, 20*:3805 (1981).

33. Bojesen, E., *Nature (London), 299*:276 (1982).

34. Lange, Y., Molinaro, A. L., Chauncey, T. R., and Steck, T. L., *J. Biol. Chem., 258*:6920 (1983).

35. Lund-Katz, S., Hammerschlag, B., and Phillips, M. C., *Biochemistry, 21*:2964 (1982).

36. Giraud, F., and Claret, M., *FEBS Lett., 103*:186 (1979).

37. Patzer, E. J., Shaw, J. M., Moore, N. F., Thompson, T. E., and Wagner, R. R., *Biochemistry, 17*:4192 (1978).

38. Lange, Y., *Fed. Proc.*, *41*:1280 (1982).

39. Lange, Y., and Ramos, B., *J. Biol. Chem.*, *258*:15,130 (1983).

40. Lange, Y., and Matthies, H. J. G., *J. Biol. Chem.*, *259*:14,624 (1984).

41. Smith, R. J. M., and Green, C., *FEBS Lett.*, *42*:108 (1974).

42. Lange, Y., Cohen, C. M., and Poznansky, M. J., *Proc. Natl. Acad. Sci. U.S.A.*, *74*:1538 (1977).

43. Kirby, C. J., and Green, C., *Biochem. J.*, *168*:575 (1977).

44. Poznansky, M. J., and Lange, Y., *Biochim. Biophys. Acta*, *506*:256 (1978).

45. Bloj, B., and Zilversmit, D. B., *Biochemistry*, *16*:3943 (1977).

46. Lenard, J., and Rothman, J. E., *Proc. Natl. Acad. Sci. U.S.A.*, *73*:391 (1976).

47. Sefton, B. M., and Gaffney, B. J., *Biochemistry*, *18*:436 (1979).

48. Patzer, E. J., Wagner, R. R., and Barenholz, Y., *Nature (London)*, *274*:394 (1978).

49. Backer, J. M., and Dawidowicz, E. A., *J. Biol. Chem.*, *256*:586 (1981).

50. Lange, Y., Dolde, J., and Steck, T. L., *J. Biol. Chem.*, *256*: 5321 (1981).

51. Op den Kamp, J. A. F., *Annu. Rev. Biochem.*, *48*:47 (1979).

52. Zambrano, F., Fleischer, S., and Fleischer, B., *Biochim. Biophys. Acta*, *380*:357 (1975).

53. Caspar, D. L. D., and Kirschner, D. A., *Nature (London)*, *231*:46 (1971).

54. Makowski, L., Caspar, D. L. D., Phillips, W. C., and Goodenough, D. A., *J. Cell Biol.*, *74*:629 (1977).

55. Fisher, K. A., *Proc. Natl. Acad. Sci. U.S.A.*, *73*:173 (1976).

56. Steck, T. L., in *Methods in Membrane Biology* (Korn, E., ed.), Vol. 2, Plenum Press, New York, 1974, pp. 245–281.

57. Sheetz, M., and Singer, S. J., *Proc. Natl. Acad. Sci. U.S.A.*, *71*:4457 (1974).

58. Lange, Y., and Slayton, J. M., *J. Lipid Res.*, *23*:1121 (1982).

59. DeKruyff, B., Van Dijck, P. W. M., Demel, R. A., Schuijff, A., Brants, F., and Van Deenen, L. L. M., *Biochim. Biophys. Acta*, *356*:1 (1974).

60. Demel, R. A., Jansen, J. W. C. M., Van Dijck, P. W. M., and Van Deenen, L. L. M., *Biochim. Biophys. Acta, 465*:1 (1977).

61. Lange, Y., d'Alessandro, J. S., and Small, D. M., *Biochim. Biophys. Acta, 556*:388 (1979).

62. Calhoun, W. I., and Shipley, G. G., *Biochemistry, 18*:1717 (1979).

63. Chapelle, S., and Gilles-Baillien, M., *Biochim. Biophys. Acta, 753*:269 (1983).

64. Stroeve, P., and Miller, I., *Biochim. Biophys. Acta, 401*:157 (1975).

65. Robenek, H., Jung, W., and Gebhardt, R., *J. Ultrastruct. Res., 78*:95 (1982).

66. Pearse, B. M. F., *Proc. Natl. Acad. Sci. U.S.A., 73*:1255 (1976).

67. Steer, C. J., Bisher, M., Blumenthal, R., and Steven, A. C., *J. Cell Biol., 99*:315 (1984).

68. Mason, W. T., Fager, R. S., and Abrahamson, E. W., *Biochemistry, 12*:2147 (1973).

69. Schroeder, F., Perlmutter, J. F., Glaser, M., and Vagelos, P. R., *J. Biol. Chem., 251*:5015 (1976).

70. Colbeau, A., Nachbaur, J., and Vignais, P. M., *Biochim. Biophys. Acta, 249*:462 (1971).

71. Wibo, M., Thines-Sempoux, D., Amar-Costesec, A., Beaufay, H., and Godelaine, D., *J. Cell Biol., 89*:456 (1981).

72. Wattenberg, B. W., and Silbert, D. F., *J. Biol. Cehm., 258*:2284 (1983).

73. Slayton, J. M., Steck, T. L., and Lange, Y., unpublished observations.

74. Farquhar, M. G., and Palade, G. E., *J. Cell Biol., 91*:775 (1981).

75. Rothman, J., *Science, 213*:1212 (1981).

76. DeSilva, N. S., and Siu, C. H., *J. Biol. Chem., 256*:5845 (1981).

77. Sleight, R. G., and Pagano, R. E., *J. Biol. Chem., 258*:9050 (1983).

78. Brown, M. S., and Goldstein, J. L., *Science, 191*:150 (1976).

79. Attie, A. D., Pittman, R. C., and Steinberg, D., *Hepatology*, *2*:269 (1982).

80. Stein, Y., Glangeaud, M. C., Fainaru, M., and Stein, O., *Biochim. Biophys. Acta*, *380*:106 (1975).

81. Poznansky, M. J., and Czekanski, S., *Biochim. Biophys. Acta*, *685*:182 (1982).

82. DeGrella, R. F., and Simoni, R. D., *J. Biol. Chem.*, *257*:14,256 (1982).

83. Dempsey, M. E., in *Subunit Enzymes* (Ebner, K., ed.), Marcel Dekker, New York, 1975, pp. 267–306.

84. Tai, H. H., and Bloch, K., *J. Biol. Chem.*, *245*:1670 (1970).

85. Srikantaiah, M. V., Hansbury, E., Loughran, E. D., and Scallen, T. J., *J. Biol. Chem.*, *251*:5496 (1976).

86. Ritter, M. C., and Dempsey, M. E., *Proc. Natl. Acad. Sci. U.S.A.*, *70*:265 (1973).

87. Caras, I. W., Friedlander, E. J., and Bloch, K., *J. Biol. Chem.*, *255*:3575 (1980).

88. Friedlander, E. J., Caras, I. W., Lin, L. F. H., and Bloch, K., *J. Biol. Chem.*, *255*:8042 (1980).

89. Ishibashi, T., and Bloch, K., *J. Biol. Chem.*, *256*:12,962 (1981).

90. Yago, N., and Tchii, S., *J. Biol. Chem. (Tokyo)*, *65*:215 (1969).

91. Jefcoate, C. R., Simpson, E. R., Boyd, G. S., Brownie, A. C., and Orme-Johnson, W. H., *Ann. N.Y. Acad. Sci.*, *212*:243 (1973).

92. Chanderbhan, R., Noland, B. J., Scallen, T. J., and Vahouny, G. V., *J. Biol. Chem.*, *257*:8928 (1982).

93. Privalle, C. T., Crivello, J. F., and Jefcoate, C. R., *Proc. Natl. Acad. Sci. U.S.A.*, *80*:702 (1983).

94. Conneely, O. M., Headon, D. R., Olson, C. D., Ungar, F., and Dempsey, M. E., *Proc. Natl. Acad. Sci. U.S.A.*, *81*:2970 (1984).

8

Glycolipid Dynamics in Serum Lipoproteins

GLYN DAWSON The Pritzker School of Medicine, The University of Chicago, Chicago, Illinois

INTRODUCTION

Human serum lipoproteins contain a mixture of neutral lipids, phospholipids, and glycosphingolipids, organized together with a variety of peptides to form a series of apparently stable particles. Glycosphingolipids (Fig. 1) can be demonstrated to be present on the surface of all types of human serum lipoprotein particles, and although the average number may be as few as one to five molecules per particle, they appear to confer specific biological properties on the lipoproteins.

GLYCOLIPID CHEMISTRY

The most abundant glycosphingolipids in human serum lipoproteins are of the globo series (Table 1; Fig. 2) (1–6), comprising glucosylceramide, lactosylceramide, trihexosylceramide ($GbOse_3Cer$) (7), and tetrahexosylceramide ($GbOse_4Cer$) in declining order of concentration. The hydrophobic ceramide core consists of sphingosine [a long-chain (C_{18}) amino-alcohol] N-acylated at C_2 with a fatty acid of varying chain length (C_{16} to C_{24}) and degree of hydroxylation (Fig. 1). The unsaturated C_4–C_5 bond in sphingosine is of trans configuration—D-erythro-1,3-dihydroxy-2-amino-4-*trans*-octadecene—and determines the characteristic spade shape of monoglycosylceramides. The C_1 hydroxyl group of sphingosine is β-linked O-glycosidically to the first sugar of the carbohydrate chain (glucose or galactose).

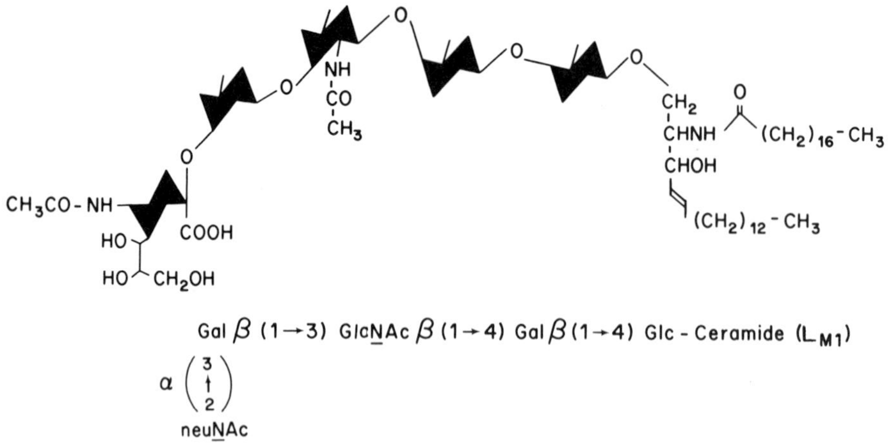

Gal β (1→3) GlcNAc β (1→4) Galβ(1→4) Glc - Ceramide (L_{M1})

α (3 ↑ 2) neuNAc

Fig. 1 Schematic representation of the major complex glycosphingolipid associated with human serum lipoproteins, IV[3]NeuAcLnOse$_4$Cer (IUPAC-IUB nomenclature), also known as sialoparagloboside or LM1 ganglioside.

Trace amounts of fucosylated glycosphingolipids expressing blood group antigens of the ABH or Lewis a or b type have been associated with serum lipoproteins (8), the oligosaccharide units being of the lactoneotetraose (7) (Galβ(1–4)GlcNAcβ(1–4)Gal(β1–4)Glc-ceramide) type in contrast to the GalNAcβ(1–3)Galβ(1–4)Galβ(1-4)Glc-ceramide of the globo (GbOse$_3$) series. The major monosialoganglioside associated with lipoproteins (approximately 35% of the total glycolipid) is G_{M3} (hematoside; II[3]NeuAcLacCer), (Fig. 3) (3). Recently, Kundu et al. (9) have shown that 54% of gangliosides are monosialo; in addition to G_{M3}, these were found to have the structure corresponding to II[3]NeuAcGgOseCer (more commonly referred to as GM_2), IV[3]NeuAcLnOse$_4$Cer [or sialoparagloboside (SPG), or Lm1] (Fig. 1), IV[6]NeuAcLnOse$_4$Cer, and the more complex sialosyllacto-N-*nor*-hexaosylceramide and sialosyllacto-N-*iso*-octaosylceramides (Table 2). Megaglycolipid with 20 or more repeating [Gal-GlcNAc] units (10) may also be associated with lipoproteins. Polysialogangliosides are mainly of the ganglio-N-tetraose type (e.g., SPG) (Fig. 3) found in high concentration in brain such as G_{D3}, G_{D1a}, G_{D1b}, G_{T1b}, and G_{Q1b} (Fig. 3), but the quantities are immensely small. Since LDL contains only 5 mol of glycolipid/particle (3) and HDL only 1 to 2 mol/particle (3), there is obviously tremendous heterogeneity among lipoprotein particles. Thus far, it has not been possible to isolate glycolipid-enriched lipoprotein

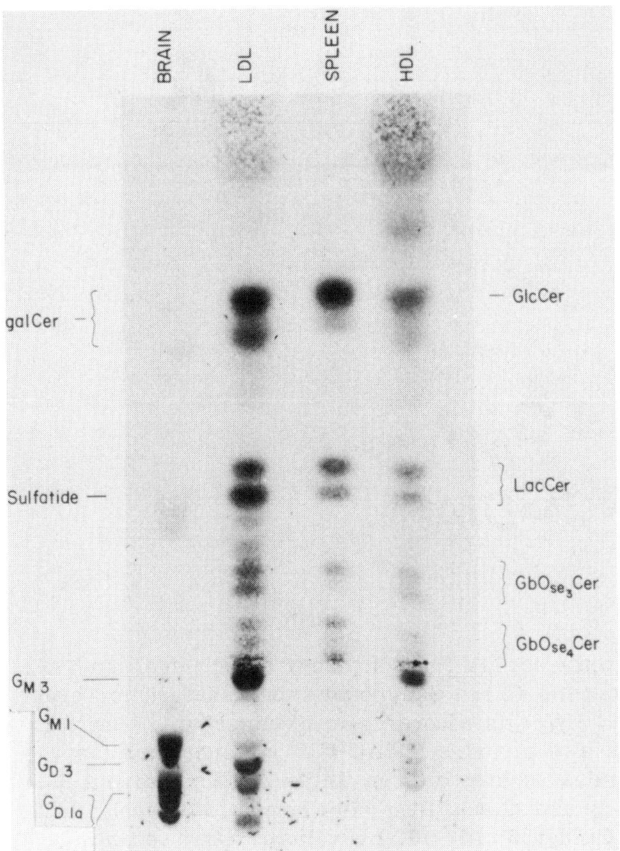

Fig. 2 Thin-layer chromatogram of the neutral glycolipids associated with the major human serum lipoproteins LDL and HDL. Neutral glycolipid nomenclature is according to the globo series in IUPAC-IUB nomenclature. Solvent system used was $CHCl_3$:CH_3OH:H_2O (100:42:6, by volume). Glycolipids were visualized by the orcinol method.

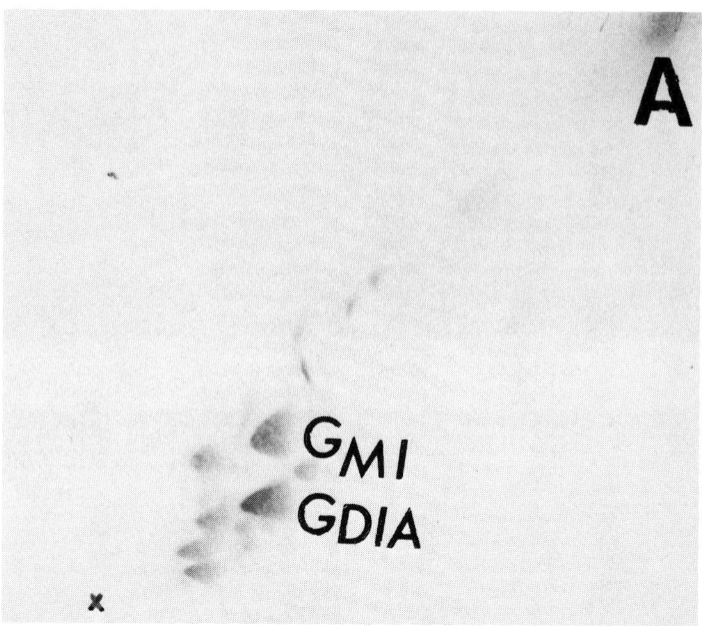

Fig. 3 Sialoglycosphingolipids (gangliosides) of human brain (A), plasma (B), and red cells (C). Ganglioside nomenclature for brain gangliosides G_{M1} and G_{D1A} is according to Svennerholm; that for plasma and red cells also includes IUPAC-IUB nomenclature for lacto-series gangliosides as identified in Table 2. The solvent system used for A, B and C was first development (vertical), $CHCl_3$:CH_3OH:0.2% $CaCl_2$(55:-45:-10, by volume); and second development (horizontal), $CHCl_3$:CH_3OH:2.5 *M* NH_4OH in 0.2% KCl (50:40:10, by volume). Gangliosides were visualized by the resorcinol method.

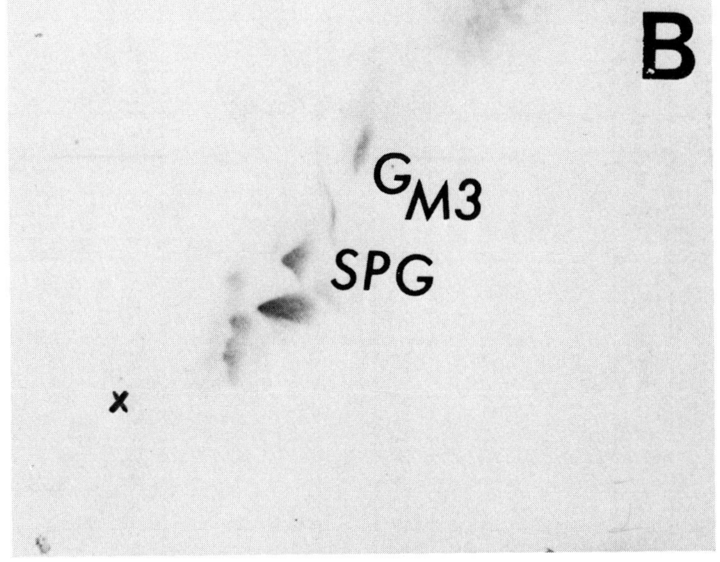

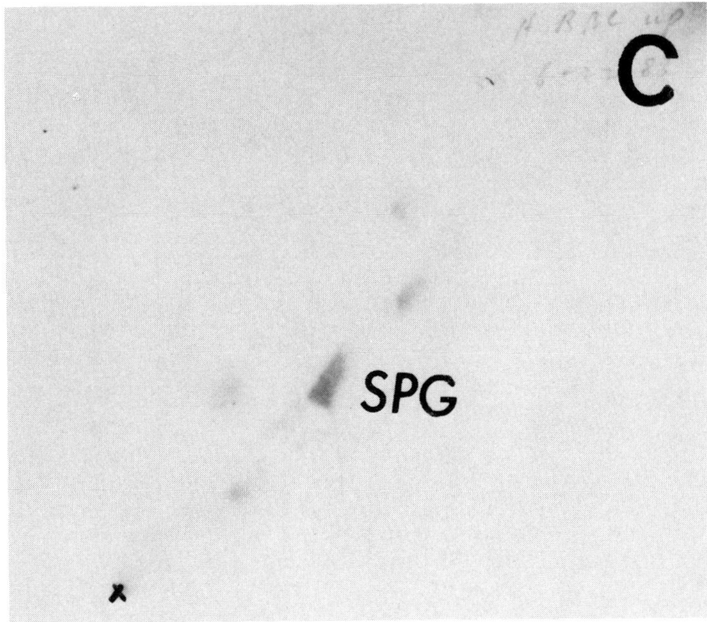

Fig. 3 (Continued)

Table 1 Major Glycolipids of Human Plasma, Erythrocytes, Platelets, and Plasma

		mol %				
		GlcCer	LacCer	$GbOse_3Cer$	$GbOse_4Cer$	G_{M3}
Plasma[a]		22	17	6	5	50
Erythrocytes		7	13	10	67	3
Platelets		3	64	17	16	ND
Leukocytes		5	48	0	0	47
Fatty Acid Chain Length Distribution						
Total fatty acid (%)						
Plasma	C_{16-18}	57	62	61	60	ND
	C_{22-24}	43	38	39	40	ND
Erythrocytes	C_{16-18}	27	45	31	20	ND
	C_{22-24}	73	55	69	80	ND

[a]Similar ratios in VLDL, LDL, and HDL: an average of 1 GSL/VLDL particle, 5 GSL/LDL particle, and 1.5 GSL/HDL particle.

Table 2 Structure of Lipoprotein-Associated Glycolipids

Type	Structure	Designation
Globo	Glc-Cer	
	Gal-Glc-Cer	
	Gal-Gal-Glc-Cer	$GbOse_3$
	GalNAc-Gal-Gal-Glc-Cer	$GbOse_4$(globotetraosyl-)
Lacto	Gal(1–4)GlcNAc(1–3)Gal-Glc-Cer	$LcnOse_4$(lactoneotetraosyl-)
	[Gal-GlcNAc]$_2$Gal-Glc-Cer	$LcOse_6$(lacto-nor-hexaosyl-)
	Gal-GlcNAc(1–6) > Gal-GlcNAc-Gal-Glc-Cer	
	Gal-GlcNAc(1–3)	$LcOse_8$(lacto-n-iso-octaosyl-)
	Fuc-[Gal-GlcNAc]$_2$Gal-Glc-Cer	Blood group antigens (A, B, H, Le, etc.)
	NeuAc 2–3 $LcnOse_4$Cer	SPG
	NeuAc 2–6 $LcnOse_4$Cer	SPG
Gala	GalCer	$GaOse_1$
Ganglio	NeuAc-Gal-Glc-Cer	G_{M3}
	GalNAc[NeuAc]Gal-Glc-Cer	G_{M2}
	Gal-GalNAc[NeuAc]Gal-Glc-Cer	G_{M1}
	NeuAc-NeuAc-Gal-Glc-Cer	G_{D3}
	NeuAc-Gal-GalNAc[NeuAc]Gal-Glc-Cer	G_{D1a}
	Gal-GalNAc[NeuAc-NeuAc]Gal-Glc-Cer	G_{D1b}
	NeuAc-Gal-GalNAc[NeuAc-NeuAc[Gal-Glc-Cer	G_{T1b}
	NeuAc-NeuAc-Gal-GalNAc[NeuAc-NeuAc]Gal-Glc-Cer or II^3(NeuAc)$_2$, IV^3(NeuAc)$_2$GgOse_4-Cer	G_{Q1b}

particles but these, if they in fact exist, could have important functional significance. The minor fucoglycosphingolipid (blood group active) and sialoglycosphingolipid (ganglioside) species appear to be the most biologically active glycolipids. As examples of this, red cells can acquire blood group specificity (e.g., B glycolipid) from serum (18), and cholera toxin-insensitive cells can acquire gangliosides such as G_{M1} (II^3NeuAcGgOse$_4$Cer with the structural sequence Gal-GalNAc-[NeuAc]Gal-Glc-ceramide) from serum lipoproteins (11) and thereby acquire full adenylate cyclase sensitivity to cholera toxin. Similarly, Sendai virus (SV)-insensitive cells can acquire G_{D1a} from serum and become fully sensitive to SV (12).

GLYCOLIPID STRUCTURE

The glycolipids found in serum lipoproteins range from the hydrophobic glucosylceramide, with a closely packed hydrophobic core and three-dimensional structure very similar to sphingomyelin, to hydrophilic gangliosides that can exist in aqueous solution at concentrations below 1 μM (the critical micelle concentration for most gangliosides) (13). The properties of individual gangliosides will therefore depend on both the number of sugar residues present and the stereochemical arrangement of the individual sugars; both are believed to confer biological specificity (14–16). The ceramide moiety can function as both a hydrogen bond donor and acceptor because of the hydroxyl (always unsubstituted) and amino groups in the sphingosine moiety. Recent studies (17) have attributed some biological specificity to the ceramide moiety in terms of enzyme (glycosyltransferase) recognition. Both the trans double bond between C_4 and C_5 of the sphingosine and the 2-D-hydroxyl fatty acid found in some glycolipids promote condensation of the ceramide packing at air-liquid interfaces (Fig. 4). Hydroxyl groups appear to be important for lateral interactions between individual glycolipids involving hydrogen bonding. Those tissues that are exposed to physical stress, such as erythrocytes, intestinal membranes, and kidney renal tubules, are heavily hydroxylated on both C_4 of sphingosine (phytosphingosine) and the α-position of the fatty acid (18), whereas serum lipoprotein glycolipids are not and α-hydroxy fatty acids are rarely found. In view of their structural properties, glycosphingolipids appear to be ideally suited to function as integral membrane components that interact with surface proteins, such as apoB, and as boundary lipids (18).

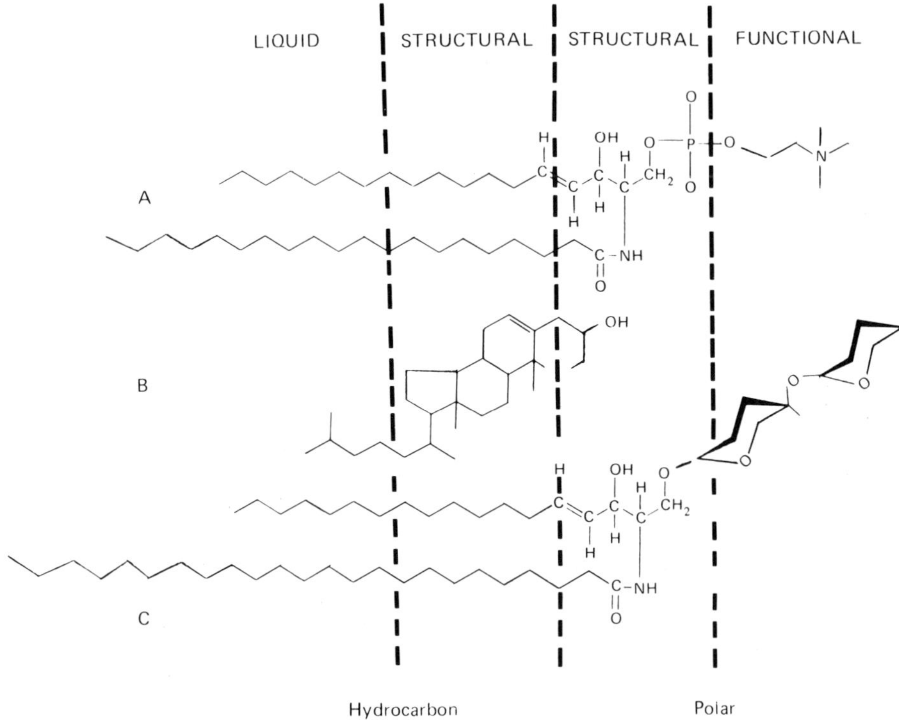

Fig. 4 Schematic representation of the orientation of sphingomyelin (A), cholesterol (B), and lactosylceramide (C) in a membrane or lipoprotein particle surface. Sphingomyelin (A) contains C_{18}-sphingosine and $C_{18:0}$ fatty acid; the glycosphingolipid lactosylceramide (C) contains C_{18}-sphingosine and $C_{24:0}$ fatty acid. Liquid, structural and functional regions are ascribed according to Ref. 18.

PHYSICAL PROPERTIES

Phase transition describes a state in which the hydrocarbon chains of a lipid such as ceramide undergo structural changes from gel to liquid phase. At low molar concentrations, both neutral glycolipids such as glucosylceramide and sialoglycolipids such as G_{M1} are readily miscible with phospholipids and in fact help to stabilize phospholipid dispersions (15,16). At higher G_{M1} concentrations (above 24 mol %), the transition temperature increases, suggesting the same type of stabilizing role for glycolipids as previously observed with cholesterol and membrane proteins. It is also possible that transient changes in the glycolipid-phospholipid ratio can induce the formation of nonbilayer structures (19), which could facilitate cell fusion or membrane transport of lipoproteins.

When spin-labeled gangliosides (labeled in the polar head group) were incorporated into egg PC unilamellar vesicles (at 2 mol %), the ESR readings were consistent with high mobility and a concentration-dependent cooperative interaction as a result of hydrogen bonding between the oligosaccharide units. These intermolecular reactions could be disrupted by either calcium ions or N-acetylhexosamine-specific lectins. Thus, the physical properties of glycolipids are to a large extent determined by the nature of the oligosaccharide units. Recent studies (20) with glycolipids and egg phosphatidylcholine multilamellar liposomes using freeze-etch electron microscopy suggest that, below the main transition temperature, neutral glycolipids (up to tetrahexosylceramides) form domains in linear patterns between the phospholipid ridges. In contrast, dimyristoylphosphatidylcholine (DMPC) liposomes containing up to 10 mol % of sialoglycosphingolipid such as G_{M1} ganglioside, and quenched below the main transition temperature, showed only a random distribution (as judged by ferritin-cholera toxin labeling). Above the main phase transition, neutral glycolipid showed a clustered arrangement, whereas G_{M1} again appeared to be organized in an evenly dispersed manner in both DMPC and POPC liposomes. However, the dispersion of G_{M1} can be specifically altered by the addition of G_{M1}-specific proteins such as cholera toxin. Thus, cholera toxin induces capping of fluorescent-labeled anti-G_{M1} antibodies in lymphocytes, but shows no affinity for G_{M1}-deficient lymphocytes—unless they have acquired G_{M1} following preincubation with human serum lipoproteins. It is also probable that the physical properties of glycolipids can be modified by interaction with membrane proteins.

GLYCOLIPIDS OF SERUM

Human serum contains approximately 20 μg/ml of glycolipid, virtually all of which is associated with the lipoprotein fractions. In normal males, most of the glycolipid is associated with the LDL (d = 1.006 to 1.063 g/ml) fraction rather than the HDL (d = 1.063 to 1.21 g/ml) fraction, but the relative amounts of the major glycolipids in each lipoprotein fraction are the same (3). In homozygous familial hypercholesterolemia, the elevation of serum glycolipids was directly proportional to the elevation of serum LDL, and isolated LDL had a normal glycolipid composition (3). However, in abetalipoproteinemia, the virtual absence of LDL was not accompanied by a dramatic reduction in serum glycolipid. This was explained by purifying HDL from these patients and showing it to be greatly enriched in glycolipid (3). Such studies suggested a role for plasma glycolipid homeostasis and that the role of glycolipid in HDL was different from that in LDL. At present, this role is hard to define. Clarke et al. (21) studied the turnover (clearance rate) of ^{125}I-labeled normal human LDL and ^{131}I-labeled glycolipid-enriched (human Fabry) LDL in dogs and found no significant differences. Dawson and Sweeley (22) administered [^{14}C]glucose intravenously to a pig (whose blood glycolipids are very similar to those of humans) and followed the appearance and disappearance of label from plasma and erythrocytes. They observed rapid incorporation into plasma glycolipids, reaching a maximum in all species after 24 hr, followed by a rapid decline with a half-life of 4 to 6 days, similar to that of human apo B (4 to 5 days). This presumably represents hepatic synthesis of glycolipid packaged into LDL. Erythrocyte glycolipids were not labeled maximally until 8 days, apart from glucosylceramide, where the label appeared exchangeable with the lipoprotein pool. Label in $GbOse_4Cer$ and $GbOse_3Cer$ remained high for 50 to 70 days, the normal erythrocyte life span in pigs, after which a rapid decline was apparent. This loss of label was concomitant with a rise in previously unlabeled plasma glycolipids, suggesting that some plasma lipoprotein glycolipid is derived from senescent erythrocyte membranes. Because of the tremendous species variation in the type and quantity of serum glycolipids, it is not possible to generalize on the role of serum glycolipids (23). However, similar studies carried out on pigs and rabbits have yielded essentially the same results and have suggested further that lipoprotein glycolipids are taken up and metabolized, at least in part, by vascular tissue.

GLYCOLIPIDS OF CELLS

As with plasma lipoprotein particles, cellular glycolipids can be shown to be expressed on the surface by labeling with the galactose oxidase-NaB^3H_4 technique, which specifically labels terminal galactose and GalNAc residues. Studies with erythrocytes showed that right-side-out ghost preparations contained exposed glycolipids, whereas inside-out ghost preparations could not be labeled by this technique (24). Subsequent studies on other types of cells suggested that most glycolipids are exposed on the outer surface of the plasma membrane and therefore come into direct contact with serum lipoproteins. Erythrocytes, platelets, lymphocytes, and monocytes have characteristic glycolipid compositions that also differ from those of serum lipoproteins (Table 1). At least 80 different glycosphingolipids have been identified in human tissues, many of them detectable in only fetal or transformed (tumor) cells. The glycolipid composition of nervous tissue changes with age, but similar age-related changes have not been reported for other tissues or for serum.

GLYCOLIPID DYNAMICS

Synthesis

Glycolipids appear to be synthesized in the endoplasmic reticulum-Golgi complex by the stepwise addition of sugars from activated nucleotide sugar donors (such as uridine diphosphate glucose, galactose, GlcNAc or GalNAc, CMP-NeuAc, and GDP-Fuc) (Fig. 5) by complexes of glycosyltransferase enzymes (25). There is no evidence for the involvement of polyisoprenoid (dolichol) intermediates, although structural studies indicating the occurrence of double inversions as in the synthesis of $GbOse_cCer$ (GalαGalβGlc-ceramide) remain to be explained. Rosenberg et al. (26) have recently used monensin, a calcium ionophore that appears to block vesicle transfer from endoplasmic reticulum to Golgi, to show separate sites of synthesis of neutral and sialoglycosphingolipids. Thus, monensin blocked ganglioside synthesis (implying that GalNAc transferase and sialotransferase are Golgi enzymes), but enhanced de novo synthesis of glucosyl- and lactosylceramide (implying that these transferases are ER localized). Similarly, monensin has been observed by us to block sulfogalactosylceramide synthesis, but not galactosylceramide synthesis in oligodendroglioma cells, implying that the former is a Golgi enzyme and the latter an endoplasmic reticulum enzyme—in common with the phospholipid and neutral lipid synthesizing enzymes (36). Others have presented evidence for the cell surface localization of some glycosyltransferases, especially sialotransferases (which are generally believed to be trans-Golgi localized), but interpretation of these data is complicated by various technical problems such as the availability of nucleotide sugars for cell surface synthesis.

There is good evidence that glycolipid synthesis is cell-cycle dependent, reaching a maximum in S/G_2 phase just prior to cell division (27). In certain tissues, such as brain and kidney, some glycolipid synthesis is under the control of hydrocortisone and testosterone, respectively. For example, sulfogalactosylceramide synthesis can be shown to be dramatically enhanced in oligodendroglioma cells by the addition of hydrocortisone to the culture medium (28). Furthermore, normal fatty acid (Nfa)-GalCer, Nfa-$GaOse_2Cer$, and α-hydroxy fatty acid (Hfa)-$GaOse_2Cer$ are all synthesized in the kidneys of male C57BL/6J mice, but not in female mice unless

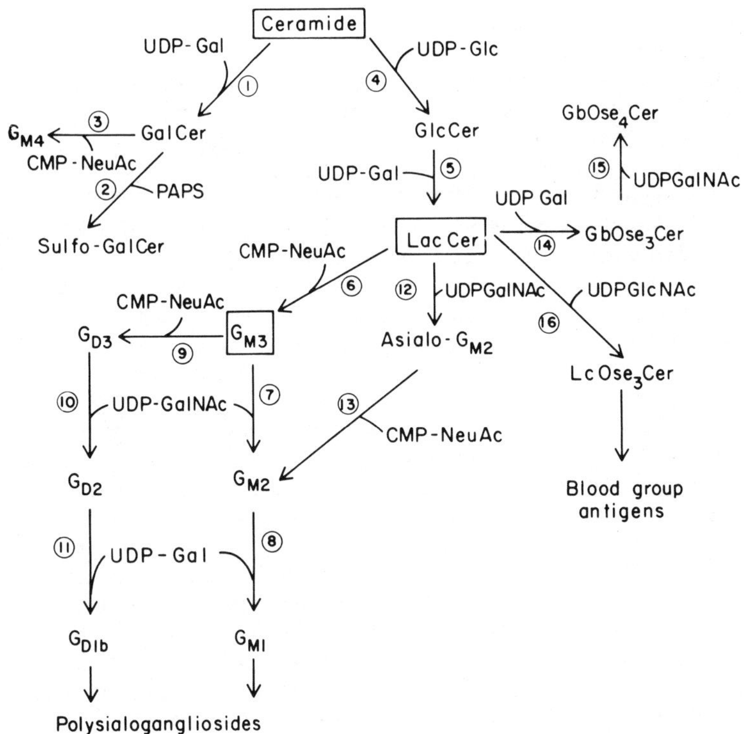

Fig. 5 Biosynthetic pathway for the major lipoprotein-associated glycolipids. Transferases 1 to 3 are expressed mainly in myelinating tissue, but the glycolipids are detectable in small amounts in lipoproteins. Transferases 4, 5, 7 to 9, and 14 to 16 are expressed in liver, bone marrow intestine, etc., and are responsible for synthesis of the major lipoprotein glycolipids. Transferases 10 to 13 appear to be neuron-specific.

testosterone is given (29–31). Female kidney compensates somewhat with a higher rate of HfaGlcCer synthesis, but digalactosylceramide is only synthesized following testosterone administration. Although we find small differences in glycolipid content between male and female lipoprotein glycolipids, it is not clear that these are statistically significant. They may simply represent the different LDL to HDL ratios observed in males and females or be of dietary origin.

Certain glycosyltransferases such as UDP GalNAc:G_{M3}:N-acetylgalactosaminyltransferase have been shown to be highly active in nervous tissue and almost undetectable in extraneural tissues such as liver; to be inactivated following cell transformation with DNA and RNA viruses (32); and to be cyclic AMP sensitive (33). The latter implies regulation by a cyclic AMP-dependent protein kinase and there is an increasing amount of circumstantial evidence in favor of this idea. Compounds such as prostaglandins and cholera toxin, which elevate cyclic AMP levels, as well as cyclic AMP analogs such as Bt_2cAMP and 8BrcAMP tend to stimulate ganglioside synthesis, whereas inhibitors inhibit synthesis (33,34). In vitro studes of G_{M3} and G_{M2} synthesis show activation by A-kinase and inactivation by alkaline phosphatase (35), but better purified enzyme preparations are needed. Although there is no evidence that lipoprotein apoproteins in any way regulate adenylate cyclase activity, we have previously shown that human serum high-density lipoprotein-3 (HDL_3) specifically stimulated glycosphingolipid and sphingomyelin synthesis in both human granulocytes and cultured skin fibroblasts, whereas LDL had no effect (37). The mechanism of this biosynthetic stimulation is not clear, but was accompanied by the specific degradation of apo A-II, recently shown (38) to be the result of the release of a specific elastaselike proteolytic activity from granulocytes.

Glycolipid Catabolism

Glycosphingolipids are catabolized within lysosomes by the sequential action of a group of highly specific glycosidases with an acidic pH optimum (Fig. 6). The lysosomal hydrolases are glycoproteins bearing specific mannose-6-phosphate-terminal sugar residues that function as a targeting device to direct the enzymes, following vesicle acidification, to the lysosome organelle (39). Most glycolipid hydrolases require the co-presence of a specific activator protein (essentially a glycolipid-binding protein) for effective hydrolysis (40). Inherited mutations result in failures of hydrolase synthesis, defective post-translational modifications, defective activator proteins, or premature degradation by proteases, and are expressed clinically as neurovisceral storage diseases—the sphingolipidoses (Fig. 6) and related oligosaccharidoses and mucopolysaccharidoses. Inherited defects of glucocerebrosidase (Gaucher disease) and $GbOse_3Cer$ α-galactosidase

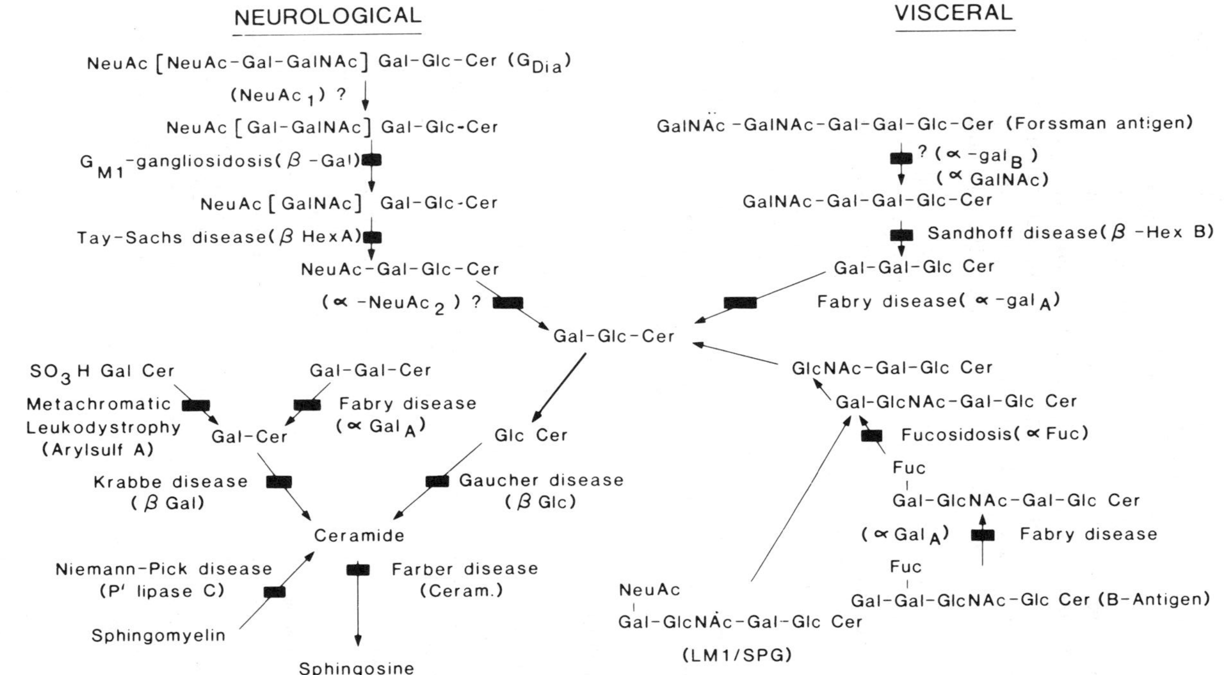

Fig. 6 Catabolic pathway for the major lipoprotein-associated glycolipids showing the site of inherited genetic defects of specific lysosomal hydrolases. Enzymes involved are indicated in parentheses; e.g., in Gaucher disease, the defective enzyme is β-glucosidase (βGlc), and the stored glycolipid is GlcDer. A question mark indicates that a genetic defect has been postulated but not described.

(Fabry disease) result in lipoprotein abnormalities and will be discussed more fully in the section on pathogenesis.

Glycolipids are intrinsic components of plasma membranes, especially the coated pits, and are thus being continually internalized, acidified, and either recycled or degraded. Chatterjee et al. (41) have shown that LDL, taken up through the "receptor-independent" pathway in homozygous familial hypercholesterolemic (HFH) fibroblasts, promotes the storage of $GbOse_3Cer$ in granular perinuclear intracytoplasmic fluorescent bodies and contributes to cellular abnormalities in HFH and possibly other forms of atherosclerosis. Patel et al. (42) have shown by the use of monensin (which at 10 μM disrupts normal intracellular proton gradients and hence the translocation of receptor-bound ligand, e.g., LDL from endosomes to lysosomes) that internalized sphingolipids (in pino-, endo-, or receptosomes) are normally catabolized by lysosomes. Thus, lipoprotein-associated glycolipid is a major source of viscerally stored glycolipid in lysosomal storage diseases, and many groups have attempted to show that reduced serum glycolipid levels are proof of effective enzyme replacement therapy in diseases such as Gaucher and Fabry.

Glycolipid Exchange

We previously showed that HDL_3 promoted de novo glycosphingolipid synthesis and that HDL_3 was able to acquire some of this newly synthesized glycolipid (37). The transfer of glycolipid from egg phosphatidylcholine liposomes to HDL_3 in an HDL_3 concentration-dependent manner (saturating at 60 to 70% transfer) was also observed with these synthetic vesicles (43,44). The time for exchange of 50% of the glycolipid [either neutral (GalCer) or acidic (G_{M1})] was in the range of 3 to 6 hr, which is in the same time frame as reported for phospholipid exchange between PC-cholesterol-mixed vesicles and bovine HDL. Efficient transfer of GSL from GSL-coated hydrophobic glass beads to HDL was also achieved, but similar silicone-bead treatment disrupted the LDL complex and caused denaturation (45). However, we were able to show that [^{3}H]GSL introduced into HDL_3 in this manner could be reversibly exchanged with LDL. Since HDL, rather than LDL, appears to be a mediator of GSL transport and synthesis, LDL (with a 4-day half-life) offers a readily available source of GSL for the HDL particle. Our data suggest that a net movement of GSL from LDL to HDL occurs in vivo. In contrast to phosphatidylcholine, which is totally exchangeable, the major sphingolipids (sphingomyelin and glycolipids) are only partially exchangeable (45) (about one-third of the total pool), suggesting that some protein, perhaps apo B or apo A-II, is regulating the exchange. In the past few years, a number of laboratories have purified both specific and nonspecific "glycolipid transport proteins" from serum and tissues. Thus, the 20- to 25-kDa protein purified by Metz and Radin (46) from spleen appeared specific for glucosylceramide, whereas a similarly sized protein purified by Bloj and Zilversmit (47) from liver stimulated phospholipid transfort as well. Wong et al. (48) have recently reported the purification of an 18.2-kDa glycolipid-specific transfer protein from bovine brain which does not enhance phospholipid transfer under conditions where both donor and acceptor matrix phospholipids were in the liquid crystalline phase. Apo A-I, the major apoprotein component of HDL, with a molecular weight of 27 kDa (49) has been shown to be able to acquire GSL from both LDL- and GSL-coated glass beads, as well as to displace endogenous apo A-I from HDL particles. Thus, it is possible that the apo A-I acts as a GSL exchange protein in human serum and may have a key role in cell-GSL-lipoprotein dynamics.

What could be the purpose of GSL exchange proteins in serum? We have previously discussed that cells can acquire new receptors and antigens from serum lipoproteins rich in apo A-I. Exogenous glycolipids can also inhibit cell growth and modify DNA synthesis. Thus, Bremer et al. (50) have shown that exogenously derived G_{M1} was able to inhibit the growth of 3T3 cells by inhibiting platelet-derived growth factor (PDGF)-stimulated DNA synthesis (but not PDGF binding) by inhibiting PDGF-stimulated kinase activity. In contrast, G_{M3} ganglioside inhibited both PDGF and epidermal growth factor (EGF)-stimulated DNA synthesis and both protein kinases. The G_{M3} (and not a wide variety of other gangliosides) could reduce EGF-stimulated in vitro tyrosine kinase activity in A431 cell membranes. None of the glycolipids tested bound directly to either of the growth factors.

GLYCOLIPIDS AND PATHOGENESIS

Storage Diseases

As discussed previously, Fabry disease and Gaucher disease are characterized by excess plasma glycolipid ($GbOse_3Cer$ and GlcCer, respectively) (51), which is distributed among the various serum lipoprotein fractions in the same relative proportions as normal individuals. This means that most of the "storage" glycolipid is associated with the LDL fraction (3,52,53). In neither disease is an elevated level of glycolipid seen in erythrocytes, whereas all cells containing functional lysosomes accumulate the specific glycolipid within these organelles. The two- to eight-fold elevation of serum glucosylceramide in Gaucher disease (52) was observed in patients who had previously undergone a splenectomy and, since

LDL is the major GSL transport particle, most of this excess GlcCer was on the surface of the LDL particle and was packaged into LDL either in hepatocytes (following exchange with GlcCer-engorged Kupffer cells) or by exchange with circulating cells such as leukocytes, which are also enriched in GlcCer. Glycolipids may therefore play a significant role in the aortic degeneration and other circulatory problems associated with Gaucher disease.

Hyperlipoproteinemias

As discussed previously, the GSL content of LDL isolated from homo- or heterozygous familial hypercholesterolemic serum appeared normal, but serum GSL levels were elevated in direct proportion to the elevation of serum LDL. Chatterjee et al. (54) have observed increased urinary excretion of GSL in HFH patients, suggesting lysosomal accumulation in renal tissues. Their data indicated a defect in GSL metabolism in familial hypercholesterolemia and that plasma exchange therapy was able to decrease urinary GSL excretion. The role, if any, of glycosphingolipids in atherosclerotic plaque formation is not clear at the present time, although the high affinity of the sphingolipid, phosphorylcholine-ceramide (sphingomyelin) for cholesterol is well documented from studies on Niemann-Pick tissue (55), acanthyocytic red cells (56), and hairy-cell leukemic cells (57). The high SM/PC [and GSL/PC (3)] ratio in HDL of acanthocytic patients probably determines the ratio in red cells since LDL is virtually absent in these patients (3). Glycosphingolipids are known to have a profound effect on both cell growth and differentiation, and an excess amount of exchangeable GSL on excess LDL particles in homozygous familial hypercholesterolemia could be one additional triggering factor in atherogenesis.

Hypolipoproteinemias

In the hypolipoproteinemias, GSL is enriched in the HDL fractions so that serum GSL levels are only slightly lower than the normal range. One of the main pathological hallmarks of abetalipoproteinemia is demyelination of peripheral nerves, suggesting that serum LDL is a source of cholesterol for maintaining peripheral myelin. However, since demyelination can be prevented clinically by administration of tocopherols (believed to stabilize membranes and retard oxidative degradation), the mechanism of this is somewhat obscure (58). Recent clinical trials aimed at establishing the therapeutic benefits of gangliosides (claimed to promote neurite formation in vitro) in treating patients with peripheral neuropathies may indicate a role for lipoprotein gangliosides in maintaining nerve function. In addition, there have been reports (59), which we have confirmed, that certain patients with Waldenstrom's macroglobulinemia produce a monoclonal antibody (in serum), which is directed against the carbohydrate of myelin-associated glycoprotein (MAG) and a peripheral nerve-specific ganglioside, causing a peripheral neuropathy. There is no evidence as yet that loss of glycolipid is of primary pathogenic importance, although glycolipids typically constitute 25% of the lipid of the myelin sheath, a much greater proportion than the 2 to 5% in typical cell membranes. The presence of antiglycolipid antibodies in serum is being actively sought in a whole range of demyelinating diseases, and may eventually indicate an additional important role for lipoprotein glycolipids.

REFERENCES

1. Svennerholm, E., and Svennerholm, L., *Nature (London)*, *198*:688 (1963).
2. Vance, D. E., and Sweeley, C. C., *J. Lipid Res.*, *8*:621 (1967).
3. Dawson, G., Kruski, A. W., and Scanu, A. M., *J. Lipid Res.*, *17*:125 (1976).
4. Clarke, J. T. R., Stoltz, J. M., and Mulcahey, M. R., *Biochim. Biophys. Acta*, *431*:317 (1976).
5. Van den Bergh, F. A. J. T. M., and Tager, J. M., *Biochim. Biophys. Acta*, *441*:391 (1976).
6. Chatterjee, S., and Kwiterovich, P. O., *Lipids*, *11*:462 (1976).
7. IUPAC-IUB Commission on Biochemical Nomenclature, *Hoppe-Seyler's Z. Physiol. Chem.*, *358*:617 (1977).
8. Marcus, D. M., and Cass, L. E., *Science*, *164*:553 (1969).
9. Kundu, S. K., Diego, I., Osovitz, S., and Marcus, D. M., *Fed. Proc.*, *43*:859 (1984).
10. Koscielak, J., Maslinski, W., Zielenski, J., Zdebska, E., Brudzynski, T., Miller-Podraza, M., and Cedergen, B., *Biochim. Biophys. Acta*, *530*:385 (1978).
11. Fishman, P. H., Bradley, R. M., Moss, J., and Manganiello, V. C., *J. Lipid Res.*, *19*:77 (1978).
12. Holmgren, J., Svennerholm, L., Elwing, H., Fredman, P., and Stanngard, O., *Proc. Natl. Acad. Sci. U.S.A.*, *77*:1947 (1980).
13. Yohe, M. C., Roark, D. E., and Rosenberg, A., *J. Biol. Chem.*, *251*:7083 (1976).

14. Pascher, I., and Sundell, S., *Chem. Phys. Lipids*, *20*:175 (1977).

15. Barenholz, Y., and Thompson, T. E., *Biochim. Biophys. Acta*, *604*:129 (1980).

16. Maggio, B., Cumar, F. A., and Caputto, R., *Biochim. Biophys. Acta*, *650*:69 (1981).

17. Hakomori, S. I., *Ann. Rev. Biochem.*, *50*:733 (1981).

18. Karlsson, K. A., in *Structure of Biological Membranes*, (Abrahammson, S., and Pascher, I., eds.), Plenum Press, New York, 1977, pp. 245–274.

19. DeKruijff, B., Cullis, P. R., and Verkleij, A. J., *Trends in Biochem. Sci.*, *5*:79 (1980).

20. Tillack, T. W., Brown, R. E., Allietta, M., and Thompson, T. E., *Fed. Proc.*, *43*:856 (1984).

21. Clarke, J. T. R., Stoltz, J. M., and Garner, J. B., *Atherosclerosis*, *35*:155 (1980).

22. Dawson, G., and Sweeley, C. C., *J. Biol. Chem.*, *245*:410 (1970).

23. Clarke, J. T. R., *Can. J. Biochem.*, *59*:412 (1981).

24. Steck, T. L., and Dawson, G., *J. Biol. Chem.*, *245*:2139 (1974).

25. Dawson, G., in *The Glycoconjugates*, Vol. 2, Academic Press, New York, 1978, pp. 255–286.

26. Saito, M., Saito, M., and Rosenberg, A., *Biochemistry*, *23*:1043 (1984).

27. Scheideler, M. A., Lockney, M. W., and Dawson, G., *J. Neurochem.* *42*:1175 (1984).

28. Dawson, G., and Kernes, S. M., *J. Biol. Chem.*, *254*:163 (1979).

29. Coles, L., Hay, J. B., and Gray, G. M., *J. Lipid Res.*, *11*:158 (1970).

30. McCluer, R. H., Williams, M. A., Gross, S. K., and Meisler, M. H., *J. Biol. Chem.*, *256*:13,112 (1981).

31. Gross, S. K., and McCluer, R. H., *Fed. Proc.*, *43*:869 (1984).

32. Brady, R. O., and Fishman, P. H., *Biochim. Biophys. Acta*, *355*:121 (1974).

33. McLawhon, R. W., Schoon, G. S., and Dawson, G., *J. Neurochem.*, *37*:132 (1981).

34. McLawhon, R. W., Schoon, G. S., and Dawson, G., *Eur. J. Cell. Biol.*, *25*:353 (1981).

35. Burczak, J. D., Fairley, J. L., and Sweeley, C. C., *Fed. Proc.*, *43*:873 (1984).

36. Pelech, S. L., and Vance, D. E., *J. Biol. Chem.*, *257*:14,198 (1982).

37. Kwok, B. C. P., Dawson, G., and Ritter, M. C., *J. Biol. Chem.*, *256*:92 (1981).

38. Byrne, R., Polacek, D., Gordon, J. I., and Scanu, A. M., *J. Biol. Chem.*, *259*:14537 (1984).

39. Sly, W. S., and Fischer, M. D., *J. Cell Biochem.*, *18*:67 (1983).

40. Li, S. C., Hirabayashi, Y., and Li, Y.-T., *J. Biol. Chem.*, *256*:6234 (1982).

41. Chatterjee, S., Gupta, P., and Kwiterovich, Jr., P. O., *Fed. Proc.*, *43*:867 (1984).

42. Patel, S. C., Das, P. K., Sorrell, S. H., and Barranger, J. A., *Fed. Proc.*, *43*:868 (1984).

43. Kwok, B. C. P., Shen, B. W., and Dawson, G., *J. Biol. Chem.*, *256*:9698 (1981).

44. Shen, B. W., Kwok, B. C. P., and Dawson, G., *J. Biol. Chem.*, *256*:9705 (1981).

45. Loeb, J. A., and Dawson, G., *J. Biol. Chem.*, *257*:11,982 (1982).

46. Metz, R. J., and Radin, N. S., *J. Biol. Chem.*, *255*:4463 (1980).

47. Bloj, B., and Zilversmit, D. B., *J. Biol. Chem.*, *256*:5988 (1981).

48. Wong, M., Brown, R., Barenholz, Y., and Thompson, T. E., *Fed. Proc.*, *43*:864 (1984).

49. Scanu, A. M., Edelstein, C., and Keim, P., in *The Plasma Proteins* (Putnam, F. W., ed.), Academic Press, New York, 1975, pp. 317–391.

50. Bremer, E. G., Hakomori, S. I., Bowen-Pope, D. F., Raines, E., and Ross, R., *Fed. Proc.*, *43*:866 (1984).

51. Vance, D. E., Krivit, W., and Sweeley, C. C., *J. Lipid Res.*, *10*:188 (1969).

52. Dawson, G., and Oh, J. Y., *Clin. Chim. Acta*, *75*:149 (1977).

53. Clarke, J. T. R., Stoltz, J. M., and Mulcahey, M. R., *Biochim. Biophys. Acta, 431*:317 (1976).

54. Chatterjee, S., Sekerke, C. S., and Kwiterovic, Jr., P. O., *J. Lipid Res., 23*:513 (1982).

55. Brady, R. O., in *The Metabolic Basis of Inherited Disease* (Stanbury, J. B., Wyngaarden, J. B., and Fredrickson, D. S., eds.), McGraw-Hill, New York, 1978, p. 718.

56. Barenholz, Y., Yechiel, E., Cohen, R., and Deckelbaum, R. J., *Cell Biophys., 3*:115 (1981).

57. Golomb, H. M., Saffold, C. W., Nathans, A. M., and Dawson, G., *Clin. Chim. Acta, 116*:311 (1981).

58. Illingworth, D. R., Orwoll, E. S., and Connor, W. E., *J. Clin. Endocrinol. Metab., 50*:977 (1980).

59. Ilyas, A. A., Quarles, R. H., MacIntosh, T. D., Dobersen, M. J., Trapp, B. D., Dalakas, M. C., and Brady, R. O., *Proc. Natl. Acad. Sci. U.S.A., 81*:1225 (1984).

9

Lecithin Cholesterol Acyltransferase and Cholesteryl Ester Transfer/Exchange Proteins

JAMAL FAROOQUI and ANGELO M. SCANU The Pritzker School of Medicine, The University of Chicago, Chicago, Illinois

INTRODUCTION

The largest percentage of cholesterol in plasma is in the form of cholesteryl esters. Under normolipidemic conditions, these esters are generated by the action of the enzyme lecithin-cholesterol acyltransferase (LCAT), which acts in concert with carrier proteins to insure the transfer/exchange of these esters between HDL and the other lipoproteins. The purpose of this chapter is to provide a short overview of the subject with a major emphasis on the events occurring in human systems, which are the ones studied most thus far.

LCAT

Source

The enzyme LCAT catalyzes the transfer of the fatty acid from the C-2 position of phosphatidylcholine to the 3-hydroxy group of cholesterol (Fig. 1). The enzyme is mainly extracellular and is secreted into plasma by the liver (1,2). In 1968, Glomset (4) postulated the mechanism to explain the role of LCAT in plasma cholesterol esterification (Fig. 2).

Perfusion studies have provided evidence that hepatocytes are involved in the production and secretion of LCAT (1–3). These experiments were performed using isolated rat liver perfused with various media: rat blood, heat-inactivated rat plasma with human erythrocytes or synthetic media containing electrolytes, albumin, and human red blood cells. After 24 hours of perfusion, the LCAT

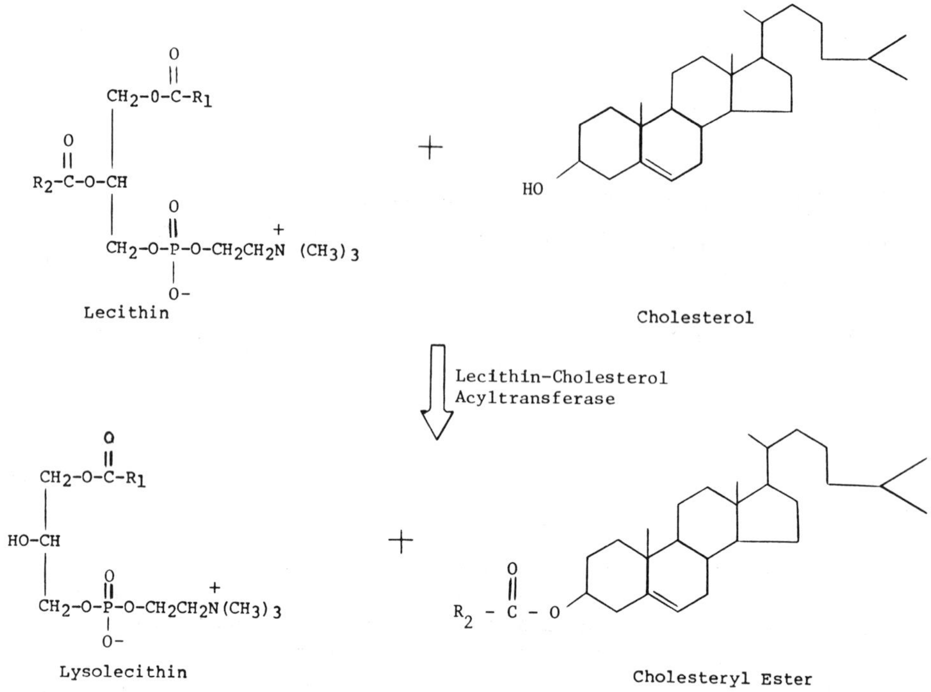

Lecithin + Cholesterol

Lecithin-Cholesterol Acyltransferase

Lysolecithin + Cholesteryl Ester

Fig. 1 Reaction of LCAT.

activity was detected regardless of the type of perfusate used, although the synthetic ones consistently contained the lowest activity. The liver was also shown to actively take up LCAT from the medium. The occurrence of this process has prevented accurate quantification of the enzyme production rate by the hepatocytes. In the plasma, LCAT is associated predominantly with the high-density lipoproteins (4,5), particularly with the smaller subspecies (6), which may be viewed as both substrate and regulators of LCAT activity. In fact, it has been suggested that LCAT may be secreted from liver cells in association with nascent discoidal HDL and may assist in the conversion of these discoidal structures into spherical particles by promoting the esterification of free cholesterol to esterified cholesterol (7).

Purification

The plasma concentration of LCAT is around 6 μg/ml as determined by radioimmunoassay (8,9); thus the mass ratio of the enzyme to all

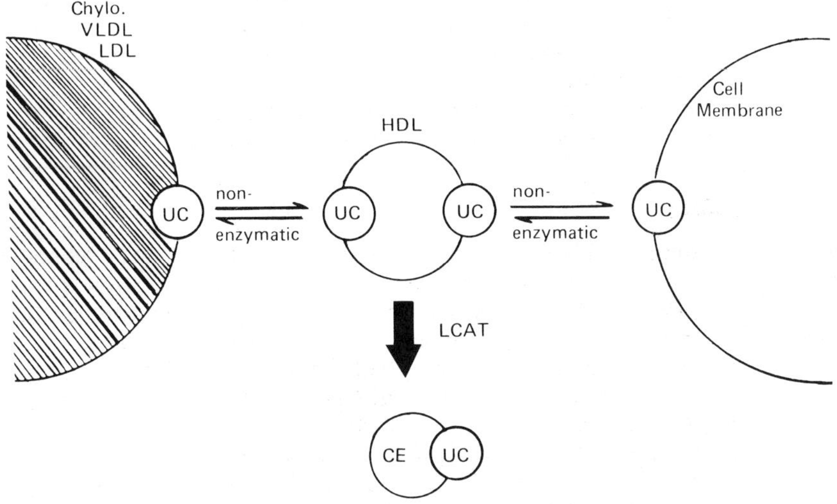

Fig. 2 Schematic presentation of role of LCAT in esterification of cholesterol. The enzyme reduces the unesterified cholesterol (UC) of other lipoproteins apparently because these lipids equilibrate readily among lipoproteins and transfer nonenzymatically to HDL that have been reacted by LCAT.

other plasma proteins is about $1:10^4$. This low plasma level of the enzyme combined with its instability has long hampered the efforts directed at the isolation of LCAT and thus the definition of its molecular properties. The first attempts to isolate LCAT were based on a multistep process involving the use of hydroxyapatite adsorption, salt precipitation, ultracentrifugation, and affinity column chromatography (5,10–12). The preparations so obtained were only partially pure and were contaminated mainly by apo A-I, apo A-II, apo D, and albumin (5,9). Subsequently, methods for obtaining highly purified preparations of the enzyme were also developed by using a multistep process. Commonly, sequential ultracentrifugation is used in the first phase of the preparation scheme, and this results in a middle, clear zone of d 1.21 to 1.25 g/ml (12–15) and is then subjected to chromatographic procedures. However, these time-consuming and expensive ultracentrifugation steps can be replaced by a chemical step in which the active fraction of the plasma is precipitated by either ammonium sulfate (16), a combination of ammonium sulfate and butanol (17), dextran sulfate in the presence of Ca^{+2} or polyethyleneglycol, 6000 mol wt (18,19). A combination of precipitation and ultracentrifugation methods has also been proposed (17,20). In the most recently developed purification scheme, specific use is made of either HDL-Sepharose affinity columns (13), phenyl-Sepharose (9), dodecylamine-agarose (21), or anti-apo D antibody-Sepharose (13,20). The final enzyme preparation is free from apoprotein contaminants inclusive of apo D and is pure by chromatographic and electrophoretic criteria (13).

Enzyme Stability

Pure preparations of LCAT undergo rapid inactivation (15). The period of stability of the pure enzyme varies from a few hours (15) to over a few days (20) and up to several weeks (21,22), depending upon the conditions of storage chosen. The enzyme is labile at 57°C (4) and is also affected by the ionic strength of the medium. It is rapidly inactivated in phosphate buffer of pH 7.4, ionic strength 0.1; at a lower ionic strength, the stability of the enzyme increases, and in 0.01 *M* phosphate buffer, pH 7.4, the enzyme activity remains unchanged for 6 hours at 37°C (23). Thus, to preserve LCAT function, it is important to store the enzyme preferably in high concentrations in media of very low ionic strength and low temperature, e.g., 4°C, under N_2, in order to minimize its exposure to the air-water interface. Inactivation of the enzyme can effectively be prevented by apo A-I. This protective action may relate to a competitive action of apo A-I for the air-water interface, thus reducing the possibility of enzyme unfolding at the surface. The lecithin-cholesterol vesicles used as a substrate can also stabilize the enzyme, but to a lesser extent than that exhibited by apo A-I.

Partially purified preparations of LCAT are comparatively more stable than the pure enzyme. This can be taken advantage of for storage purposes. For instance, fractions separated on hydroxyapatite remain stable for 4 weeks. Dialyzed dextran-sulfate-active supernatant fractions remain stable for up to 6 months (22).

Enzyme Activators (See Table 1)

Fielding et al. (11), using sonicated mixtures of lecithin and unesterified cholesterol, found that LCAT is activated by apo A-I, the principal apolipoprotein of HDL. Apo A-II, the second major apolipoprotein in HDL, has been shown to either block, be inert, or activate LCAT depending upon the in vitro system used. The inhibitory effect has been shown to occur in an apo-A-I-containing system following the displacement of apo A-I by apo A-II. By itself, apo A-II has no effect on the LCAT reaction. In turn, if the lipid substrate contains both apo A-I and apo A-II, apo A-II can enhance apo A-I activation. This activation of enzyme activity was also demonstrated for apo C-I (25,26), while apo C-II, apo C-III, and

Table 1 Activators and Inhibitors

Activators	Inhibitors
Apo A-I	Apo C-II, apo A-II in an apo-A-I-containing system
Apo C-I	Apo C-III
Apo E_2 and Apo E_3	Apo D
apo A-IV	
Synthetic peptides	Reversible inhibition by DTNB, high concentration of dithiothreitol and β-mercaptoethanol:
Low concentration of dithiothreitol and β-mercaptoethanol	p-Hydroxymercuribenzoate p-Chloromercuriphenyl sulfonic acid N-ethyl maleimide, iodoacetate DFP, diethylnitrophenylphosphate, Phenyl sulfonyl chloride
	Divalent cations such as Ag^{+2}, Zn^{+2}, Cu^{+2}, Mg^{+2}
	Cysteine, penicillamine, thioglucose, thiourea
	Certain organic phosphorus insecticides
	Local anesthetics such as dibucaine, benzocaine, tetracaine, and lidocaine, guanine, xanthine, and hypoxanthine, deoxycholate, detergents, dicarboxylic, lecithins, neutral lysolecithin, as well as enantiomeric lysolecithins

apo D inhibited the reaction (14). In 1984, Chen et al. (27) studied the activation of LCAT by apo E and apo A-IV. Apo E was purified from a dysbetalipoproteinemic patient (genotype E_2E_2) and from a hypertriglyceridemic subject (genotype E_3E_3); apo A-IV was purified from normolipidemic plasma. These apolipoproteins were then incorporated into lecithin-cholesterol liposomes that were used as substrate for LCAT. The activation by apo E_2 and apo E_3 was 40 ± 3% and 32 ± 2%, respectively, of that of apo A-I at a concentration of 0.5 nmol. The activation by apo A-IV was 25 ± 2% of that of apo A-I at a comparable apoprotein concentration. Yokoyama et al. (28) and Pownall et al. (29) recently prepared synthetic peptides of 20 or 22 amino acid residues capable of producing amphiphilic helixes upon binding to phospholipid vesicles. These synthetic peptides activated the LCAT reaction and it was speculated that this activation was the result of an induced change in the conformation of the lecithin molecules in the substrate particles. The mechanism of activation by apo A-I is still disputed. Apo A-I has been suggested to exert its cofactor activity by interacting reversibly with the enzyme at water-vesicle interface. Alternatively, apo A-I may control the degree of penetration of the enzyme into the substrate and facilitate its optimal orientation for the transferase reaction.

Inhibitors (See Table 1)

LCAT can be inhibited by a number of agents. A reversible inhibition by a sulfhydryl blocking agent dithiobis (2-nitrobenzoic acid) has been widely used for the enzyme assay in plasma. Although low concentrations of β-mercaptoethanol or dithiothreitol enhance the enzyme activity by preventing the oxidation of the sulfhydryl groups, high concentrations of the reducing agents cause a decline in the LCAT activity (23). This has been attributed to the cleavage of the intramolecular disulfide bridges. A serine protease inhibitor, diisopropylfluorophosphate (DFP), has also been shown to inhibit enzyme activity (4). Based on the nature of these inhibitory studies, it appears that cysteine and serine are the residues involved in the LCAT-catalyzed acyltransferase reaction. The rapid inhibition of the enzyme activity by DFP cannot be prevented by preincubating LCAT with either the substrate or DTNB, indicating that the reactive sites for DFP and DTNB in the enzyme are not close to each other.

In 1977, Nakagawa et al. (30) reported that LCAT can be inhibited by heavy metal cations such as Ag^{+2}, Cd^{+2}, and Zn^{+2} and that the inhibition by Zn^{+2} can be reversed by EDTA. Calcium ions that are known to inhibit LCAT activity in the plasma (4) have been shown to have no effect on the activity of purified enzyme (20,31). The inhibitory effect of Cu^{+2}, Hg^{+2}, and complexing agents (cysteine, mercaptoethanol, penicillamine, thioglucose, thiourea, etc.) on LCAT activity in vitro has also been reported (32). The activity of LCAT in vitro is also inhibited by certain organic-phosphorus insecticides (33,34), local anesthetics such as dibucaine, benzocaine, tetracaine, and lidocaine (35), guanine, xanthine, and hypoxanthine, various penicillins, etc. For all of these compounds, the mechanism of inhibition is unknown. In the case of inhibitor action by deoxycholate, detergents (4), dicarboxylic lecithins (36), natural lysolecithins (37), and enantiomeric lysolecithins (38), the inhibitory site of action appears to be at the level of the phospholipid substrate rather than the enzyme itself.

General Properties (See Table 2)

The apparent molecular weight of LCAT, estimated from polyacrylamide gel electrophoretic patterns in SDS, was found to be in the range of 65,000 to 69,000 (13,15,20,22). A somewhat lower value was obtained from sedimentation equilibrium centrifugation, and this discrepancy may be related to the anomalous behavior of LCAT in polyacrylamide gels being a glycoprotein reported to contain 24% carbohydrate by weight (31 mol mannose, 30 mol galactose, 17 mol glucosamine, and 13 mol sialic acid per mole of enzyme). The enzyme is heterogeneous by isoelectric focusing in polyacrylamide gels, exhibiting five or more bands with isoelectric points ranging from 3.8 to 5.5 (43). This microheterogeneity appears to be related to sialic acid content since, upon treatment with neuraminidase, the multiple bands converge into a single one with an isoelectric point of 5.2. The reasons for this microheterogeneity are unknown. Many serum sialoglycoproteins are known to be recognized by specific hepatic receptors only after their desialylation, which exposes the terminal galactose (24) or mannose residue (25). If a similar process applies to LCAT, the different forms of the enzyme reflect different stages of its catabolism.

The in vitro reduction in the sialic acid content of LCAT by neuraminidase treatment was found to be accompanied by an increase in the enzyme activity (42). It is possible that the decrease in the sialic acid content increases the affinity of the enzyme for the substrate through either a reduction in surface charge of the enzyme or its hydrophilicity.

The reported amino acid composition indicates that LCAT has a relatively high content of aspartic and glutamic acid, proline, glycine, valine, and leucine (18). Recent studies have also shown that the N-terminal region of LCAT has an unusually strong hydrophobic character that may favor the binding of the enzyme to hydrophobic lipid substrates.

Table 2 Properties of LCAT

Methods and conditions	Observed value	References
Molecular weight		
Sedimentation equilibrium in 1 m*M* phosphate, pH 7.2	59,000	15
Sedimentation equilibrium in 6 *M* guan Hcl	60,700	39
SDS gel electrophoresis	65,000–69,000	13,15,22
Isoelectric point	4.28–4.37 (4 bands)	40
	4.1–5.5 (5 bands)	14
	4.2–4.5 (4 bands)	39
Partial specific volume	0.712 ml/g	15
	0.708 ml/g	39
Sedimentation coefficient ($S°_{20}W$)	3.9 S	43
Stoke's radius	40 Å	43

Circular dichroism	α-helix (24%)	39
	β-sheet (27%)	39
	Remainder of structure (49%)	39
Carbohydrate content	24%	15
Mannose	31 mol/59,000 g	15
Galactose	30 mol/59,000 g	15
Glucosamine	17 mol/59,000 g	15
Sialic acid	13 mol/59,000 g	15
Amino acid sequence		
	1 2 3 4 5 6 7 8 9 Phe-Trp-Leu-Leu-X-Val-Leu-Phe-Pro	41
	Phe-Trp-Leu-Asn-Val-Leu-Phe-Pro	42
	Phe-Trp-Leu-Phe-Asn-Val-Leu-Phe-Pro	
	10 11 12 13 14 15 16 17 Pro/His-Tyr-Asn-Tyr-( )-Ile-Tyr-Glu	(Farooqui and Scanu, unpublished observation)

Immunological Properties

Polyclonal antibodies against LCAT have been raised both in the goat and in the rabbit. Anti-LCAT antisera totally inhibit LCAT activity in whole plasma and interact equally well against isolated LCAT and lipoprotein-bound enzyme. Moreover, the reactivity of these antibodies for LCAT does not appear to be affected by the presence of lipids. The immunoreactivity of LCAT remains unchanged after storage at 4°C for at least 2 months.

Recently, a monoclonal antibody against the purified LCAT has been developed in our laboratory using conventional hybridoma techniques (44). Out of three clones that survived after subcloning and expansion, only one clone exhibited a high titer and specificity against the pure enzyme. Interestingly, this antibody was found to react (by ELISA) with one acidic phospholipase A_2 from *Agkistrodon halys pallas*, two basic phospholipases A_2 from *A.P. poscivorus*, and a new K-49 phospholipase A_2 found in this venom (45). No difference in the reactivity was observed between acidic and basic phospholipases. Modification of the active site of the basic D-49 phospholipase from *A.P. piscivorus* with phenacylbromide inactivated the enzyme and inhibited the reactivity with the clone. These immunological results indicate that LCAT and the enzymes of the phospholipase A_2 family may have an antigenic determinant in common and also suggest that this determinant may be located at or near the active site.

Functions

LCAT, by promoting the formation of cholesteryl esters, performs several unique functions within the circulating plasma: (1) participate in the process of cholesterol efflux from cells, (2) maintain the balance between free and esterified cholesterol, (3) contribute to the stabilization and maturation of the plasma lipoproteins, and (4) contribute to the action of the cholesteryl ester exchange/ transfer proteins. In general, the action of LCAT may be viewed as creating the gradient necessary for the transfer of free cholesteryl esters to tissue where they undergo hydrolysis with generation of free cholesterol available for the buildup or reconstruction of cellular membranes.

Enzyme Regulation

Currently, nothing is known on the factors controlling enzyme synthesis, cellular export, and sites of degradation. Information on the subject is likely to be soon forthcoming.

CHOLESTERYL ESTER TRANSFER/EXCHANGE PROTEINS

Mode of Action

Contrary to previous assumptions, it is now well established that an active transfer/exchange of cholesteryl esters takes place among plasma lipoproteins (46,47). If plasma is incubated at 37°C in the absence of LCAT, an exchange of cholesteryl esters among individual lipoprotein classes takes place without a change in the lipoprotein mass distribution. Using lipoproteins radiolabeled in their cholesteryl ester moiety, it has been demonstrated that transfer/exchange of cholesteryl esters occurs from LDL to VLDL (46), from LDL to HDL (48,49) from VLDL to HDL and LDL (50), and from HDL or HDL_3 to LDL (51) (see Fig. 3). It is now established that this exchange/transfer of cholesteryl esters in the plasma is mediated by the cholesteryl ester/triglyceride exchange/transfer protein. The first indication of an involvement of this protein in the transport of nonpolar lipids was obtained in 1975 in studies showing that a factor in the lipoprotein-free fraction of rabbit plasma promotes an exchange of esterified cholesterol between VLDL and LDL (46). Subsequently, a comparable factor was found to be present in human plasma (49) and shown to promote not only an exchange of cholesteryl esters among all plasma lipoprotein fractions (50), but also a net mass transfer from HDL to VLDL (52). The transfer factor in rabbit plasma was partially purified and characterized as a high M_r globulin with a pI of 5.2 (46). Prepara-

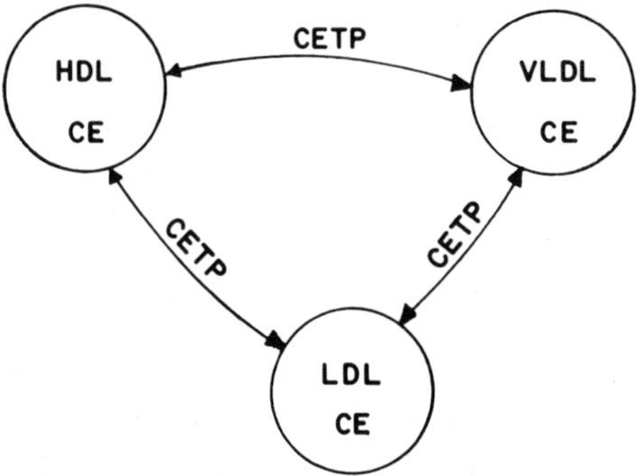

Fig. 3 Schematic view of transfer/exchange of cholesterol esters (CE) among various groups of lipoproteins by cholesterol ester transfer protein (CETP).

tions of this protein with a higher degree of purity have since been obtained from human lipoprotein-free plasma and identified as a glycoprotein with an apparent M_r of 80,000 and a pI of 5.0 (49). More recently, the transfer/exchange protein was found to bind to HDL (53).

In earlier studies it had been suggested that apolipoprotein D, a minor HDL apoprotein, promoted the irreversible transfer of esterified cholesterol from human HDL to both VLDL and LDL (54). Other groups, however, were unable to confirm this observation (56). Subsequently, apo D and LCAT in association with apo A-I were proposed to exist physiologically as components of a small molecular complex with the ability to esterify free cholesterol and transfer the esters to the major lipoprotein classes. These interesting and provocative suggestions await further experimental details.

Localization

Recently, the localization of the cholesteryl ester transfer activity in plasma was studied after fractionation by a single-step density ultracentrifugal method (57). Before analysis, each fraction was subjected to delipidation and the activity measured in an in vitro system containing a standard mixture of [3H] CE-HDL and CE-LDL. The bulk of cholesteryl ester transfer activity was detected in the HDL fraction of d 1.125 to 1.21 g/ml. In turn, the activity was located in the "lipoprotein-free" fraction of d 1.25 g/ml when the lipoproteins were separated by ultracentrifugal flotation.

Purification and Properties

Plasma Lipid Transfer Proteins

The cholesteryl ester transfer or exchange protein has been purified from both human (58–63) and rabbit plasma (64). This protein, recently designated lipid transfer protein I (LTP-I), has a molecular weight of 63,000 to 69,000, is heat stable, and retains 95% of its transfer activity after incubation for 15 min at 62°C (58) or 1 hr at 58°C (63). A second lipid transfer protein, LTP-II of M_r 55,000, has been purified from human plasma. Both of these proteins facilitate the transfer of radiolabeled cholesteryl ester, triacylglycerol, and phosphatidylcholine among plasma lipoproteins. The progressive addition of antibodies raised against human LTP-I to either a highly purified mixture of human LTP-I and LTP-II or highly purified rabbit lipid transfer protein results in the specific immunoprecipitation of proportional amounts of up to 100% of cholesteryl ester, triacylglycerol, and phosphatidylcholine transfer activities. However, similar precipitation studies on human and rabbit lipoprotein-free plasma resulted in the progressive removal of all cholesteryl ester and triacylglycerol transfer activities, but only 30% (human) or 20% (rabbit) of phosphatidylcholine transfer activity. These results indicate that LTP-I and LTP-II have antigenic sites in common, allowing precipitations of both proteins by specific antibody to LTP-I. As suggested by Morton and Zilversmit (59), it is possible that LTP-II is a degradation product of LTP-I formed during the purification process.

Another plasma protein(s) that facilitates approximately 50% of the transfer of radiolabeled phosphatidylcholine, but none of the transfer of cholesteryl ester or triacylglycerol between lipoproteins, has been identified in human plasma (62). This protein, not yet purified, is heat sensitive, clearly different from LTP-I, and has a molecular weight of 41,000. Furthermore, several investigators (50,58,65) have observed that rat plasma is deficient in cholesteryl ester and triacylglycerol transfer activity, but contains phospholipid transfer activity (58,65). Rat plasma, thus, does not appear to contain a protein homologous to LTP-I, but does contain a temperature-sensitive phosholipid transfer protein similar to LTP-II.

The physiological role of these phosphatidylcholine transfer proteins as speculated by Tall et al. (60) would be to enhance the mass transfer of phosphatidylcholine to HDL and also to facilitate transfer of phospholipids from cell membranes into HDL. Since the movement of phosphatidylcholine into HDL tends to be followed by that of cholesterol (81), the action of phosphatidylcholine transfer protein could result in augmented cholesterol efflux from the cells.

Intracellular Lipid Transfer Proteins

The properties of various intracellular lipid transfer proteins have been listed in Table 3. The cytosolic fraction of both beef and rat liver contains a transfer protein that is specific for the transfer of phosphatidylcholine. Although the molecular weights of these two proteins are the same, their isoelectric points differ considerably. The primary structure of transfer protein from beef liver has been determined (79) and the lipid binding site has been identified (80). A transfer protein that specifically transfers phosphatidylinositol and phosphatidylcholine has been purified from beef strain or beef heart cytosol (66,68). These two proteins are identical in molecular weights, isoelectric points, and lipid specificities. Nonspecific transfer proteins have been isolated from rat (77) and beef (71) liver, as well as from rat hepatomas (73). These nonspecific transfer proteins accelerate the transfer of phosphatidylcholine, phosphatidylethanolamine, phosphatidylinositol, phosphatidylserine, phosphatidic acid, phosphatidylglycerol, sphingomyelin, cholesterol, neutral glycosphingolipids, and gangliosides. They do not appear to accelerate the transfer of cholesterol ester, triglycerides, or

Table 3 Properties of Lipid Transfer Proteins

Source	Mol wt	Isoelectric point	Lipid involved in transfer/exchange	Reference
Plasma lipid transfer proteins				
Human				
Plasma I	63,000–69,000	5.0	CE, TG, PC	58–63
II	55,000	—	CE, TG, PC	63
III	41,000	—	PC	63
Rabbit				
Plasma	68,000	—	CE, TG, PC	64
Intracellular lipid transfer proteins				
Beef				

	Brain I	32,300	5.3	PI, PC	66,67
	II	32,800	5.6		
	Heart I	33,500	5.3	PI, PC	68
	II	33,500	5.6		
	Liver	28,000	5.8	PC	69,70
	I	14,500	9.55	PC, PE, SPM, PA	71,72
	II	14,500	9.75	PG, PS, cholesterol, GMI, $GbOSe_4Cer_4$	
Rat					
	Hepatoma	11,200	5.2	SPM, PC, PE, PI + PS	73
	Liver	28,000	8.5	PC	74–76
		12,500	8.8	PE, PC, PI, PS, SPM, cholesterol	77,78

Abbreviations: CE, cholesteryl ester; $GbOSe_4Cer$, globotetraglycosylceramide; GMI, II^3-N-acetylneuramino-syl-gangloiotetraglycosylceramide; PA, phosphatidic acid; PC, phosphatidylcholine; PE, phosphatidylethanolamine; PG, phosphatidylglycerol; PI, phosphatidylinositol; PL, phospholipid, PS, phosphatidylserine; SPH, sphingomyelin; TG, triglycerides.

diphosphatidylglycerol. The nonspecific lipid transfer proteins have relatively lower molecular weights, between 13,500 and 14,500, and higher isoelectric points. They are also more heat stable.

GENERAL COMMENTS

The importance of LCAT in cholesteryl ester formation in plasma and lipoprotein metabolism has emerged particularly from the studies of patients with LCAT deficiency, a familial disorder first described by Norum and Gjone in 1967 in three Norwegian sisters (82). All of these patients had high plasma levels of unesterified cholesterol and lecithin and low values of lysolecithin and cholesteryl esters. These and other patients described later had hypertriglyceridemia; the presence of LP-X particles in their plasma and in their serum α_1-lipoprotein behaved atypically in several ways (83,84). Both the LDL and the HDL classes were found to be highly heterogeneous in density and size and to contain a percentage of unesterified cholesterol, phosphatidylcholine, and triglycerides higher than their normal counterparts (84). Of the particles comprising HDL, the majority of them were found to be disc shaped, 150 to 200 Å in diameter, and organized in stacks with a periodicity of 50 to 55 Å and a variable length (85). A smaller percentage consisted of comparably smaller structures 45 to 60 Å in diameter with flotation rates, F (1.20) of 0 to 3, and electrophoretic migration in the pre-albumin region with slightly more unesterified cholesterol and phosphatidylcholine than normal HDL (86). The dependence of these lipoprotein abnormalities on LCAT deficiency became particularly evident from the results of the experiments showing the total reversal either in vitro when purified LCAT preparations were added to serum, or in vivo when LCAT-deficient subjects were transfused (87–89). These and subsequent studies (89) in patients with either primary or secondary LCAT deficiencies have led to the notion that the largest percentage of cholesteryl esters in the plasma is derived from the LCAT reaction that in turn influences HDL biogenesis (90). Because of the complex series of remodeling events that the lipoproteins undergo in the plasma, it is still difficult to ascertain the role played by LCAT on nascent lipoproteins, although it has been suggested that the smaller HDL are those having the highest affinity for the enzyme (90). The other observed lipoprotein abnormalities (i.e., large LDL and HDL, LP-X) may be secondary to the low levels of HDL particles and their attending inability to serve as acceptors for the surface components of the triglyceride-rich lipoproteins after lipolysis by lipoprotein lipase. The real basis for the genetic abnormality is still undetermined and must await the developments of current studies directed at obtaining sufficient information of primary structure of LCAT to generate efficient oligonucleotide probes and cDNA clones to examine the DNA of the LCAT-deficient patients. Moreover, it must be established whether these patients exhibit intrinsic abnormalities in the biosynthesis and processing of proapo A-I and proapo A-II and their export mechanisms. Information is also needed on the cholesteryl ester transfer/exchange mechanism; the total reversibility of the lipoprotein abnormalities induced in LCAT-deficient patients by LCAT suggests that this system is normal, however, a direct documentation is needed. Ultimately, it will be important to establish whether these two proteins recognize common regulatory mechanisms.

Until now, no deficiency states of cholesteryl ester transfer proteins have been reported in human subjects. The anticipated development of sensitive and specific methods for their quantification should facilitate the search for primary or secondary abnormalities. Considerable variations, however, in the activity of the plasma cholesteryl ester transfer protein have been reported among various species such as man, rabbit, guinea pig, rat, and pig (91). The different species have been divided into low, intermediate, and high transfer activity groups. Species like rat, dog, pig, cow, and sheep exhibit very low levels whereas guniea pig, chicken, turkey, lizard, toad, snake, and man show intermediate levels of transfer activity, and possum, rabbit, and trout contain high levels of activity. In species where the activity is very low, there are marked differences in the fatty acid composition of cholesteryl esters in the different lipoproteins (91). By contrast, in the species with higher transfer activity, including man (92), rabbit (91), and trout (93), the cholesteryl ester fatty acid composition is virtually identical in all postabsorptive lipoprotein fractions. The information available indicates that both LCAT and the cholesteryl transfer proteins interact with HDL. In neither case, however, is the site of interaction known. As indicated above, the smaller HDL particles are the preferred substrate for LCAT. Whether these HDL particles also preferentially interact with the cholesteryl ester proteins remains to be established.

Overall, much remains to be established on the physicochemical and biochemical events attending the plasma transport of cholesteryl esters. This also applies to the issue of reverse cholesterol transport in which cholesterol transfers from plasma membranes to HDL. The LCAT mediation in the latter process was postulated by Glomset in 1968. This postulate appears still to be valid today, except that the cholesteryl ester proteins have entered into the picture. This transport process is highly dynamic and requires that a suitable gradient be established to permit the cholesterol to transfer from the cell membrane to the plasma. As new cholesteryl ester molecules are generated by the action of LCAT, they must be transferred from HDL to suitable acceptors, mainly triglyceride-rich particles via the cholesteryl ester/triglyceride exchange process. It should be pointed out that the HDL particles are just a component of this dynamic system and are, per se, unable to promote the removal of cholesterol from the cells. When the extracellular concentration of HDL is sufficiently high, a transfer of cholesterol from the plasma to the cell can occur, as recently shown in a lymphoblastoid cell line in culture. In the case of liver and steroidogenic cells, HDL has been shown to act as a cholesterol donor to these cells. The precise mechanism for this uptake remains to be established.

REFERENCES

1. Osuga, T., and Portman, O. W., *Am. J. Physiol.*, *220*:735–741 (1971).
2. Simon, J. B. and Boyer, J. L., *Biochim. Biophys. Acta.* *218*:549-551 (1970).
3. Marsh, J. B., and Kashub, E., *Fed. Proc.* *29*:673 (1970).
4. Glomset, J. A., *J. Lipid Res.*, *9*:155–167 (1968).
5. Akanuma, Y., and Glomset, J. A., *Biochem. Biophys. Res. Commun.*, *32*:639–643 (1968).
6. Fielding, C. J., and Fielding, P. E., *FEBS Lett.*, *15*:355–358 (1971).
7. Hamilton, R. L., Williams, M. C., Fielding, C. J., and Havel, R. J., *J. Clin. Invest.*, *58*:667–680 (1976).
8. Albers, J. J., Adolphson, J. L., and Chen, C.-N., *J. Clin. Invest.*, *67*:141–148 (1981a).
9. Albers, J. J., Chen, C.-H, and Adolphson, J. L., *J. Lipid Res.*, *22*:1206–1213 (1981b).
10. Glomset, J. A., and Wright, J. L., *Biochim. Biophys. Acta,* *89*:266–276 (1964).
11. Fielding, C. J., Shore, V. G., and Fielding, P. E., *Biochim. Biophys. Acta,* *270*:513–518 (1972b).
12. Lacko, A. G., Rutenberg, H. L., and Soloff, L. A., *Atherosclerosis,* *19*:297–305 (1974).
13. Albers, J. J., Cabana, V. G., and Stahl, Y. D. B., *Biochemistry,* *15*:1984–1987 (1976).
14. Albers, J. J., Lin, J. T., and Roberts, G. P., *Artery,* 5:61–75 (1979).

15. Chung, J. A., Abano, D. A., Fless, G. M., and Scanu, A. M., *J. Biol. Chem.*, *254*:7456–7464 (1979).

16. Varma, K. G., and Soloff, L. A., *Biochem. J.*, *155*:583–588 (1976).

17. Soutar, H. J., Pownall, H. J., Hu, A. S., and Smith, L. C., *Biochemistry*, *13*:2828–2836 (1974).

18. Doi, Y., and Nishida, T., *Methods Enzymol.*, *71*:753–767 (1981).

19. Chong, K. S., Davidson, L., Huttash, R. G., and Lacko, A., *Arch. Biochem. Biophys.*, *211*:119–124 (1981).

20. Aron, L., Jones, S., and Fielding, C. J., *J. Biol. Chem.*, *253*:7220–7226 (1978).

21. Chen, C.-H., and Albers, J. J., *Biochem. Med.*, *25*:215–226 (1981).

22. Kitabatake, K., Piran, U., Kamio, Y., Doi, Y., and Nishida, T., *Biochim. Biophys. Acta*, *573*:145–154 (1979).

23. Furukawa, Y., and Nishida, T., *J. Biol. Chem.*, *254*:7213–7219 (1979).

24. Fielding, C. J., Shore, V. G., and Fielding, P. E., *Biochem. Biophys. Res. Commun.*, *46*:1493–1498 (1972a).

25. Soutar, A. K., Garner, C. W., Baker, H. N., Sparrow, J. T., Jackson, R. L., Gotto, Jr., A. M., and Smith, L. C., *Biochemistry*, *14*:3057–3064 (1975).

26. Sigler, G. F., Soutar, A. K., Smith, L. C., Gotto, Jr., A. M., and Sparrow, J. T., *Proc. Natl. Acad. Sci. U.S.A.*, *73*:1422–1426 (1976).

27. Chen, C.-H, and Albers, J. J., *Arteriosclerosis Council Abstr.*, *519a* (1984).

28. Yokoyama, S., Murase, T., and Akanuma, Y., *Biochim. Biophys. Acta*, *530*:258 (1978).

29. Pownall, H. J., Hu, A., Gotto, Jr., A. M., Albers, J. J., and Sparrow, J. J., *Proc. Natl. Acad. Sci. U.S.A.*, *77*:3154–3158 (1980).

30. Nakagawa, M., Takamura, M., and Kojima, S., *J. Biochem. (Tokyo)*, *81*:1011–1016 (1977).

31. Piran, U., and Nishida, T., *J. Biochem.*, *80*:887–889 (1976).

32. Nakagawa, M., Motojima, S., Fujimato, Y., Furusawa, K., Murata, K., and Kojima, S., *Chem. Pharm. Bull.*, *30*:1884–1888 (1982b).

33. Nakagawa, M., and Uchiyama, M., *Biochem. Pharmacol.*, *23*:1641–1646, (1974).

34. Nakagawa, M., Kobayashi, H., Katsua, M., Takada, N., and Kojima, S., *Chem. Pharm. Bull.*, *30*:214–218 (1982c).

35. Bell, F. P., and Hubert, E. V., *Lipids*, *15*:811–814 (1980).

36. Douset, N., Douset, J. C., Soula, G., and Douste-Blazy, L., *Scand. J. Clin. Lab. Invest.*, *38*:21–25 (1978).

37. Nakagawa, M., and Nishida, T., *J. Biochem.*, *74*:1263–1266 (1973).

38. Smith, N. B., and Kuksis, A., *Can. J. Biochem.*, *58*:1286–1291 (1980).

39. Chong, K. S., Hara, S., Thomson, R. E., and Lacko, A. G., *Arch. Biochem. Biophys.*, *222*:553–560 (1983).

40. Utermann, G., Manzel, H. J., Adler, G., Dieker, P., and Weber, W., *Eur. J. Biochem.*, *107*:225–241 (1980).

41. Doi, Y., and Nishida, T., *Fed. Proc.*, *40*:1695 (1981).

42. Yang, C.-Y., Gotto, Jr., A. M., and Pownall, H. J., *Arteriosclerosis Council Abstr.*, *535a* (1984).

43. Doi, Y., and Nishida, T., *J. Biol. Chem.*, *258*:5840–5846 (1983).

44. Khalil, A., Farooqui, J., Maraganore, J., Lester, E., Heinrikson, R. L., and Scanu, A. M., *Fed. Proc.*, *44*:6097 (1985).

45. Maraganore, J. M., Merutka, G., Cho, W., Welches, W., Kezdy, F. J., and Heinrikson, R. L., *J. Biol. Chem.*, *259*:13,839–13,843 (1984).

46. Zilversmit, D. B., Hughes, L. B., and Balmer, J., *Biochim. Biophys. Acta*, *409*:393–398 (1975).

47. Janiak, M. L., Small, D. M., and Shipley, G. G., *J. Lipid Res.*, *20*:183–199 (1979).

48. Barter, P. J., and Jones, M. E., *Atherosclerosis*, *34*:67–74 (1979).

49. Pattnaik, N. M., Montes, A., Hughes, L. B., and Zilversmit, D. B., *Biochim. Biophys. Acta*, *530*:428–438 (1978).

50. Barter, P. J., and Lally, J. I., *Biochim. Biophys. Acta*, *531*:233–236 (1978a).

51. Sniderman, A., Teng, B., Vezina, C., and Marcel, Y. L., *Atherosclerosis*, *31*:327–333 (1978).

52. Marcel, Y. L., Vezina, C., Teng, B., and Sniderman, A., *Atherosclerosis, 35*:127–133 (1980).

53. Pattnaik, N. M., and Zilversmit, D. B., *J. Biol. Chem., 254*:2782–2786 (1979).

54. Chajek, T., and Fielding, C. J., *Proc. Natl. Acad. Sci. U.S.A., 75*:3445–3449 (1978).

55. Morton, R. E. and Zilversmit, D. B., *Biochim. Biophys. Acta, 663*:350–355 (1981a).

56. Albers, J. J., Cheung, M. C., Ewens, S. L., and Tollefson, J. H., *Atherosclerosis, 39*:395–409 (1981).

57. Groener, J. E. M., Van Rozen, A. J., and Erkelens, D. W., *Atherosclerosis, 50*:261–271 (1984).

58. Ihm, J., Ellsworth, J. L., Chataing, B., and Harmony, J. A. K., *J. Biol. Chem., 257*:4818–4827 (1982).

59. Morton, R. E., and Zilversmit, D. B., *J. Lipid Res., 23*:1058–1067 (1982).

60. Tall, A. R., Abbreu, E., and Shuman, J., *J. Biol. Chem., 258*:2174–2180 (1983).

61. Calvert, G. D., and Abbey, M., in *Atherosclerosis VI* (Schettler, G., Gotto, Jr., A. M., Middelhoff, G., Habenicht, A. J. R., and Jurutka, K. R., eds.), Springer-Verlag, Berlin, pp. 428–431 (1983).

62. Albers, J. J., Tollefson, J. H., Chen, C.-H., and Steinmetz, A., *Atherosclerosis, 4*:49–58 (1984).

63. Abbery, S., Bastiras, and Calvert, D., *Biochim. Biophys. Acta, 833*:25–33 (1985).

64. Abbey, M., Calvert, G. D., and Barter, P. J., *Biochim. Biophys. Acta, 793*:471–480 (1984).

65. Barter, P. J., Gooden, J. J. M., and Rajaram, O. V., *Atherosclerosis, 33*:165–169 (1979).

66. Helmkamp, G. M., Jr., Harvey, M. S., Wirtz, K. W. A., and Van Deenen, L. L. M., *J. Biol. Chem., 249*:6382–6389 (1979).

67. Demel, R. A., Kalsbeek, P., Wirtz, K. W. A., and Van Deenan, L. L. M., *Biochim. Biophys. Acta, 446*:10–15 (1977).

68. Dicorleto, P. E., Warach, J. B., and Zilversmit, D. B., *J. Biol. Chem., 254*:7795–7802 (1979).

69. Kamp, H. H., Wirtz, D. W. A., and Van Deenen, L. M., *Biochim. Biophys. Acta, 318*:310–313 (1973).

70. Moonen, P., Akeroyd, R., Werterman, J., Puyk, W. C., Smits, P., and Wirtz, K. W. A., *Eur. J. Biochem.* *106*:279–290 (1980).

71. Crain, R. C., and Zilversmit, D. B., *Biochemistry*, *19*:1433–1439 (1980).

72. Bloj, B., and Zilversmit, D. B., *J. Biol. Chem.*, *256*:5988–5991 (1981).

73. Dyatlovitskaya, E. V., Timofeeva, N. G., and Bergelson, L. D., *Eur. J. Biochem.*, *82*:463–471 (1978).

74. Lutton, C., and Zilversmit, D. B., *Biochim. Biophys. Acta*, *441*:370–379 (1976).

75. Lumb, R. M., Kloosterman, A. D., Wirtz, K. W. A., and Van Deenen, L. L. M., *Eur. J. Biochem.*, *69*:15–22 (1976).

76. Poorthuis, B. J. H. M., Van der Krift, T. P., TeerLink, T., Akeroyd, R., Hostetler, K. Y., and Wirtz, K. W. A., *Biochim. Biophys. Acta*, *600*:376–386 (1984).

77. Bloj, B., and Zilversmit, D. B., *J. Biol. Chem.*, *252*:1613–1619 (1977).

78. Poorthuis, B. J. H. M., Glatz, J. F. C., Akeroyd, R., and Wirtz, K. W. A., *Biochim. Biophys. Acta*, *665*:256–261 (1981).

79. Akeroyd, R., Moonen, P., Westerman, J., Puyk, W. C., and Wirtz, K. W. A., *Eur. J. Biochem.*, *114*:385–391 (1981).

80. Wirtz, K. W. A., in *Lipid-Protein Interactions* (Jost, P. C., and Griffith, O. H., eds.), Wiley Interscience, New York, 1982, p. 151.

81. Tall, A. R., and Green, P. H. R., *J. Biol. Chem.*, *256*: 2035–2044 (1981).

82. Norum, K. R., and Gjone, E., *Scand. J. Clin. Lab. Invest.*, *20*:231–243 (1967).

83. Torsvik, H., Berg, K., Magnani, H. N., McConathy, W. J., Alaupovic, P., and Gjone, E., *FEBS Lett.*, *24*:165–168 (1972).

84. Torsvik, H., *Scand. J. Clin. Lab. Invest.*, *24*:188–196 (1969).

85. Norum, K. R., Glomset, J. A., Nichols, A. V., and Forte, T., *J. Clin. Invest.*, *50*:1131–1140 (1971).

86. Forte, T., Norum, K. R., Glomset, J. A., and Nichols, A. V., *J. Clin. Invest.*, *50*:1141–1148 (1971).

87. Glomset, J. A., Norum, K. R., Nichols, A. V., Forte, T., King, W. C., Labers, J. J., Mitchell, C. D., Applegate, K. R.,

and Gjone, E., *Scand. J. Clin. Lab. Invest.*, *33(Suppl. 37)*: 165–172 (1974).

88. Norum, K. R., Glomset, J. A., Nichols, A. V., Forte, T., Albers, J. J., King, W. C., Mitchell, C. D., Applegate, K. R., Gong, E. L., Cabana, V., and Gjone, E., *Scand. J. Clin. Lab. Invest.*, *35(Suppl. 142)*: 31–55 (1975).

89. Norum, K. R., and Gjone, E., *Scand. J. Clin. Lab. Invest.*, *22*: 339–342 (1978).

90. Glomset, J. A., Janssen, E. T., Kennedy, R., and Dobbins, J., *J. Lipid Res.*, *7*: 639–648 (1966).

91. Ha, Y. C., and Barter, P. J., *Comp. Biochem. Physiol.*, *71B*: 265–269 (1982).

92. Goodman, D. S., and Shiratori, T., *J. Lipid Res.*, *5*: 307–313 (1964).

93. Chapman, M. J., Goldstein, S., Mills, G. L., and Leger, C., *Biochemistry*, *14*: 4455–4465 (1978).

10

Plasma Albumin as a Lipoprotein

ARTHUR A. SPECTOR College of Medicine, University of Iowa, Iowa City, Iowa

PHYSIOLOGICAL FUNCTIONS OF ALBUMIN

Albumin is the most abundant protein in the extracellular fluid. Human albumin consists of a single polypeptide chain containing 584 amino acid residues and has a molecular weight of 66,250 (1). Human blood plasma contains 42 ± 8 g/l of albumin, or 0.63 mmol/l (2). The albumin content in the interstitial fluid varies in different tissues, the values ranging from 15 to 30 g/l, or 0.23 to 0.45 mmol/l (2).

Albumin is known to perform three important physiological functions. One is to provide most of the colloid osmotic pressure in the circulatory system. Another is to bind ions such as calcium. This reduces the concentration of the unbound ion, the form that determines the chemical activity. At the same time, it provides a reservoir of bound ions that are available for rapid dissociation if there is a need for additional unbound material. The third function is to bind small organic molecules that have a low water solubility and thereby facilitate their movement through the circulation. This is called the transport function of albumin. Among the substances that are transported by albumin in this way are fatty acids, bilirubin, amino acids such as tryptophan, and hormones such as thyroxine and cortisol (1,2). Many commonly prescribed drugs have a low solubility in water and also are transported through the circulation by albumin, e.g., salicylate, penicillin, diphenylhydantoin, and chlorothiazide (1).

Lipid Transport Function

The role of albumin as a lipoprotein concerns the fact that it serves as the transport protein for fatty acid. The fatty acid that is transported by albumin is present in unesterified form and is called free fatty acid, the commonly used abbreviation being FFA. When albumin is referred to as a lipoprotein, the distinction between it and other plasma lipoproteins should be recognized. There are four main classes of plasma lipoproteins: chylomicrons, very-low-density lipoproteins, low-density lipoproteins, and high-density lipoproteins. Each of these has a micellar structure consisting of a complex mixture of lipids. One or more proteins, called apolipoproteins, are embedded in the mixed micelle, with a segment of the polypeptide chain exposed at the surface. Even in the class of lipoproteins having the highest protein content—high-density lipoproteins—lipid comprises about 50% of the structure. At the other extreme, chylomicrons contain about 98% lipid. By contrast, the albumin-lipid complex is primarily a globular protein containing only a tiny amount of physically bound lipid. Even at the highest reported plasma FFA concentrations in humans, 2.5 mmol/l (3), lipid accounts for only 1.5% of the complex. This basic compositional and structural difference should be kept in mind when referring to plasma albumin as a lipoprotein. It functions, however, as a true lipoprotein: a protein that contains lipid and serves to transport the lipid through the circulation.

PLASMA FREE FATTY ACID

The plasma FFA is derived from two sources. During fasting and in response to stress or exercise, fatty acid is released from adipocytes in the form of FFA (4–7). The fatty acid is hydrolyzed from the triacylglycerols stored in adipocytes, passes out of these cells and into the plasma, and is transported by albumin for utilization by other tissues. FFA becomes the main metabolic substrate under these conditions. The fatty acid released into the plasma as a result of the mobilization of fat from adipocytes is what is commonly referred to by the term FFA.

What is not generally recognized is that fatty acid also enters the plasma in the form of FFA in the fed state, although in lesser amounts than during fasting, exercise, or stress. In the fed state, the FFA is derived from the hydrolysis of triacylglycerols contained in chylomicrons or very-low-density lipoproteins (8,9). These triacylglycerols are hydrolyzed by lipoprotein lipase bound to the endothelial surface (10). Most of the fatty acid released in this catabolic process passes through the capillary wall and directly into the cells of the organ where the hydrolysis occurs. For example

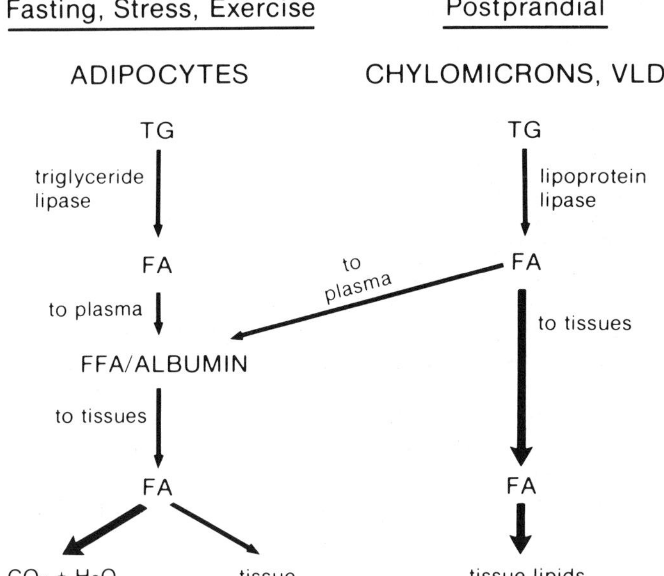

Fig. 1 Schematic representation of the origin and transport of plasma FFA. TG, triacylglycerol; FA, fatty acid; FFA, plasma free fatty acid; VLDL, plasma very-low-density lipoproteins.

most of the fatty acid that is hydrolyzed in the microcirculation of the heart is taken up and utilized by the myocardial cells. A small amount escapes into the circulation however, and becomes part of the plasma FFA pool. Fig. 1 illustrates schematically the origins and metabolism of the plasma FFA.

Concentration

In humans, the plasma FFA concentration can vary from 0.09 to 1.20 mmol/l under normal conditions (11). The lowest values occur after a meal rich in carbohydrates; the higher values occur after a period of fasting. After stopping prolonged strenuous exercise, FFA values as high as 2.5 mmol/l can be reached (3). In the basal state, the plasma FFA concentration is usually between 0.3 and 0.5 mmol/l (11). The most important factor regulating the availability of FFA to the tissues is the molar ratio of FFA to plasma albumin (12,13). Assuming that the albumin concentration is 0.63 mmol/l (2), the molar ratio of FFA to albumin ordinarily will vary between

0.14 and 1.9, with a basal value of about 0.6. After strenuous exercise, the ratio may reach 4.

Composition

The plasma FFA consists of a very complex mixture of fatty acids. Analysis by gas-liquid chromatography of the FFA extracted from human albumin indicates the presence of 43 separate fatty acids, 26 of which have been identified (14). Many of these are present in only very small amounts, and five long-chain fatty acids account for about 90% of the plasma FFA (9,15–18). The amounts of these fatty acids, palmitic, palmitoleic, stearic, oleic, and linoleic, together with several others of special biological importance, are listed in Table 1. Although the variations in these values make generalizations tenuous, a rough estimate is that human plasma FFA contains about 35% saturated, 40% monounsaturated, and 25% polyunsaturated fatty acid. There is little variation in plasma FFA composition with increasing age or between males and females (17).

Table 1 Composition of the Plasma Fatty Free Acids in Humans

Fatty acid		Composition range (%)
Name	Structure[a]	
Palmitic	16:0	23–30
Palmitoleic	16:1Δ9	2–7
Stearic	18:0	4–13
Oleic	18:1Δ9	31–43
Linoleic	18:2Δ9, 12	9–24
Linolenic	18:3Δ9, 12, 15	0–1.8
Arachidonic	20:4Δ5, 8, 11, 14	0–4.7

[a]Number of carbon atoms to number of double bonds. The numbers after the Δ refer to the positions of the double bonds, counting from the carboxyl group.

Solubility in Plasma

The long-chain fatty acids that comprise the plasma FFA have a very low solubility in water. In the physiological concentration range of 0.09 to 1.2 mmol/l, the solubility of these long-chain fatty acids would be exceeded by far if all of the fatty acid in plasma were freely dissolved. If such were the case, the circulating FFA concentration probably would not exceed 10 to 20 μmol/l. Through its ability to bind fatty acids, albumin enables a much higher FFA concentration to be present in the plasma: concentrations that are far above the maximum solubility of long-chain fatty acids in aqueous solutions. These relatively high plasma FFA concentrations allow the tissues to have more rapid access to a substantial quantity of energy-producing substrate when the metabolic need arises.

Turnover and Metabolism

Because plasma FFA is present in relatively small amounts, its metabolic significance went unrecognized for many years. Subsequent radioisotope infusion studies demonstrated that the half-life of the plasma FFA was only 1 to 2 min (19). When the rapidity of the turnover was realized, the metabolic importance became apparent. A simple calculation, contained in Table 2, illustrates this point. This calculation indicates that about 75% of the caloric need can be met by the plasma FFA, assuming that all of the FFA turnover is utilized for oxidation. The estimate will vary depending on how much the plasma FFA concentration deviates during a 24-hour period from the average value of 0.5 mmol/l used in this calculation. Likewise, the estimate will decrease if a significant amount of the FFA turnover enters other metabolic pathways such as membrane synthesis, lipoprotein production, or intracellular storage as triacylglycerol. Even when these alternate metabolic fates are taken into account, the main point remains clear. A sizable portion of the total energy requirement can be supplied if necessary by the plasma FFA.

Since the plasma FFA consists of a mixture of fatty acids, it is likely that not all components are utilized for energy purposes. Certain fatty acids probably are targeted to specific tissues where they are used for the synthesis of membrane lipids or intracellular storage lipids such as triacylglycerols and cholesteryl esters (20). The liver utilizes FFA for ketone body synthesis (21). Endothelial cells and platelets take up arachidonic acid contained in the plasma FFA to supply storage pools that are subsequently used for prostaglandin synthesis (22–25). These cells appear to have special mechanisms for incorporating arachidonic acid; a separate acyl CoA synthase has been demonstrated in the case of platelets (26).

Table 2 Estimate of the Contribution of Plasma Free Fatty Acid to Energy Metabolism in Humans

Parameter	Value
Weight	70 kg
Plasma volume	3 l
Plasma FFA (average value)	0.5 mmol/l
Average FFA molecular weight	280
$t_{\frac{1}{2}}$ of plasma FFA	1.5 min
Turnover of plasma FFA	10 mmol/l·hour 720 mmol/day 201.6 g/day
Caloric value of turnover (9 cal/g)	1818 cal/day
Caloric requirement (moderate activity)	2350 cal/day
Maximum contribution from plasma FFA turnover to caloric requirement[a]	77%

[a]This estimate assumes that all of the FFA turnover is utilized for fatty acid oxidation.

Cells in the nervous system probably depend on the plasma FFA for a supply of linolenic acid or its derivatives, the n-3 class of polyunsaturated fatty acids that are abundant in neural membranes (27). These additional uses emphasize the considerable physiological importance of the plasma FFA.

ALBUMIN STRUCTURE

When the plasma FFA is in the ordinary concentration range—0.09 to 1.2 mmol/l—more than 99% of the fatty acid is bound to albumin (28). Since the plasma albumin concentration is about 0.63 mmol/l, a single albumin molecule must be able to transport more than one molecule of fatty acid. As seen in Fig. 2, which illustrates data for the binding of oleic acid to albumin in the form of a Scatchard plot, albumin actually has the capacity to bind 10 or more long-chain fatty acid molecules (29). Even larger binding capacities can be demonstrated for fatty acids of medium-chain length such as decanoate, laurate, and myristate (29–31). This multiple binding process is extremely complex because the fatty acid binding sites of albumin

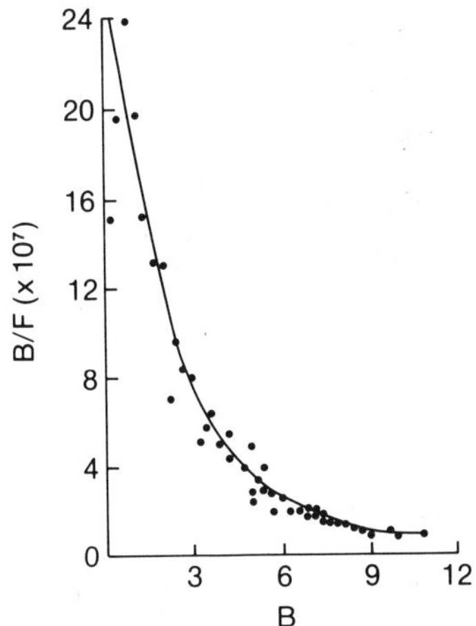

Fig. 2 Binding of oleic acid to human plasma albumin. The results are presented in the form of a Scatchard plot. B, molar ratio of bound oleic acid to albumin; F, unbound oleic acid concentration.

are not equivalent, as suggested by the curvilinearity of the Scatchard plot in Fig. 2. To obtain an understanding of this complicated process, it is necessary to examine the structure of albumin, the factors involved in the interaction between fatty acids and albumin, and the nature of the molecular interaction.

The complete amino acid sequence of plasma albumin is known, and a tertiary structure that is consistent with many different types of experimental findings has been proposed (32). Fig. 3 is a schematic representation of the tertiary structure, emphasizing important considerations regarding the lipid transport function of albumin. Human and bovine albumin, the two plasma albumins that have been studied extensively, have very similar sequences and structures.

Even though albumin consists of a single polypeptide chain, it is folded in such a way that the protein behaves as if it were composed of three nearly identical globular subunits (32). The functional subunits, indicated as I, II, and III in Fig. 3, contain 186, 192, and 206 amino acids, respectively, and are called domains. In each domain, the polypeptide chain is folded into three looped regions. The looped regions are numbered 1 to 9 in Fig. 3, beginning with the first domain, which contains loops 1 to 3. There is a considerable amount of sequence homology in the three domains, suggesting that albumin evolved from a primordial gene for a single domain through gene

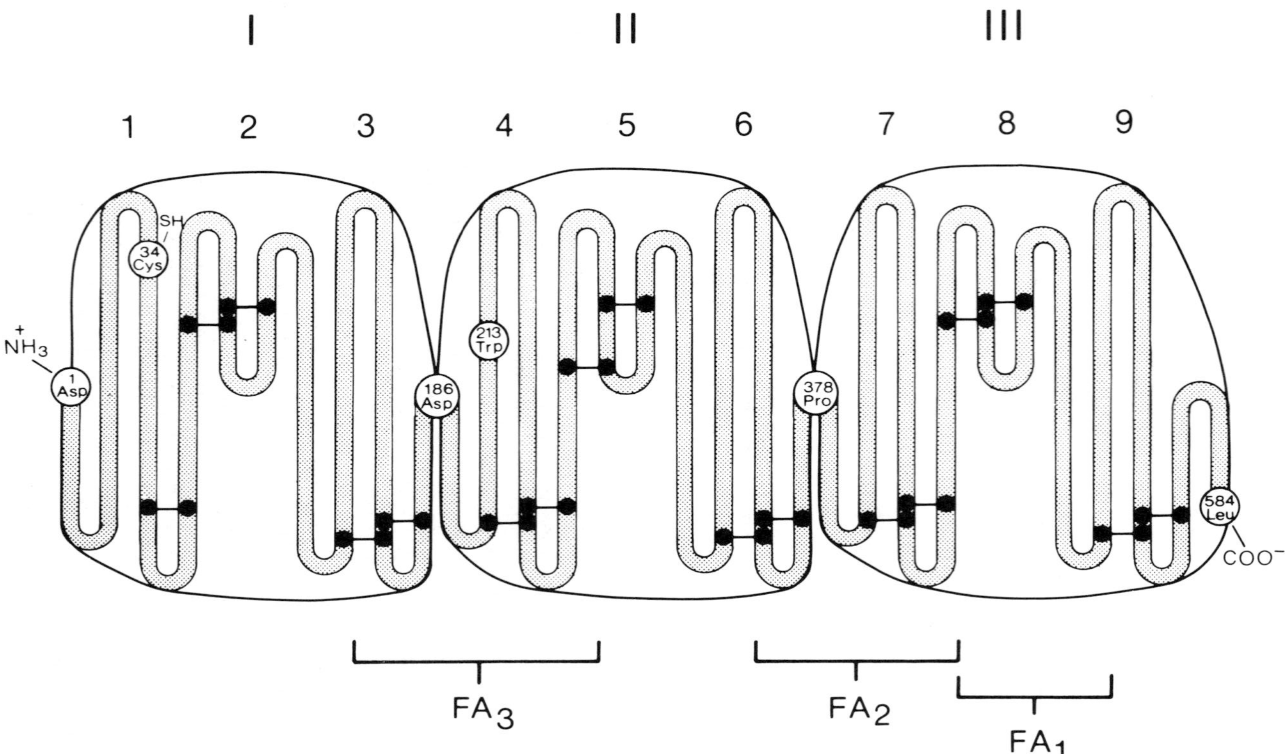
I
II
III
1
2
3
4
5
6
7
8
9
+NH3
1 Asp
SH
34 Cys
213 Trp
186 Asp
378 Pro
584 Leu
COO−
FA3
FA2
FA1

duplication (32). Most of the looped regions of the polypeptide chain are held together by disulfide bonds, six of these linkages being present in the second and third domains and five in the first domain.

There are 35 cysteine residues in albumin, 34 of which are oxidized to form the 17 disulfide bonds. The only reduced cysteine residue is contained in the first domain, 34 residues from the amino-terminal aspartate. Human albumin contains only one tryptophan residue, located in the second domain in loop 4. In the three-dimensional structure, the tryptophan residue is located in the crevice between the first and second domain, a region that contains a binding site for fatty acids and other organic anions (33). The location of the tryptophan is important because most spectroscopic studies of albumin involve ultraviolet absorbance or fluorescence properties. One of the main structural differences between human and bovine albumin is that the latter contains two tryptophan residues (1). The second tryptophan of bovine albumin is located in the first domain in loop 3 at amino acid residue 134 (1). The fluorescence of this tryptophan residue is quenched when fatty acids bind to bovine albumin (28,34). This property makes bovine albumin especially useful for spectroscopic investigations of fatty acid binding.

Location of Fatty Acid Binding Sites

The three strongest fatty acid binding sites have been localized within the albumin structure to a reasonable degree of certainty. Through limited proteolysis the albumin chain was cut into defined

---

Fig. 3 Structure of human serum albumin. This representation has been adapted from work reported by Brown (32) and Peters (1). The curvilinear structure is a representation of the folded polypeptide chain. This begins at the amino-terminal end with aspartate and continues to the carboxyl-terminal amino acid, leucine. Numbers above the amino acids refer to their position in the polypeptide sequence. The polypeptide chain is grouped into three globular domains that are designated as I, II, and III. Each domain contains three folded loops of the polypeptide chain. These looped regions are numbered consecutively, 1 to 9, beginning at the amino-terminal end, as indicated above the structure. Each dark, round structure within the polypeptide chain represents a half-cysteine residue, and the solid connection between each pair indicates the disulfide bond that joins them. The symbols FA_1, FA_2, and FA_3 refer to the locations of the three strongest fatty acid-binding sites.

fragments (35,36), and binding studies revealed which of these fragments can combine tightly with fatty acids (37). This work indicated that the strongest binding site, designated FA_1 in Fig. 3, is present in the third domain in the region of loops 7 and 8. The second strongest site, FA_2, is located between the second and third domain in the region of loops 6 and 7. These two sites are specific for long-chain fatty acids (1,28,38). The third site, FA_3, is located in the cleft between the first and second domains, between loops 3 and 4 (1). This site also can bind drugs, organic dyes, and fluorescent compounds (1,33,39,40). Studies with fluorescent and spin-labeled fatty acids give a somewhat similar picture, except that both of the strongest albumin binding sites, FA_1 and FA_2, are localized by this method to the third domain in the region of loops 7 and 8 (41,42).

Structural Requirements for Binding

The main structural features of albumin required for fatty acid binding are illustrated in Fig. 4. These results were obtained for palmitic acid binding to bovine albumin (43). When the tertiary structure of the protein is disrupted with 6 M urea, the binding

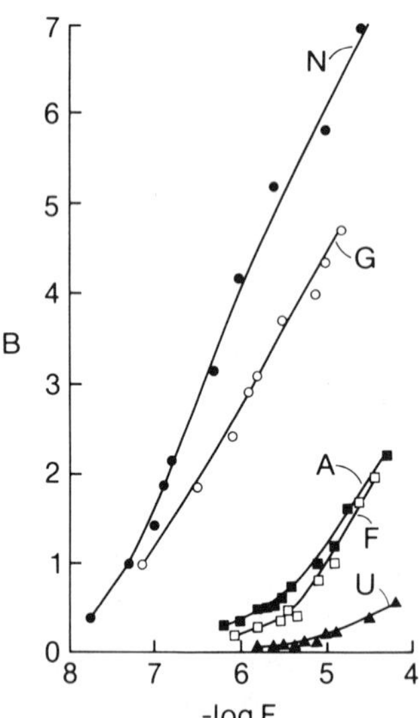

Fig. 4 Effect of structural modifications on the binding of palmitic acid to bovine albumin. N, native albumin; G, guanidated with O-methyl isourea; A, acetylated with acetic anhydride; F, treated with formaldehyde; U, denatured with 6 M urea.

affinity is reduced greatly, and the maximum binding capacity is only about 0.5 mol/mol. By contrast, native albumin binds at least 7 mol/mol of palmitate. Acetylation of lysine groups or addition of formaldehyde to arginine groups also reduces the binding affinity greatly and lowers the maximum binding capacity to 2 mol/mol. These treatments abolish the positive charges on the lysine and arginine groups. By contrast, guanidation of the lysine residues, which does not remove the positive charge, reduces binding only slightly. These findings indicate that two processes are involved in fatty acid binding. One is ionic interaction between the carboxylate group of the fatty acid and positively charged lysine or arginine groups of the protein. The other are hydrophobic interactions between the fatty acid hydrocarbon chain and nonpolar amino acid chains in the interior of the globular protein structure (28,43). Disruption of the native tertiary structure reduces binding by destroying the conformation of hydrophobic pockets into which the fatty acid hydrocarbon chain burrows. In addition, it probably displaces positively charged lysines or arginines that ordinarily are located near the entrance to the pocket and interact with the ionized carboxyl group.

FATTY ACID BINDING TO ALBUMIN

Fatty Acid Structure

Binding data obtained with structurally modified fatty acids also support a mechanism involving both ionic and hydrophobic interactions. Table 3 shows the effects of modifying or removing the carboxyl group on palmitic acid binding to bovine albumin (43). Conversion of the carboxyl group to a methyl ester, alcohol, or methyl group greatly reduces the extent of palmitic acid binding and the binding affinity. Since the pK_a of a fatty acid is about 4.8, most of the fatty acid in biological fluids of pH 7 to 7.5 is in anionic form. The reduction in binding that occurs when the anionic group is removed supports the idea that the interaction involves electrostatic attraction of the carboxylate group to positively charged amino acid residues of albumin. ^{13}C-NMR studies confirm that the anionic form of the fatty acid binds to albumin (44); furthermore, they indicate that the microenvironment of the anionic group is different at many of the fatty acid binding sites.

The other factor that regulates binding is the length and structure of the fatty acid hydrocarbon chain. This is illustrated in Table 4, which shows the magnitude of the first binding constant for a series of fatty acids and human albumin (29). K_1 increases by about 5 log units when the length of a saturated fatty acid increases from 6 to 18 carbon atoms. This indicates that a great deal of the binding energy comes from hydrophobic

Table 3 Effect of Modifying the Carboxyl Group on Palmitic Acid Binding to Bovine Albumin

		Binding parameters	
Compound	Structure[a]	n_{max}[b]	$K_1 \times 10^5$ (M^{-1})
Palmitic acid	$R—COO^-$	7	700
Methyl palmitate	$R—CO—O—CH_3$	2.4	0.3
Palmitoyl alcohol	R—CHOH	1.2	2
Hexadecane	$R—CH_3$	2	0.3

[a]$R = Cl_{15}H_{31}$.
[b]Maximum amount bound (mol/mol).

Table 4 Effect of Fatty Acid Chain Length on the Highest Energy-Binding Constant[a]

Fatty acid		$K_1 \times 10^6$
Name	Structure	(M^{-1})
Hexanoic	6:0	0.015
Octanoic	8:0	0.34
Decanoic	10:0	0.10
Lauric	12:0	2.4
Myristic	14:0	21
Palmitic	16:0	62
Stearic	18:0	150
Oleic	18:1	260
Linoleic	18:2	79

[a]Human plasma albumin, 37°C, pH 7.4.

interactions between the hydrocarbon chain and nonpolar amino acid chains that line the binding pockets. The introduction of one cis double bond in the middle of the hydrocarbon chain of an 18 carbon atom fatty acid increases K_1 threefold. A second cis double bond introduced between it and the methyl terminus, however, reduces K_1 to a lower value than for the corresponding saturated fatty acids. These findings indicate that a tighter fit with the binding pocket occurs when the hydrocarbon contains a single fixed angulation in the middle of the chain, but that additional angulations further down the hydrocarbon chain reduce the strength of the interaction.

Rate of Binding

Fatty acid binding to albumin is extremely rapid. Stopped-flow measurements of the change in dipole vector have been used to measure the rate of this process (45). Binding occurs through a two-step mechanism. First, a very fast step occurs in which the fatty acid anions are transferred from the unbound state to sites on or near the surface of the albumin molecule. This process probably is diffusion controlled, is fairly nonspecific, and has a weak binding interaction. These weak, nonspecific sites may be the tertiary class of binding sites detected in equilibrium binding experiments. They have an association constant for long-chain fatty acids in the range of 1×10^3 M^{-1} (28,41). A much slower step follows, with a rate of 3 sec^{-1} at 0°C, in which the fatty acid moves to highly specific pockets in the interior of the globular protein structure (45). These probably are the primary and secondary sites detected by equilibrium binding measurements, with association constants in the range of 1×10^8 to 1×10^6 M^{-1} (28,38). The kinetics of the rearrangement are first order, and it is rate-limited by a negative entropy of activation (45). The rearrangement is accompanied by a small conformational change that causes the tertiary structure of albumin to open up slightly. This conformational change enables the binding pocket to mold to the shape of the incoming fatty acid hydrocarbon chain, a process that is called configurational adaptability (46).

This kinetic model of rapid association with nonspecific surface sites, followed by a slower internalization into tightly binding pockets, is consistent with certain FFA utilization results. Based on studies of palmitate uptake by the perfused rat liver, it was concluded that the fatty acid carried by plasma albumin exists in two pools (47). One was available for uptake by the liver very rapidly, the other only slowly. These kinetically distinguishable pools may represent fatty acid bound to the surface and internal sites, respectively. However, physical measurements give only a single value for the dissociation constant, k_d. For palmitic acid, the measurements are 3×10^{-3} sec^{-1} at 1°C and 4.2×10^{-2} sec^{-1} at 25°C (48,49).

Unbound Fatty Acid

The fatty acid anions bound to albumin are in equilibrium with a small amount of unbound fatty acid (28,38). Almost all of the dissociated fatty acid should also be in anionic form at physiological pH values. Unbound fatty acid usually accounts for no more than 0.1 to 0.2% of the total FFA and ranges between 0.005 and 1 μmol/l. Accurate measurement of the unbound FFA concentration is necessary for two reasons. First, in order to calculate the important binding parameters, N_i, the number of binding sites, and K_i, the binding constant for each site, both the bound and unbound FFA concentrations must be measured (28,38). Second, it is likely that the utilization of albumin-bound FFA by tissues occurs at least partly through the unbound pool (12,13,50).

What is usually done is to measure the unbound FFA concentration at a pH of about 7.4 and, because the fatty acid pK_a is about 4.8, to assume that all of the unbound material is in anion monomer form. This should be a good approximation as long as the critical micelle concentration of the fatty acid is not exceeded. Experiments of fatty acid distribution between a buffer solution and heptane indicate, however, that this assumption probably is not correct (51). There appears to be a premicellar association of unbound fatty acid, forming either anion dimers, acid-anion dimers, or higher associated forms (52–54). This becomes even more complicated because the extent of association depends on the unbound fatty acid concentration and the type of fatty acid present. Association becomes greater as the unbound concentration increases. Furthermore, the question is muddled by the fact that no premicellar association was detected by electron spin resonance using spin-labeled stearic acid (55). Therefore, the observed association may be an artifact of the heptane-aqueous buffer systems used to measure fatty acid partition. This issue must be resolved in order to obtain a complete understanding of fatty acid binding to albumin and the mechanism of its subsequent uptake by tissues.

Analysis of Binding to Albumin

A set of binding data consists of values of fatty acid bound to albumin in mol/mol, designated B, and corresponding values for the unbound fatty acid concentration in mol/l, designated F. These results usually are graphed in the form of a Scatchard plot, B/F versus B, as shown in Fig. 2. Two things are evident from such a plot. First, there are many fatty acid binding sites on each albumin molecule. Second, the binding sites are either heterogeneous or negative cooperativity occurs during the binding process. This complexity has necessitated the development of detailed models to analyze fatty acid binding data.

Scatchard Model

The Scatchard analysis is formulated as

$$B = \frac{n_1 k_1 F}{1 + k_1 F} + \frac{n_2 k_2 F}{1 + k_2 F} + \cdots \frac{n_n k_n F}{1 + k_n F} \qquad (1)$$

where B is the molar ratio of fatty acid to albumin; F is the unbound fatty acid concentration; n is the number of binding sites in a given class; and k is the average association constant for the binding sites of that class. Each term represents a different class of binding sites. The simplest model that will fit fatty acid-albumin binding results such as those in Fig. 2 contains three terms. This has been interpreted to indicate that albumin contains three different classes of fatty acid binding sites: primary, secondary, and tertiary. Table 5 illustrates the parameters of the three-class Scatchard binding model which have been reported as the best fits for the binding of palmitic acid to human albumin; they are generally similar (28,38,56). These models contain 2 or 3 primary sites with a k_1 between 10^8 and 10^7 M^{-1}, 3 to 5 secondary sites with a k_2 of about 10^6 M^{-1}, and from 20 to 60 tertiary sites with a k_3 of about 10^3 M^{-1}.

Table 5 Scatchard Analysis of Palmitic Acid Binding to Human Albumin

Binding parameters	Values		
	23°C, pH 7.4[a]	25°C, pH 8.5[b]	37°C, pH 7.4[c]
n_1	2	2	3
$k_1 \times 10^6$ (M^{-1})	60	80	50
n_2	5	5	3
$k_2 \times 10^6$ (M^{-1})	3	4	3
n_3	20	30	63
$k_3 \times 10^6$ (M^{-1})	0.001	0.002	0.0004

[a]Ref. 38.
[b]Ref. 56.
[c]Ref. 28.

The widespread interpretation of this model in physiological terms is that albumin contains two very strong binding sites that are specific for long-chain fatty acids, several moderately strong binding sites that are available to all types of fatty acids, drugs, and other organic compounds, and a large number of very weak sites that have little importance regarding actual transport but may be involved in the mechanism of binding (38).

Multiple Binding Model

Another analytical method that has been employed is to consider fatty acid binding as occurring through a series of multiple equilibria:

$$B = \frac{K_1F + 2\,K_1K_2F^2 + \cdots + N\,K_1K_2 \cdots K_nF^n}{1 + K_1F + K_1K_2\,F^2 + \cdots + K_1K_2 \cdots K_nF^n} \qquad (2)$$

where B and F are the same terms as in Eq. 1, and K_i is the equilibrium constant for each association. This analysis has been called the stepwise equilibrium model (57). Table 6 shows the stepwise equilibrium analysis for binding to human albumin of the four most prevalent FFA found in plasma. These data were obtained at 37°C, pH 7.4 (29). Since the binding constants for each fatty acid

Table 6 Multiple Binding Analysis for Fatty Acids and Human Albumin

	$K_i \times 10^6$ (M^{-1})			
N_i	Palmitate	Oleate	Stearate	Linoleate
1	62	260	150	79
2	23	94	53	8.7
3	12	29	19	5.1
4	3.1	22	5.6	3.1
5	1.5	11	4.5	0.68
6	0.96	2.4	3.7	0.34

occur in a generally descending order, there is no evidence from this analysis for any positive cooperativity in the binding process.

An advantage of the multiple binding analysis is that values are obtained for each mol/mol of fatty acid that binds, not an average value for several mol/mol of fatty acid that bind to a group of similar binding sites, as is provided by the Scatchard analysis. In the Scatchard analysis, the value for k_i is entirely dependent on the value selected for n_i, and this is often a somewhat arbitrary assignment. The fact that the selection of n_i values is arbitrary is evident from the values for K_i in Table 6. These values do not group in any obvious way. For example, it is impossible to say with assurance whether the n_1 class contains two or three binding sites. The value of k_1 for palmitate binding to human albumin has been shown to vary from 5.2×10^7 to 2.0×10^7, depending on whether n_1 is taken as 2 or 3 (43). Furthermore, the value of n_2 depends on the value selected for n_1. If $n_1 = 2$, the best fit requires that $n_2 = 4$. By contrast, if $n_1 = 3$, the best fit requires that $n_2 = 3$. As in the case of k_1, k_2 depends on the value selected for n_2 (43). These kinds of uncertainties are obviated by use of the multiple binding analysis.

A disadvantage of the multiple binding model is that a computer is required to analyze the results (58). While the most precise fits of the binding results are also obtained for the Scatchard model when a computer analysis is employed (57), reasonably good estimates of n_i and k_i in the Scatchard model can be obtained by inspection if the binding data are presented in the graphical form shown in Fig. 2.

Distribution Analysis

One might expect that when 1 mol of fatty acid and 1 mol of albumin are available, all of the fatty acid binds to the strongest albumin binding site, designated FA_1 in Fig. 3; when the second mole of fatty acid is added, all of it binds to the second strongest albumin binding site, FA_2; etc. The stepwise equilibrium analysis, however, is not consistent with this interpretation (50,59). The successive values of K_i in the stepwise model (Table 6) are not sufficiently separated for binding to occur only at single sites. Instead, each mole of fatty acid probably is spread over two or three binding sites having K_i that differ from one another by only 5- to 10-fold. The distribution is given by the equation:

$$P_i = \frac{[PF_i]}{[P_T]} = \frac{K_1 K_2 \cdots K_i F^i}{1 + K_1 F + K_1 K_2 F^2 + \cdots + K_1 \cdots K_n F^n} \qquad (3)$$

Table 7 Distributional Analysis of Oleic Acid Binding to Human Albumin[a]

Oleic acid bound to albumin (mol/mol)	Number of albumin molecules (%)
0	30.8
1	43.1
2	22.1
3	3.6
4	0.4

[a]This calculation is based on a solution containing 0.58 mmol/l oleic acid and 0.58 mmol/l albumin at 37°C, pH 7.4, and having physiological ionic strength.

where P_i is the fraction of the albumin that has i molecules of attached fatty acid; PF_i is the albumin containing bound fatty acid; P_T is the total albumin; and K_i and F are the same as in Eq. 2. Table 7 shows the surprising conclusion concerning how fatty acid is distributed among the population of albumin molecules when the concentrations of oleic acid and albumin are 0.58 mmol/l, both in the physiological range, so that the molar ratio of total FFA to albumin is 1. Not all of the albumin molecules in the solution contain one bound oleate molecule—only 43% do. A variety of other albumin species are present in the solution; 31% contain no fatty acid, 22% contain two oleate molecules, 3.6% contain three, and 0.4% contain four.

Interpretation of the distributional analysis is even more complicated because it does not specify which albumin binding sites are involved in any of the fatty acid-albumin complexes. For example, the analysis does not indicate that those albumin complexes containing one fatty acid ligand have this fatty acid bound only at the FA_1 site. Actually, the fatty acid probably is distributed over several different sites in this population of albumin molecules. Because FA_1 has the highest energy-binding constant, however, the probability is greater that the fatty acid is located at the FA_1 site. Likewise, in albumin complexes containing two fatty acid ligands, the likelihood is that the fatty acid is contained predominantly at the FA_1 and FA_2 binding sites.

Functional implications. The concept of distribution is important in interpreting several properties of the fatty acid-albumin complex. First, a moderate amount of fatty acid will be distributed over weaker binding sites in a small percentage of the albumin molecules even when the molar ratio of FFA to albumin is between 0.5 and 2, the usual physiological range. As indicated in Table 7, four binding sites become involved in the transport process even under ordinary physiological conditions. When the molar ratio begins to exceed 2, a fifth and sixth site become involved in binding (50). Therefore, the n_2 sites of the Scatchard model are not superfluous with regard to physiological FFA transport. Second, some competitive binding between FFA and other organic compounds, such as drugs that do not bind to the FA_1 and FA_2 sites, is likely to occur even when the molar ratio of FFA to albumin does not exceed 2. Indeed, some displacement of drugs by fatty acids has been observed experimentally when there are less than 2 molecules of fatty acid per molecule of albumin (39). Finally, spectroscopic studies indicate that the fluorescence of the tryptophan residues of human and bovine albumin is affected even when the molar ratio of fatty acid to albumin is less than 2 (28,39,41,50). This has been explained on the basis of a fatty-acid-induced protein conformational change because, as seen in Fig. 3, the FA_1 and FA_2 fatty acid binding sites are distant from the tryptophan residue. While conformational changes involving the region of the protein that contains the tryptophan residue undoubtedly occur when fatty acids bind (39,60), some of the effects observed with relatively small amounts of bound fatty acid may not be due only to conformational changes. An additional contributing factor probably is the presence of some fatty acid at the secondary binding sites in a small percentage of the albumin molecules, as indicated by the distributional analysis.

Spectroscopic Studies

Several different spectroscopic approaches confirm the general picture obtained from the physical binding measurements. A ^{13}C-NMR study demonstrates the heterogeneity of the individual fatty acid binding sites (41) as predicted by the stepwise equilibrium analysis (29). This study shows that the anionic form of the fatty acid is bound (34). Furthermore, it provides some support for the distributional hypothesis because at least two carboxyl carbon peaks are observed even when the molar ratio of FFA to albumin is less than 1 (41). Electron spin resonance studies with spin-labeled stearic acid indicate that the fatty acid binding sites are heterogeneous and that albumin contains seven strong fatty acid binding sites (55), in good agreement with the sum of n_1 and n_2 predicted by the Scatchard analysis. They also show that the middle of the fatty acid hydrocarbon chain interacts most tightly with the binding site (61). Studies with fluorescent fatty acid analogs indicate that albumin contains five strong binding sites, which also is in reasonably good agreement with the Scatchard analysis. Unlike the studies with albumin fragments (35–37), however, the fluorescence data suggest that the two strongest sites, FA_1 and FA_2 in Fig. 3, lie side by side in an antiparallel fashion in the third structural domain (39,62).

Basis for the Curvilinear Scatchard Plot

There are two possible explanations for the curvilinear Scatchard plot obtained for FFA binding to albumin, as shown in Fig. 2. One is that the fatty acid binding sites are heterogeneous. This has been implied in the interpretation of the binding results according to the Scatchard analysis (Eq. 1), where the binding sites are separated in n_1, n_2, and n_3 classes. Another interpretation is that fatty acid binding is associated with negative cooperativity. The simplest formulation of the negative cooperativity model is that all of the fatty acid binding sites are equivalent, although binding to each succeeding site becomes more difficult as additional molecules of fatty acid are bound. This could occur as a result of either conformational changes in the protein structure, or stearic hindrance. Since binding data are equilibrium measurements, they do not indicate whether heterogeneity or negative cooperativity is the basis for the curvilinear plot. The ^{13}C-NMR studies help to resolve this question. They support heterogeneity because they demonstrate that different types of interactions occur between the fatty acid and protein at the various binding sites (41). Therefore, an explanation based solely on negative cooperativity can be excluded. What remains questionable, however, is whether negative cooperativity still may be involved even though the sites are heterogeneous. In summary, the curvilinearity is due to either heterogeneity or a combination of heterogeneity and negative cooperativity, not negative cooperativity alone.

Competition for Transport

Since albumin binds drugs, bilirubin, thyroxine, and steroid hormones, it is important to consider whether these substances might interfere with its capacity to transport fatty acids. The presently available information indicates that they do not have a major inhibitory effect. Albumin contains at least six relatively strong binding sites for organic anions (28,38). Two of these, designated FA_1 and FA_2 in Fig. 3, are specific for fatty acids. Drugs and other organic anions bind to sites that are secondarily involved in FFA transport, those designated the n_2 class in the Scatchard analysis of fatty acid binding (Table 5). Furthermore, most drugs and metabolites that bind to albumin are present in concentrations of less than 1 mol/mol of protein, and the molar ratio of FFA to albumin rarely exceeds 2 under physiological conditions. Except in the case of bilirubin, the K_1 for drug and hormone binding to albumin is 100 to 1000 times smaller than the K_1 and K_2 for fatty acid binding (1,28,30). For these reasons, drugs and other compounds do not effectively compete with fatty acids under physiological conditions, and FFA transport by albumin is not appreciably reduced.

Through conformational effects, however, some slight displacement of fatty acid may occur when albumin must transport additional ligands (63). Likewise, some competition with distributed fatty acid may occur at the drug binding sites (39). Even when such effects occur, there are enough auxiliary binding sites to take up any fatty acid that may be displaced, and the capacity of albumin to transport physiological amounts of FFA is not seriously compromised.

UTILIZATION OF ALBUMIN-BOUND FATTY ACID

Half of the albumin-bound FFA in the circulation leaves the plasma every 1 to 2 min. The transfer of albumin between the plasma and interstitial fluid is 140 g/day in a 70-kg human (2), or 2.11 mmol/day. The average plasma FFA concentration is 0.5 mmol/l. Assuming a plasma albumin concentration of 0.63 mmol/l (2), the average molar ratio of FFA to albumin is 0.79. Therefore, only 1.68 mmol/day of FFA can leave the plasma in association with the albumin efflux. As shown in Table 2, however, 720 mmol/day of FFA leaves the plasma, or about 430 times more than can be accounted for by albumin turnover. This indicates that most of the FFA must dissociate from albumin when it passes from the circulatory system into the tissues. Since about 0.1% of the FFA is unbound and the rate of FFA dissociation from albumin is rapid (48,49), the requirement for dissociation poses no special problem. The interstitial fluid contains 0.23 to 0.45 mmol/l albumin (2), enough to serve as an acceptor for the FFA that dissociates from plasma albumin and exits from the capillary.

How FFA crosses the capillary wall is not known. Because the dissociated fatty acid is predominantly in anionic form, it is likely that the fatty acid anion is the species that moves across. The fatty acid anion probably passes through channels between adjacent endothelial cells or vesicular networks that traverse the cell. Endothelial cells also rapidly take up FFA and incorporate them into membrane phospholipids and intracellular triacylglycerols (22–24).

The newly incorporated fatty acid can be hydrolyzed from these intracellular lipid esters and released from the endothelial cell in the form of FFA (24). These findings suggest an alternative mechanism for fatty acid passage through the capillary wall. It is possible that fatty acids are esterified into endothelial lipids after uptake at the capillary luminal surface, and that this is followed by hydrolysis and release as FFA after these lipid esters move to the antiluminal surface of the endothelial cell. Such a process, which is entirely conjectural at this time, could serve as a mechanism for moving fatty acid across the endothelium.

Cellular Uptake

Almost all of the FFA that leaves the capillary and enters the extracellular space probably binds initially to the albumin present in the interstitial fluid. It is then rapidly taken up by the cells, where it is utilized either as an oxidative substrate or for the synthesis of complex lipids. A schematic overview of this process is illustrated in Fig. 5. An important question is whether albumin plays a direct role in the entry of the fatty acid into the cell. Uptake studies in which both the fatty acid and albumin are radioactive indicate that cellular fatty acid incorporation exceeds albumin incorporation by 150- to 200-fold (64). Therefore, as was concluded for passage across the capillary wall, FFA must dissociate from the albumin contained in the extracellular fluid during the process of cellular uptake.

Albumin has been found to increase the rate of palmitic acid uptake by cultured cardiac cells and hepatocytes (65), suggesting that it plays a direct role in the cellular uptake mechanism. In agreement with this idea, receptors for plasma albumin have been found in liver, and they are thought to mediate the transfer of fatty acid into the hepatocytes (66). According to this view, the fatty acid-albumin complex binds to these plasma membrane receptors, and the receptor then removes the fatty acid and facilitates its entry into the cell interior. As the receptor removes the fatty acid, the albumin is released from the cell surface into the extracellular fluid. Such a mechanism is consistent with the result of the double-label experiment mentioned above because in this formulation, the albumin involved in delivering the fatty acid to the receptor does not remain associated with the cells. While a mechanism involving albumin receptors may operate in the liver, other tissues apparently do not require the presence of albumin for fatty acid uptake. For example, Ehrlich ascites cells have been shown to take up fatty acid in the unbound form in the absence of albumin (64). Cells also can take up fatty acid when it is available as a complex with other proteins, including β-lactoglobulin (68) and plasma lipoproteins (69). Furthermore, a small reduction in pH, which increases FFA dissociation from

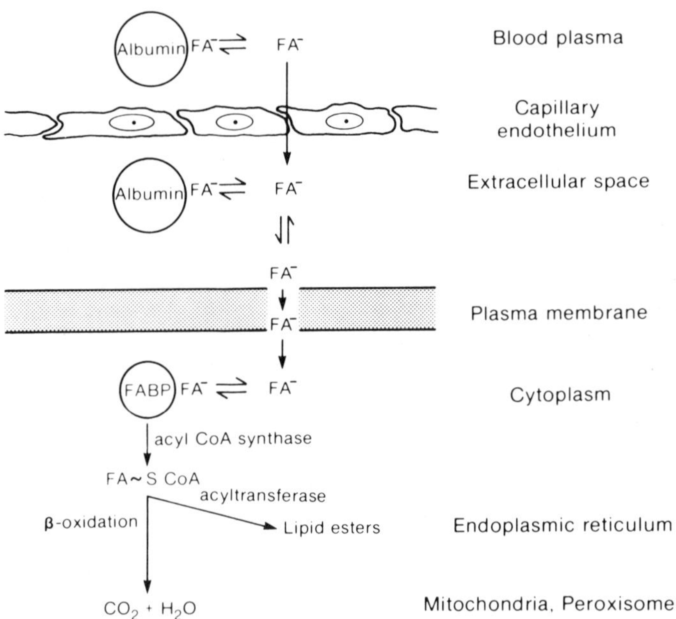

Fig. 5 Schematic representation of FFA utilization. FABP, fatty acid binding protein; FA^-, fatty acid anion; FA∿SCoA, fatty acyl CoA.

albumin, increases FFA uptake by cells (70). These findings do not exclude the involvement of an albumin receptor in the hepatic uptake process, but they suggest that such a receptor may not be essential for FFA uptake by all cells.

An alternative mechanism for FFA uptake, which does not involve the presence of an albumin receptor in the plasma membrane, is illustrated in Fig. 5. According to this view, the unbound form of fatty acid combines with the cell membrane, and albumin plays no direct role in the uptake process (12,13). Instead, albumin provides a reservoir of fatty acid in close proximity to the cell surface, thereby facilitating diffusion of the unbound form by reducing the diffusion path length. The rapid fatty acid dissociation rate insures that when the unbound form is taken up, it is replaced quickly by fatty acid from the albumin reservoir.

The unbound form of the fatty acid either binds to a fatty acid receptor in the plasma membrane or enters the membrane lipid bilayer directly. Since the fatty acid anion is the predominant unbound form, it is likely that the anionic form is the species that initially binds to the cells. After binding, at least some of the fatty acid anions enter the membrane lipid bilayer and align themselves parallel to the phospholipid fatty acyl chains, with the ionized carboxyl group pointing outward so that it is located in the region of the phospholipid head groups (71). It is likely that saturated fatty acids are taken up into solidlike membrane lipid domains, whereas unsaturated fatty acids enter fluid domains (72). The existence of two types of membrane fatty acid binding sites has been detected by equilibrium distribution experiments (31). They could represent two different types of membrane receptors, one membrane receptor and one type of lipid bilayer binding site, or two types of lipid bilayer sites, such as the solid and fluid lipid bilayer domains. More work is needed to sort out these possibilities.

Due to considerable technical problems, it is not yet possible to perform the proper kinetic experiments to determine which of the two general mechanisms—albumin-mediated uptake or uptake of the unbound fatty acid—is correct (64).

Membrane Transport

After combining with the cell membrane, the fatty acid is internalized and utilized by the cell (73). Four mechanisms have been proposed for the membrane permeation process. These proposals are illustrated in Fig. 6. The albumin receptor mechanism assumes that this receptor mediates the transfer of the fatty acid across the membrane (66). Albumin is thought to dissociate from the carrier either after delivering the fatty acid or as the fatty acid is translocated.

Another type of protein carrier that facilitates the transfer of fatty acids across the membrane has been identified in adipocytes (74). This carrier, which is strongly inhibited by phoretin, utilizes the unbound form of fatty acid. A saturable, carrier-mediated fatty acid transport process also has been observed in cultured cardiac cells (75).

Phosphatidylcholine has been proposed as a transmembrane carrier of fatty acid in the liver (76). Phosphatidylcholine contained in the hepatocyte plasma membrane exhibits a rapid turnover rate (76), as has been reported in other cells (77). According to this idea, the fatty acid is esterified to lysophosphatidylcholine, forming phosphatidylcholine in the outer leaflet of the membrane lipid bilayer. The phosphatidylcholine so formed somehow moves to the inner leaflet where it is hydrolyzed by a phospholipase, releasing the fatty acid into the cytoplasm. As opposed to the two carrier-mediated mechanisms, a lysophosphatidylcholine-phosphatidylcholine cycle requires energy. This is required to form the acylcoenzyme A intermediate needed to esterify lysophosphatidylcholine. Such a mechanism requiring metabolic energy is difficult to reconcile with the finding that fatty acid movement across the cell membrane can operate effectively in the presence of metabolic inhibitors (64,78).

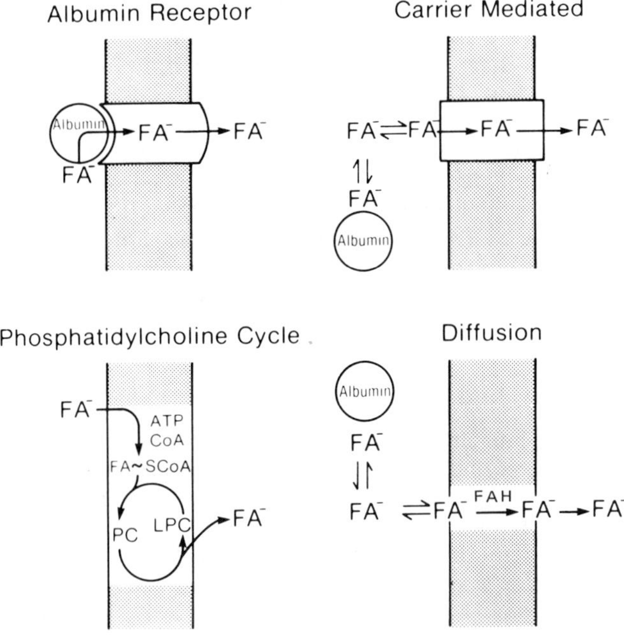

Fig. 6 Mechanisms proposed for membrane transport of fatty acid. PC, phosphatidylcholine; LPC, lysophosphatidylcholine, FA^-, fatty acid anion; FAH, fatty acid; FA∿SCoA, fatty acyl CoA.

The fourth mechanism proposed is that fatty acids diffuse through the lipid bilayer without any carrier mediation or energy requirement (64,67,68). This is consistent with the observation that the process of fatty acid uptake, as opposed to subsequent activation and utilization, is not saturable (64,67). Even in studies demonstrating carrier mediation of fatty acid uptake, a nonsaturable component has been observed (74,75). Physical measurements also indicate that diffusion plays an important role in the membrane transport of amphipathic compounds (79). The difficulty with the diffusion hypothesis is explaining how the anionic form of the fatty acid crosses the hydrophobic interior of the membrane lipid bilayer. By contrast, the major advantage of the carrier-mediated hypotheses is that they can explain the transmembrane movement of the anionic form. One possibility is that the fatty acid anion is not the form that crosses the membrane. It has been observed that two uncharged fatty acid analogs, methyl palmitate and palmitoyl alcohol, enter cells even more effectively than fatty acids (80,81). Furthermore, fatty acid uptake increases as pH decreases from 7.4 to 6.0 (70). Since the pKa of a fatty acid is about 4.8, such a reduction in pH increases the amount of the undissociated acid form relative to anionic form. These considerations suggest that the protonated form of fatty acid may be the actual species that crosses the membrane lipid bilayer. It is not clear, however, how the necessary proton would be supplied for such a process.

There are no difficulties in formulating mechanisms for the desorption of fatty acid anions from the cytoplasmic surface of the plasma membrane. Fatty acid binding protein (FABP), a low molecular weight protein, is present in the cytoplasm and tightly binds 1 mol/mol of fatty acid (82). Binding to FABP followed by ATP-dependent conversion to acylcoenzyme A insures continued flux of fatty acid from the plasma membrane to the cytoplasm as shown in Fig. 5.

Protection Against Cellular Injury

Fatty acid anions are amphipathic substances at physiological pH: they have an ionized carboxyl group and a long nonpolar tail. Therefore, they have the properties of a detergent. Were it not for binding to albumin, FFA would be extremely toxic to blood cells, blood vessels, and tissues in the physiological concentration range of 0.09 to 1.2 mmol/l. The toxic form is the unbound anion. Albumin, by tightly binding more than 99% of the total FFA, reduces the unbound form to the concentration range of 0.005 to 1 μmol/l, a nontoxic level (28). This allows an appreciable amount of total FFA to be present in the plasma and thereby be immediately available to the tissues without causing any toxicity. The tissues can have ready access to the bound FFA because the dissociation rate is so rapid (48,49). An appropriate analogy is to consider the lipoprotein form of albumin as a buffer for the fatty acid in the circulation. The fatty acid dissociates as required to make FFA immediately available to tissues, but the unbound FFA anion concentration is maintained at a low level because the released fatty acid is quickly taken up by the tissues. The process can be formulated as:

$$PF_n^- \rightleftharpoons PF_{n-1}^- + F^- \qquad (4)$$

where PF_n^- is albumin containing n moles of fatty acid anions; PF_{n-1}^- is albumin after 1 mol of bound fatty acid anion has dissociated; and F^- is the dissociated fatty acid anion.

Various kinds of toxicity occur when the FFA concentration rises to a level where binding to albumin cannot keep the unbound fatty acid anion concentration low enough to prevent detergent effects. This usually occurs when the molar ratio of FFA to albumin exceeds 4, at which point the unbound fatty acid concentration begins to increase above 10 μmol/l. For example, adenosine diphosphate-induced platelet aggregation is greatly enhanced by the saturated fatty acids, palmitate and stearate, when the molar ratio reaches 4 to 6 (83). Myocardial arrhythmias, especially in the presence of ischemia, are produced by FFA concentrations in this range (84–86). High palmitic acid concentrations also increase lactate dehydrogenase release from the ischemic heart (87). Arachidonic acid in high concentrations will produce stroke and sudden death (88,89). These effects are thought to occur because cells accumulate large quantities of free fatty acid under these conditions, with saturated fatty acids accumulating in the greatest amount (64,73,90,91). Much of this free fatty acid is associated with the cell membrane (12,13,92), and there are effects on membrane enzymes when fatty acids build up to high concentrations. These include inhibition of the Na^+/K^+-ATPase (93), modulation of adenylate cyclase (94,95), and stimulation of membrane-bound guanylate cyclase (96). Presumably, the anionic form of the fatty acid accumulates in the membrane lipid bilayer, thereby perturbing membrane structure and the function of macromolecules embedded in the membrane. Albumin prevents this by binding the fatty acid and reducing the unbound concentration to nontoxic levels, provided that the capacity of the strong albumin binding sites is not exceeded.

SUMMARY AND CONCLUSIONS

Plasma albumin is the transport protein for FFA, the unesterified form of fatty acid in the circulation. In this context it can be considered a lipoprotein. Fatty acid, which physically binds to albumin in anionic form, usually accounts for less than 1% of the complex. Therefore, this lipoprotein is predominantly a globular protein containing one or at most a few fatty acid anions. This structure is much different from that of the typical plasma lipoproteins, which are mixed micelles composed of 50 to 98% lipid.

Albumin contains many binding sites for amphipathic compounds. At least 6 of these sites can bind fatty acids very tightly, with association constants in the range of 2×10^8 to $1 \times 10^6\ M^{-1}$. Fatty acids are bound more strongly than most other organic ligands, and only long-chain fatty acids are able to bind to the two highest energy sites. Because of this and the large number of sites available, the capacity of albumin to transport fatty acid is not seriously compromised by the presence of other organic ligands.

Even though fatty acids are bound tightly, about 0.1% of the total FFA is present in unbound form. Exchange between the bound and unbound forms of FFA occurs rapidly. The half-life of the plasma FFA is only 1 to 2 min, and FFA is a major source of lipid for the tissues. In order to pass from the plasma into the extracellular space, FFA must dissociate from albumin. Likewise, FFA must dissociate from the albumin present in the interstitial fluid in order to enter cells. Whether albumin actually delivers the fatty acid to cell surface receptors or merely serves as a reservoir for fatty acid in the interstitial fluid is not known. It is almost certain, however, that albumin does not function as a carrier that moves fatty acid across the cell membrane.

The most likely physiological role of albumin as a lipoprotein is to maintain, through physical binding, FFA concentrations in the plasma and extracellular fluid which far exceed the solubility of fatty acids in these aqueous solutions. Therefore, one can think of albumin as a buffer for the FFA present in the circulation. This enables hundreds of times more FFA to be transported at any given time than would be possible if all of the fatty acid were in unbound form. Since so much of the fatty acid is bound, the tissues are protected against damage from high unbound fatty acid concentrations. Finally, the ability of the bound fatty acid to rapidly dissociate from albumin provides the tissues with a fairly high concentration of immediately available substrate for energy production and complex lipid synthesis when the need arises.

ACKNOWLEDGMENT

The preparation of this review was supported by Arteriosclerosis Specialized Center of Research grant HL14230 from the National Heart, Lung, and Blood Institute, National Institutes of Health.

REFERENCES

1. Peters, T., Jr., in *The Plasma Proteins. Structure, Function and Genetic Control* (Putnam, F. W., ed.), Vol. 1, Academic Press, New York, 1975.

2. Peters, T., Jr., and Reed, R. G., in *Transport by Proteins* (Blauer, G., and Sund, H., eds.), Walter de Gruyter & Co., Berlin, 1978.

3. Havel, R. J., Ekelund, L.-G., and Holmgren, A., *J. Lipid Res.*, *8*:366 (1967).

4. Dole, V. P., *J. Clin. Invest.*, *35*:150 (1956).

5. Gordon, R. S., and Cherkes, A., *J. Clin. Invest.*, *35*:206 (1956).

6. Gordon, R. S., Jr., *J. Clin. Invest.*, *36*:810 (1957).

7. Laurell, S., *Acta Physiol. Scand.*, *41*:156 (1957).

8. Eaton, R. P., Berman, M., and Steinberg, D., *J. Clin. Invest.*, *48*:1560 (1969).

9. Heimberg, M., Dunn, G. D., and Wilcox, H. G., *J. Lab. Clin. Med.* *83*:393 (1974).

10. Nilsson-Ehle, P., Garfinkel, A. S., and Schotz, M. C., *Ann. Rev. Biochem.*, *49*:667 (1980).

11. Spector, A. A., and Fletcher, J. E., in *Nutrition and Drug Interrelations* (Hathcock, J. N., and Coon, J., eds.), Academic Press, New York, 1978.

12. Spector, A. A., *Ann. N. Y. Acad. Sci.*, *149*:768 (1968).

13. Spector, A. A., *Prog. Biochem. Pharm.*, *6*:130 (1971).

14. Saifer, A., and Goldman, L., *J. Lipid Res.*, *2*:268 (1961).

15. Dole, V. P., James, A. T., Webb, J. P. W., Rizak, M. A., and Sturman, M. F., *J. Clin. Invest.* *38*:1544 (1959).

16. Havel, R. J., Carlson, L. A., Ekelund, L.-G., and Holmgren, A., *J. Appl. Physiol.*, *19*:613 (1964).

17. Rogiers, V., *J. Lipid Res.*, *22*:1 (1981).

18. McDaniel, H. G., Papapietro, S. E., Rogers, W. J., Mantle, J. A., Smith, L. R., Russell, R. O., Jr., and Rackley, C. E., *Am. Heart J.*, *102*:10 (1981).

19. Fredrickson, D. S., and Gordon, R. S., Jr., *J. Clin. Invest.*, *37*:1504 (1958).

20. Spector, A. A., Mathur, S. N., Kaduce, T. L., and Hyman, B. T., *Prog. Lipid Res.*, *19*:155 (1981).

21. McGarry, J. D., and Foster, D. W., *Ann. Rev. Biochem.*, *49*:395 (1980).

22. Spector, A. A., Kaduce, T. L., Hoak, J. C., and Fry, G. L., *J. Clin. Invest.*, *68*:1003 (1981).

23. Spector, A. A., Kaduce, T. L., Hoak, J. C., and Czervionke, R. L., *Arteriosclerosis* *3*:323 (1983).

24. Denning, G. M., Figard, P. H., Kaduce, T. L., and Spector, A. A., *J. Lipid Res.*, *24*:993 (1983).

25. Needleman, S. W., Spector, A. A., and Hoak, J. C., *Prostaglandins*, *24*:607 (1982).

26. Wilson, D. B., Prescott, S. M., and Majerus, P. W., *J. Biol. Chem.*, *257*:3510 (1982).

27. Hyman, B. T., and Spector, A. A., *J. Neurochem.*, *37*:60 (1981).

28. Spector, A. A., *J. Lipid Res.*, *16*:165 (1975).

29. Ashbrook, J. D., Spector, A. A., Santos, E. C., and Fletcher, J. E., *J. Biol. Chem.*, *250*:2333 (1975).

30. Ashbrook, J. D., Spector, A. A., and Fletcher, J. E., *J. Biol. Chem.*, *247*:7043 (1972).

31. Spector, A. A., Ashbrook, J. D., Santos, E. C., and Fletcher, J. E., *J. Lipid Res.*, *13*:445 (1972).

32. Brown, J. R., *Fed. Proc.*, *35*:2141 (1976).

33. Swaney, J. B., and Klotz, I. M., *Biochemistry* *9*:2570 (1970).

34. Spector, A. A., and John, K. M., *Arch. Biochem. Biophys.* *127*:65 (1968).

35. Peters, T., Jr., and Feldhoff, R. C., *Biochemistry*, *14*:3384 (1975).

36. Reed, R. G., Feldhoff, R. C., and Peters, T., Jr., *Biochemistry* *15*:5394 (1976).

37. Reed, R. G., Feldhoff, R. C., Clute, O. L., and Peters, T., Jr., *Biochemistry* *14*:4578 (1975).

38. Goodman, D. S., *J. Am. Chem. Soc.*, *80*:3892 (1958).

39. Spector, A. A., Santos, E. C., Ashbrook, J. D., and Fletcher, J. E., *Ann. N.Y. Acad. Sci.*, *226*:247 (1973).

40. Santos, E. C., and Spector, A. A., *Mol. Pharmacol.*, *10*:519 (1974).

41. Berde, C. B., Hudson, B. S., Simoni, R. D., and Sklar, L. A., *J. Biol. Chem.*, *254*:391 (1979).

42. Hsia, J. C., En, S. R., Tan, C. T., and Tinker, D. O., *J. Biol. Chem.*, *257*:1724 (1982).

43. Spector, A. A., John, K., and Fletcher, J. E., *J. Lipid Res.*, *10*:56 (1969).

44. Parks, J. S., Cistola, D. P., Small, D. M., and Hamilton, J. A., *J. Biol. Chem.*, *258*:9262 (1983).

45. Scheider, W., *Proc. Natl. Acad. Sci. U.S.A.* *76*:2283 (1979).

46. Karush, R., *J. Am. Chem. Soc.*, *76*:5536 (1954).

47. Soler-Argilaga, C., Infante, R., and Polonovski, J., *J. Lipid Res.*, *16*:116 (1975).

48. Scheider, W., *Biophys. J.*, *24*:260 (1978).

49. Svensson, A., Holmer, E., and Andersson, L. O., *Biochim. Biophys. Acta*, *342*:54 (1974).

50. Spector, A. A., and Fletcher, J. E., in *Disturbances in Lipid and Lipoprotein Metabolism* (Dietschy, J. M., Gotto, A. M., Jr., and Ontko, J. A., eds.), Am. Physiol. Soc., Washington, D.C., 1978.

51. Goodman, D. S., *J. Am. Chem. Soc.*, *80*:3887 (1958).

52. Mukerjee, P., *J. Phys. Chem.*, *69*:2821 (1965).

53. Smith, R., and Tanford, C., *Proc. Natl. Acad. Sci. U.S.A.* *70*:289 (1973).

54. Simpson, R. B., Ashbrook, J. D., Santos, E. C., and Spector, A. A., *J. Lipid Res.*, *15*:415 (1974).

55. Rehfeld, S. J., Eatough, D. J., and Plachy, W. Z., *J. Lipid Res.*, *19*:841 (1978).

56. Arivdsson, E. O., Green, F. A., and Laurell, S., *J. Biol. Chem.*, *246*:5373 (1971).

57. Fletcher, J. E., and Spector, A. A., *Comput. Biomed. Res.*, *2*:164 (1968).

58. Fletcher, J. E., Spector, A. A., and Ashbrook, J. D., *Biochemistry*, *9*:4580 (1970).

59. Wosilait, W. D., and Soler-Argilaga, C., *FEBS Lett.*, *73*:72 (1977).

60. Hsia, J. C., and Kwan, N. H., *J. Biol. Chem.*, *256*:2242 (1981).

61. Perkins, R. C., Jr., Abrumrad, N., Balasubramanian, K., Dalton, L. R., Beth, A. H., Park, J. H., and Park, C. R., *Biochemistry* *21*:4059 (1982).

62. Sklar, L. A., Hudson, B. S., and Simoni, R. D., *Biochemistry*, *16*:5100 (1977).

63. Spector, A. A., and Soboroff, J. M., *Proc. Soc. Exp. Biol. Med.*, *137*:945 (1971).

64. Spector, A. A., Steinberg, D., and Tanaka, A., *J. Biol. Chem.*, *240*:1032 (1965).

65. Paris, S., Samuel, D., Jacques, Y., Gacke, C., Franchi, A., and Ailhaud, G., *Eur. J. Biochem.* *83*:235 (1978).

66. Weisiger, R., Gollan, J., and Ockner, R., *Science*, *211*:1048 (1981).

67. DeGrella, R. F., and Light, R. J., *J. Biol. Chem.*, *255*:9731 (1980).

68. Spector, A. A., and Fletcher, J. E., *Lipids*, *5*:403 (1970).

69. Spector, A. A., and Soberoff, J. M., *J. Lipid Res.*, *12*:545 (1971).

70. Spector, A. A., *J. Lipid Res.*, *10*:207 (1969).

71. Mabrey, S., and Sturtevant, J. M., *Biochim. Biophys. Acta*, *486*:444 (1977).

72. Klausner, R. D., Kleinfeld, A. M., Hoover, R. L., and Karnovsky, M. J., *J. Biol. Chem.*, *255*:1286 (1980).

73. Spector, A. A., and Steinberg, D., *J. Biol. Chem.*, *240*:3747 (1965).

74. Abrumrad, N. A., Perkins, R. C., Park, J. H., and Park, C. R., *J. Biol. Chem.*, *256*:9183 (1981).

75. Samuel, D., Paris, S., and Ailhaud, G., *Eur. J. Biochem.*, *64*:583 (1976).

76. Wright, J. D., and Green, C., *Biochem. J.*, *123*:837 (1971).

77. Spector, A. A., and Steinberg, D., *J. Biol. Chem.*, *242*:3057 (1967).

78. DeGrella, R. F., and Light, R. J., *J. Biol. Chem.*, *255*:9739 (1980).

79. Wang, J., Rich, G. T., Galey, W. R., and Solomon, A. K., *Biochim. Biophys. Acta*, *255*:691 (1972).

80. Kuhl, W. E., and Spector, A. A., *J. Lipid Res.*, *11*:458 (1970).

81. Spector, A. A., and Soboroff, J. M., *J. Lipid Res.*, *13*:780 (1972).

82. Ockner, R. K., and Manning, J. A., *J. Clin. Invest.*, *54*:326 (1974).

83. Hoak, J. C., Spector, A. A., Fry, G. L., and Warner, E. D., *Nature* (London), *228*:1330 (1970).

84. Kurien, V. A., and Oliver, M. F., *Lancet*, *1*:813 (1970).

85. Hoak, J. C., Warner, E. D., and Connor, W. E., in *Myocardiology* (Bajusz, E., and Rona, G., eds.), University Park Press, Baltimore, Md., 1972.

86. Miller, N. E., Mijos, O. D., and Oliver, M. F., *Clin. Sci. Mol. Med.* *51*:209 (1976).

87. deLeiris, J., Opie, L. H., and Lubbe, W. F., *Nature (London)*, *253*:746 (1975).

88. Silver, M. J., Hoch, W., Kocsis, J. J., Ingerman, C. M., and Smith, J. B., *Science*, *183*:1986 (1974).

89. Furlow, T. W., Jr., and Bass, N. H., *Science*, *187*:658 (1975).

90. Spector, A. A., *Cancer Res.*, *27*:1587 (1967).

91. Spector, A. A., Hoak, J. C., Warner, E. D., and Fry, G. L., *J. Clin. Invest.*, *49*:1489 (1970).

92. Hoak, J. C., Spector, A. A., Fry, G. L., and Barnes, B. C., *Blood*, *40*:16 (1972).

93. Ahmed, K., and Thomas, B. S., *J. Biol. Chem.*, *246*:103 (1971).

94. Fain, J. N., and Shepherd, R. E., *J. Biol. Chem.*, *250*:6586 (1975).

95. Orly, J., and Schramm, M., *Proc. Natl. Acad. Sci. U.S.A.*, *72*:3433 (1975).

96. Wallach, D., and Pastan, I., *J. Biol. Chem.*, *251*:5802 (1976).

11

Apo B-Dependent and -Independent Cellular Cholesterol Homeostasis

ANDREW A. KANDUTSCH The Jackson Laboratory, Bar Harbor, Maine

INTRODUCTION

Cholesterol has four different essential functions in vertebrates: it is a component of cellular membranes; as the free and esterified sterol to fatty acids, it is a structural component of lipoproteins; and it is the precursor of both bile acids and steroid hormones. The several requirements for cholesterol may be met either by synthesis within cells to meet their specific needs, or by unidirectional uptake from blood plasma or interstitial fluids. In addition, the unesterified cholesterol molecules in lipoproteins are in equilibrium with those in the plasma membranes of cells. Equilibrium between the various cellular and lipoprotein compartments containing cholesterol is influenced by the ratio of cholesterol to phospholipid and by the types of phospholipids in the compartments. Although high levels of dietary cholesterol may raise the cholesterol to phospholipid ratio in lipoproteins, red cells, and platelets, the extent to which the exchange mechanism contributes to the net flux of cholesterol in nucleated cells under normal conditions of cellular excess or deficiency is presently not clear. Net uptake of both free and esterified cholesterol by cells and tissues occurs when lipoproteins are internalized and degraded. Most lipoprotein degradation occurs in the liver which plays a unique and critical role in cholesterol homeostasis in the entire organism. To a lesser and variable degree, other tissues and organs may internalize and degrade LDL and HDLc by mechanisms that involve the binding of apo B or apo E to a cell surface receptor. Excess cholesterol within the cell may be esterified and stored in droplets, released to an exogenous acceptor, or converted into other products (i.e., bile acids).

However, the concentration of free cholesterol in cells does not fluctuate widely.

The regulation of receptor-mediated uptake of lipoproteins, as well as mechanisms for controlling the intracellular synthesis of cholesterol, has been studied intensely during the last decade. However, the literature dealing with these subjects is confusing, with different or contradictory hypotheses and disparate interpretations of experimental results. This chapter presents an overview of current knowledge of the mechanisms that modulate the concentrations of cholesterol in cells and tissues. Obviously, cholesterol homeostasis in an entire organism involves other complex control systems. The most important of these are controls over bile acid synthesis, bile secretion, absorption of sterols and bile acids in the intestine, and synthesis and degradation of various lipoprotein species.

THE CHOLESTEROL BIOSYNTHETIC PATHWAY

The pathway for the biosynthesis of cholesterol from acetyl-CoA is complex, involving more than 24 reactions. The pathway also gives rise, via branches at the level of the intermediate farnesyl pyrophosphate, to two other isopentenoid compounds, dolichol and coenzyme Q (CoQ). In addition to these end products, isopentenyl units are found in serine tRNAs as substituents on adenine residues and a farnesyl unit is attached to cytochrome oxidase. The different products of the pathway have different roles in a rather wide variety of cellular processes, including such major ones as the production and functioning of plasma membranes and glycoproteins and in energy metabolism.

All living cells have either the entire biosynthetic pathway or at least that part of it capable of giving rise to polyprenyl compounds that function like dolichol in oligosaccharide assembly or as the polyprenyl side chain of coenzyme Q (Fig. 1). Some organisms (e.g., bacteria, a few algae) do not synthesize sterol and do not have any

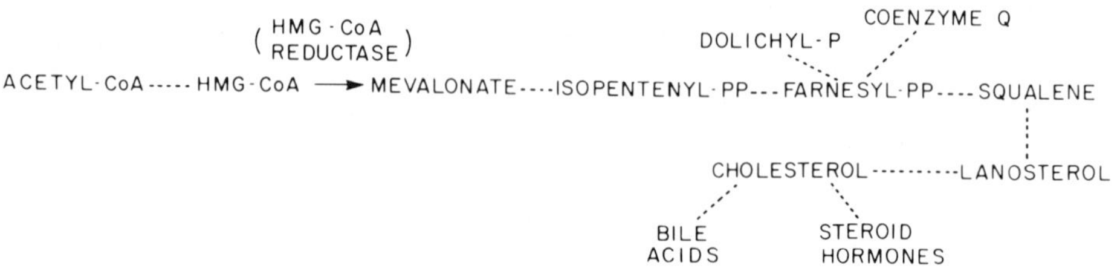

Fig. 1 Partial pathway for the biosynthesis of polyprenyl compounds.

of it in their membranes. Some amebas and most arthropods, including insects, do not synthesize sterols, but sterols must be ingested and taken up by cells for use in the production of cellular membranes and for metabolism to hormones. The cells of all vertebrate animals are capable of making cholesterol. However, in vivo, cholesterol is present in the blood and extracellular fluid; presumably, cellular cholesterol requirements could be met either by intracellular biosynthesis or by uptake. In culture, growing vertebrate cells are capable of synthesizing all of the cholesterol they require. If cholesterol synthesis is blocked, they can derive all, or nearly all, of their requirement from an exogenous source. In cells growing in culture medium containing serum, HMG-CoA reductase is partially repressed and the cells derive part of their cholesterol from synthesis and part from the serum lipoproteins. The extent to which various cells in vivo meet their cholesterol requirements by intracellular biosynthesis or by uptake from the extracellular fluid is an important question that bears heavily upon current concepts of the regulation of cholesterol synthesis.

Cholesterol is an end product in most vertebrate cells, except for the reduction of a small fraction to cholestanol. Its major—perhaps only—functional role in these cells is as a component of the plasma membrane and intracellular membranes. Cell replication requires the production of new membranes and, in synchronized cell cultures, the synthesis of cholesterol increases dramatically during the G_1 phase of the cell cycle, falling again to low levels by the beginning of the S phase. In vivo, high rates of cholesterol synthesis are associated with rapid cell division in skin, intestine, developing brain, hemopoietic tissues, and malignant tumors, whereas low rates of sterol synthesis are found in quiescent cells, e.g., those of mature brain, muscle, kidney, and lungs. Liver has few dividing cells; however, it utilizes large amounts of cholesterol for bile acid production and for incorporation into lipoproteins. The amount of cholesterol required by the liver for these purposes increases with the ingestion of food and is influenced by the nature of the diet. Endocrine organs also have special requirements for cholesterol as the precursor of steroid hormones. Utilization of cholesterol for this purpose changes in response to specific, discontinuous physiological signals.

REGULATION OF THE PATHWAY

It is apparent from the preceding brief description of the pathway, its products, and their functions, that the requirements of various differentiating, replicating, and quiescent cells for each of the several products of the pathway (e.g., dolichol, CoQ, cholesterol) may differ temporally and quantitatively. Thus, regulation of the pathway in a single cell must allow for differential rates of synthesis of the various products. There is clear evidence that in the liver in vivo and in cells in culture the regulation of cholesterol synthesis is *quantitatively* different from the regulation of dolichol and CoQ synthesis. Furthermore, the mechanism that regulates dolichol synthesis in some differentiating tissues appears to be *qualitatively* different from, and independent of, the mechanism that controls cholesterol synthesis (1). It is also apparent that a requirement for increased synthesis of cholesterol for bile acid or lipoprotein production in the liver is independent of a requirement for steroid hormone production in endocrine glands or of a need for membrane production by dividing cells. Thus, cholesterol synthesis for these different purposes must be regulated independently.

The Major Site of Regulation over Cholesterol Biosynthesis: Reduction of 3-Hydroxy-3-Methylglutaryl-Coenzyme A (HMG-CoA) to Mevalonic Acid

Under most conditions, the rate-limiting reaction in the biosynthetic pathway is that catalyzed by HMG-CoA reductase. The level of this enzyme activity, and consequently the rate of cholesterol synthesis, is altered in response to a variety of stimuli (Table 1). In vivo, the hepatic and intestinal enzyme, but not enzyme in other tissues, exhibits a diurnal cycle. Hepatic HMG-CoA reductase is depressed by

Table 1 Tissue Rates of Cholesterol Synthesis

High		Low
Liver	↔[a]	Liver
Adrenal gland	↔[a]	Adrenal gland
Testes (spermatogenic)		Large bowel
Ovary		Kidney
Small bowel		Lungs
Skin (epidermis)		Spleen
Hematopoietic tissues		Mature brain
Developing brain		Muscle
Malignant tumors		

[a]Regulated between high and low rates.

dietary sterols or fasting and is stimulated by factors that increase the excretion of bile acids and cholesterol by interfering with their reabsorption in the intestine (e.g., cholestyramine, plant sterols). Administration of a large dose of mevalonic acid, the product of the reaction catalyzed by HMG-CoA reductase, suppresses the reductase, presumably by increasing the concentration of a regulatory metabolite further along the pathway. Various hormones, especially insulin, glucagon, and thyroxine, also may effect the level of enzyme activity (Table 2). The rate of cholesterol synthesis in the intestine is inhibited by whole bile but not by cholesterol or bile acids. Certain oxysterols (e.g., 25-hydroxycholesterol, 7-ketocholesterol) suppress intestinal cholesterol synthesis when they are fed with the diet but cause only transient suppression in liver. HMG-CoA reductase in endocrine glands increases when steroid hormone production is stimulated by trophic hormones.

In cell cultures there is a burst of HMG-CoA reductase activity and sterol synthesis in the G_1 phase of the cell cycle, and levels of reductase activity are positively correlated with rates of culture growth. Addition of serum, LDL, HDLc, VLDL, or certain oxygenated sterols to the culture medium suppresses HMG-CoA reductase. In contrast, purified cholesterol or other monohydroxy sterols have no effect, providing that an antioxidant is present in the medium (6). High concentrations of mevalonic acid suppress HMG-CoA reductase in cell cultures as they do in liver in vivo. Two similar fungal metabolites, compactin and mevinolin, act as analogs of HMG-CoA to competitively inhibit HMG-CoA reductase. These competitive inhibitors cause HMG-CoA reductase levels to increase in liver and in cell cultures, while at the same time cholesterol synthesis is inhibited. Similar increases in HMG-CoA reductase are seen in cells deficient in cytosolic acetyl-CoA as a result of treatment with (−)hydroxycitrate, or in cells genetically deficient in HMG-CoA synthetase (7). In these cases, where increased HMG-CoA reductase is associated with blockage of the pathway at, or prior to, the production of mevalonate, addition of mevalonate to the medium causes the elevated levels of reductase to decline to normal or lower levels.

HMG-CoA reductase is a microsomal glycoprotein, of molecular weight ∿97,000, with N-linked, high-mannose oligosaccharide chains. Dolichol is essential to N-linked glycoprotein assembly and is, therefore, involved in the production of HMG-CoA reductase. Recently, the mRNA coding for the reductase has been sequenced and the amino acid sequence of HMG-CoA reductase has been deduced (8). HMG-CoA reductase has a short half-life, about 1.5 hours, so extensive changes in the amount of the enzyme can be brought about in a matter of a few hours by altering the rate of its synthesis and/or the rate of its degradation. Essentially all of the major regulatory changes in HMG-CoA reductase activity that have been observed in vivo or in

Table 2 Factors That Influence HMG-CoA Reductase Activity and Cholesterol Synthesis[a]

Factor	Effect on HMG reductase	Effect on cholesterol synthesis
Liver in vivo		
Diurnal cycle in food intake and light	Cycle	Cycle
Food deprivation	Decrease	Decrease
Dietary sterols (e.g., cholesterol, cholest-4-en-3-one, cholic acid)	Decrease	Decrease
Mevalonic acid (bolus)	Decrease	Increase
Dietary cholestyramine or plant sterols	Increase	Increase
Compactin or mevinolin	Increase	Decrease
Triton WR 1339 (i.p.)	Increase	Increase
Cell cultures		
Cell replication	Cycle (G_1 phase)	Cycle
VLDL, LDL, HDLc	Decrease	Decrease
Mevalonic acid	Decrease	Increase
Oxysterols	Decrease	Decrease
Insulin (surviving hepatocytes)	Activation	?
Glucagon (surviving hepatocytes)	Inactivation	?
Compactin or mevinolin	Increase	Decrease
(−) Hydroxy citrate	Increase	Decrease

[a]See references 2 to 5 for relevant reviews.

vitro are slow enough to be mediated by this mechanism. However, short-term regulation of the activity of HMG-CoA reductase by reversible phosphorylation has been demonstrated and is proposed as an additional, physiologically important control.

Although HMG-CoA reductase is the rate-limiting enzyme for cholesterol synthesis under normal conditions, many of the other enzymes in the pathway are coordinately regulated with the reductase. Thus, when the concentration of HMG-CoA reductase increases or decreases, corresponding changes—although slower and less extensive—occur in enzyme activities along the entire pathway. These secondary changes in other enzyme activities increase the capacity for large alterations in the rate of cholesterol synthesis, and tend to maintain the status of HMG-CoA reductase as the rate-limiting enzyme in the pathway.

Regulation of HMG-CoA Reductase Synthesis/Degradation

The mechanism by which major regulatory changes in sterol synthesis are brought about in vivo or in cultured cells involves a change in the rate of synthesis of HMG-CoA reductase. In some cases, a change in the rate of degradation of the reductase has also been observed. These changes in the rate of HMG-CoA reductase synthesis are accompanied by corresponding changes in the level of its mRNA. It is generally accepted that some or all of these changes are due to feedback repression of HMG-CoA reductase by a sterol product of the pathway. However, there is considerable disagreement in the published literature as to the source of the regulatory sterol (whether extra- or intracellular) and its nature, whether it is cholesterol or a related oxysterol.

Apo B (Apo E)-dependent regulation of HMG-CoA reductase and cholesterol synthesis. The hypothesis that HMG-CoA reductase and sterol synthesis is regulated by lipoprotein cholesterol has its roots in the striking observation that dietary cholesterol can repress hepatic HMG-CoA reductase and sterol synthesis nearly completely within hours after its ingestion. The hypothesis is easy to accept because we anticipate that a feedback system regulating the rate of cholesterol synthesis will monitor the concentration of cholesterol. It should, however, be kept in mind that high rates of cholesterol synthesis in intestine, developing brain, skin, and blood-forming tissues are virtually unaffected by changes in blood cholesterol concentrations or by dietary cholesterol. Furthermore, the effect of dietary cholesterol upon HMG-CoA reductase in liver is not specific, since other dietary sterols that are not metabolized to cholesterol (e.g., cholic acid, cholest-4-en-3-one) can influence the hepatic enzyme in the same way as cholesterol. Therefore, repression of hepatic HMG-CoA reductase by dietary cholesterol does not indicate that cholesterol is itself the regulatory molecule in liver.

A model for the general regulation of cholesterol synthesis by LDL, proposed by Brown and Goldstein (9), has gained wide recognition and is presented without qualification in many current reviews and books. The essential features of the model are as follows:

1. LDL binds to a cell surface receptor via apo B.
2. The receptor-LDL complex localizes in coated pits.
3. The complex is endocytosed and lysosomal degradation of LDL occurs with release of free cholesterol to the cytoplasm.
4. The released cholesterol fulfills the sterol requirements of the cell, increases cholesterol esterification by stimulating acyl-CoA:cholesteryl acyltransferase (ACAT), down-regulates the LDL receptor, and represses HMG-CoA reductase.

However, some of the basic assumptions that underlie the model appear to be incorrect and recent evidence indicates that LDL does not play a major—or general—role in the regulation of cholesterol synthesis in vivo.

The basic observations that support the hypothesis were made with cultures of normal human fibroblasts and fibroblasts from patients with familial hypercholesterolemia (FH) type II. The addition of serum or LDL to the medium of normal fibroblast cultures resulted in all of the changes indicated by the model. In contrast, LDL does not bind specifically to fibroblasts homozygous for FH, and none of the changes that follow binding to normal fibroblasts occurs. The LDL receptor revealed by these results has been isolated as a glycoprotein, of molecular weight 160,000, and shown to be present on the surfaces of most cell types (10).

Although LDL depresses the concentration of HMG-CoA reductase and of cell surface LDL receptors while increasing the esterification of cholesterol by fatty acids, these changes are not causally related. Thus, under other conditions, HMG-CoA reductase can be repressed while the synthesis and concentration of cholesterol esters decline (11), or while the concentration of surface LDL receptors increases (12). The apparent increase in ACAT activity in cells incubated with LDL seems to be largely or entirely due to increases in the concentrations of cholesterol substrate available to the microsomal enzyme.

It may be noted here that all of the changes found in cultured cells treated with LDL are also induced by relatively very low concentrations of certain oxygenated sterols. The obvious possibility that the effects attributed to LDL cholesterol are, in fact, due to small amounts of oxygenated sterols is discussed further later.

Uptake of LDL cholesterol vs. de novo cholesterol synthesis in nonhepatic cells in vivo. As is discussed more fully in the following chapter, LDL (apo B) receptors also bind apo E (HDL_c) and are more correctly designated as apo B,E receptors. There appear to be some species differences in receptor specificity. However, apo B,E receptors are present upon the surfaces of mammalian cell cultures of many cell types. The physiological relevance of the receptor-dependent uptake of LDL observed with cultured cells has been tested by two kinds of experiments: (1) those aimed at determining the extent of LDL uptake by various tissues in vivo, and (2) experiments to determine the source of cholesterol present in various cells and tissues; i.e., what proportion of the total is derived by uptake from the plasma lipoproteins and what proportion by local synthesis. The methodology and the species of animal used in different investigations vary, and there are appreciable differences in the results obtained and the conclusions drawn. However, some specific statements and generalizations can be made, based largely upon the extensive studies of Dietschy and co-workers (13,14).

1. There are important species differences in rates of hepatic cholesterol synthesis, the rate in rat liver being exceptionally high. In the rat and monkey, a large proportion of the cholesterol of the adrenal gland and spleen, but not that of any other nonhepatic tissue, is derived from extracellular fluids. In other species (hamster, guinea pig, rabbit), only a minor part of the cholesterol present in extrahepatic tissues is taken up from the circulation; instead, nearly all of it is synthesized locally.
2. There are corresponding important species differences in the uptake and degradation of LDL. The proportion of total LDL degradation that takes place in the livers of rats, pigs, and hamsters has been reported to be 52, 39, and 73%, respectively. Not all of the LDL taken up by the liver involves binding to the LDL receptor. Receptor-mediated uptake in the rat accounts for about 67% of the total; in the hamster, the proportion is about 90%. In the rat, appreciable uptake of LDL, based upon tissue weight, occurs in the adrenal gland, ovary, and spleen. In the hamster, the intestine accounts for about 7% of the total LDL uptake, whereas only minor amounts are taken up by other tissues. These measurements of LDL uptake, in vivo, are generally consistent with those obtained by measuring the proportion of cholesterol in different organs, which is derived from extracellular sources.

Evidence that receptor-mediated LDL uptake does not regulate cholesterol synthesis in extrahepatic tissues in vivo. Since only a minor proportion of the cholesterol present in most extrahepatic tissues is taken up from extracellular fluids, it seems clear that cholesterol synthesis in these cells is not regulated by the uptake of LDL cholesterol. Certainly high rates of sterol synthesis in organs such as developing brain, skin, intestinal mucosa, or hematopoietic tissues in vivo are essentially independent of dietary cholesterol or of blood levels of LDL or cholesterol. Regulation of sterol synthesis in brain is especially significant in this regard, because it is physically separated by the blood-brain barrier from circulating lipoproteins and cholesterol. In developing brains, with many replicating and differentiating cells, the rate of sterol synthesis is high. In mature brains, sterol synthesis can hardly be detected and cholesterol turnover is extremely slow. The low rate of cholesterol turnover in mature brain shows that quiescent cells may require very little additional cholesterol for maintenance and repair. Measurements of LDL uptake and rates of sterol synthesis in rat intestine (15) and in hamster liver (16) indicate that these two parameters are not correlated and are regulated independently. Under most circumstances wherein the supply of exogenous cholesterol available to the liver is altered (e.g., by dietary cholesterol) or the demand for secretion of sterol products is changed (e.g., by cholestyramine feeding), the rate of LDL uptake remains constant, while the rate of cholesterol synthesis varies (13). However, increased numbers of hepatic LDL-like receptors and increased uptake of LDL were observed when the adaptive increase in HMG-CoA reductase to a bile acid sequestrant was blocked by mevinolin (17). Further evidence that cholesterol synthesis is not normally regulated in vivo by receptor-mediated uptake of LDL comes from studies of receptor-negative FH patients (FH, homozygous) and receptor-negative rabbits (WHHL) with extremely high levels of LDL, and of patients with abetalipoproteinema (absence of LDL). Whole-body cholesterol synthesis rates and rates of cholesterol synthesis in various tissues and organs of receptor-deficient humans and rabbits and in patients with abetalipoproteinemia are normal (18–20). Moreover, the numbers of LDL receptors on the cells of abetalipoproteinemia patients are approximately normal, although fully induced levels of receptor might be expected in the absence of LDL (21).

All of the results obtained with genetic variants lacking LDL or the LDL receptor are consistent with the idea that receptor-mediated uptake of LDL is not responsible, in a major or direct way, for the regulation of cholesterol synthesis in vivo. At the same time, it is clear from studies with FH patients and WHHL rabbits that receptor-mediated LDL uptake is important for the degradation of LDL. When the receptors are absent, the fractional rate of LDL turnover is decreased and LDL accumulates to very high concentrations in the blood. Despite evidence that hepatic rates of cholesterogenesis are not increased in LDL receptor-deficient rabbits, it seems apparent that suppression of hepatic sterol synthesis by ingested cholesterol is mediated by lipoproteins that deliver cholesterol to the liver. These lipoproteins include chylomicron and VLDL remnants, HDL, and LDL.

Regulation of sterol synthesis by oxysterol metabolites. The hypothesis that it is the cholesterol component of LDL that regulates cellular cholesterol synthesis is based upon a few early reports that preparations of cholesterol (or some related C_{27}-sterols) suppressed cholesterol synthesis and HMG-CoA reductase activity when they were added at a high concentration (66 to 130 μM) to the media of cell cultures. However, subsequent investigations showed that, unlike aged preparations, freshly purified cholesterol did not have any effect on HMG-CoA reductase when the incubation time was short or when an antioxidant was present in the culture medium. When the incubation was prolonged and antioxidants were omitted, inhibition developed after a lag of about 6 hours. They also showed that a number of oxysterols produced from cholesterol by autoxidation reactions (e.g., 7-ketocholesterol, 25-hydroxycholesterol) suppressed sterol synthesis and HMG-CoA reductase when they were present in culture media at concentrations as low as 0.05 μM. Thus, it appears that the inhibitory activity attributed to crystalline cholesterol in various publications can be accounted for by contaminant oxysterols that were present in the initial preparation or generated during incubation in the absence of an antioxidant (5). Potent oxysterol repressors of the reductase have been identified in commercial samples of fetal calf serum, in freshly isolated human serum, and in human serum lipoproteins, including LDL (22). Most of the oxysterols found in serum or lipoproteins are probably products of cholesterol autoxidation (e.g., 7-ketocholesterol, 7α-hydroxycholesterol, 25-hydroxycholesterol). However, the 26-hydroxycholesterol found in serum lipoproteins probably originates in the liver where it is produced as a bile acid metabolite. The combined inhibitory activities of these oxysterols initially present in human serum or in lipoprotein preparations may be sufficient to inhibit sterol synthesis in cell cultures under usual culture conditions. Furthermore, autoxidation of cholesterol to give rise to inhibitory oxysterols is facilitated by unsaturated fatty acids that are present in high concentrations in serum and lipoproteins. Since a potent oxysterol such as 25-hydroxycholesterol produces the same effects as LDL in cell culture, these observations are consistent with the possibility that the effects of LDL are, in fact, due to free or esterified oxysterols contained therein. Studies with mutant cell cultures provide further evidence that LDL and oxysterols act through a common mechanism. A number of independent, mutant cell lines selected for resistance to the effects of one oxysterol (25-hydroxycholesterol) are all resistant to the effects of LDL as well as to the effects of all other oxysterols tested.

Structural features of cholestanol and lanostanol derivatives that have been shown to be potent suppressors of HMG-CoA reductase in cell cultures are illustrated in Fig. 2. All of the sterols have a hydroxyl function at position 3, and a second hydroxyl or keto function at

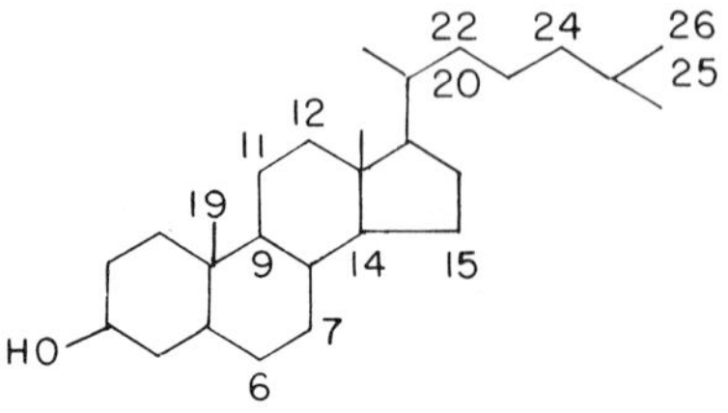

5α-CHOLESTAN-3β-OL

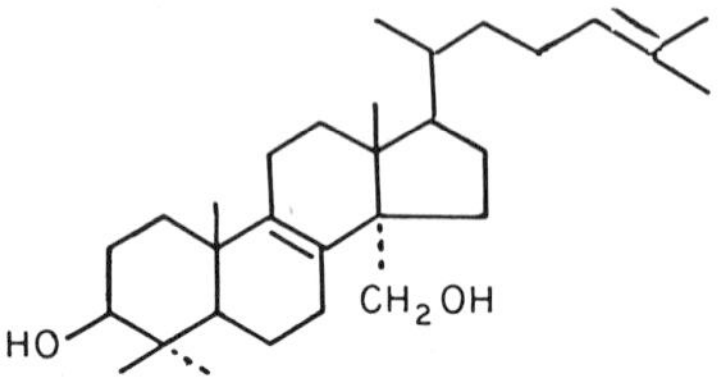

32-HYDROXYLANOSTEROL

Fig. 2 Oxysterol repressors of HMG-CoA reductase.

one of the numbered positions. The potencies of the sterols vary widely, cholestanol derivatives with an oxygen function located on the side chain or on carbon-15 being the most potent. Culture medium concentrations that are required to suppress the reductase are in the range of 10^{-6} to 10^{-8} M.

The mechanism by which sterols suppress the synthesis of HMG-CoA reductase. As mentioned previously, all of the major regulatory fluctuations in HMG-CoA reductase activity that have been examined in detail involve alterations in the rate of synthesis of the reductase (23–25). In vivo, these include changes in the hepatic reductase: during the diurnal cycle, in response to fasting, or to the administration of cholesterol, mevalonate, cholestyramine, or compactin (or mevinolin). In cultured cells, LDL, mevalonate, and oxysterols suppress the synthesis of HMG-CoA reductase, whereas mevinolin elevates it. There is some indication that the rate of reductase degradation in cell cultures may be inhibited by mevinolin and increased by oxysterols or LDL under some—but not all—conditions. These changes in the synthesis of HMG-CoA reductase are associated with corresponding changes in the concentration of reductase mRNA, indicating that the major site of regulation is either gene transcription or inhibition of the degradation of the mRNA. It is of some interest that 25-hydroxycholesterol does not suppress HMG-CoA reductase activity in enucleated cells (cytoplasts), consistent with regulation at the level of gene transcription (26). However, the concentration of HMG-CoA reductase activity is stable in the cytoplasts, suggesting that degradation of the reductase ceased shortly after enucleation. The apparent short half-life of the degradative system suggests the possibility of control at this level over HMG-CoA reductase.

A number of oxygenated sterols, which suppress HMG-CoA reductase when added to cell cultures, are natural precursors of cholesterol or products of its metabolism to bile acids or steroid hormones. These sterols include the bile acid intermediates 7α- and 26-hydroxycholesterol, the steroid hormone precursors 20α- and 22R-hydroxycholesterol, and the obligate cholesterol precursors 32-hydroxylanosterol and 32-oxolanosterol. 24(S)24-Hydroxycholesterol (cerebrosterol) has been found in bovine brains (5). Evidence obtained in vitro suggests that other oxysterol metabolites capable of repressing the reductase may also be produced. In the presence of inhibitors of 2,3-oxidosqualene cyclase, squalene 2,3:22,23-diepoxide is produced and metabolized to 24(S),25-epoxycholesterol (27). Unidentified polar sterols capable of suppressing HMG-CoA reductase activity are present in extracts of cultured cells. Inhibitory oxysterols are, therefore, produced in all cells that synthesize cholesterol as an end product, as well as in cells that synthesize cholesterol and metabolize it to other steroid products.

A proposed scheme (Fig. 3) for the feedback regulation of HMG-CoA reductase by an intracellular sterol metabolite is based upon models for bacterial induction-repression regulatory systems and models for the regulation of protein synthesis by steroid hormones. The scheme postulates intracellular production of a regulatory oxysterol and specific binding of the oxysterol to a soluble protein.

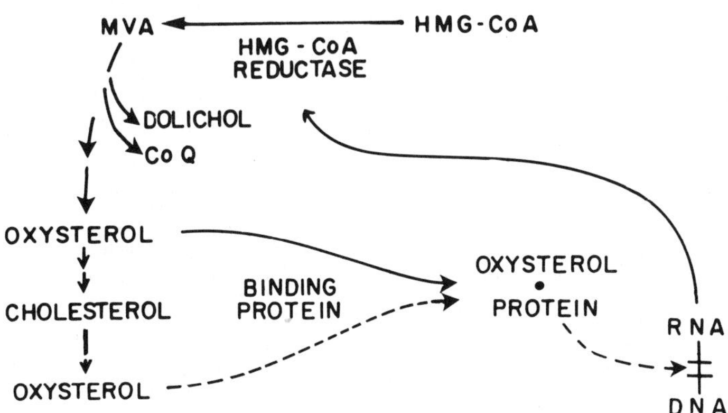

Fig. 3 Model for the regulation of HMG-CoA reductase by oxysterols.

The sterol-protein complex inhibits transcription or translation of the gene for HMG-CoA reductase. In support of this model, a cytosolic binding protein specific for oxysterols has been identified (28,29). The binding protein is present in all cells and tissues tested, including a variety of cell cultures, liver, kidney, spleen, and brain. It binds 25-hydroxycholesterol with high affinity (K_d 10^{-9} *M*) and other oxysterols with an affinity that is generally proportional to their activities as repressors of HMG-CoA reductase (Table 3). The binding protein does not bind cholesterol, estradiol, dexamethasone, cortisone, or testosterone. The uncomplexed binding protein (molecular weight ∿236,000) appears to be composed of at least three subunits. Upon binding of an oxysterol, a subunit is lost to give a sterol-protein complex of about 169,000 daltons. Under appropriate conditions, a smaller polypeptide (molecular weight ∿97,000) with sterol-binding activity is obtained. The sterol-binding characteristics (K_d and kinetics) of the protein are generally similar to those of steroid hormone-receptor interactions, and the polymeric structure of the

Table 3 Comparison of Relative Affinities of Some Oxysterols for the Binding Protein with Their Potencies as Repressors of HMG-CoA Reductase

Sterol	Repression of HMG-CoA reductase (μM)[a]	Relative binding affinities (μM)[b]
25-Hydroxycholesterol	0.17	0.03
(25R)26-Hydroxycholesterol	0.26	0.11
20α-Hydroxycholesterol	0.30	0.06
5α-Lanost-8-ene-3β,32-diol	0.70	0.45
24-Ketocholesterol	1.0	0.33
7-Ketocholesterol	1.7	1.4
7α-Hydroxycholesterol	2.5	1.1
22R-Hydroxycholesterol	8.2	3.8

[a]Concentration required for 50% repression of reductase in cell cultures.
[b]Concentration required to displace 50% of tritiated 25-hydroxycholesterol.
Source: Ref. 28.

protein seems to be somewhat analogous with the general structure of steroid hormone receptors (30).

Taken together, the specificity of the effect of the oxysterols upon the synthesis of HMG-CoA reductase, their high potencies, and the existence of a specific oxysterol-binding protein provide strong support for the model in Fig. 3 and for its biological relevance. However, direct evidence that oxysterol metabolites do regulate the reductase is still lacking. Until such evidence is obtained, further speculation may be of little value. Nevertheless, it may be worthwhile to suggest a means, consistent with the model, by which independent regulation of cholesterol synthesis in different tissues for different purposes might be achieved. In replicating cells that do not catabolize cholesterol but employ it for membrane production, HMG-CoA reductase may be regulated by a precursor sterol (i.e., 32-hydroxycholesterol). In liver, regulation of cholesterol synthesis for bile acid production may be regulated by bile acid precursors such as 7α- or 26-hydroxycholesterol. In endocrine glands, 20α-hydroxycholesterol could regulate cholesterol synthesis for hormone production. Regulation of the reductase by a product of cholesterol catabolism presupposes that regulation by an obligate cholesterol precursor such as 32-hydroxylanosterol is inoperative. Regulation by a precursor oxysterol could be obviated by increasing the threshold concentration of oxysterol required for repression of the reductase beyond levels attained by the precursor. Cholesterol catabolites, present in relatively high concentrations, might then provide feedback regulation of the reductase. Such a situation may exist in liver since primary liver cell cultures are about 10 times more resistant to oxysterols than are other cell cultures. These cultures, and liver in vivo, contain a relatively nonspecific cytosolic protein that binds both cholesterol and 25-hydroxycholesterol (31). Possibly the nonspecific binding protein competes with the oxysterol-binding protein for regulatory oxysterols, essentially inactivating low concentrations of a cholesterol precursor and increasing the effective dose of oxysterol to levels that can only be met by a product of cholesterol catabolism.

The scheme in Fig. 3 for regulation of cholesterol synthesis by oxysterols can be employed to explain all established examples of regulation of HMG-CoA reductase by sterols in vivo or in cultured cells. It is, however, incomplete in that it does not indicate how levels of cellular regulatory oxysterols are modulated or what the effectors are. The availability of exogenous cholesterol for bile acid production in liver may determine the concentration of a regulatory oxysterol. In endocrine glands, signals governing the concentration of oxysterols might be initiated by tropic hormones. At the present time, there seem to be no clear ideas regarding the signals that initiate and terminate the cycle of HMG-CoA reductase in replicating cells. It should be clear from the above discussion that detailed knowledge of the feedback regulation of HMG-CoA reductase is incomplete and that current models are still largely speculative.

Other Proposed Regulatory Systems

Although there is little doubt that feedback regulation by sterols is a physiologically relevant control process, it seems unlikely that all regulation of HMG-CoA reductase observed in vivo is accomplished through this mechanism. For example, levels of many enzyme activities change during fasting, during feeding or light cycles, and during the cell cycle. Hormones alter the synthesis of many proteins and many metabolic activities. Changes induced in levels of HMG-CoA reductase by such factors may be a result of other, more general, mechanisms that control the synthesis of selected groups of proteins. On the other hand, since definitive evidence is not available, the possibility that a regulatory sterol is ultimately involved in each of these mechanisms cannot be excluded. A few other mechanisms for regulating HMG-CoA reductase have been proposed, but there is no clear or undisputed evidence that any of them are important under conditions in vivo.

Ancillary Effect of an Unidentified Metabolite of Mevalonate in Repression of HMG-CoA Reductase

As was discussed previously, when a large dose of mevalonate is administered intragastrically to rats, the synthesis of hepatic HMG-CoA reductase and the level of its mRNA decline. Similar results are obtained when mevalonate is added at high concentration to the media of cultured cells. These observations can be explained in terms of the increased production of a regulatory oxysterol resulting from an abnormally large flow of mevalonate metabolites. Under very special conditions an unidentified metabolite of mevalonate may depress HMG-CoA reductase activity through another mechanism. Reductase levels in various cell cultures growing in serum-containing or serum-free medium can be almost completely repressed by 25-hydroxycholesterol alone. However, if mevalonate synthesis is blocked by a genetic deficiency of HMG-CoA synthetase, or by the addition of high concentrations of mevinolin (or compactin) to the medium, HMG-CoA reductase activity rises several-fold. The addition of 25-hydroxycholesterol or LDL to these blocked cultures results in a marked decline in HMG-CoA reductase from its elevated level; however, appreciable reductase activity remains. The residual reductase activity is resistant to the further addition of oxysterol (or LDL), but declines rapidly when mevalonate is added to the culture medium (7,32). This observation has been taken to indicate that some unidentified product of mevalonate metabolism, other than a regulatory sterol, is required for full repression of the reductase.

Regulation of HMG-CoA Reductase Activity by Reversible Phosphorylation

It has been shown that HMG-CoA reductase in cell homogenates is inactivated when the homogenates are incubated with ATP and Mg^2, and that activity is regained upon reincubation with a phosphatase. An HMG-CoA reductase kinase (which phosphorylates and activates reductase) and a phosphatase have been identified in liver (33). One indication that phosphorylation of the enzyme may be of physiological significance is the observation that in liver, intesting, developing brain, and L-cell cultures, a major portion of the total HMG-CoA reductase present appears to be inactive and can be activated by preincubating a cell homogenate before assaying the enzyme. NaF, a phosphatase inhibitor, blocks activation of the enzyme. However, many other tissues and cell cultures have little of the inactive form of the enzyme. Other support for a physiological role is the observation that in surviving rat hepatocytes insulin causes activation, and glucagon some inactivation, of the reductase. Smaller corresponding changes in response to these hormones in vivo have been reported, but these reports have been contradicted by others. Whether or not reversible phosphorylation is employed in vivo for rapid regulation of HMG-CoA reductase activity and sterol synthesis is open to question. Marked regulatory changes in the level of HMG-CoA reductase in liver in vivo, or in cultured cells that occur over a period of hours in response to sterols or other environmental factors, do not involve any appreciable change in the ratio of active to inactive enzyme.

CONCLUSIONS

The organism has at least four different independent requirements for cholesterol: as a component of both cell membranes and circulating lipoproteins, and as a precursor of both bile acids and steroid hormones. Cholesterol required by various cells and tissues for these purposes can be taken up from the plasma or extracellular fluids, or it can be synthesized locally. Excess cholesterol within the cell can be stored as fatty acid esters or secreted by an equilibrium diffusion process. Liver, endocrine tissues, and intestine, which use cholesterol to produce secreted products, may take up high proportions of their total cholesterol from the plasma. These organs may also have high rates of cholesterol synthesis. By increasing or decreasing the rate of cholesterol synthesis, liver responds to changes in the amounts of cholesterol provided to it by the plasma. In other organs and cells, rates of cholesterol synthesis are largely independent of dietary cholesterol or levels of blood cholesterol. With the exception of liver and (in some species) the adrenal gland, most of the cholesterol present in cells and tissues is synthesized locally.

Many cell types have surface receptors that bind LDL or HDLc. Apo B-dependent, receptor-mediated uptake and degradation of LDL accounts for about two-thirds of total LDL uptake in the organism; most of the LDL is taken up and degraded in the liver and intestine. Under normal circumstances in vivo, there seems to be little regulation of the number of LDL receptors on cell surfaces or of LDL uptake; the changing requirements of cells and tissues for cholesterol are met by alterations in the rate of cholesterol synthesis.

The mechanisms by which the rate of cellular cholesterol synthesis is regulated are not yet clear. A major control system involves feedback repression of the synthesis of HMG-CoA reductase by a sterol product of the biosynthetic pathway. Current evidence suggests that the regulatory sterols are not cholesterol, but are oxysterols with more than one hydroxyl or keto function. Oxysterols repress the synthesis of the reductase by altering the level of its mRNA through a process that involves binding of the oxysterol to a specific cytosolic protein. It is thought that regulation of cholesterol synthesis for the production of bile acids or steroid hormones may be modulated by oxysterols produced from cholesterol as intermediates in these pathways. Regulation of cholesterol synthesis for membrane production in dividing cells that do not catabolize cholesterol may be modulated by a cholesterol precursor. Oxysterol feedback repression of HMG-CoA reductase could account for all of the major regulatory fluctuations in enzyme activity that have been observed in vivo; however, this remains to be demonstrated. Modulation of HMG-CoA reductase activity by reversible phosphorylation could provide for rapid, short-term changes in cholesterol synthesis. However, there is no clear evidence that such regulation occurs in vivo.

ACKNOWLEDGMENTS

The writing of this chapter and the author's work were supported by grants CA02758 (from the National Cancer Institute) and GM29241 (from the National Institutes of Health, DHHS).

REFERENCES

1. James, M. J., Potter, J. E. R., and Kandutsch, A. A., in *Regulation of HMG-CoA Reductase* (Sabine, J. R., ed.), CRC Press, Boca Raton, Fla., 1983.

2. Gibbons, G. F., Metropoulous, K. A., and Myant, N. B., *Biochemistry of Cholesterol*, Elsevier Biomedical Press, New York, 1982.

3. Schroepfer, G. J., Jr., *Annu. Rev. Biochem.*, *50*:585 (1981).

4. Dugan, R. E., in *Biosynthesis of Isoprenoid Compounds* (Porter, J. W., and Spurgeon, S. L., eds.), John Wiley & Sons, New York, 1981, p. 95.

5. Kandutsch, A. A., Chen, H. W., and Heiniger, H.-J., *Science*, *201*:498 (1978).

6. Kandutsch, A. A., and Chen, H. W., *J. Biol. Chem.*, *252*:409, (1977).

7. Sinensky, M., Torget, R., Schnitzer-Polokoff, R., and Edwards, P. A., *J. Biol. Chem.*, *257*:7284 (1982).

8. Chin, D. J., Gil, G., Russell, D. W., Liscum, L., Luskey, K. L., Basu, S. K., Okayama, H., Berg, P., Goldstein, J. L., and Brown, M. S., *Nature (London)*, *308*:613 (1984).

9. Brown, M. S., and Goldstein, J. L., *Ann. Rev. Biochem.*, *46*:897 (1977).

10. Schneider, W. J., Beisiegel, U., Goldstein, J. L., and Brown, M. S., *J. Biol. Chem.*, *257*:2664 (1982).

11. Goldstein, J. L., Faust, J. R., Dygos, J. H., Chorniat, R. G., and Brown, M. S., *Proc. Natl. Acad. Sci. U.S.A.*, *25*:1877 (1978).

12. Fung, C. H., and Khachadurian, A. K., *J. Biol. Chem.*, *255*: 676 (1980).

13. Dietschy, J. M., Spady, D. K., and Stange, E. F., *Biochem. Soc. Trans.*, *11*:639 (1983).

14. Turley, S. D., Anderson, J. M., and Dietschy, J. M., *J. Lipid. Res.*, *22*:551 (1981).

15. Stange, E. F., and Dietschy, J. M., *Proc. Natl. Acad. Sci. U.S.A.*, *80*:5739 (1983).

16. Spady, D. K., Turley, S. D., and Dietschy, J. M., *Biochim. Biophys. Acta*, *735*:381 (1983).

17. Kovanen, P. T., Bilheimer, D. W., Goldstein, J. L., Garamillo, G. G., and Brown, M. S., *Proc. Natl. Acad. Sci. U.S.A.*, *78*: 1194 (1981).

18. Dietschy, J. M., Kita, T., Suckling, K. E., Goldstein, J. L., and Brown, M. S., *J. Lipid Res.*, *24*:469 (1983).

19. Jackson, R. L., Smith, L. C., Taunton, O. D., and Gotto, A. M., Jr., *Life Sci.*, *21*:1395 (1977).

20. Goodman, D. S., Deckelbaum, R. J., Palmer, R. H., Dell, R. B., Delpre, R. R. G., Beigel, Y., and Cooper, M., *J. Lipid Res.*, *24*:1605 (1983).

21. Illingworth, D. R., Alam, N. A., Sundberg, E. E., Hagemenas, F. C., and Layman, D. L., *Proc. Natl. Acad. Sci. U.S.A.*, *80*:3475 (1983).

22. Chen, H. W., *Fed. Proc.*, *43*:126 (1984).

23. Chin, D. J., Luskey, K. L., Faust, J. R., McDonald, R. J., Brown, M. S., and Goldstein, J. L., *Proc. Natl. Acad. Sci. U.S.A.*, *79*:7704 (1982).

24. Faust, J. R., Luskey, K. L., Chin, D. G., Goldstein, J. L., and Brown, M. S., *Proc. Natl. Acad. Sci. U.S.A.*, *79*:5205 (1982).

25. Clarke, C. F., Edwards, P. A., Lan, S.-F., Tanaka, R. D., and Fogelman, A. M., *Proc. Natl. Acad. Sci. U.S.A.*, *80*:3305 (1983).

26. Cavenee, W. K., Chen, H. W., and Kandutsch, A. A., *J. Biol. Chem.*, *256*:2675 (1981).

27. Nelson, J. A., Steckbeck, S. R., and Spencer, T. A., *J. Am. Chem. Soc.*, *103*:6974 (1981).

28. Taylor, F. R., Saucier, S. E., Shown, E. P., Parish, E. G., and Kandutsch, A. A., *J. Biol. Chem.*, *259*:12382 (1984).

29. Kandutsch, A. A., Taylor, F. R., and Shown, E. P., *J. Biol. Chem.*, *259*:12388 (1984).

30. Sherman, M. R., *Annu. Rev. Physiol.*, *46*:83 (1984).

31. Kandutsch, A. A., and Thompson, E. B., *J. Biol. Chem.*, *255*:10,813 (1980).

32. Brown, M. S., and Goldstein, J. L., *J. Lipid Res.*, *21*:505 (1980).

33. Ingebritsen, T. S., and Gibson, D. M., in *Molecular Aspects of Cellular Regulation* (Cohen, P., ed.), Vol. 1, Elsevier/North-Holland Press, Amsterdam, 1980, p. 63.

12

The Role of Apo E in Cholesterol Metabolism

KARL H. WEISGRABER Gladstone Foundation Laboratories for Cardiovascular Disease, University of California, San Francisco, California

INTRODUCTION

Cholesterol Metabolism

Cholesterol is an essential component in the maintenance of cellular membrane integrity. It also serves as a precursor for the synthesis of steroid hormones and bile acids. However, as is the case with many essential compounds, an excess of cholesterol can have devastating effects. This is best exemplified by the deposition of cholesterol in atherosclerotic plaques and the resultant clinical consequences of restricted arterial blood flow. Therefore, proper cholesterol homeostasis must be maintained in the body for normal function. Plasma lipoproteins play an important role in this homeostatic process, both in transporting or redistributing cholesterol to organs or cells requiring it for normal function and in transporting excess cholesterol from overloaded cells to the liver for elimination from the body. The roles that lipoprotein receptors and apolipoprotein (apo) B play in these processes are treated in other chapters in this book and will only be discussed briefly. For a more comprehensive review on lipoprotein receptors and cholesterol metabolism, the reader is referred to references 1 to 4. This chapter will focus on apo E and its role in both the delivery and removal of cholesterol from cells.

A simplified scheme of lipoprotein cholesterol metabolism emphasizing the delivery and removal of cholesterol from various tissues and organs is presented in Fig. 1. Dietary cholesterol and triglyceride enter the plasma as a component of chylomicrons. These triglyceride-rich lipoproteins are formed from the absorbed dietary lipids in intestinal epithelial cells and are secreted into the mesenteric lymph.

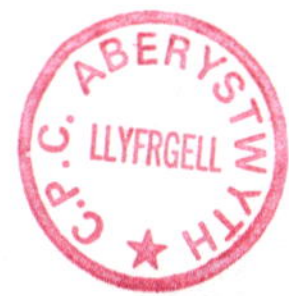

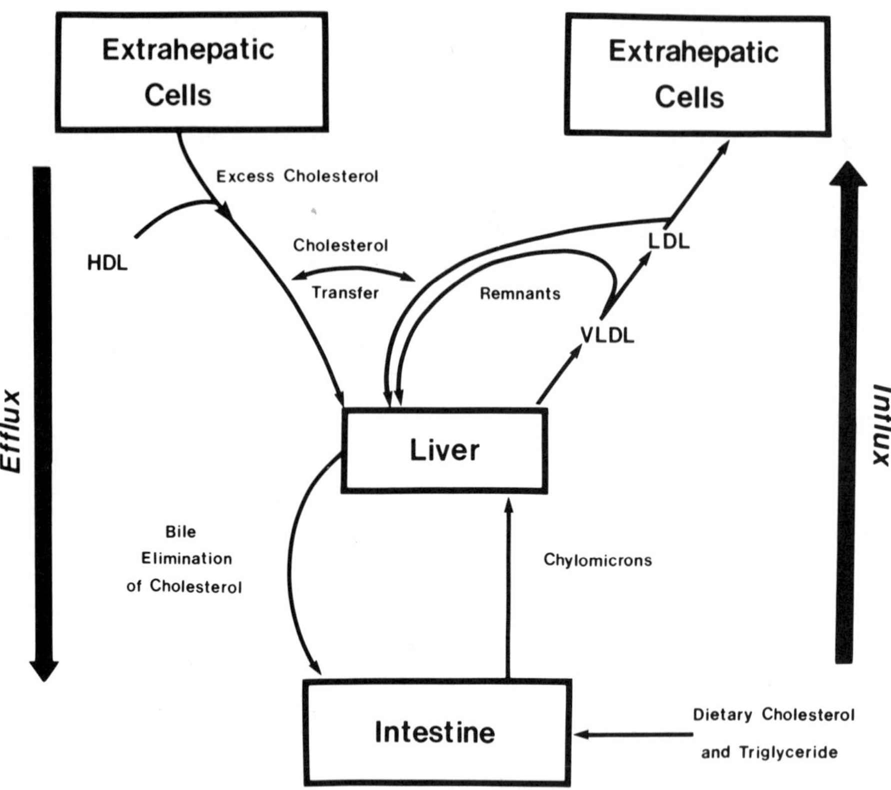

Fig. 1 Simplified schematic representation of lipoprotein-mediated cholesterol transport. The pathways on the right represent cholesterol influx into the body and the pathways on the left represent efflux from the body. The liver plays a central role in modulating the influx and efflux pathways as it is the only organ capable of eliminating cholesterol from the body. This elimination is accomplished through bile production.

The triglyceride core of circulating chylomicrons is hydrolyzed by the enzyme lipoprotein lipase, and the released fatty acids are used by cells for energy production or are stored in the form of triglycerides. This lipolytic process produces a remnant particle that is recognized and taken up by hepatic lipoprotein receptors. By this route, dietary cholesterol is delivered to the liver by a receptor-dependent process. (A discussion of these receptors will be presented in a later section.) The liver, in turn, is capable of synthesis and excretion of very-low-density lipoproteins (VLDL), which contain both triglyceride and cholesterol. It should be mentioned at this point that cells are capable of de novo synthesis of cholesterol. Thus, the cholesterol transported by the various lipoproteins shown in Fig. 1 represents cholesterol derived from both exogenous and endogenous sources. Cellular synthesis of cholesterol is a highly regulated process in which the uptake of lipoproteins by lipoprotein receptors plays a major role. A detailed discussion of this topic is presented in Chapter 13.

The VLDL secreted by the liver are also subjected to hydrolysis by lipoprotein lipase, and in this process a VLDL remnant is produced that is either taken up by the liver or converted to low-density lipoprotein (LDL) particles (Fig. 1). The LDL produced by the depletion of the triglyceride core of VLDL are cholesterol-rich lipoproteins. Depending on the species, differing proportions of VLDL remnants are converted to LDL. For example, in the rat, only ~10% is converted, whereas in man, a larger proportion is converted to LDL (5,6). The basis for this species distinction is not known. The LDL are capable of delivering cholesterol in a regulated manner to hepatic and extrahepatic cells via the LDL receptor. This receptor system has been delineated in a series of elegant studies by Goldstein and Brown and their associates (for a review see references 2 to 4 and Chapter 14). As will be discussed in the next section, apo E also binds to the LDL receptor. Therefore, the LDL receptor will be referred to as the apo B,E(LDL) receptor. The receptor has been demonstrated in a variety of cells and tissues, both hepatic and extrahepatic, including fibroblasts, smooth muscle cells, adrenal glands, testes, and ovaries. The Brown and Goldstein studies have established the central role that the apo B,E(LDL) receptor plays in lipoprotein metabolism and provided the stimulus that led to the description of other lipoprotein receptor systems. The cholesterol delivered to peripheral (extrahepatic) cells can be used for membrane synthesis or for specialized needs, as is the case with adrenal cells where the cholesterol is used for steroid hormone production.

The lipoprotein transport routes on the right-hand side of Fig. 1 can be viewed as an influx of cholesterol to various tissues and organs in the body, with the liver playing a central modulating role. To provide a balance for the influx of cholesterol, a mechanism must exist to provide a route for cholesterol efflux—the so-called reverse cholesterol transport process, which maintains cholesterol homeostasis. The efflux pathways are illustrated on the left-hand side of Fig. 1. It has been demonstrated in vitro that several cell types with an excess of cholesterol have the ability to secrete the excess cholesterol if the appropriate acceptor molecules are present (7). High-density lipoproteins (HDL) function as efficient acceptors. The cholesterol is secreted in the unesterified form and is esterified on the acceptor HDL particles by the plasma enzyme lecithin:cholesterol acyltransferase (LCAT), and the cholesteryl ester is incorporated into the core of the HDL. The cholesteryl ester can then be transported to the liver directly by HDL or transferred by a cholesteryl ester transfer protein to remnant particles (VLDL or LDL) and, thereby, be indirectly targeted to the liver. The liver, which plays a central role in cholesterol efflux, is the major organ capable of eliminating cholesterol from the body. This elimination is accomplished when the liver secretes either cholesterol or cholesterol that has been converted to bile acids into the bile. The bile is eliminated via the intestine.

In the following sections, the generalized lipoprotein transport routes shown in Fig. 1 and the lipoprotein receptors that are involved in these routes will be discussed in more detail. This chapter will focus on the role that apo E plays in these processes.

Apo E

Apolipoprotein E is an apolipoprotein component of several lipoprotein classes. As shown in Fig. 2, apo E migrates as a M_r = 35,000 protein as determined by SDS–gel electrophoresis and is contained in chylomicrons and their remnants, VLDL and a subclass of HDL, referred to as HDL with apo E (8,9). LDL is the only major lipoprotein class that does not contain apo E. The protein was first described in the early 1970s (10) and was originally referred to as the "arginine-rich" apolipoprotein because of its high arginine content (10 to 12%) relative to other apolipoproteins. It has been demonstrated in several species, including man, rat, rabbit, swine, guinea pig, mouse, and a variety of monkey species (8). The major site of apo E synthesis is the liver (11). However, apo E mRNA is also present in several peripheral tissues and cells, including the brain, kidney, testis, muscle, adrenal, and macrophages (12,13). The protein is synthesized with an 18-residue presegment that is cotranslationally cleaved, and it does not contain a prosegment (14). The gene encoding apo E has been mapped to chromosome 19 (15), and the complete nucleotide sequence, including putative regulatory elements, has been determined (16).

Human apo E has a molecular weight of 34,000 and is a single polypeptide chain containing 299 amino acids. The sequences of

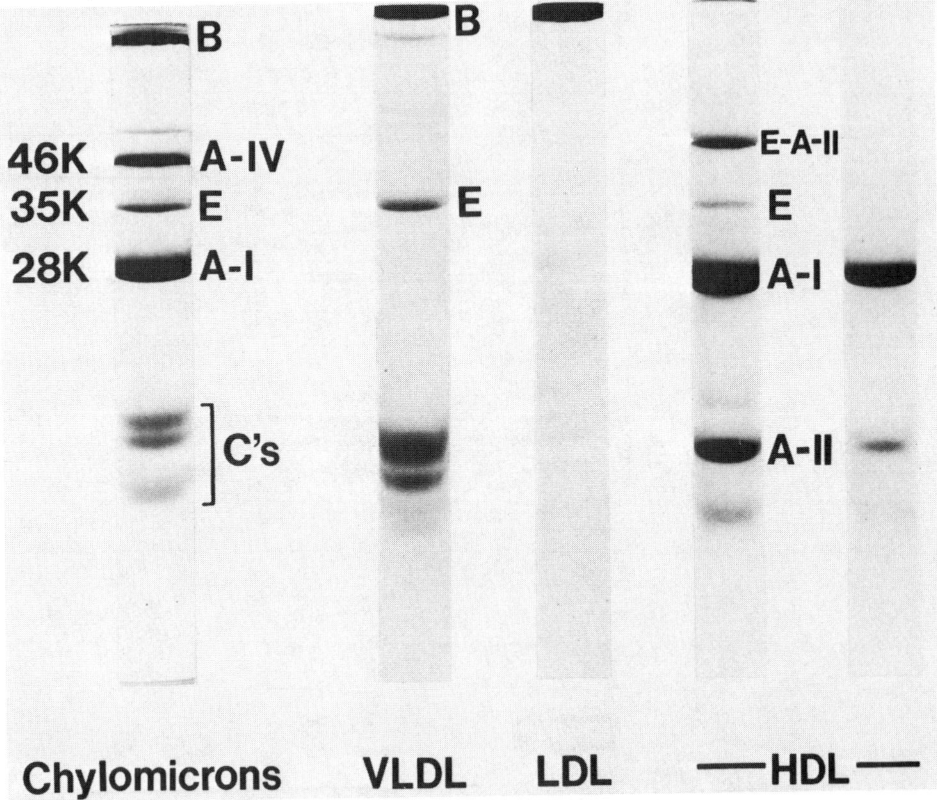

Fig. 2 Sodium dodecyl sulfate–polyacrylamide gels of chylomicrons VLDL, LDL, and HDL, showing the apolipoprotein composition of these lipoprotein classes. (From Ref. 1. Reproduced with permission.)

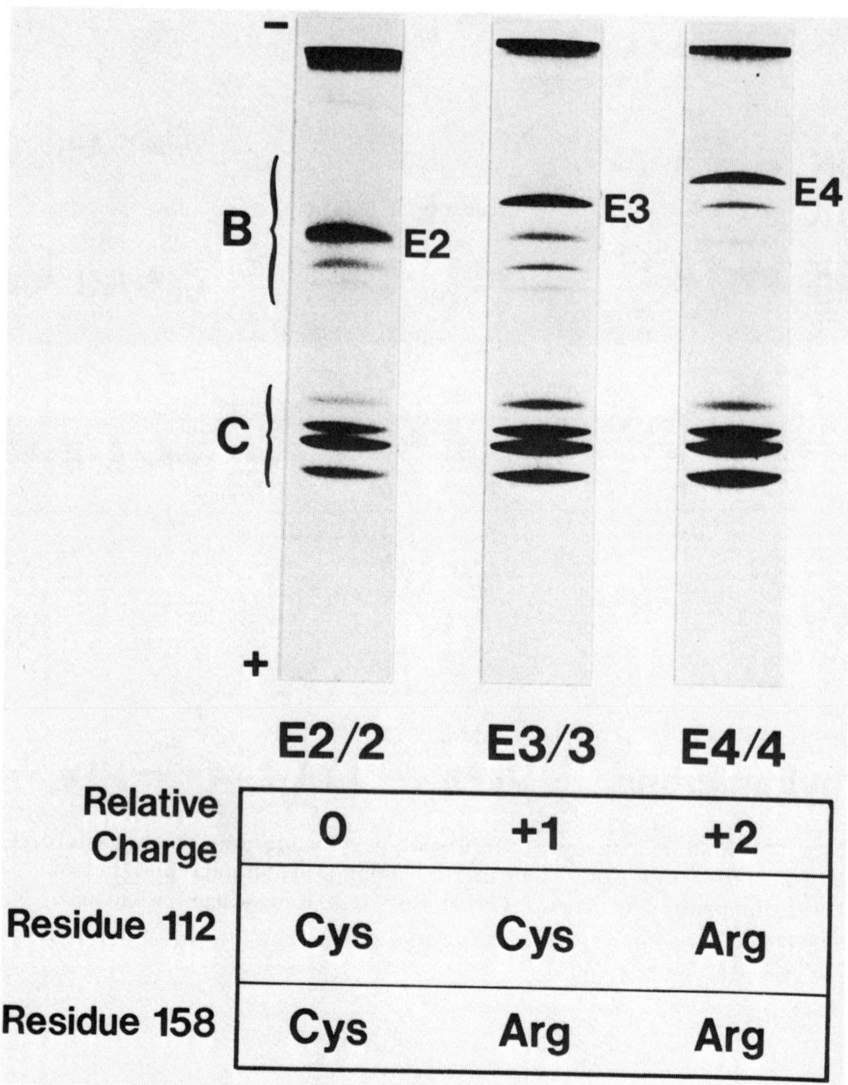

Fig. 3 Isoelectric focusing on polyacrylamide gels of the VLDL from subjects with homozygous phenotypes E2/2, E3/3, and E4/4. The major isoforms differ progressively from each other by one unit of positive charge. The minor isoforms have been demonstrated to arise by posttranslational addition of sialic acid. The basis for the charge heterogeneity of the major isoforms arises as the result of cysteine-arginine interchanges at residues 112 and 158. (From Ref. 19. Reproduced with permission.)

human (17) and rat apo E (18) are known (see Appendix for human sequence). Human apo E exhibits a charge polymorphism on isoelectric focusing gels (Fig. 3) that is the result of (1) a genetically determined polymorphism at the level of the structural gene (single locus) and (2) a variable content of sialic acid, which is added in a posttranslational glycosylation step. Most commonly, three major isoforms are observed and are designated by their focusing position on isoelectric focusing gels: E2, E3, and E4 (see Ref. 20 for nomenclature). Thus, as a result of the single genetic locus for apo E and the three major isoforms, six common phenotypes are observed: three homozygous (E2/2, E3/3, E4/4) and three heterozygous (E4/3, E4/2, E3/2). The results of screening studies from several laboratories around the world indicate the following approximate frequencies for the six common phenotypes: E4/4, 3%; E3/3, 60%; E2/2, 1%; E4/3, 22%; E4/2, 2%; and E3/2, 12%.

Isoelectric focusing gels of VLDL from three subjects demonstrating the three homozygous focusing patterns are shown in Fig. 3. The minor, more acidic apo E isoforms represent sialylated derivatives of the major isoform. The three major isoforms progressively differ from each other by one unit of charge. For the apo E shown in Fig. 3, this charge heterogeneity was determined to be the result of arginine-cysteine interchanges at two sites in the protein, residues 112 and 158, with the interchange of neutral cysteinyl residues and positively charged arginyl residues accounting for the charge differences (21).

Originally, it was assumed that only three alleles existed, each coding for one of the major isoforms: E2, E3, and E4. However, the heterogeneity of apo E has proved to be more complex. It is now known that structurally different forms of apo E can have identical total charges and thus focus in identical positions on isoelectric focusing gels. Also, apo E isoforms have now been observed that do not focus in one of the three common positions (E2, E3, or E4). The information currently available on the focusing position and structure of the known apo E variants is summarized in Table 1. As apo E3 is the most common isoform observed in the population, the structure of the variants is given relative to it. The receptor binding properties of the apo E variants are also listed in Table 1.

INTERACTION OF APO E WITH APO B,E(LDL) RECEPTORS

In addition to interacting with the apo B on LDL, lipoproteins containing apo E but not apo B also bind. These apo E-containing lipoproteins are generally referred to as HDL with apo E; they often contain apo A-I in addition to apo E (8). The HDL with

Table 1 Summary of Apo E Variants

Focusing position	Charge relative to apo E-3	Structure relative to apo E-3	Receptor binding activity relative to apo E-3	Ref.
E3	—	—	—	22
E4	+1	$Cys_{112} \to Arg$	100%	22
E2	-1	$Arg_{158} \to Cys$	<2%	22
E2	-1	$Arg_{145} \to Cys$	45%	23
E2	-1	$Lys_{146} \to Gln$	40%	24
E3	0	$Cys_{112} \to Arg$, $Arg_{142} \to Cys$	<20%	a
E3	0	$Ala_{99} \to Thr$, $Ala_{152} \to Pro$	Unknown	14
E1	-2	$Gly_{127} \to Asp$, $Arg_{158} \to Cys$	4%	25
E5	+2	Unknown	Unknown	26
E7	+4	Unknown	Unknown	27

[a]S. C. Rall, Jr., unpublished observations.

apo E are a heterogeneous class of lipoproteins that span the density range from d = 1.006 to approximately d = 1.10 g/ml. They have been demonstrated in a variety of species, including man (8). At the lower densities, they are enriched in apo E relative to apo A-I, while at the higher densities, the inverse is the case. A canine HDL with apo E subclass with unique characteristics was used to establish the fact that apo E also interacted with apo B,E(LDL) receptors. This lipoprotein, referred to as apo E HDL_c, is isolated from the d = 1.006–1.02 g/ml density fraction of plasma from dogs fed a cholesterol-fat-enriched diet. The apo E HDL_c contain apo E as their only apolipoprotein component. In addition, apo E HDL_c are of a similar size and have a similar chemical composition to that of LDL. Thus, the receptor binding properties of apo E HDL_c and

LDL can be compared directly, without the typical concerns resulting from comparing particles of different size or chemical composition. In either direct binding assays or in competition assays with LDL, apo E HDL_c were demonstrated to bind effectively to apo B,E(LDL) receptors (28). In fact, apo E HDL_c bind with a much higher affinity (~20- to 25-fold) than do LDL. The equilibrium dissociation constant (K_d) and maximum amount bound (B_{max}) were determined by Scatchard analysis of direct binding data for apo E HDL_c and LDL. The K_d for the apo E HDL_c and LDL were ~1×10^{-10} and 2.8×10^{-9} M, respectively (29). In addition, the B_{max} data demonstrated that approximately four times the number of LDL particles compared to apo E HDL_c particles were required to saturate the receptor sites. As will be discussed below, the higher binding affinity of apo E HDL_c and the difference in saturation levels between apo E HDL_c and LDL were interpreted to be the result of apo E HDL_c binding to multiple receptor sites, whereas apo B-containing lipoproteins do not bind to multiple receptor sites.

The chemical modification of specific amino acid residues contained in proteins has proved to be a useful approach in establishing that receptor binding is mediated through the protein moiety of the lipoprotein complex, i.e., either apo B or apo E, and in identifying amino acids important in the binding of apo B and apo E to the apo B,E(LDL) receptor. Modification of a limited number of arginyl (30) or lysyl residues (31) on apo B or apo E abolished receptor binding activity, implying that these residues were important in receptor interaction. Modification of glutamyl, aspartyl, or cysteinyl residues on apo B had no effect. These studies also suggested that the receptor binding domain on apo B and apo E might be similar, as lysyl and arginyl residues appeared to be important for the binding of both ligands.

Recently, much has been learned regarding the structure of the apo B,E(LDL) receptor. Using the technique of radiation inactivation, the functional molecular weight has been determined to be ~100,000 (32). This value agrees closely with the calculated molecular weight of the protein sequence predicted from the nucleotide sequence of a receptor cDNA (33). The receptor is known to be highly glycosylated with the mature receptor having an apparent molecular weight of approximately 160,000 on SDS-polyacrylamide gel electrophoresis. Apparently, the radiation inactivation technique is only sensitive to the contribution of the protein moiety to the molecular weight of the receptor molecule. Based on the Scatchard analysis of the HDL_c and LDL binding data and molecular weight of the receptor determined by radiation inactivation, the model depicted in Fig. 4 was proposed (32). It is consistent with the known binding differences between apo E HDL_c and LDL. According to the model, each receptor has a molecular weight of ~100,000 daltons (protein contribution only) and

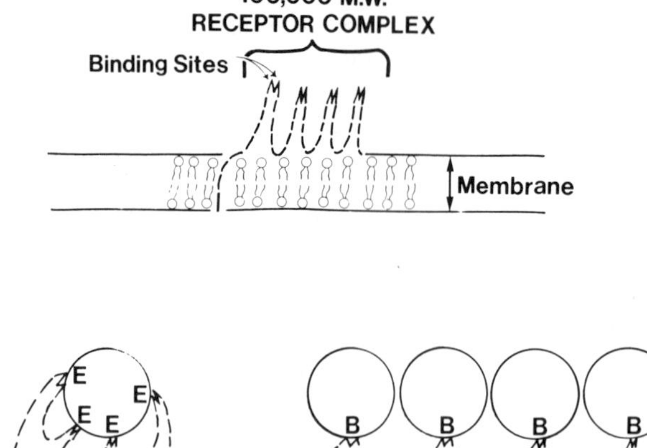

Fig. 4 Schematic model of the apo B,E(LDL) receptor unit illustrating the multiple binding sites. The M_r = 100,000 receptor unit is capable of binding one apo E HDL_c particle or four LDL particles. (From Ref. 32. Reproduced with permission.)

contains multiple binding sites. In the simplest case, each receptor can bind one apo E HDL_c particle by the interaction of four binding sites with four apo E molecules on an apo E HDL_c particle. In comparison, four LDL particles are bound per receptor, with each particle bound by one binding site. Presumably, this difference in the mode of binding of the two particles is because the apo B binding site(s) is spaced such that multiple interactions with a single receptor are not possible or that there is only one binding site on apo B per LDL particle. Receptor saturation studies have also been carried out using apo E-phospholipid recombinants. As discussed below, apo E must be bound to lipid to exhibit receptor binding properties. Such phospholipid recombinants contain four molecules of apo E per particle. Using a mixture of apo E and apo E that has been chemically modified to abolish its receptor binding ability, a phospholipid recombinant particle that contains only one molecule of a receptor-active apo E per particle has been produced (34). At receptor saturation, eight times the number of these recombinant particles bind versus the number of apo E HDL_c particles, and two times the number of recombinant particles bind versus LDL. These results indicate that the receptor unit shown in Fig. 4 actually contains eight binding sites. It is noteworthy that in the putative lipoprotein binding region of the apo B,E(LDL) receptor there are eight repeating units of ~40 amino acids each (33). Presumably, these repeating units represent the multiple binding sites predicted from the direct binding studies and results of radiation inactivation, which also predicts that the receptor unit responsible for both LDL and HDL_c binding is the same size, i.e., $M_r \sim 100,000$ (32). As a consequence of the multiple interactions, apo-E-containing lipoproteins bind with a higher affinity and are more effective competitors than LDL for apo B,E(LDL) receptors. This is an important distinction between these two lipoprotein classes.

Binding of LDL to the cell surface apo B,E(LDL) receptors leads to internalization of the lipoprotein particles and their delivery to lysosomes. In the lysosome, the lipoprotein is degraded and the released lipoprotein cholesterol participates in the mediation of a series of intracellular events that regulate cholesterol metabolism (for review see Refs. 2 to 4 and Chapter 13). Hydroxymethyl glutaryl-CoA reductase, the rate-limiting step in cholesterol biosynthesis, is suppressed. Acyl CoA:cholesterol acyltransferase, an enzyme that esterifies cholesterol intracellularly, is activated. This results in conversion of the cholesterol to cholesteryl ester, which is a storage form of cholesterol. Finally, the expression of the surface apo B,E(LDL) receptors is down-regulated. Through these regulatory processes, cholesterol homeostasis in the cell is maintained. It has been shown that the cholesterol contained in HDL with apo E and delivered to the cell by the interaction of apo E with the apo B,E(LDL) receptor is also capable of participating in the same regulatory events. Thus, apo E-containing lipoproteins not only bind to apo B,E(LDL) receptors, but also regulate intracellular cholesterol metabolism.

It is important to point out that apo E must bind to lipid in order to interact with the apo B,E(LDL) receptor (35); the free protein will not bind. Combination with phospholipid vesicles producing an apo E-phospholipid recombinant is sufficient (35), and dimyristoylphosphatidylcholine (DMPC) is commonly used. As do most of the other apolipoproteins, apo E displays an increase in α-helical content when combined with phospholipid (36). Presumably, this change in helical content is reflective of conformational changes in the molecules that are associated with lipid binding. Thus, the apo E-lipid interaction is responsible for conferring the proper conformation on apo E for effective receptor interaction. The presence of apo E on a lipoprotein particle does not in itself insure that the particle will bind to receptors: it has been demonstrated that in certain types of VLDL, all of the apo E present is not available for receptor interaction (37). In these cases, lipid appears to play a modulating role.

Because apo B,E(LDL) receptors are present on both hepatic and extrahepatic cells, they participate in both the cholesterol influx and efflux pathways schematized in Fig. 1. As we have just discussed, the B and E apolipoproteins mediate the interaction with these receptors and are, therefore, responsible for the targeting and delivery of cholesterol to cells expressing receptors.

HEPATIC APO E RECEPTOR

In addition to apo B,E(LDL) receptors, the liver has been shown to contain a second distinct lipoprotein receptor. In contrast to apo B,E(LDL) receptors, this receptor interacts with only apo E-containing lipoproteins and not LDL and is, therefore, referred to as the apo E receptor (38). The receptor was discovered when the binding of canine apo E HDL_c and LDL to canine hepatic membranes was compared. In these studies, membranes prepared from the livers of adult dogs display little specific binding of LDL but high levels of apo E HDL_c binding. This specific binding satisfied the criteria for receptor binding: it was saturable, high affinity ($K_d = 2.3 \times 10^{-10}$ M), calcium dependent, and sensitive to proteolytic digestion with pronase. Furthermore, chemical modification of the arginyl or lysyl residues of apo E HDL_c abolished specific binding. These observations indicated that the specific binding of apo E HDL_c to adult liver membranes was via a distinct hepatic receptor. An important characteristic of this receptor is that it appears to occur only in the liver. A receptor with identical characteristics has also been observed on hepatic membranes prepared from adult humans and swine (39). Presumably, the apo E receptor represents the chylomicron remnant receptor that has been postulated to exist in various studies.

An interesting observation was made when binding of canine apo E HDL_c and LDL were compared (38). With membranes from the livers of young dogs, apo E HDL_c and LDL were bound, indicating that apo B,E(LDL) receptors were expressed in these immature animals. Further studies demonstrated a linear correlation of expression of apo B,E(LDL) receptors with age, while the apo E receptor level remained relatively constant (39). The binding of LDL decreased with increasing age of the animals. Fetal swine liver membranes also displayed high LDL binding activity, whereas in the adult animal, LDL binding was markedly reduced. In adult human membranes, only low levels of LDL binding were detectable, whereas high levels of apo E HDL_c bound (38,39).

Because the expression of apo B,E(LDL) receptors is known to be highly regulated and responsive to the cholesterol requirements of the cell, a series of studies were conducted to determine if the

Table 2 Regulation of the Expression of Canine Hepatic Apo B,E (LDL) and Apo E Receptors

Source of hepatic membranes	Receptor[a]	
	Apo B,E	Apo E
Adult animals		
Control	±	++
Cholestyramine-treated	+++	++
Prolonged fasted	+++	++
Cholesterol-fed	±	++
Enhanced bile acid synthesis (interruption of enterohepatic circulation)	++	++
Decreased bile acid synthesis followed by bile acid infusion	±	++
Young animals		
Control	+++	++
Cholesterol-fed	±	++
Infusion of lipoprotein cholesterol	±	++

[a]+, Receptor detected at significant levels; ±, receptor barely detectable by assay.

apo E receptor was similarly regulated (40,41). The results of these studies conducted in dogs are summarized in Table 2. Two strategies were employed. The first was designed to increase the cholesterol requirements of the liver. This was experimentally accomplished by removing bile acids (using cholestyramine or by surgical interruption of the enterohepatic circulation) or by prolonged fasting. The second approach was to lower the cholesterol requirements of the liver by saturating the system through an increase in the cholesterol content of the diet (cholesterol-fed). Each of the approaches had the predicted effect on the expression of the apo B,E(LDL) receptors. In cholesterol-deprived states, the expression of these receptors was increased, and in states where cholesterol was not in demand, they were down regulated (Table 2).

Note that in young animals, cholesterol feeding down-regulated the normal expression of apo B,E(LDL) receptors, and in adults, cholesterol deprivation resulted in expression of the receptors (Table 2). In marked contrast to the regulation of the apo B,E(LDL) receptors, expression of the apo E receptors was relatively constant. This suggests that the expression of hepatic apo E receptors is relatively refractory to changes in metabolic states, whereas the expression of hepatic apo B,E(LDL) receptors, as has been demonstrated in other cells and tissues, is not. Uniquely, however, the regulation of hepatic apo B,E(LDL) receptors is very rapid, going from high levels of expression to barely detectable levels of lipoproteins or bile acid infusion within 2 to 4 hr.

METABOLIC ROLES OF APO E

Intracellular Regulation of Cholesterol Metabolism

As was discussed in the section on the interaction of apo E with apo B,E(LDL) receptors, apo E-containing lipoproteins are capable of delivering cholesterol to cells that express apo B,E(LDL) or apo E receptors. These apo E-containing lipoproteins also elicit the same responses regarding the intracellular regulation of cholesterol metabolism as do LDL (28). The fact that apo E-containing lipoproteins can function in place of LDL in vivo is illustrated by the lipoprotein disorder, abetalipoproteinemia. In subjects affected with this disorder, apo B is not present in detectable levels in the plasma. The basis for this lack of apo B is not understood; however, as a consequence of its absence, VLDL and LDL are not present, and triglyceride metabolism and transport are grossly affected. However, intracellular cholesterol homeostasis does not appear to be significantly affected, suggesting that apo E-containing lipoproteins are capable of carrying out the normal function of LDL in regulating intracellular cholesterol metabolism (42,43). Abetalipoproteinemic subjects have been demonstrated to have increased circulating levels of HDL with apo E (43).

Chylomicron Remnant Clearance

A second metabolic role of apo E is associated with chylomicron remnant clearance. These remnants are known to be rapidly and efficiently cleared from plasma by hepatic receptors (44). Several lines of evidence indicate that the apo E on these remnants is the recognition signal responsible for their uptake (45,46). Again, the canine apo E HDL_c proved useful in establishing this role for apo E. When compared on a particle basis, the cholesterol of both apo E HDL_c and chylomicron remnants is cleared with nearly identical kinetic parameters by perfused rat livers (46). In addition, the apo E HDL_c can compete with chylomicron remnants for hepatic binding sites and retard the uptake of remnants in perfused livers (46). These data indicate that apo E HDL_c and chylomicron remnants bind to the same receptor and that apo E mediates the interaction. More recent studies, using a variety of methods including apo E monoclonal antibodies, demonstrate that the apo E, and not the apo B48, is responsible for the binding of chylomicron remnants to receptors (46).

However, as we have discussed in a previous section, the liver contains two receptors, apo B,E(LDL) and apo E, both of which are capable of interacting with apo E. Thus, both receptor systems have the potential for mediating the clearance of chylomicron remnants. However, two lines of evidence indicate that the apo B,E(LDL) receptors may not represent the major clearance mechanism. First, subjects homozygous for the lipid disorder familial hypercholesterolemia do not have an impaired clearance of chylomicron remnants. However, these subjects do not have normally functioning apo B,E (LDL) receptors that are capable of internalizing lipoprotein particles (2–4). Second, as discussed above, in several species including man there appears to be an age dependency for the expression of apo B,E(LDL) receptors, with low levels expressed at maturation. Thus, in adults there appears to be a need for an alternative mechanism. Although the evidence is clear that a second receptor system distinct from the apo B,E(LDL) is responsible for the clearance of the major portion of chylomicron remnants, it has not been established that this "remnant receptor" is the hepatic apo E receptor. However, two points suggest that this may be the case: (1) apo E is the recognition factor responsible for chylomicron remnant clearance, and (2) unlike the hepatic apo B,E(LDL) receptors, the apo E receptor does not appear to be regulated. This is an ideal property for a remnant receptor.

Reverse Cholesterol Transport

As has been discussed, the canine apo E HDL_c has proved to be valuable as a probe used to gain insight into the metabolic characteristics of apo E. Studies on the in vivo properties of apo E HDL_c have also proved useful and have suggested an additional metabolic role for apo E, namely, a role in the so-called reverse cholesterol transport process. As shown in Fig. 5, ^{125}I-apo E HDL_c is rapidly cleared from plasma with less than 25% of the injected dose remaining at 20 min, and the major portion of the apo E HDL_c cleared by the liver (47). In fact, for the first 20 min, greater than 90% of the injected dose can be accounted for by the radioactivity in the plasma and liver. Hepatocytes have been demonstrated to be the cell type in the liver responsible for this rapid uptake of the apo E HDL_c (47).

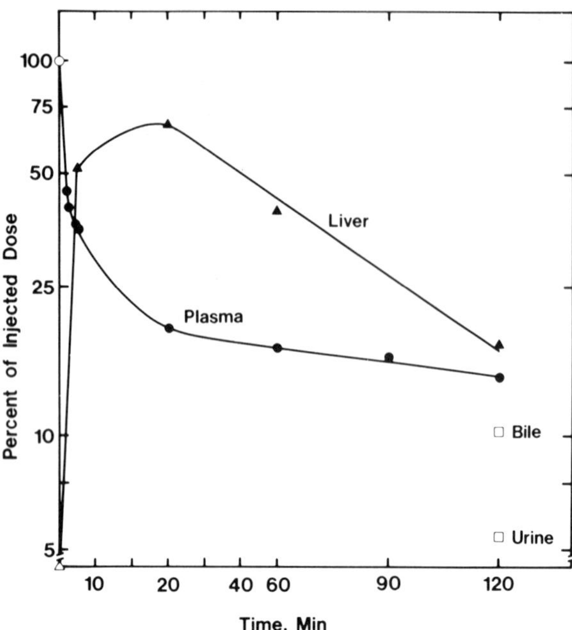

Fig. 5 In vivo metabolism of canine apo E HDL_c. ^{125}I-labeled apo E HDL_c was injected into a dog, and the radioactivity was determined at various time intervals in the plasma and liver. At the end of the experiment (120 min), the radioactivity in the bile and urine was measured. (From Ref. 47. Reproduced with permission.)

The rapid clearance of these cholesterol-rich lipoproteins, which are targeted to the major organ in the body capable of eliminating cholesterol from the body, suggested that this mechanism might be of physiological significance. (Recall from the Introduction that the cholesterol influx pathways in Fig. 1 must be balanced by an efflux pathway from the body to maintain cholesterol homeostasis.)

It has been demonstrated in vitro that extrahepatic or peripheral cells containing an excess amount of cholesterol can release this cholesterol to an appropriate acceptor. One such acceptor is HDL. Many of the studies demonstrating this role have been performed using cholesterol-loaded macrophages. It is pertinent to note that macrophages have also been demonstrated to synthesize and secrete apo E (48). Also important in this regard is that several peripheral tissues have been demonstrated to contain significant levels of apo E mRNA (12,13). Thus, important components necessary for reverse cholesterol transport have been demonstrated: peripheral cells can secrete excess cholesterol and can synthesize apo E, a ligand recognized by the hepatic apo E receptor.

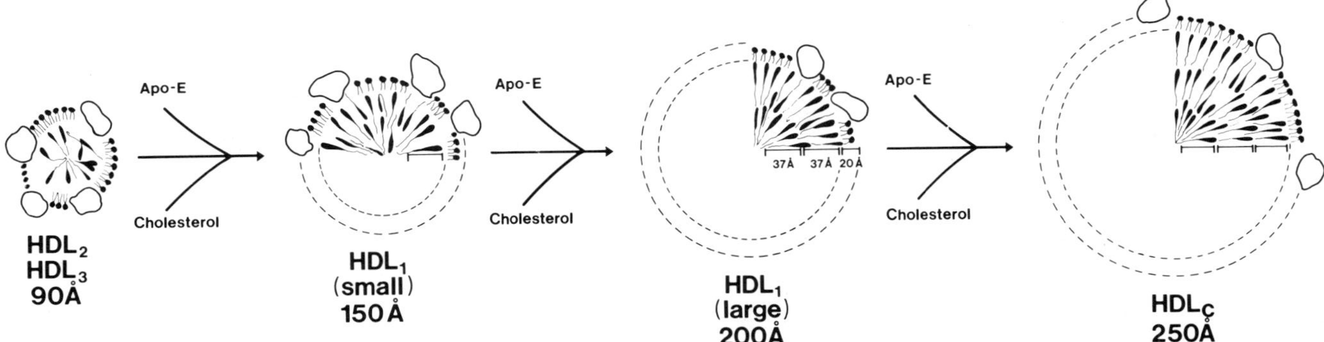

Fig. 6 Model of the core expansion of HDL_2 and HDL_3 with the addition of cholesteryl ester to the core and apo E to the surface of the particle. The cholesteryl ester is produced by the action of LCAT on the acquired surface cholesterol, which is obtained from cells. The expansion occurs in incremental steps of approximately 37 Å as the cholesteryl ester is added in ordered layers. Both the smaller HDL_3 (90 Å) and the larger HDL_2 particles are capable of this core expansion. (From Ref. 49. Reproduced with permission.)

Additional in vitro studies provide insight into how the reverse cholesterol transport process might be operating in vivo. The HDL accepting cholesterol from an inert support (Celite) or from cholesterol-loaded macrophages have been shown to undergo a series of remodeling changes (49). Provided that there is a source of active LCAT and apo E, these loaded HDL are converted into a series of HDL particles of increasing size. The accepted cholesterol first becomes associated with the surface of the HDL particle. This surface-associated cholesterol is then converted to cholesteryl esters by LCAT, and the cholesteryl esters are shifted to the hydrophobic core of the HDL particle, resulting in an increase in particle size. The expansion of the core appears to occur in a stepwise manner with the addition of incremental layers of ordered cholesteryl ester molecules, and is accompanied by an enrichment of these particles with apo E (49). A schematic diagram of this incremental core expansion is shown in Fig. 6. The spectrum of HDL-containing apo E particles that are produced in these in vitro experiments is very similar to the spectrum of HDL particles that is observed in cholesterol-fed animal models (8). In fact, particles with characteristics very similar to those of apo E HDL_c have been produced in in vitro experiments (49). Thus, these experiments provide strong evidence that similar processes may be operating in vivo, with the HDL with apo E participating in the direct elimination of cholesterol from the body.

Several species, including man, contain a plasma cholesteryl ester transfer protein that is capable of net transfer of cholesteryl ester from high- to lower-density lipoproteins, such as LDL or remnants of VLDL and chylomicrons. Thus, in these species, a second or indirect elimination of cholesterol may also be operating (50,51).

TYPE III HYPERLIPOPROTEINEMIA: CONSEQUENCE OF THE RECEPTOR-DEFECTIVE FORMS OF APO E

Studies of the lipoprotein disorder type III hyperlipoproteinemia have provided many interesting and important insights into the metabolic properties of apo E (for a complete review of this disorder see Refs. 19,52, and 53). Patients affected with this relatively rare familial lipid disorder are characterized by elevated plasma levels of cholesterol and triglyceride, each typically greater than 300 mg/dl. Also, plasma apo E levels are elevated three- to eight times. Clinically, affected subjects are prone to premature atherosclerosis and display cholesterol deposits in the form of xanthomas in various locations of the body. A characteristic class of lipoproteins, referred to as β-VLDL, accumulates in the plasma of these patients and distinguishes the disorder. The β-VLDL are a heterogeneous class of cholesterol-rich lipoproteins that contains lipoprotein remnants derived from both hepatic and intestinal sources (54), suggesting a remnant removal defect in these patients. Apo E is a major apolipoprotein component of the β-VLDL. The LDL levels in these subjects are also reduced, suggesting a defect in the conversion of VLDL to LDL.

A major advance in the understanding of type III hyperlipoproteinemia was made when it was recognized that type III disease is frequently associated with the E2/2 phenotype (55,56), although some cases of apo E2 heterozygosity have been reported. Because of the accumulation of hepatic and intestinally derived remnants and elevated plasma apo E levels, it was postulated that the apo E2 might have a defective ability to interact with lipoprotein receptors. Consistent with this hypothesis were the results from in vitro (57,58) and in vivo (59) studies, which indicated that the receptor binding activity and metabolism of apo E2 were altered. With the demonstration that the structural basis for the apo E heterogeneity was a series of amino acid substitutions at various sites in the protein, it became possible to test directly the effect of these substitutions on receptor binding activity.

The apo E2, E3, and E4 that were first tested had the structure shown in Fig. 3. The binding activities are listed in Table 1 and were determined in assays using the apo B,E(LDL) receptors on cultured fibroblasts. In many cases, similar results have been obtained using hepatic apo E receptors (60). The binding activity of apo E3 is normalized to 100% and is assumed to represent normal activity. As shown in Table 1, the apo E3 and apo E4 (Cys_{112}→Arg) have identical receptor binding activities, indicating that the arginine for cysteine substitution at residue 112 does not affect receptor binding activity. In marked contrast, the apo E2 (Cys_{158}→Arg), which was obtained from a type III patient, had a greatly reduced binding activity: 1% of apo E3. This indicated that the cysteine for arginine substitution at residue 158 alters normal binding activity, and confirmed the hypothesis that type III apo E2 has a receptor binding defect. Study of additional type III subjects led to the discovery that the apo E2 was structurally heterogeneous. Importantly, these additional apo E2 variants, apo E2(Arg_{145}→Cys) and apo E2(Lys_{146}→Glu), also have reduced binding activity. The apo E3(Cys_{112}→Arg, Arg_{142}→Cys) and apo E1(Gly_{127}→Asp, Arg_{158}→Cys) variants are also defective and were also obtained from either confirmed type III patients or subjects displaying several features of the disease. The apo E2 (Arg_{158}→Cys) appears to be the most commonly occurring apo E2 variant. It is important to note that in all studies of type III subjects in which the characterization of the apo E has included receptor binding activity, at least one of the apo E alleles has been demonstrated to code for a receptor-defective variant. Thus, rather than restricting the definition of type III disease as being associated with a particular apo E phenotype, the definition should be expanded to indicate that the important feature is the association of the disorder with the presence of a receptor-defective form of apo E.

It is well known that all subjects with the E2/2 phenotype do not display clinical features of type III hyperlipoproteinemia. In fact, many have lower than normal levels of plasma cholesterol and triglyceride. When the structure of the apo E2 was examined in several of these subjects, it was determined that the apo E2 was the apo E2($Arg_{158} \rightarrow Cys$) variant, the most severely defective form of the protein. However, it is important to note that these subjects have β-VLDL as well as low LDL levels. They have the lipoprotein abnormalities that characterize the diseased state, but they do not accumulate the remnants to the degree that occurs in type III hyperlipoproteinemia. The presence of these lipoprotein abnormalities without clinical expression of type III disease is commonly referred to as familial dysbetalipoproteinemia (61). Thus, while the presence of a receptor-defective apo E variant predisposes a subject to the dyslipoproteinemia, it does not necessarily predispose the subject to the massive accumulation of β-VLDL and clinical features associated with type III hyperlipoproteinemia. It is clear that additional factors modulate the expression of type III hyperlipoproteinemia. These factors appear to be both genetic and environmental in nature and include dietary, age, and hormonal influences. It is well known that type III patients are very responsive to dietary and drug therapy and that age, diabetes, and hypothyroidism exacerbate the disease (for a more complete discussion of these factors and type III hyperlipoproteinemia see Refs. 19,52, and 53).

Let us now examine in more detail how the presence of a receptor-defective form of apo E could account for the lipoprotein abnormalities in type III hyperlipoproteinemia and dysbetalipoproteinemia. These potential mechanisms are schematically summarized in Fig. 7. (1) The removal of chylomicron remnants (intestinally derived β-VLDL) by hepatic receptors could be impaired by the presence of a receptor-defective apo E. (2) The regulation of hepatic receptors [apo B,E(LDL) and apo E receptors] may contribute to the build-up of chylomicron and VLDL remnants. Recall that the expression of the hepatic apo B,E(LDL) receptors appears to be age dependent. If the hepatic apo B,E(LDL) receptors are down-regulated, then it is possible that the apo E receptors cannot handle the overload and effectively remove remnants with a defective apo E. In this regard, it is important to note that type III hyperlipoproteinemia is rarely expressed before maturity and thus may correlate with the down-regulation of hepatic apo B,E(LDL) receptors. (3) In the event of inadequate delivery of cholesterol to the liver due to defective remnant clearance, the liver may be stimulated to increase synthesis

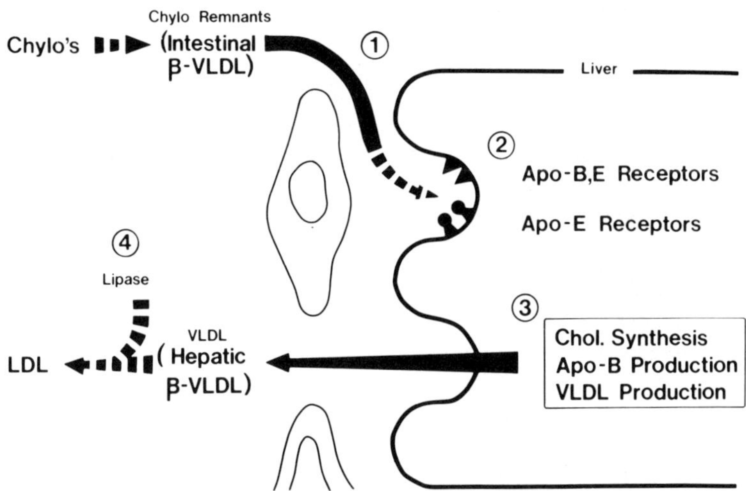

Fig. 7 Potential mechanisms accounting for the lipoprotein abnormalities observed in type III patients and dysbetalipoproteinemic subjects. (1) Impaired removal of chylomicron (chylo) remnants; (2) down-regulation of hepatic apo B,E(LDL) receptors; (3) stimulation of hepatic cholesterol synthesis and secretion of VLDL; (4) impaired conversion of hepatic VLDL to LDL. (From Ref. 19. Reproduced with permission.)

of cholesterol and secretion of VLDL, leading to the overproduction of VLDL and the accumulation of VLDL remnants in the plasma. (4) The presence of a receptor-defective apo E may result in an impaired conversion of VLDL to LDL by lipases. It is not presently known if there is a receptor component to this conversion process. However, recent in vitro studies have demonstrated that VLDL particles (from type III patients) that contain apo E2 ($Arg_{158} \rightarrow Cys$) are not converted to particles in the LDL density range unless apo E3 is present (62). It has been postulated that the apo E3 is capable of interacting with an unidentified plasma component that results in the remodeling of the VLDL remnants, which allows or promotes their conversion to particles in the LDL density range (62).

LIPOPROTEIN RECEPTOR BINDING DOMAIN OF APO E

Because of the importance of apo E interactions with the apo B,E(LDL) and apo E receptors, much attention has been focused on determining the region of the apo E molecule responsible for this interaction. The first important clues that further delineated the receptor binding domain were provided by studying the receptor binding properties of the naturally occurring apo E variants listed in Table 1.

As discussed in the preceding sections, apo E3 and apo E4 (Cys_{112}→Arg) have essentially identical receptor binding properties, indicating that the arginine for cysteine substitution at residue 112 does not affect receptor binding activity. However, variants with cysteine for arginine substitutions at residues 158, 145, and 142, as well as glutamine for lysine substitution at residue 146, all have reduced receptor binding activity. It is significant that all the substitutions that adversely affect receptor binding involve the substitution of a basic amino acid with a neutral one, confirming the chemical modification studies (30,31). Because the binding activity of the apo E2 (Arg_{158}→Cys) and apo E1(Asp_{127}→Gly, Arg_{112}→Cys) variants are similar, one would conclude that the glycine for aspartic acid at residue 127 is without effect. Thus, the structure-function studies of the apo E variants indicate that the region of apo E in the vicinity of residues 142 to 158 is involved in receptor binding and that basic amino acid residues in this region are involved.

Two additional independent lines of evidence also confirm that this central portion of apo E is the receptor binding domain. The first verification was obtained when the receptor binding activity of thrombolytic and cyanogen bromide fragments of apo E were determined (63). The proteolytic enzyme thrombin cleaves apo E at a limited number of sites, producing two major fragments: an amino-terminal fragment (residues 1 to 191) and a carboxyl-terminal fragment (residues 216 to 299) (Fig. 8). When the fragments were combined with phospholipid and tested for receptor binding, it was found that only the amino-terminal fragment possessed receptor binding activity (63). Cyanogen bromide digestion of apo E yielded eight cyanogen bromide fragments (17), and the largest fragment, designated CNBr-II (residues 126 to 218) (Fig. 8), was the only fragment that displayed any significant activity. Taken together, the results of the binding studies of the apo E fragments indicate that the receptor binding domain is located between residues 126 and 191 (highlighted region in Fig. 8). Note that this region overlaps with the amino acid substitution sites known to adversely affect receptor binding.

The second independent verification that the receptor binding domain is located in the center of the apo E molecule was obtained in studies with apo E monoclonal antibodies (64). The strategy was to screen apo E monoclonal antibodies to identify one that interfered with the receptor binding activity of apo E, and then to determine the epitope or antigenic determinant of the inhibiting antibody. A basic assumption of this approach is that an antibody that inhibits receptor binding activity is interacting with an epitope at or in

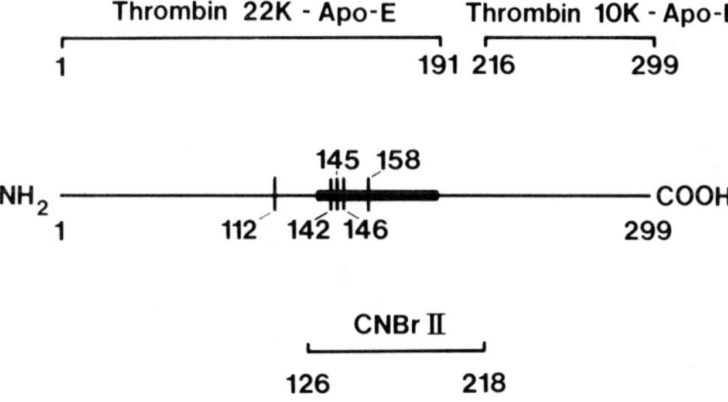

Fig. 8 Linear schematic representation of apo E and the major thrombolytic and cyanogen bromide (CNBrII) fragments. Various sites where amino acid substitutions have been demonstrated are indicated on the apo E representation (center). Residues 126 to 191 (highlighted) represent the receptor binding domain of apo E postulated from studies of thrombolytic and cyanogen bromide fragments of apo E.

close proximity to the receptor binding domain, whereas an antibody interacting with a noncritical region of apo E will not inhibit receptor binding activity. Of the five antibodies that were screened, only one, designated 1D7, was an effective inhibitor of the receptor binding activity of apo E, inhibiting greater than 95% of the activity. The other four antibodies added at equal immunoreactive amounts to 1D7 had no significant effect.

Using the thrombolytic and cyanogen bromide fragments of apo E shown in Fig. 8, as well as synthetic fragments of apo E and several of the apo E variants listed in Table 1, it was possible to narrow the 1D7 epitope to residues 140 to 150 (64). Thus, the monoclonal antibody studies also indicated that the central region of apo E is the receptor binding domain. Based on the Chou-Fasman algorithm, residues 131 to 150 are predicted to exist in an alpha-helix that is flanked by beta-turns. A schematic representation of this region is shown in Fig. 9. Note that the helical region is enriched in basic residues and contains three amino acid substitution sites that affect receptor binding. Recent evidence indicates that Arg_{158} is not directly involved in the interaction with lipoprotein receptors but that the positive charge at this position is required to maintain the proper conformation of the binding domain (65).

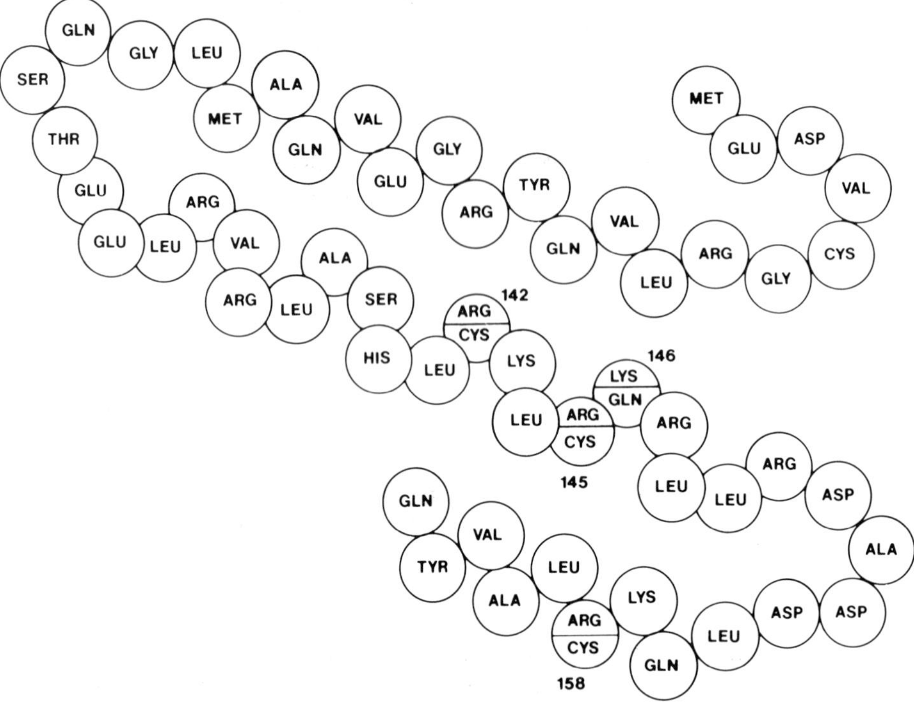

Fig. 9 Schematic representation of the predicted secondary structure of the central portion of the apo E molecule. The amino acid substitution sites and nature of the amino acid interchanges are indicated by double residues. (From Ref. 1. Reproduced with permission.)

SUMMARY

Apo E is an important component of cholesterol homeostasis. It is the ligand responsible for the recognition and uptake of chylomicron remnants by hepatic receptors. Through this process, apo E directs dietary cholesterol to the liver, from which it is eventually redistributed to extrahepatic peripheral cells that require it for membrane synthesis or for more specialized needs such as hormone synthesis. Because of the ability of apo E to interact with apo B,E(LDL) receptors of extrahepatic peripheral cells, apo E can also participate in the lipoprotein-mediated distribution of cholesterol to these cells. In addition to participating in the pathways that lead to an influx of cholesterol into the body and to cholesterol redistribution, apo E also appears to play a prominent role in the reverse cholesterol transport pathway. In this pathway, the excess cholesterol of peripheral cells is targeted and transported by an apo E-mediated process to the liver for elimination from the body via the bile.

Several genetic variants of apo E have been identified, and the structures of most have been determined. The structural basis of these variants has been shown to be a series of amino acid substitutions. Comparison of the receptor binding properties of these variants has demonstrated that several have a defective ability to bind to lipoprotein receptors. The defective forms have a neutral amino acid substituted for a basic amino acid. These defective variants are the underlying cause of the genetic lipid disorder type III hyperlipoproteinemia. In this disorder, plasma cholesterol, triglyceride, and apo E levels are elevated. The plasma accumulation of hepatic and intestinally derived remnants are, in part, the result of the presence of a functionally defective apo E molecule with an impaired ability to bind to lipoprotein receptors. Knowledge of the substitution sites in the functionally defective apo E variants, in conjunction with other biochemical studies, has led to the delineation of the lipoprotein receptor binding domain of apo E. This domain is located near the center of the protein molecule and is enriched in basic amino acids that presumably interact with the clusters of acidic residues located in the putative lipoprotein binding region of the apo B,E(LDL) receptor.

ACKNOWLEDGMENTS

The author would like to express his appreciation to Drs. Robert W. Mahley, Stanley C. Rall, Jr., and Thomas L. Innerarity for reading the chapter and offering helpful suggestions. Thanks are also extended to Barbara Allen and Sally Gullatt Seehafer for editorial assistance, James X. Warger and Norma Jean Gargasz for graphic arts, and Kerry Humphrey and Debbie Morris for manuscript preparation.

REFERENCES

1. Mahley, R. W., and Innerarity, T. L., *Biochim. Biophys. Acta*, *737*:197–222 (1983).

2. Goldstein, J. L., and Brown, M. S., *Annu. Rev. Biochem.*, *46*:897–930 (1977).

3. Brown, M. S., Kovanen, P. T., and Goldstein, J. L., *Science*, *212*:628–635 (1981).

4. Brown, M. S., Anderson, R. G. W., Basu, S. K., and Goldstein, J. L., *Cold Spring Harbor Symp. Quant. Biol.*, *46*:713–721 (1982).

5. Sigurdsson, G., Noel, S.-P., and Havel, R. J., *J. Lipid Res.*, *19*:628–634 (1978).

6. Eisenberg, S., Bilheimer, D. W., Levy, R. I., and Lindgren, F. T., *Biochim. Biophys. Acta*, *326*:361–377 (1973).

7. Brown, M. S., Ho, Y. K., and Goldstein, J. L., *J. Biol. Chem.*, *255*:9344–9352 (1980).

8. Mahley, R. W., in *Disturbances in Lipid and Lipoprotein Metabolism* (Dietschy, J. M., Gotto, A. M., Jr., and Ontko, J. A., eds.), American Physiological Society, Bethseda, Md., 1978, pp. 181–197.

9. Mahley, R. W., Innerarity, T. L., Rall, S. C., Jr., and Weisgraber, K. H., *J. Lipid Res.*, *25*:1277–1294 (1984).

10. Shore, V. G., and Shore, B., *Biochemistry*, *12*:502–507 (1973).

11. Wu, A.-L., and Windmueller, H. G., *J. Biol. Chem.*, *254*:7316–7322 (1979).

12. Blue, M.-L., Williams, D. L., Zucker, S., Khan, S. A., and Blum, C. B., *Proc. Natl. Acad. Sci. U.S.A.*, *80*:283–287 (1983).

13. Elshourbagy, N., Boguski, M. S., Liao, W. S., Jefferson, L. S., Gordon, J. I., and Taylor, J., *Proc. Natl. Acad. Sci. U.S.A.*, *82*:8242–8246 (1985).

14. McLean, J. W., Elshourbagy, N. A., Chang, D. J., Mahley, R. W., and Taylor, J. M., *J. Biol. Chem.*, *259*:6498–6504 (1984).

15. Olaisen, B., Teisberg, P., Gedde-Dahl, T., Jr., *Human Genet.*, *62*:233–236 (1982).

16. Paik, Y.-K., Chang, D. J., Reardon, C. A., Davies, G. E., Mahley, R. W., and Taylor, J. M., *Proc. Natl. Acad. Sci. U.S.A.*, *82*:3445–3449 (1985).

17. Rall, S. C., Jr., Weisgraber, K. H., and Mahley, R. W., *J. Biol. Chem.*, *257*:4171–4178 (1982).

18. McLean, J. W., Fukazawa, C., and Taylor, J. M., *J. Biol. Chem.*, *258*:8993–9000 (1983).

19. Mahley, R. W., and Angelin, B., *Adv. Intern. Med.*, *29*:385–411 (1984).

20. Zannis, V. I., Breslow, J. L., Utermann, G., Mahley, R. W., Weisgraber, K. H., Havel, R. J., Goldstein, J. L., Brown, M. S., Schonfeld, G., Hazzard, W. R., and Blum, C., *J. Lipid Res.*, *23*:911–914 (1982).

21. Weisgraber, K. H., Rall, S. C., Jr., and Mahley, R. W., *J. Biol. Chem.*, *256*:9077–9083 (1981).

22. Weisgraber, K. H., Innerarity, T. L., and Mahley, R. W., *J. Biol. Chem.*, *257*:2518–2521 (1982).

23. Rall, S. C., Weisgraber, K. H., Innerarity, T. L., and Mahley, R. W., *Proc. Natl. Acad. Sci. U.S.A.*, *79*:4696–4700 (1982).

24. Rall, S. C., Jr., Weisgraber, K. H., Innerarity, T. L., Bersot, T. P., Mahley, R. W., and Blum, C. B., *J. Clin. Invest.*, *72*:1288–1297 (1983).

25. Weisgraber, K. H., Rall, S. C., Jr., Innerarity, T. L., Mahley, R. W., Kuusi, T., and Ehnholm, C., *J. Clin. Invest.*, *73*:1024–1033 (1984).

26. Yamamura, T., Yamamoto, A., Hiramori, K., and Nambu, S., *Atherosclerosis*, *50*:159–172 (1984).

27. Yamamura, T., Yamamoto, A., Sumiyoshi, T., Hiramori, K., Nishioeda, Y., and Nambu, S., *J. Clin. Invest.*, *74*:1229–1237 (1984).

28. Innerarity, T. L., and Mahley, R. W., *Biochemistry*, *17*: 1440–1447 (1978).

29. Pitas, R. E., Innerarity, T. L., Arnold, K. S., and Mahley, R. W., *Proc. Natl. Acad. Sci. U.S.A.*, *76*:2311–2315 (1979).

30. Mahley, R. W., Innerarity, T. L., Pitas, R. E., Weisgraber, K. H., Brown, J. H., and Gross, E., *J. Biol. Chem.*, *252*: 7279–7287 (1977).

31. Weisgraber, K. H., Innerarity, T. L., and Mahley, R. W., *J. Biol. Chem.*, *253*:9053–9062 (1978).

32. Innerarity, T. L., Kempner, E. S., Hui, D. Y., and Mahley, R. W., *Proc. Natl. Acad. Sci. U.S.A.*, *78*:4378–4382 (1981).

33. Yamamoto, T., Davis, C. G., Brown, M. S., Schneider, W. J., Casey, M. L., Goldstein, J. L., and Russell, D. W., *Cell*, *39*:27–38 (1984).

34. Pitas, R. E., Innerarity, T. L., and Mahley, R. W., *J. Biol. Chem.*, *255*:5454–5460 (1980).

35. Innerarity, T. L., Pitas, R. E., and Mahley, R. W., *J. Biol. Chem.*, *254*:4186–4190 (1979).

36. Roth, R. I., Jackson, R. L., Pownall, H. J., Gotto, A. M., Jr., *Biochemistry*, *16*:5030–5036 (1977).

37. Gianturco, S. H., Gotto, A. M., Jr., Hwang, S.-L. C., Karlin, J. B., Lin, A. H. Y., Prasad, S. C., and Bradley, W. A., *J. Biol. Chem.*, *258*:4526–4533 (1983).

38. Hui, D. Y., Innerarity, T. L., and Mahley, R. W., *J. Biol. Chem.*, *256*:5646–5655 (1981).

39. Mahley, R. W., Hui, D. Y., Innerarity, T. L., and Weisgraber, K. H., *J. Clin. Invest.*, *68*:1197–1206 (1981).

40. Angelin, B., Raviola, C. A., Innerarity, T. L., and Mahley, R. W., *J. Clin. Invest.*, *71*:816–831 (1983).

41. Angelin, B., Raviola, C. A., and Mahley, R. W., in *Bile Acids and Cholesterol in Health and Disease* (Paumgartner, G., Stiehl, A., and Gerok, W., eds.), MTP Press, Boston, 1983, pp. 139–150.

42. Blum, C. B., Deckelbaum, R. J., Witte, L. D., Tall, A. R., and Cornicelli, J., *J. Clin. Invest.*, *70*:1157–1169 (1982).

43. Innerarity, T. L., Bersot, T. P., Arnold, K. S., Weisgraber, K. H., Davis, P. A., Forte, T. M., and Mahley, R. W., *Metabolism*, *33*:186–195 (1984).

44. Sherrill, B. C., and Dietschy, J. M., *J. Biol. Chem.*, *253*: 1859–1867 (1978).

45. Hui, D. Y., Innerarity, T. L., Milne, R. W., Marcel, Y. L., and Mahley, R. W., *J. Biol. Chem.*, *259*:15,060–15,068 (1984).

46. Sherrill, B. C., Innerarity, T. L., and Mahley, R. W., *J. Biol. Chem.*, *255*:1804–1807 (1980).

47. Funke, H., Boyles, J., Weisgraber, K. H., Ludwig, E. H., Hui, D. Y., and Mahley, R. W., *Arteriosclerosis* *4*:452–461 (1984).

48. Basu, S. K., Brown, M. S., Ho, Y. K., Havel, R. J., and Goldstein, J. L., *Proc. Natl. Acad. Sci. U.S.A.* *78*:7545–7549 (1981).

49. Gordon, V., Innerarity, T. L., and Mahley, R. W., *J. Biol. Chem.*, *258*:6202–6212 (1983).

50. Barter, P. J., Hopkins, G. J., and Calvert, G. D., *Biochem. J.*, *208*:1–7 (1982).

51. Fielding, C. J., and Fielding, P. E., *Med. Clin. North Am.*, *66*: 363–373 (1982).

52. Brown, M. S., Goldstein, J. L., and Fredrickson, D. S., in *The Metabolic Basis of Inherited Disease* (Stanbury, J. B., Wyngaarden, J. B., Fredrickson, D. S., Goldstein, J. L., and Brown, M. S., eds.), McGraw-Hill, New York, 1983, pp. 655–671.

53. Mahley, R. W., Innerarity, T. L., Rall, S. C., Jr., and Weisgraber, K. H., *Ann. N.Y. Acad. Sci.*, *454*:209–221 (1985).

54. Fainaru, M., Mahley, R. W., Hamilton, R. L., and Innerarity, T. L., *J. Lipid Res.*, *23*: 702–714 (1982).

55. Utermann, G., Hees, M., and Steinmetz, A., *Nature (London)*, *269*: 604–607 (1977).

56. Zannis, V. I., and Breslow, J. L., *Biochemistry*, *20*: 1033–1041 (1981).

57. Havel, R. J., Chao, Y.-S., Windler, E. E., Kotite, L., and Guo, L. S. S., *Proc. Natl. Acad. Sci. U.S.A.* *77*: 4349–4353 (1980).

58. Schneider, W. J., Kovanen, P. T., Brown, M. S., Goldstein, J. L., Utermann, G., Weber, W., Havel, R. J., Kotite, L., Kane, J. P., Innerarity, T. L., and Mahley, R. W., *J. Clin. Invest.*, *68*: 1075–1085 (1981).

59. Gregg, R. E., Zech, L. A., Schaefer, E. J., Brewer, H. B., Jr., *Science*, *211*: 584–585 (1981).

60. Hui, D. Y., Innerarity, T. L., and Mahley, R. W., *J. Biol. Chem.*, *259*: 860–869 (1984).

61. Havel, R. J., *Med. Clin. North Am.*, *66*: 411–454 (1982).

62. Ehnholm, C., Mahley, R. W., Chappell, D. A., Weisgraber, K. H., Ludwig, E., and Witztum, J. L., *Proc. Natl. Acad. Sci. U.S.A.*, *81*: 5566–5570 (1984).

63. Innerarity, T. L., Friedlander, E. J., Rall, S. C., Jr., Weisgraber, K. H., and Mahley, R. W., *J. Biol. Chem.*, *258*: 12,341–12,347 (1983).

64. Weisgraber, K. H., Innerarity, T. L., Harder, K. J., Mahley, R. W., Milne, R. W., Marcel, Y. L., and Sparrow, J. T., *J. Biol. Chem.*, *258*: 12,348–12,354 (1983).

65. Innerarity, T. L., Weisgraber, K. H., Arnold, K. S., Rall, S. C., Jr., Mahley, R. W., *J. Biol. Chem.*, *259*: 7261–7267 (1984).

13

Biological and Clinical Implications of LDL Receptors

WIELAND GEVERS, GERHARD A. COETZEE, and
DENEYS R. van der WESTHUYZEN University of Cape Town
Medical School, Observatory, South Africa

INTRODUCTION

The evolution of generalized eukaryotic cellular life, particularly in multicellular organisms, has brought with it a large number of molecular or supramolecular adaptations that facilitate communication and cooperation between cells. Cell surface macromolecules have participated in an especially significant manner in these evolutionary developments because they uniquely straddle the extra- and intracellular worlds. They are well positioned to receive "messages," which in chemical terms means that they can undergo reversible transmembrane conformational changes when they bind or release, in a concentration-dependent manner, specific regulatory molecules in the environment. Alternatively, they can be cleaved to release biologically active molecules into their surroundings, or they can "piggyback" other molecules into or out of cells, either by the creation of specific molecular "pores" or by bulk membrane translocation into the cellular interior. Specialization and refinement of such functions have given rise to the panoply of chemically and functionally differentiated macromolecules that occupy the cell surfaces of individual cells in a given organism, and this forms much of the basis of organ cooperation and overall homeostatic control.

Among the cell surface molecules of particular interest are those known as "receptors." Although this term has come to have an apparently specific application in the biological sciences, it is worth noting that the functions of many cell surface entities called "receptors" may actually be better described by other terms such as "perceptors," "sensors," or "signal transducers." This etymological problem is not trivial, since the principal physiological functions of cell components can come to be misleadingly represented or inadequately circumscribed by the words we choose to associate with them.

In this chapter, the focus is on the LDL receptor, which since its discovery in 1973 has been exceptionally well characterized, first in functional terms and then by chemical and molecular-genetic analysis. This receptor has a high and selective affinity for lipoprotein particles in which certain protein components are suitably exposed at the surface. In this case, "receptor" simply refers to a specific recognition and binding capacity, since there is no evidence that conformational changes that may accompany binding link up with any intracellular effector systems; the receptor also does not appear to be a precursor of any active signal molecules inside or outside the cell. The main consequence of the binding of a lipoprotein to an LDL receptor is the transport of the particle into the cellular interior by means of the continuously occurring process of endocytosis via coated pits and vesicles. This usually results in the dispatch of the lipoprotein to a lysosome where the protein components are completely degraded and the ester bonds of the lipids hydrolyzed; the products of these processes are assimilated by the cell or released into the environment. An LDL receptor acts as a shuttle since it is recycled back to the cell surface and makes many journeys in its lifetime: it is one of the longer-lived cellular proteins.

While the study of LDL receptors in normal and mutant cells of various types and in various situations has been highly rewarding in terms of cell biological and physiological insights, there are a number of difficulties that arise when attempts are made to organize the available information into an explanatory framework for whole-body function in normal and diseased animals. While this reflects the paucity of knowledge in a number of key areas, there are also problems of perspective and interpretation. We will try to assess the significance of LDL receptors by first describing how the receptors are synthesized and how they appear to function in individual cells. The regulation of receptor function in cultured cells will be discussed next, and finally we will consider the manner in which the receptors take part in the anabolic and catabolic phases of metabolism in vivo.

LIFE CYCLE OF LDL RECEPTORS

LDL receptors are glycoproteins that make up a very tiny minority (one in many thousands) of the macromolecules populating the surfaces of animal cells. The actual number of these receptors on the surface of a particular cell can vary considerably (between 5,000 and 50,000 in the case of cultured fibroblasts); this variation is called up- and down-regulation. Irrespective of the receptor numbers, however, and whether or not a lipoprotein ligand has been picked up, each receptor molecule spends only a few minutes on the surface before being internalized in a specific and directed manner.

Most of our current knowledge about the molecular structure and function of the LDL receptor has come from the work of Goldstein and Brown in Dallas; this has involved purification of the receptor from the adrenal glands of cattle, now possible using a three-step procedure beginning with membrane preparations. The receptor is first solubilized by treatment with nonionic detergents, which are then removed to permit sequential ion-exchange and affinity chromatography, the latter on columns of agarose beads to which either LDL or antibodies to the LDL receptor are linked. The eluting agent is either NH_4OH or a polysulfated hydrocarbon called suramin, which inhibits binding of LDL to the LDL receptor (1). Other achievements by this group have included the preparation and analytical use of poly- and monoclonal antibodies directed against the receptor protein, and most recently the cloning of a cDNA (2), as well as the entire human gene with 18 exons (3). The receptor may vary in the details of its structure in other species, but it is likely that the information at hand will be generally applicable. Before describing the biosynthesis and placement of receptor molecules at the surface, it may be useful to summarize those structural features that have a bearing on the processes that manufacture the ligand-binding glycoprotein (Fig. 1).

The LDL receptor consists of a single, relatively large polypeptide chain (over 800 amino acids) with a relative molecular mass of about 100,000. One or two N-linked and sulfated oligosaccharide chains plus about 9 to 18 O-linked carbohydrate chains furnish approximately 10% of the molecule, which is nonprotein and which increases the total mass to about 115,000. The structure of the carbohydrate chains is not identical in the two types of human cells so far examined (4), and further variations may well be encountered in other cell types. The presence of about a dozen sialic acid residues on the oligosaccharides of each receptor molecule is one reason for a rather acidic overall charge (isoelectric point 4.6). The receptor is an asymmetric transmembrane protein. Starting at the C terminus there is a limited cytosolic domain of 50 residues, which may be concerned with the binding of the receptor to clathrin or other molecules in coated pits. The cell membrane is traversed by a succeeding hydrophobic sequence of 22 amino acids. Emerging on the external surface, the polypeptide chain becomes particularly rich in serine and threonine residues, many of which bear the clustered O-linked carbohydrate chains. The asparagines, with their N-linked chains, are also positioned close to

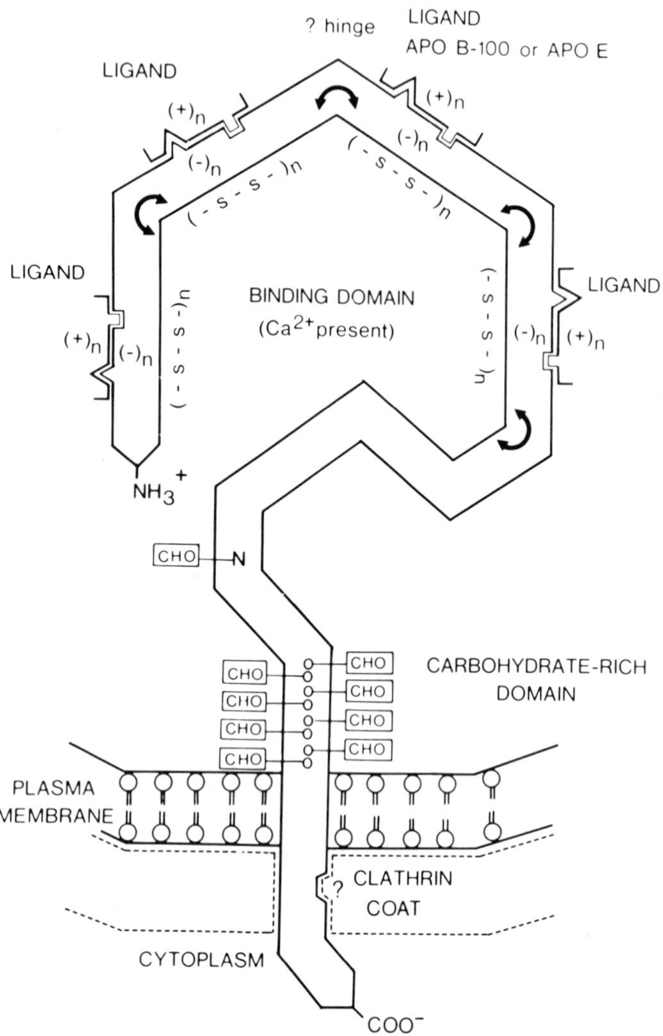

Fig. 1 Schematic representation of the various domains of the LDL receptor. The binding domain is shown speculatively as consisting of four equivalent cysteine-rich binding sites, which are joined together by random coil "hinges," and which permit the binding at saturation of four separate LDL or one apo E-containing HDL particle (four apo E ligands). The clathrin binding site on the cytoplasmic domain is also speculative. (From Refs. 2 and 3.)

this sugar-rich domain near the cell membrane. An intervening domain is followed by the lipoprotein-binding domain: this is rich in disulfide-linked cysteine residues and for this reason is likely to contain somewhat rigid subdomains. There are 8 repeating sequences of about 40 residues, each containing a group of 4 negative charges near its C-terminal end. The binding domain is rather sensitive to a number of proteases such as pronase, trypsin, or papain, and its ability to form functional ligand-binding sites depends on the presence of Ca^{2+} or Mn^{2+}. The remarkable homology of the "external" receptor sequence just distal to the carbohydrate-rich domain, with a segment of the precursor to the growth factor epidermal growth factor (EGF), is of utmost interest in terms of the evolution of cell surface molecules such as the LDL receptor (2).

The Pathway to the Cell Surface

Transcription of the structural genes for LDL receptors (which in humans are located on the autosomal chromosome pair 19) leads to the export from the nucleus of an mRNA species that encodes the complete sequence of amino acids required to form receptor protein (see Fig. 2). The rate at which new mRNA "blueprints" appear in the cytosol fluctuates in different circumstances and this is the main basis of up- and down-regulation of the receptor number in body cells. It is likely that free cytosolic ribosomes begin to translate the LDL receptor-encoding mRNAs, synthesizing hydrophobic "signal sequences" that permit the docking of the relevant ribosomes on specific sites of the rough endoplasmic reticulum. Here, further extension of the polypeptide chains occurs with cotranslational proteolytic removal of the N-terminal "signal sequences." The nascent proteins fold and acquire disulfide bonds, plus the immature, mannose-rich form of the N-linked oligosaccharide chains. Completion of the polypeptides means that the membrane-spanning sequences have been synthesized, and it is possible that these parts of the receptor molecules have already become anchored in the reticulum membrane in the correct topographic position, i.e., with the C-terminal domains exposed to the cytoplasmic compartment of the cell.

While "anchoring" may suggest a rather static condition of the receptors at this stage of their formation, this is not the case since translocation to the Golgi apparatus soon occurs, either by "membrane flow" from the reticulum or, more likely, by a system of directed vesicular transport. In the complex enzymatic "processing factory" of the Golgi plates and vesicles, the O-linked oligosaccharides are added in stages and the immature N-linked chains are remodeled and extended, both types of chains acquiring sialic acid residues (4). These modifications, which occur within 30 min after the synthesis of the polypeptides, are somehow closely associated with, and may be necessary for, the next movement of the receptor molecules to their

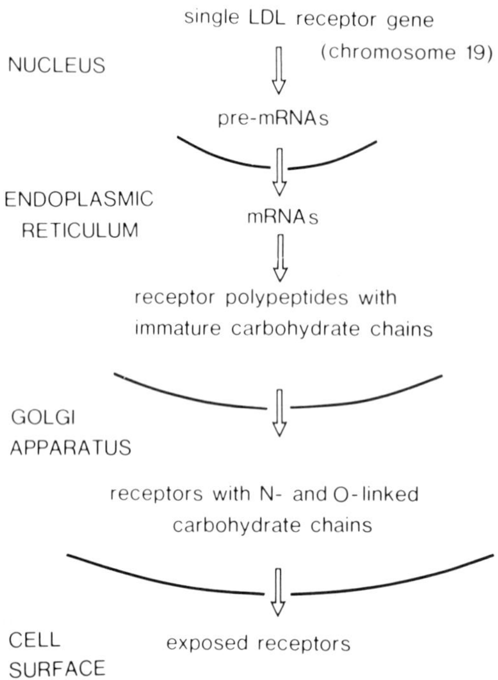

Fig. 2 Biosynthesis of LDL receptors in mammalian cells.

functionally important position on the cell surface. Again, the precise mechanism for incorporation of the new LDL receptors at sites in the cell membrane is not known; it will become apparent later that existing receptors recycle to the cell membrane after engaging in endocytosis via coated pits, and a common vesicular pool in transit could be one of the mechanisms bringing about randomization of life cycles for the whole population.

There is some direct evidence that the receptor molecules exist as monomers in the cell membrane, since the technique of radiation inactivation applied to intact membranes gives an estimate of molecular size that is in close agreement with the biochemical information already provided above (5).

Studies of the binding of certain HDL particles containing only apo E as protein components have indicated that the external domain of an LDL receptor can bind 4 molecules of apo E, probably located on a single lipoprotein particle, with very high affinity (Kd about 10^{-10} M) (5). The same sites can also bind 4 apo B molecules located on separate LDL particles, with appreciably lower but still high affinity (Kd about 3×10^{-9} M). Binding studies are facilitated by the use of certain organic polyanions, such as heparin or dextran sulfate, which displace bound LDL when added in excess to incubated cells. More information is needed on the molecular aspects of the binding reactions, since there are indications that binding constants determined under equilibrium conditions at 0°C may give misleading impressions of the true operational "affinity" of the LDL receptors for their various ligands at body temperatures and under conditions where the internalization of the receptors via the coated pits occurs more rapidly than the "off reactions" of ligands from receptors on the cell surface (6).

It will have become apparent from the above that the ligand specificity of the LDL receptor extends to lipoproteins that can offer two apparently rather different apolipoproteins at the particle surface—apo E and apo B. The former is an arginine-rich protein of known primary structure, which can be found in association with a variety of particles including chylomicrons, VLDL of β or pre-β mobility, a variety of ill-defined intermediates of intravascular lipoprotein lipolysis, and certain species of HDL. The limited sequence of amino acids responsible for binding of apo E has been defined by Mahley and colleagues partly on the basis of human mutations affecting binding to the LDL receptor (7). The clustering of positive charges in this part of apo E is indicative of the important role played by electrostatic interactions in the strength and specificity of the interaction between the two proteins. Apo B is a protein that appears to have a much larger relative molecular mass; its structure is still unknown but the existence of at least two isoforms, most commonly called apo B-100 and apo B-48, has been established by immunological mapping and polyacrylamide gel electrophoresis under denaturing conditions (8). Apo B-48 has been the only isoform so far detected in any particles that have been produced by the intestinal mucosa, while the majority (and in some animal species all) of the apo B present in particles produced by the liver has been of the apo B-100 type. Specifically, apo B-100 is the only isoform present in LDL (and in the lipoproteins called Lp(a) present in the plasma of most individuals at much lower concentrations) and there is no doubt that this protein is the natural ligand for the LDL receptor apart from apo E. Apo B-48 does not bind to the receptor and may lack the sequences required for binding. Nevertheless, the factors that govern the availability of apolipoproteins present in various types and sizes of lipoproteins are not yet fully understood, and there may be other explanations for the many data which presently support the notion that intestinally derived apo B is not a ligand for the LDL receptor.

It will have become clear that there are good reasons why many workers refer to the LDL receptor as the apo B-100,E or apo B,E receptor, terms that better define the specificity and probably the functions of this particular lipoprotein receptor.

Clustering and Internalization of LDL Receptors (9)

Once on the cell surface, the LDL receptors rapidly become concentrated in membrane specializations called coated pits (Fig. 3). The coating that gives rise to this name is present on the cytoplasmic side of the indented cell membrane and consists largely of a special structural protein called clathrin (monomeric relative molecular mass about 180,000). These coated pits represent only about 2% of the surface, yet the majority of the ligand-binding sites is found here at any given moment. A number of other receptors and proteins share

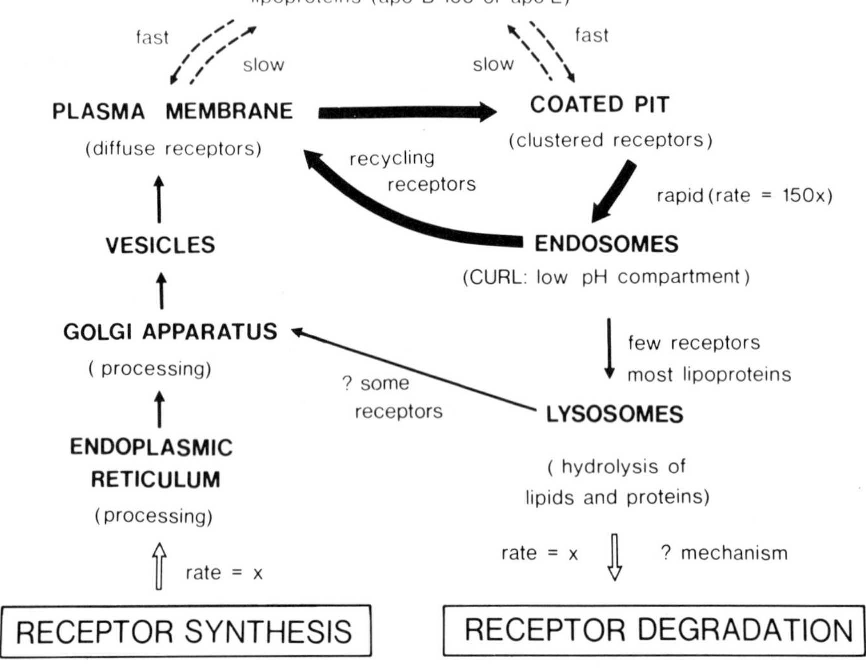

Fig. 3 Cyclic function and turnover of LDL receptors. Long-lived LDL receptors recycle continuously from the cell surface, picking up lipoproteins if available and sharing the coated pit-based endocytosis mechanism with other similar "carriers." Most receptors recycle to the surface by means of a "short loop" (prelysosomal), while others may return via a lysosome- or Golgi-based "long loop." The rate of receptor biosynthesis equals the rate of receptor degradation in the steady state: each receptor cycles approximately 150 times. CURL, compartment of uncoupling of receptor and ligand.

this location and in the case of some receptors, probably including the LDL receptor, clustering is not dependent on the prior binding of the appropriate ligands. Continuous internalization of the coated pits and their contents occurs in a complex membranous sorting reaction that only takes place at temperatures well above 4°C. [Binding of ligands to receptors occurs at low temperatures, and use is made of this difference to quantify the sequential phases of the endocytic pathway in cultured cells (Fig. 4)]. Although transient formation of coated vesicles may occur during endocytosis, there is no doubt that uncoated vesicles appear, which coalesce to form specific structures called endocytic vesicles. The vesicles are "outside-in" so that the ligands are exposed to the lumen, which is acidified by an ATP-dependent proton pump located in the membrane. The low pH affects the tightness of the bonds between the receptors and their lipoprotein ligands, and most of them dissociate within a few minutes.

There are good reasons for believing that small "recycling vesicles" bud off tubular extensions of the larger endosomes and that these return to the cell membrane bearing most of the receptors and, for largely geometric reasons, only a minority of the ligands; obviously, any lipoproteins still bound will accompany their receptors, as will the free particles that are dissolved in the small liquid phases of the recycling vesicles (9). This apparently fruitless and "messy" aspect of the sorting process is one reasonable explanation for the phenomenon

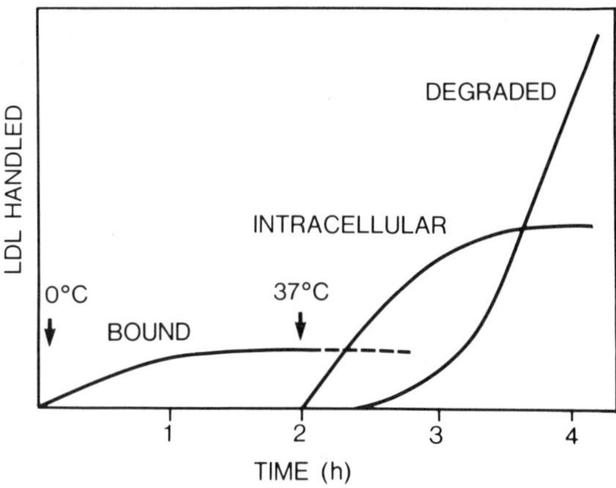

Fig. 4 Basic idealized features of receptor-mediated LDL binding, internalization, and degradation in cultured cells, illustrating the temperature and time dependence of these processes. No scale is indicated on the ordinate because different cell types give different absolute and relative levels for each process.

of retroendocytosis, which has been observed in the handling of LDL by cultured cells: receptor economy is the advantage gained in exchange for the spillage of lipoprotein back into the medium (10). The inhibition of receptor recycling by the ionophoric antibiotic monensin, which among other effects nullifies the acidification of endocytic vesicles, has been interpreted to indicate that the segregation of recycling vesicles from endosomes is somehow dependent on this aspect of vesicle function. A puzzling discrepancy, however, is the fact that retroendocytosis of LDL is markedly enhanced by monensin, especially when the pool of endocytic vesicles is large. The possibility thus remains that recycling and retroendocytic vesicles are not identical and that the latter subserve a different, as yet undescribed function in the overall process of receptor-mediated endocytosis.

The endocytic vesicles are targeted in an unknown manner to the lysosomes, with which they fuse to form secondary lysosomes with an acidic interior and a rich complement of hydrolytic enzymes. Apo B is attacked by cathepsin D, a pepsinlike endoprotease with a highly acidic pH optimum, and then joins with cathepsin B and a variety of peptidases to degrade the protein to the amino acid level (11) (the possibility of peptide fragments being released into the cytosol has not been excluded—there are some cell types where this could well happen, e.g., the liver with its biliary excretion route). The lipids are attacked by acid lipase and the lysosomal cholesterol esterase, generating free cholesterol among other products. The low molecular mass products of particle digestion are released into the cytosol, from which further redistribution occurs into various pathways of intracellular utilization or egress from the cell. Free cholesterol can be expected to partition into membranes of various kinds, to be converted to intracellular cholesterol esters by enzymatic action, or to be lost from different cells according to their biochemical specializations, such as lipoprotein secretion and bile formation in the case of hepatocytes, steroid hormone synthesis in endocrine glands, and so-called "reverse cholesterol transport" in many other cells.

Inhibition of lysosomal hydrolases by treatment of cultured cells with basic agents such as ammonium chloride, methylamine, or chloroquine raises the pH within lysosomes and other vesicles in which a low pH is maintained, including endocytic vesicles. This is associated with the enhanced release of retroendocytosed ligand lipoproteins. The reasons for the "back-up" stasis of the vesicular pathway under these conditions are not clear.

The steps of receptor-mediated endocytosis in which fusion of endosomes with lysosomes occurs are markedly slowed below 20°C, and this was used to show that recycling of the majority of internalized receptors occurred from prelysosomal structures or steps. It is feasible that LDL receptors may actually be partitioned into the lysosome-targeted route and that this may result either in receptor degradation or in a separate salvage pathway requiring that the Golgi apparatus be traversed so that the receptors can be recycled the long way round as it were, perhaps in association with new receptor molecules. The binding of specific antibodies to LDL receptors is followed by the internalization of the "illegitimate" ligands: in the case of polyclonal antibodies, nearly all the receptors are targeted to the lysosomes (and degraded), while with monoclonal antibodies, the receptors recycle efficiently. This difference relates presumably to the degree to which the different ligands dissociate at the low intravesicular pH.

LDL Receptor Degradation

Estimates have been made of the number of times that a given LDL receptor would recycle to the cell surface in cultured fibroblasts before its final destruction at a site or sites that are still uncertain (9). Approximately 12 min is required for a single cycle and 150 such cycles are undertaken—corresponding to an average lifespan of about 30 hours. These rather precise numbers should not be extrapolated to other cell types, however, and there are already indications that the rates of steps or sequences of steps are under some forms of regulation. For example, the handling of large numbers of ligands via the "piggyback" endocytotic pathway causes a temporary depletion of the hepatic surface receptors for asialoglycoproteins, and one interpretation of this situation is that the return of receptors to the surface occurs more slowly when ligands are being internalized than when unoccupied receptors are cycling. In any case, it would be very surprising indeed if the complex pathway were independent of any kind of physiological control.

The secondary lysosome presents itself as an obvious seat of receptor degradation. Here, the bulky and protease-sensitive ligand-binding domain of the receptor would be exposed to the cathepsins and other lysosomal peptidases. The enormous organizational and structural complexity of the entire Golgi-endoplasmic reticulum-lysosome region makes it likely, however, that there may be other places where the receptor molecules are degraded. All that is certain is that the necessity for effective regulation of receptor number means that degradation must occur at a rate that is appropriate for the transition from one steady state to another. It is not known, for instance, whether the degradation rate is controlled either by the susceptibility of receptor molecules to available proteases or by the rate at which receptors are partitioned into the degradation compartment.

It is clear that the number of receptor molecules actually on the surface of a given cell is a function of the following determinants inter alia:

1. The rate at which the gene is transcribed and the product RNAs processed to form translatable mRNAs

2. The balance between exposed receptors at the surface and internalized, "masked" receptor molecules, influenced by the flux along the receptor recycling route(s)
3. The rate of receptor degradation in the lysosomes or elsewhere

REGULATORY ASPECTS OF LDL RECEPTOR FUNCTION IN CULTURED CELLS

Since the role of LDL receptors is apparently entirely concerned with the facilitated unidirectional uptake of lipid-rich particles, there is a clear need for coordinate regulation of this function in terms of cellular homeostasis. Because most of the earlier studies on this regulatory aspect have involved the uptake of LDL (a lipoprotein rich in cholesterol esters and poor in triglycerides) in cultured fibroblasts, a great deal of emphasis has been given to receptor regulation in relation to cholesterol supply and demand in dividing cells.

Cholesterol Homeostasis in Cultured Skin Fibroblasts (12)

Studies of dividing human fibroblasts in culture have provided consistent and convincing evidence for the intimate involvement of LDL receptors in a system of interdependent processes that provide cells with just enough cholesterol to satisfy their requirements, most of which related to the processes associated with cell proliferation and the required formation of new cellular membranes (Fig. 5). Fibroblasts do not synthesize steroid hormones in significant amounts, if at all, nor do they form bile acids; they also do not manufacture and secrete lipoproteins or make specialized membranes such as myelin. In addition, they do not have to play a role in the bulk transport of cholesterol from one body compartment to another. All these processes are carried out by other cell types in the body; perhaps it is just as well that the initial attack on the problems of cellular cholesterol homeostasis was conducted on cells that have a simpler view of the need for an adequate supply of cholesterol.

The basic finding in fibroblasts has been that cholesterol derived from endocytosed lipoproteins exerts powerful effects on the endogenous enzymatic pathway by which the cells can synthesize the cholesterol they need from readily available two-carbon fragments. In practice, this is brought about by repression of the synthesis of the flux-generating enzyme, hydroxymethylglutaryl-CoA reductase (HMG-CoA reductase), and by enhancement of enzyme degradation. Cultured cells thus opt for the external source of cholesterol in preference to their own product. Another repressive effect involves the gene for the LDL receptor itself, so that the formation of new receptors is cut back, leading in the course of 1 to 2 days to a new and down-regulated steady state. The third component of the homeostatic system is the activation of acyl-CoA cholesterol acyl-transferase

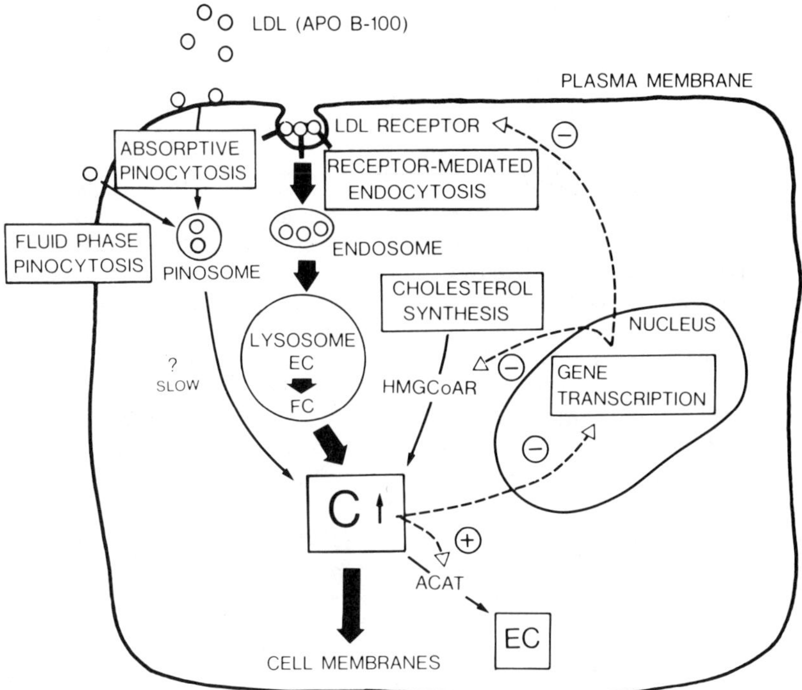

Fig. 5 Cholesterol homeostasis in dividing fibroblasts. The scheme shows a down-regulated cell adapting to the presence in the surrounding fluid of large amounts of LDL. C in the central square depicts a pool of cholesterol and its metabolites that produce regulatory effects at the sites indicated by dotted arrows. EC, esterified cholesterol; FC, free cholesterol; HMGCoAR, hydroxymethylglutaryl-CoA reductase; ACAT, acyl-CoA cholesterol acyltransferase.

(ACAT) by the increased supply of one of its substrates and, possibly, by another form of activation. The latter reaction removes "excess" cholesterol into a cellular storage pool from which the cholesterol needs of the cell can be met on a short-term basis.

It is important to note that the three homeostatic responses are tightly coupled in dividing cultured cells and that they appear to give a "driver's seat" role to exogenous lipoproteins in providing cholesterol for new membranes. In most of the cellular studies, however, no accurate measurements have been made of the *actual* net contribution made by the exogenous and endogenous sources of cholesterol, respectively, under the various conditions tested. The marked changes in the LDL receptor numbers and in the HMGCoA reductase actually observed during down-regulation, however, have strongly suggested a cellular preference for exogenous supplies of cholesterol.

LDL Receptors in the Liver, Intestine, and Endocrine Glands

Recent interest has shifted to the regulation of receptor numbers in those cell types where the metabolism of cholesterol is both more complex and quantitatively more significant than in peripheral fibroblasts. Cell culture systems in the case of the liver, intestine, and adrenal cortex are not yet well standardized from the standpoint of defined growth phases, and satisfactory human cell systems present problems of a particularly serious kind. Nevertheless, primary cultures of hepatocytes from a variety of species have been studied in terms of receptor physiology, and use has also been made of well-differentiated transformed cells that can be propagated in culture. Cultured hepatocytes from rabbits and neonatal pigs and HEP G2 cells derived from a human liver tumor all show the features of regulable LDL receptors coupled to changes in HMGCoA reductase activities; primary rat liver cell cultures do not, for reasons that are not yet clear (6). Cell isolates from the adrenal glands take up LDL via apo B,E receptors, while freshly isolated intestinal epithelial cells have also been studied with some success in this manner. Nevertheless, the existence of a tightly coupled regulatory network has not been shown in these two interesting cell types in vitro.

LDL Receptor-Independent Uptake of Cholesterol-Rich Lipoproteins

It is appropriate at this stage to introduce the notion of receptor-unrelated cellular assimilation of lipoproteins such as LDL. Various studies of cultured cells have revealed the ability of cells to take up LDL (often heterologous in terms of the species of origin) by non-saturable, Ca^{2+}-independent processes that may reflect a variety of membrane events, ranging from fluid-phase pinocytosis of whole micro-droplets of medium to ill-defined but somewhat more selective adsorptive endocytosis of high capacity but low affinity (6). There are also equilibrative exchanges of lipid components between cell membranes and lipoproteins in which no net uptake takes place (unless intracellular esterification of cholesterol maintains the gradient across the cell membrane). In the case of cells lacking LDL receptors because of mutations in the gene for this protein, a remarkably effective and apparently normal pattern of intracellular cholesterol metabolism can be maintained in virtually all body cells, dependent on the presence of sufficiently high ambient LDL concentrations. While this may partly reflect the lack of dependence of peripheral cell types such as fibroblasts on the LDL receptor pathway, there is every indication that cells exposed to high LDL concentrations do internalize the particles by alternative mechanisms.

The acquisition of cholesterol by adsorptive endocytosis is less effective in producing the "classical" counterregulatory responses than is that which follows the involvement of the high-affinity, low-capacity LDL receptors via the coated pits. This may be because the destruction of the apoprotein surface of the particles is less efficient than it is in the aggressive lysosomal environment, although it is not yet certain that lysosomes do not participate in the steps that follow on the as yet poorly understood uptake process. Steinberg and colleagues have established that the degradation of apo B internalized by nonreceptor-mediated endocytosis in cultured hepatocytes is not sensitive to chloroquine or leupeptin treatment of the cells, suggesting noninvolvement of acidified vesicles or lysosomes, while colchicine is also without its usual inhibitory effect as observed in the case of the LDL pathway (6). The suggestion has accordingly been made that the proteolytic attack is carried out in the cytoplasm by systems that are believed to be responsible for the basal turnover of short-lived cellular proteins. To the extent that the cholesterol esters released from the LDL particles by this kind of pathway may not be readily available to the regulatory pool of cholesterol or its oxidized metabolites, the responses of HMG-CoA reductase and LDL receptor modulation or changed ACAT activity may be attenuated or slow or even absent. It would be interesting to know whether the adsorptive low-affinity mechanism is also regulated in some kind of responsive cellular network; its activity may carry a significance that cannot presently be assessed. Interestingly, there is evidence that liver cells take up iron from transferrin both by receptor-mediated endocytosis and by an absorptive process in which the ligand is not internalized but delivers its iron load at the surface.

Modulation of LDL Receptors by Factors Other than Cholesterol Demand and Supply

One of the less well-ploughed areas of receptor research has been the search for factors or determinants that are not directly related to lipoproteins, but which may influence receptor number or other aspects of receptor function. One physical factor is temperature; for unknown reasons, the number of binding sites at 37°C is roughly twice that detectable at 4°C (the apparent affinity, however, is lower). Senescent cells express fewer receptors when fibroblasts are subjected to serial culture, corresponding to lessened mitotic activity and vitality. Confluent, nondividing cultured cells have very low receptor numbers, endothelial cells being a prime example. The hormone insulin has protein synthesis-dependent effects on the receptor activity, which seems to represent processes that are not related to growth stimulation and the associated need for membrane cholesterol. Ascorbic acid exerts a similar clear-cut effect on the number of binding sites at the surfaces of cultured smooth muscle but not fibroblastic cells; the effect is transient and depends on protein synthesis for its expression. The regulation of liver-cell receptors by thyroid hormones (in humans) and by estrogens (in rats) also indicates that LDL receptors will be found to fall within the bounds of pleiotropic responses to hormonal and metabolic signals.

ROLE OF LDL RECEPTORS IN WHOLE-BODY LIPID METABOLISM

The preceding sections have dwelt on molecular and cellular events in the life histories of LDL receptors, and there is little reason to doubt that there is a broad generality of these mechanisms in all nucleated cells of mammals. The fact that the number of receptor molecules actually present on individual cell surfaces is regulated in response to cellular activities or environmental changes is also beyond dispute, although the tightness of such controls may vary in different cases or situations.

What remains to be assessed is the quantitative contribution made in a given intact animal body by LDL receptors to anabolic and catabolic phases of whole-body lipid metabolism. It is sometimes difficult for molecular scientists to convert their data and thoughts into models that make metabolic sense; at the other extreme, represented by mathematically based compartmental analysis, problems are often encountered in going beyond abstract concepts such as "rapidly exchanging pools" and "rate constants connecting subsets of molecules," into the real world of organ-dependent metabolism.

A systematic metabolic approach to these problems starts off by recognizing that organs or tissues of measurable mass are made up of one or more cell types in measurable proportions. Receptor numbers can be estimated by direct ligand-binding experiments on isolated membrane preparations (or their fractionated components) or by quantitative single- or double-antibody-binding techniques applied to similar types of material; the data can be assumed to represent, or be at least proportional to, the number of receptors actually available on the surfaces of the cells. In some cases, free cells can be isolated and used for direct binding studies in vitro (e.g., lymphocytes). Plasma lipoprotein concentrations can be measured and, in most cases, the availability of lymph concentrations and some knowledge of the properties of the endothelia of the particular capillary beds concerned would allow the concentrations of lipoprotein ligands for LDL receptors to be "guessed at" and related to the known affinity constants and V_{max} values for receptor-mediated LDL uptake. In principle, the information thus obtained can be worked into an estimate of the likely flux through the LDL receptor pathway in an organ or tissue in defined circumstances. The same considerations would apply to the assessment of nonreceptor-mediated LDL uptake into the cells. While the above approach is rational, the reader will be left in no doubt as to the probable accuracy of the final estimates and the uncertainties that would remain!

Another concern is the problem of quantifying the relative use made by a given set of cells of endogenously synthesized cholesterol vis-á-vis that taken up via the LDL receptors. In animal models, use can be made of the incorporation of tritiated water into cholesterol as an accurate and simple measure of de novo synthesis, and this can be compared with the uptake of LDL cholesterol assessed by methods that are free of assumptions or indirect inferences. This comparison has an important bearing on the accuracy of one perspective, which essentially sees the LDL receptor as a catabolic device concentrated in the liver and present elsewhere as a back-up, and another which ascribes anabolic roles to the receptor pathway that go beyond the single clear-cut instance of the steroidogenic endocrine glands.

Cholesterol Homeostasis in the Cells of a Living Organism

One of the difficulties in assessing cellular regulatory responses to LDL is that while tissue lymph contains these particles at a concentration that is approximately 10 times lower than that in the plasma, even this amount would saturate the LDL receptors in most tissues and cause them to be permanently down-regulated. Another problem is that uncritical extension of the "cultured fibroblast" model to other cell types would lead one to suppose that one of the main functions of the LDL receptor is the supply of cholesterol to cells that prefer not to make their own. However, certain compounds needed by all cells at all times, such as ubiquinone and dolichol, are also synthesized via HMG-CoA reductase, and the supply of cholesterol from LDL leaves these requirements unsatisfied. The nature of the "signal" molecules supposedly giving rise to the regulatory phenomena has yet to be unraveled, and studies of a variety of cell types other than fibroblasts have revealed numerous examples where uncoupling of the expression of LDL receptors from the rates of endogenous cholesterol synthesis appears to be the rule. Persuasive evidence has been assembled by Kandutsch and colleagues indicating that certain oxidized derivatives of cholesterol may be natural transcriptional regulators acting in the general manner of steroid hormones via cytoplasmic and nuclear receptors (see Chapter 11). Finally, direct measurements of endogenous cholesterol biosynthesis in intact tissues throughout the bodies of experimental animals, representing a wide range of species, combined with estimates of the rates of actual "LDL transport" or uptake, have allowed Dietschy and co-workers to postulate that most tissues, including the liver in its pivotal role, largely rely on their own biosynthetic capacity to satisfy their needs in vivo (13). The most striking findings indicate that tissues cope primarily with variations in their cholesterol requirements by appropriately varying their rate of cholesterol synthesis, rather than by up- or down-regulating their LDL receptors. Thus, modulation of the receptors appears to be a secondary device that is called upon only in circumstances when the biosynthetic "peak" effort cannot meet the cellular demand because of inherent phenotypic limitations or the presence of an inhibitor (13). On the other hand, there is evidence which suggests that specialized cells may be influenced significantly by LDL availability; an example is the enhancement of human lymphocyte growth responses by LDL acting on the high-affinity LDL receptor. Measurement of LDL receptor numbers in freshly isolated mononuclear cells from human subjects, and the finding of marked upward changes in these numbers following culture in lipoprotein-deficient media, have also indicated that marked repression of receptor synthesis occurs as expected in intact bodies, at least in some cell types.

Liver cells occupy a central position in the regulation of the synthesis, transformation, and clearance of lipoproteins. LDL receptors in the liver are coded for by the same gene as that which is responsible for LDL receptors in fibroblasts in the skin; this has been proved in human receptor mutants suffering from the homozygous form of familial hypercholesterolemia and in rabbits, bred by Watanabe, which have essentially the same defect [Watanabe heritable hyperlipemia (WHHL) rabbits] (14). The LDL concentration in the vicinity of liver cells is probably as high as that in the plasma, and it is difficult to imagine that the saturation of the receptors will ever be less than complete, especially when one bears in mind the preferential claim that apo E-bearing particles are likely to have vis-á-vis LDL in binding to the receptors.

The metabolism of cholesterol in liver cells takes place in a highly complicated and interlocking series of processes that represent a large daily flux (Fig. 6). On the outflow side, cholesterol is irreversibly biotransformed into bile acids and secreted into bile in the free form together with these products; this is the only quantitatively significant way by which the body can excrete the sterol in order to remain in balance over a period of time. The cells also elaborate and secrete a variety of lipoproteins containing free and esterified cholesterol as essential components. Cholesterol production occurs by de novo synthesis in the liver cells, and a large amount of cholesterol uptake occurs when the remnants of fat-rich plasma lipoproteins are taken up by endocytosis following binding either to LDL receptors or to the similar but independent apo E receptors. There are important differences in the inherent maximum capacities of livers from different species to synthesize cholesterol. For example, the maximum rate of

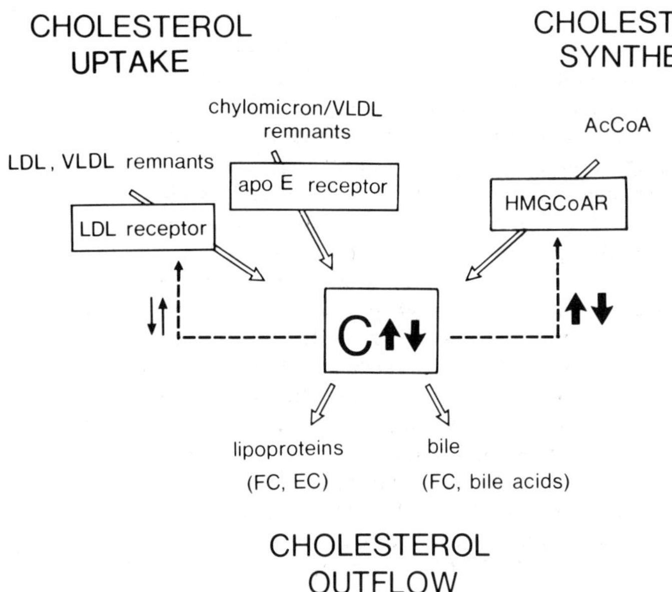

Fig. 6 Cholesterol traffic in liver cells. A balance between cholesterol synthesis and uptake, on the one hand, and the outflow of this sterol into the blood and bile, on the other, is maintained primarily by adaptive shifts in the rate of de novo cholesterol synthesis brought about by fluctuations in the activity of HMGCoA reductase. A back-up mechanism depends on appropriate shifts in LDL receptor number; this occurs when the endogenous synthetic pathway is unable to compensate because of inherent capacity limitations or pharmacological inhibition.

synthesis per gram liver in male hamsters and humans is about 40 to 50 times less than that in rats. The evidence is strong that up- or down-regulation of LDL receptors generally tends to occur in such livers only when shifts in the rate of de novo biosynthesis cannot maintain the homeostatic balance between cholesterol availability and outflow (13).

It is noteworthy in this regard that in humans the daily flux of LDL-derived cholesterol into the liver is considerably larger than the endogenous capacity of this organ for synthesizing cholesterol or the usual episodic dietary inflow. The outflow of cholesterol as a component of exported lipoproteins is also large and is likely to be somewhat more irregular than LDL catabolism.

The evolving concepts for the regulation of cholesterol metabolism in the liver developed largely by Dietschy (13), are not fully consistent with several correlations that have been made by others between the fluxes through the various in- and outflow pathways and the levels of LDL receptors. In primary hepatocyte cultures, as already mentioned, the LDL receptor number is efficiently regulated by the availability of exogenous lipoprotein cholesterol in much the same way as in fibroblasts (15); this also applies to the intracellular responses of HMGCoA reductase and ACAT. In addition, binding studies performed on isolated membrane preparations have indicated that receptor number in the liver is positively responsive to whole-body manipulations of various kinds, at least in certain species (16). These include low-cholesterol diets, infusions of bile salts, induction of hypothyroidism, and the administration of drugs that sequester bile salts in the intestine or inhibit the synthesis of cholesterol in the liver (HMG-CoA reductase inhibitors such as compactin and mevinolin). The presence of high receptor numbers has also been positively correlated with the efficient formation of bile salts and bile secretion, with the export into the blood of the larger classes of VLDL, which are not converted into LDL in the intravascular compartment, and with the absence of direct secretion of LDL into the circulation. Conversely, low or zero receptor numbers have been correlated with decreased secretion of cholesterol into the bile, and with the elaboration of smaller classes of VLDL that are efficiently converted into LDL, plus the apparent direct formation of LDL by the liver cells.

Because we lack information on the conversion of subclasses of VLDL into LDL in the vascular compartment, perhaps involving hepatic lipase on liver cell surfaces, (1) we must discover how the biosynthesis of different apolipoproteins is differentially controlled and how these elements are assembled into different kinds and sizes of particles, varying in lipid and apolipoprotein composition; (2) the regulation of bile acid formation in relation to the cholesterol supply from various sources needs to be unraveled; (3) regulated synthesis and secretion of LCAT and hepatic lipase may be important; (4) the indirect evidence for direct secretion of LDL by liver cells in certain circumstances needs to be confirmed and characterized; (5) handling of chylomicron and other apo B-48-containing remnant particles must be compared with the ways in which similar particles containing apo B-100 are internalized; and (6) the details of reverse cholesterol transport via HDL subclasses or other particles must be integrated into the entire framework. More precisely, the determinants of hepatic LDL receptor number must be established and the importance of modulations in these numbers to all the cholesterol-handling pathways must be determined. Somehow, the "classical fibroblast" homeostatic system exists within the larger cybernetic superstructure required by the liver to organize its affairs (17).

In the case of epithelial cells of the small intestine, there appears to be a complete dissociation between the rate of endogenous cholesterol synthesis and the LDL receptor number, while the ACAT system is also uncoupled from the endocytic uptake pathway (13). On the other hand, evidence from various experiments suggests strongly that steroidogenic glands make extensive use of lipoprotein-derived cholesterol through LDL receptors and efficiently regulate their surface receptor number, which in any case is the largest of any organ in the body, expressed per unit mass of tissue (10 times more than liver). These organs are small, however, and their contribution to total body disposition of cholesterol is insignificant.

Fate of LDL In Vivo

Steinberg and colleagues, through ingenious and valid shortcuts, have contributed decisive answers to many of the quantitative questions in this field (18). By synthesizing LDL derivatives containing radioactive adjuncts that are unable to readily diffuse out of the lysosomes in which endocytosed LDL particles are degraded, they have fashioned quantitative fingerprints by which the relative contributions of different organs in an animal can be compared with each other after bolus injection of the derivatized LDL. The roles of different cell types within a single organ can also be assessed using autoradiographic morphological examination. These experiments have unambiguously pointed to the liver as the principal site of LDL catabolism (60 to 80% of the total), together with the intestines and the endocrine glands. In addition and most importantly, the studies have shown the decisive importance of LDL receptors in mediating the catabolic events, although the effective use that is made in animals lacking LDL receptors of nonreceptor-dependent pathways has also been shown by this approach.

One of the problems in the assessment of LDL receptor function is the role that this receptor plays in the handling of lipoproteins other than LDL. The affinity of LDL receptors for apo E-bearing particles (provided they satisfy certain requirements) is higher than that for apo B-100-containing particles, and the former are rapidly removed by the liver and other cells within minutes or hours, rather than days, as in the case of LDL with its apo B-100 ligand. The manner in which apo E mediates receptor binding in a variety of particles is complex and apparently strongly influenced by the size of particles (mainly determined by the triacylglycerol content of the particles), by the presence of other apolipoproteins (e.g., apo C's), by the nature of the accompanying apo B and other determinants, and by the requirement of multiple copies of apo E on individual lipoproteins in order to produce the very high affinity of binding (5). Nevertheless, apo E appears to be the dominant ligand in VLDL particles rich in triacylglycerols or cholesterol esters (7). There is also a second receptor in liver cells which appears to be constitutively expressed (Fig. 6). This entity, termed the apo E receptor, shows similarities to the LDL or B,E receptor: the common features include dependence on Ca^{2+}, sensitivity to pronase digestion, elimination of receptor binding when the clustered positive charges are removed by chemical modification, depressed binding in the case of the interesting human apo E mutants in some of which, for example, the crucial arginine residue at position 158 is replaced by cysteine in the receptor binding region, and clustering of receptors in coated pits as part of the pathway of receptor-mediated endocytosis. The importance of particle-associated apo B-48 in the function of this receptor remains an unsolved problem, and it is possible that the receptor actually discriminates against apo B-100. In any case, it is this receptor that is responsible for the virtually normal handling of diet-derived lipoprotein remnants by the liver in animals devoid of functional LDL receptors.

The problem of two similar receptors, of which only the B,E receptor is subject to up- and down-regulation, is a central one in the cholesterol metabolism of the liver. The chemical specificities for the handling of different particles by one or the other of these entities need to be determined in great detail, but the availability of the WHHL rabbit and similar animal models should permit the extension of the Steinberg approach to other particles apart from LDL. It should be remembered, however, that apo E migrates rapidly from one particle to another in the plasma, and reconstitution of particles labeled only in the apo B moiety may be the only feasible solution to this problem, with attendant interpretational difficulties.

The dependence of whole-body catabolism of LDL on LDL receptors has also been assessed by comparing the fractional catabolic rate (FCR) of LDL in normal subjects (FCR 0.45 pools/day) with that in receptorless familial hypercholesterolemia patients (FCR 0.15 pools/day). In addition, the FCR of native LDL in normal subjects has been compared with that of modified particles in which high-affinity ligand binding has been eliminated by chemical modifications such as the removal of a sufficient number of arginine residues by treatment with 1,2-cyclohexanedione (a usefully reversible modification) or by alkylation of lysines with the same effect. These studies have clearly established the predominance of receptor-mediated processes in clearing LDL from the blood (60 to 90%), but they cannot reliably indicate the extent to which the occupation of existing receptors by particles other than LDL may influence a particular experimental result. Extensions of these experiments to other kinds of particles are needed but will encounter the same difficulties of migrating particle components referred to above. The turnover experiments clearly point to independent but complementary roles for LDL production and LDL catabolism in the determination of the steady-state LDL concentration in the plasma of a given individual (19).

LDL Receptor Mutants

Familial hypercholesterolemia was identified by Mueller in Norway over 50 years ago as a single gene defect. Since then, homo- and heterozygotes suffering from this metabolic disorder have been studied intensively because it became evident that the affected gene was that for the high-affinity LDL receptor in all tissues of the body. Heterozygotes remove LDL from the blood at only two-thirds of the normal rate and suffer from atherosclerotic complications in the fourth or fifth decades of their lives; homozygotes are severaly hypercholesterolemic and usually succumb to atherosclerosis in the first or second decade of life.

The existence of these relatively large numbers of LDL receptor mutants in the human population, as well as the deliberate establishment of a very similar mutant experimental animal in the form of the WHHL rabbit, has provided a useful approach to the assessment of the physiological roles of LDL receptors. It has been possible to assign virtually all known cases of FH to defective LDL receptor genes residing at a single autosomal pair of loci on chromosome 19 (Table 1). Strains of skin fibroblasts and transformed lymphoblastoid cells from these persons and their relatives have been characterized by means of standardized LDL binding and degradation studies to define the receptor defect in functional terms (20). More recently, biosynthetic studies have been conducted in which the intracellular maturation of the glycosylated receptor molecules and their placement

Table 1 Mutant Alleles for the LDL Receptor Gene on Human Chromosome Pair 19 (Familial Hypercholesterolemia)

Type	Effect
"Null allele"	Apparent absence of gene product as detected by LDL or specific antibody binding
Processing defects combined with lowered affinity for LDL	Complete failure to reach the cell surface of precursors of varying sizes (normal, larger, or smaller)
	Slowed or diminished passage of precursors to cell surface (found in South Africans and in WHHL rabbits)
Binding defects	Normal passage to cell surface of receptor molecules defective in LDL or antibody binding
Internalization defect	Defect in receptor molecules (? cytoplasmic domain) which prevents clustering in coated pits

Source: Refs. 21 and 22.

on the cell surfaces was detected and quantified by the appropriate use of mono- and polyclonal antibodies to the receptor protein (21,22). This approach has enabled Brown and Goldstein and colleagues to identify LDL receptor gene products with considerable precision; a variety of allelic mutations are associated either with the total absence of functionally active receptor protein, or with blocked or slowed intracellular maturation of receptor precursor forms of varying molecular size. The existence of apparently homozygous genetic compounds was demonstrated in homozygously defective individuals, and the occurrence of a "founder" effect in a large cohort of South African FH patients has also been documented. Interestingly, detailed investigation of one "noncompound" or true homozygote and her obligatorily heterozygotic parents suggested that the normal or "wild-type" gene products (or the products of other genes) influence the movement of receptor molecules to the cell surface (23). This may help to explain wide variations in apparent receptor gene expression in hetero- and homozygotes, a small number of whom have survived to the fifth decade of life, and may even have a bearing on the regulated expression of the receptor protein in homozygous "normal" persons.

Use has also recently been made of the fact that certain monoclonal antibodies directed at receptor determinants are internalized and degraded by tissue cells throughout the body, as though the antibodies were lipoprotein particles, so that the rates at which such labeled antibodies disappear from the circulation after injection reflect the total body "activity" of the receptors. The particular advantage of this approach is the apparent absence of competition from various lipoprotein ligands also present in the system, and this minimizes a serious source of error that appears when labeled LDL is used to assess the overall receptor contribution to LDL catabolism in intact animals.

Animals of the steady-state metabolism of FH homozygotes with severely defective or absent LDL receptors in all tissues has revealed the constant occurrence of very high LDL concentrations in the plasma coupled with low HDL levels, especially of the subclass HDL_2. The plasma also contains other lipoprotein particles that contain apo B-100 and/or apo E and that are rich in cholesterol esters (24). (In WHHL rabbits, the presence of triacylglycerols in the prevalent particles, making these animals triglyceridemic as well as hypercholesterolemic, is believed to result from the normal tendency of rabbits to secrete particles rich in these lipids.) The fractional catabolic rate of injected LDL is decreased in receptorless individuals to the extent that LDL particles survive in the blood about two to three times as long as in normal persons; this is part of the information previously discussed to establish the role of LDL receptors in LDL catabolism in vivo. Contrasting with the fractional catabolic rates, the absolute rates of LDL clearance (from the vastly expanded pool of these particles in the plasma) are higher than in normals. This massive flux is carried by LDL receptor-independent pathways, mostly in the parenchymal cells of the liver. Rates of cholesterol biosynthesis in the tissues, including the liver but excluding the adrenal cortex, are more or less normal, suggesting that the cells of all tissues are able to achieve a new steady state of cholesterol supply and demand in the presence of the particular lipoprotein pattern described above. It is likely that the saturation of low-affinity sites leading to adsorptive endocytosis is the basis of this successful compensation, together with endogenous methods of regulation of the biosynthetic pathway for cholesterol, possibly based on oxidized metabolites. In vivo, of course, the onset of premature atherosclerosis renders the compensation less than "successful." It is also worth noting that intestinal production of chylomicrons is normal in these subjects, as is the synthesis of steroid hormones.

The liver appears to secrete LDL directly into the circulation in FH patients and in WHHL rabbits, at least according to data obtained from studies in vivo of apo B-100 turnover, for which this conclusion is the best current explanation. This fact, together with defective clearance of apo E- and apo B-100-containing intermediate-density products of intravascular VLDL metabolism resulting in enhanced, so-called "shunt" formation of LDL, is responsible on the synthetic side for the raised LDL concentrations observed in FH subjects in the steady state. On the catabolic side, the slow clearance of LDL by the receptorless liver cells is the other important determinant of this situation. The overall result is a state in which very high prevailing LDL levels are associated with a tremendous flux of LDL, with enhanced absolute rates of both formation and destruction. It is interesting that the administration to FH heterozygotes of a bile salt-binding resin such as cholestyramine, together with an HMGCoA reductase inhibitor derived from fungi (mevinolin), caused their plasma LDL levels to fall by 50%, reflecting an increased production of functional LDL receptors from the single "good" gene in the liver cells. Homozygotes cannot respond in this way; some measure of success has, however, been obtained by liver transplantation in at least one subject to date, which vividly illustrates the crucial role of hepatic receptors in the regulation of the plasma LDL concentration.

The insights provided by the receptor mutants at the whole-body level confirm the need to pursue the delineation of LDL receptor function (in those organs where most of the action occurs) in terms of the pathways that somehow require the involvement of these surface proteins in their control and disposition. In addition, the superimposition of more general controls, such as age and sex, needs to be understood in order to explain why the attainment of middle age in many human populations confers the dubious status of de facto heterozygous FH (Table 2), and why this also applies to dogs but not to rats.

Finally, it remains to be emphasized that homozygous familial hypercholesterolemia is in some respects the best evidence for a "lipid

Table 2 Impairment of LDL Receptor Function with Aging in Healthy Human Subjects

Group	Plasma LDL cholesterol (mg/dl)	Fractional catabolic rate for LDL*	
		Receptor-dependent	Receptor-independent
Subjects aged 20–29	105	0.173	0.174
Subjects aged 50–59	165	0.113	0.168

*Pools per day.
Source: Ref. 25.

connection" in atherosclerosis. The devastatingly early onset of arterial disease arising from a double dose of a single mutant gene cannot be explained by the operation of any other risk factors for atherosclerosis. This fact alone makes the LDL or B,E receptors important items for detailed investigation in normal persons, FH patients, and experimental animals, and underlines the need for an understanding of receptor involvement in the pathogenesis of vascular disease precipitated by less obvious causes (26).

SUMMARY

LDL receptors represent a specific class of cell surface macromolecules whose principal activity it is to facilitate the selective uptake and internalization of certain lipoproteins from the extracellular environment of a large number of cell types. It is accepted that an important function of the receptors is to catalyze the dismemberment and disposal of particles such as LDL; receptor capacity, especially in the liver, has a definite influence on the steady-state concentration of particles in the plasma. The extent to which the provision of cholesterol to nonhepatic cells occurs via LDL receptors, which has been postulated to be their second major function, is still controversial. While cultured cells generally display a preference for exogenous lipoprotein cholesterol provided in the LDL receptor pathway, significant dependence on such a source of cholesterol has not been proved for any tissue in living animals, except in the case of steroidogenic tissues such as the adrenal cortex. It is thus likely that cholesterol homeostasis at the cellular and organismal level will turn out to be more complex than might have been expected, and innovative studies of LDL receptors in relation to these problems are needed to resolve the existing contradictions.

REFERENCES

1. Schneider, W. J., Beisiegel, U., Goldstein, J. L., and Brown, M. S., *J. Biol. Chem.*, *257*:2664 (1982).

2. Yamamoto, T., Davis, C. G., Brown, M. S., Schneider, W. J., Casey, M. L., Goldstein, J. L., and Russell, D. W., *Cell, 39*: 27 (1984).

3. Südhof, T. C., Goldstein, J. L., Brown, M. S., and Russell, D. W., *Science, 228*:815 (1985).

4. Cummings, R. D., Kornfeld, S., Schneider, W. J., Hobgood, K. K., Tolleshaug, H., Brown, M. S., and Goldstein, J. L., *J. Biol. Chem.*, *258*:15,261 (1983).

5. Mahley, R. W., and Innerarity, T. L., *Biochim. Biophys. Acta, 737*:197 (1983).

6. Attie, A. D., Pittman, R. C., and Steinberg, D., *Hepatology, 2*:269 (1982).

7. Hui, D. Y., Innerarity, T. L., and Mahley, R. W., *J. Biol. Chem.*, *259*:860 (1984).

8. Kane, J. P., *Annu. Rev. Physiol.*, *45*:637 (1983).

9. Brown, M. S., Anderson, R. G. W., and Goldstein, J. L., *Cell, 32*:663 (1983).

10. Aulinskas, T. H., Oram, J. F., Bierman, E. L., Coetzee, G. A., Gevers, W., and van der Westhuyzen, D. R., *Arteriosclerosis, 5*:45 (1985).

11. van der Westhuyzen, D. R., Gevers, W., and Coetzee, G. A., *Eur. J. Biochem.*, *112*:153 (1980).

12. Goldstein, J. L., and Brown, M. S., *Annu. Rev. Biochem.*, *46*: 897 (1977).

13. Dietschy, J. M., *Klin. Wochenschrift, 62*:338 (1984).

14. Pittman, R. C., Carew, T. E., Attie, A. D., Witztum, J. L., Watanabe, Y., and Steinberg, D., *J. Biol. Chem.*, *257*:7994 (1982).

15. Pangburn, S. H., Newton, R. S., Chang, C.-M., Weinstein, D. B., and Steinberg, D., *J. Biol. Chem.*, *256*:3340 (1981).

16. Kovanen, P. T., *Clin. Endocrinol. Metab.*, *12*:243 (1983).

17. Brown, M. S., Kovanen, P. T., and Goldstein, J. L., *Science, 212*:629 (1981).

18. Steinberg, D., *Arteriosclerosis, 3*:283 (1983).

19. Packard, C. J., and Shepherd, J., in *Atherosclerosis Reviews* (Gotto, A. M., Jr., and Paoletti, R., eds.), Vol. 11, Raven Press, New York, 1983, p. 29.

20. Goldstein, J. L., and Brown, M. S., *Annu. Rev. Genet.*, *13*:253 (1979).

21. Tolleshaug, H., Goldstein, J. L., Schneider, W. J., and Brown, M. S., *Cell*, *30*:715 (1982).

22. Tolleshaug, H., Hobgood, K. K., Brown, M. S., and Goldstein, J. L., *Cell*, *32*:941 (1983).

23. Schneider, W. J., Brown, M. S., and Goldstein, J. L., *Mol. Biol. Med.*, *1*:355 (1983).

24. Goldstein, J. L., Kita, T., and Brown, M. S., *New Engl. J. Med.*, *309*:288 (1983).

25. Miller, N. E., *Lancet*, *1*:263 (1984).

26. Goldstein, J. L., and Brown, M. S., *J. Lipid Res.*, *25*:1450 (1984).

14

Lipoprotein Receptors in Steroidogenesis

JAMES R. SCHREIBER The Pritzker School of Medicine, The University of Chicago, Chicago, Illinois

DAVID B. WEINSTEIN Sandoz Corporation, East Hanover, New Jersey

INTRODUCTION

The accumulation and utilization of cholesterol by any tissue are dependent upon a dynamic balance between those mechanisms that determine the rates of de novo cholesterol synthesis, the rates of uptake and/or removal of cholesterol from cells by plasma lipoproteins, and the synthesis and hydrolysis of stored pools of cholesteryl esters. Cholesterol is a critical structural component of mammalian membranes and is used as substrate for bile acid production by the liver and for hormone production by steroidogenic tissues. The pathways by which cells within an organ maintain an equilibrium with cholesterol carried in plasma lipoproteins have been extensively reviewed (1–3).

All organs, particularly the steroidogenic organs, maintain their cholesterol balance by regulation of the rate of de novo cholesterol synthesis and by the utilization of cholesterol acquired by the receptor-mediated lipoprotein pathways. The rates of de novo cholesterol synthesis in most peripheral tissues have been underestimated until recently due to methodological errors in the estimation of the pool dilution of radiolabeled precursors. In several animal species that have whole-body sterol synthesis rates similar to those of man, it has now been shown that the adrenal gland maintains the highest cholesterol synthetic rate per gram of tissue weight. The cholesterol synthetic rate of the ovary ranks it between second and fourth place among all organs on a per gram weight basis. Thus, at maximal rates of de novo cholesterol synthesis, the cholesterol mass available to the adrenal, ovary, and liver is up to several hundred micrograms/h/gram wet weight (4). Certainly, newly synthesized cholesterol is not utilized as a single homogeneous pool, even though intracellular transport and exchange processes are very rapid. Newly synthesized cholesterol may have multiple fates with its ultimate destiny in the pathways leading to new membrane synthesis, membrane turnover, sterol ester storage pool formation, removal from the cell via exocytotic processes, or, in the liver and steroidogenic tissues, conversion to bile acids and steroid hormones, respectively. The contribution of de novo synthesized cholesterol to the total daily substrate requirement for steroid hormone production has been a difficult parameter to evaluate quantitatively.

Recent studies in several laboratories have provided some insight into the relative contributions of receptor-dependent and receptor-independent pathways for the acquisition of lipoprotein cholesterol by various tissues (5–7). The highest rates of uptake of low-density lipoprotein (LDL) are found in the liver, adrenals, gonads, intestine, and spleen. The techniques, which utilize radiolabeled, nondegradable markers as part of the surface protein or hydrophobic lipid core of low- and high-density lipoprotein (HDL), have provided information which suggests that receptor-dependent lipoprotein clearance mechanisms in some organs, especially steroidogenic tissue, may be more important than de novo cholesterol synthesis. However, since the utilization of the cholesterol-containing lipid components of lipoproteins such as HDL may not be directly related to whole particle uptake and utilization at the cellular level (7), it is currently not possible to provide *absolute* quantitative data on cholesterol provision to steroidogenic tissues.

In view of the important role that LDL and HDL may have in regulating both cholesterol content and sterol synthesis rate in the delicate homeostatic balance of the steroidogenic organs, we have attempted to review the current status of knowledge concerning lipoprotein (LDL and HDL) interaction with the adrenal, ovary, testis, and placenta in the delivery of cholesterol substrate from the plasma compartment for steroid hormone production. The role of the lipoprotein cell surface receptors and their characteristics will be of paramount importance. An extensive and elegant review of the last decade of research efforts delineating the role of lipoproteins and de novo cholesterol synthesis in the maintenance of steroidogenesis has recently been prepared by Gwynne and Strauss (8).

ADRENAL GLAND

The adrenal cortex produces glucocorticoids in response to ACTH (adrenocorticotrophic hormone) stimulation. ACTH binds to specific membrane receptors (9), stimulates adenylate cyclase activity, and

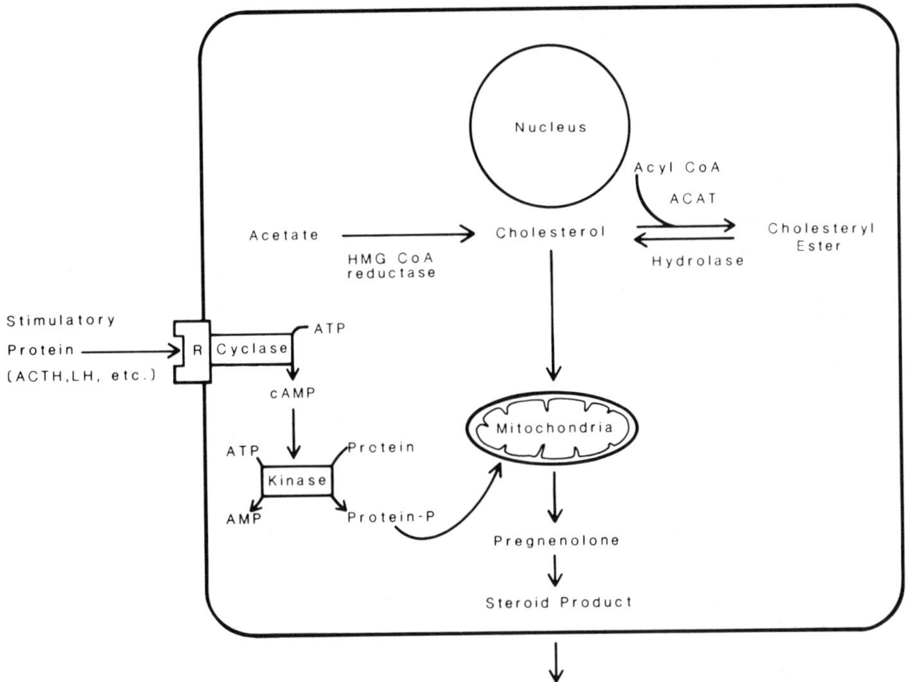

Fig. 1 Cholesterol metabolism in steroidogenic cell. R, membrane receptor; cyclase, adenylate cyclase; ATP, adenosine triphosphate; AMP, adenosine monophosphate; P, phosphate; kinase, cAMP-dependent protein kinase; hydrolase, cholesteryl ester hydrolase; ACAT, acyl CoA:cholesterol acyltransferase. (See section in text on adrenal gland for explanation.) This summary, except for the trophic hormones involved, is the same for the ovary and testis steroidogenic cells. Another source of cholesterol for the cell is LDL and/or HDL, depending on the species studied.

increases adrenal cortex intracellular cyclic adenosine monophosphate (cAMP) (10) (see Fig. 1). cAMP stimulates the activity of cAMP-dependent protein kinase, which phosphorylates proteins that mediate many, if not all, of the cellular effects of ACTH (11). ACTH stimulates cholesteryl ester hydrolase (12) and suppresses the cholesterol esterifying enzyme system including acyl-coenzyme A synthetase (13) and acyl CoA:cholesterol acyltransferase (ACAT) (14). ACTH thus increases the amount of free cholesterol available for use as substrate for glucocorticoid synthesis. ACTH acutely increases the conversion of cholesterol to pregnenolone and chronically

Table 1 Effects of Trophic Hormone (ACTH, LH, hCG, etc.) and Lipoprotein on Steroidogenic Cells

Characteristic	Trophic hormone (alone)	Lipoprotein (alone)	Both
Cholesterol ester hydrolase	↑		
Acyl CoA:cholesterol acyltransferase	↓		
Mitochondrial side-chain cleavage enzyme	↑		
Lipoprotein receptor number	↑	↓	
Lipoprotein cholesterol uptake		↑	↑↑
Cholesteryl ester content	↓	↑	
De novo cholesterol synthesis	↑	↓	
HMG-CoA reductase activity	↑	↓	
Steroidogenesis	↑	→	↑↑

↑, increase; ↑↑, large increase; ↓, decrease; →, no effect.

maintains the enzymes necessary for conversion of pregnenolone to cortisol and corticosterone (15,16) (Fig. 1 and Table 1).

LDL

Bovine Adrenal Cortex

Whole homogenates and membranes prepared from fresh bovine adrenal cortex tissue and cultured adrenocortical cells contain binding sites for bovine and human ^{125}I-LDL (17). The bovine LDL binding sites are high affinity (Kd at 4°C = 15 to 30 μg LDL protein/ml), saturable (maximum binding = 1 μg bovine LDL/mg membrane protein at 4°C and 2.5 μg bovine LDL/mg at 37°C), and specific (^{125}I-LDL is displaced >80% by bovine LDL but <10% by equal protein concentration of bovine HDL). Specific ^{125}I-bovine LDL binding requires divalent cations (e.g., Ca^{2+}, Mn^{2+}), is inhibited by EDTA (removes endogenous Ca^{2+}), and is destroyed by pronase (17). The LDL receptor was partially purified (350-fold purification) following solubilization with the nonionic detergent octyl-β-D-glucoside and chromatography on DEAE-cellulose and agarose (18). Characteristics of this solubilized acidic protein-octylglucoside complex are that it binds ^{125}I-LDL specifically and with high affinity, and has a Stokes radius of 53 Å, a sedimentation coefficient of 7.3 $S_{20,w}$, and a calculated molecular weight of 164,000 (18). The solubilized receptor was purified to homogeneity (purification factor 1050) by use of an affinity column (LDL coupled to Sepharose 4B) or an immunoaffinity column (monoclonal antibody against the LDL receptor coupled to Sepharose 4B) (19). The purified bovine adrenocortical LDL receptor appears to be a single chain, acidic (isoelectric point = 4.6) glycoprotein that binds ^{125}I-LDL with high affinity (Kd = 10 μg LDL protein/ml) and saturably (maximum binding = 1.7 mg ^{125}I-LDL/mg isolated receptor) (19).

A cDNA clone for the LDL receptor was isolated by employing a bovine adrenal cDNA library. The recombinant plasmid contains a 2.8 kilobase insert that includes a sequence corresponding to the known amino acid sequence of a 36-residue cyanogen bromide fragment of the bovine adrenal LDL receptor. The plasmid hybridizes to an mRNA of about 5.5 kilobases. Quantification of the mRNA reveals it to be ninefold more abundant in bovine adrenal than in bovine liver. Incubation of adrenocortical cells with sterols reduces LDL receptor mRNA by more than 90%, accounting for the sterol-induced down-regulation of LDL receptor number (20).

ACTH and cholera toxin minimally stimulate the production of glucocorticoids by adrenocortical cells grown in medium without LDL. Human LDL, but not human HDL, plus ACTH or cholera toxin stimulate steroid secretion four- to ninefold. LDL provides cholesterol substrate, and ACTH and cholera toxin stimulate the enzymatic conversion of cholesterol to glucocorticoid product. These adrenocortical cells bind ^{125}I-human LDL to high-affinity (Kd = 15 μg LDL protein/ml) LDL receptors. Dextran sulfate releases receptor-bound LDL. After binding, human and bovine LDL are rapidly internalized and degraded to amino acids and free cholesterol in lysosomes (a process blocked by chloroquine). Binding, internalization, and degradation of radiolabeled human LDL are blocked by excess unlabeled human LDL, but not human HDL, suggesting that the LDL receptor mediates these events (21). Added to cultured adrenal cells, bovine LDL causes a marked reduction in HMG-CoA (3-hydroxy-3-methylglutaryl coenzyme A) reductase activity (the rate-limiting enzyme in de novo cholesterol synthesis) and bovine LDL stimulates a 10-fold increase in cellular cholesteryl ester content. ACTH and cholera toxin stimulate a 2- to 3-fold increase in ^{125}I-human LDL binding, a 2- to 3-fold increase in ^{125}I-human LDL internalization, and a 2.5- to 5-fold increase in ^{125}I-human LDL degradation. Cholera toxin stimulates a 10-fold increase in the conversion of reconstituted LDL containing [^{3}H] cholesteryl linoleate to 11-[^{3}H]deoxycortisol (Table 1). In the bovine adrenal cortex, LDL, but not HDL, provides cholesterol substrate via the LDL receptor for steroidogenesis and helps regulate cellular cholesterol content by suppressing both de novo cholesterol synthesis and LDL receptor content (21). Factors that stimulate steroidogenesis, such as ACTH and cholera toxin, stimulate the acquisition of LDL cholesterol via the LDL receptor.

Rabbit Adrenal

The importance of the LDL receptor in rabbit adrenal steroidogenesis has been studied in detail with the use of the Watanabe heritable hyperlipidemic (WHHL) rabbit. The WHHL rabbits have plasma cholesterol levels of 500 to 900 mg/100 ml (of which 90% of the cholesterol is located in LDL) and an absence of detectable LDL receptors (22,23). As a consequence of the lack of LDL receptors in the WHHL rabbit, the total fractional catabolic rate (FCR) for LDL is 3.5-fold greater in the normal compared to the WHHL rabbit (24). FCR is the fraction of the total LDL plasma pool degraded per day. Using intravenous infusions of LDL, which is taken up by both LDL receptor-dependent and receptor-independent mechanisms, and methyl LDL, which is taken up by receptor-independent mechanisms only, it has been shown in the normal rabbit that 67% of total FCR of LDL is due to LDL receptor-mediated clearance and 33% is due to receptor-independent clearance. In the WHHL rabbit, the entire FCR of LDL is due to receptor-independent mechanisms (24).

Normal rabbit adrenal membranes have high-affinity (Kd = 1 μg LDL protein/ml) and saturable (maximum binding = 130 ng LDL protein/ml) binding sites for rabbit ^{125}I-LDL. Binding is inhibited by excess LDL and 2 mM EDTA (since LDL binding is calcium dependent) (25). Adrenal membranes from WHHL rabbits have no EDTA-sensitive ^{125}I-LDL binding (i.e., no detectable LDL receptors) (25). Employing rabbit [^{14}C]sucrose-LDL [the [^{14}C]sucrose remains trapped intracellularly following LDL uptake and degradation and is a cumulative measure of these processes (26)], it has been demonstrated that the FCR in normal rabbit adrenals is 10-fold that of WHHL rabbit adrenals (27). Using this method, it was estimated that 92% of LDL cholesterol enters the normal adrenal via the LDL receptor pathway, while none enters via the LDL receptor pathway in the WHHL rabbit (27). Even though the FCR of LDL in the WHHL adrenal is low, the total delivery of LDL cholesterol to the WHHL adrenal is not significantly different from that of the normal rabbit adrenal because of the greatly increased pool size of LDL in the WHHL rabbit (27). This results from the fact that cholesterol transfer is the product of FCR and pool size. In addition, de novo cholesterol synthesis is two- to five-fold greater in the WHHL adrenal compared to normal (28). Thus, the WHHL rabbit adrenal gland is able to maintain normal amounts of cholesterol for adrenal steroidogenesis, in the absence of the LDL receptor, by increasing de novo cholesterol synthesis (28) and receptor-independent uptake of LDL (27).

Mouse Adrenal

In mice given 4-aminopyrazolopyrimidine (4-APP, a purine analog that blocks hepatic lipoprotein secretion and thus lowers circulating cholesterol levels), the intravenous injection of ^{125}I-human LDL results in adrenal uptake 50 times that of intravenously administered ^{125}I-albumin. LDL uptake results in increased cellular cholesteryl ester content and decreased HMG-CoA reductase activity. Dexamethasone administration (which suppresses ACTH) results in diminished uptake of human LDL. Human ^{125}I-LDL uptake is blocked by human LDL, but not human HDL, suggesting that it is mediated by a specific LDL receptor (29). ^{125}I-LDL, but not ^{125}I-HDL, uptake is blocked by the prior injection of a rabbit antibody directed against purified bovine adrenal LDL receptor, indicating that bovine and mouse LDL receptors contain common antigenic determinants, and that LDL and HDL are taken up by separate mechanisms (30). Membranes from mice adrenals possess high-affinity (Kd = 8 to 10 μg LDL protein/ml) receptors. Binding is blocked by LDL, but not HDL, and is inhibited by EDTA, but restored by Ca^{2+}. ACTH increases maximum binding 2.1-fold, but has no effect on binding affinity for LDL. 4-APP increases LDL receptors fourfold, an action blocked by dexamethasone (31).

Mouse Y-1 adrenal tumor cells have been examined in detail. These cells contain high-affinity (Kd = 25 μg LDL protein/ml) LDL receptors. ^{125}I-LDL binding is blocked by human and mouse LDL, but not by human or mouse HDL, and is heparin-releasable (32). LDL is bound by receptor, internalized, and hydrolyzed by lysosomes to amino acids and cholesterol. Human LDL and mouse LDL increase cellular cholesterol and cholesteryl ester, and suppress HMG-CoA reductase activity and LDL receptor number (32). ACTH increases LDL receptor binding site number, LDL internalization, LDL degradation, cholesterol transport to mitochondria, and cholesterol conversion to 20-hydroxy-pregn-4-en-3-one (33). HDL, both human and mouse, has no effect on any of these parameters. Balance studies indicate that the LDL receptor pathway provides 75% of the cholesterol required for Y-1 adrenal tumor cell steroidogenesis (32).

Rat Adrenal

Rat adrenal membranes contain high-affinity (Kd = 35 μg human LDL protein/ml) and specific receptors for LDL. Binding of ^{125}I-human LDL is Ca^{2+} dependent, destroyed by pronase, and blocked by human LDL, but not by human HDL or methyl human LDL (31).

ACTH increases by two- to five-fold the number of ^{125}I-human LDL binding sites at the same time it is depleting cellular cholesteryl ester (but not free cholesterol) (31).

To test the importance of the LDL receptor, Carew et al. (26) infused ^{14}C-labeled sucrose human LDL (which measures total human LDL protein coat uptake) and ^{14}C-labeled sucrose methylated human LDL (which measures human LDL protein coat uptake via nonreceptor-mediated pathways). Following cellular uptake and degradation of the LDL particle, [^{14}C]sucrose remains trapped intracellularly as a cumulative measure of degradation. By this method, 70% of rat adrenal uptake of LDL occurs via the LDL receptor (26). Infusion of LDL results in LDL uptake followed by: (1) decreased LDL receptor number, (2) decreased LDL uptake via the LDL receptor, and (3) unchanged LDL uptake via the LDL receptor-independent pathway (26). Stein et al. (34) measured cumulative LDL cholesteryl ester uptake by various tissues by utilizing an infusion of reconstituted human LDL containing a core of cholesteryl linoleyl ether, a non-metabolizable analog of cholesteryl linoleate ester. Highest uptake of any organ on a weight basis is in the adrenal, suggesting LDL receptor-mediated uptake of the cholesteryl ester core (34).

In rats whose circulating cholesterol has been lowered by 90% with 4-APP, the adrenal gland cholesteryl ester content declines 90%, de novo cholesterol synthesis increases 30-fold, and HMG-CoA reductase activity increases 150- to 200-fold (35). The infusion of human LDL induces in these adrenals: (1) decreased de novo cholesterol synthesis, (2) decreased HMG-CoA reductase activity, and (3) increased cellular cholesterol and cholesteryl ester content (35–37) (Table 1). When ACTH secretion is blocked by the administration of dexamethasone, these effects of LDL are blocked (35). The effects of LDL are concentration dependent and saturable (Km = 61 mg LDL cholesterol/dl), which suggest receptor-mediated uptake of LDL cholesterol (37). Human LDL and rat LDL are equally effective (37). Added human LDL restores ACTH responsiveness of the cell suspensions of adrenals from hypocholesterolemic rats, presumably by providing cholesterol (38).

The issue of specificity (HDL versus LDL and rat lipoprotein versus human lipoprotein) of the lipoprotein effect on rat adrenal steroidogenesis is complex and the role of lipoprotein receptors in this interaction is far from clear. For example, at equal concentrations of infused circulating cholesterol (~10 mg/dl), human and rat LDL are 10- to 20-fold *less* effective than human and rat HDL in transferring *cholesterol* into the rat adrenal cell (37). However, when adrenal uptake in vivo of ^{125}I-lipoproteins is studied, rat HDL, human HDL, and rat LDL are equally effective and are 10-fold more effective than human LDL (39). Results seem to depend on experimental conditions and the cellular parameters chosen for study, e.g., cholesterol transport versus ^{125}I-lipoprotein uptake. What must be remembered in all this, however, is the question of the physiological significance of the LDL receptor in the rat adrenal. The great majority of cholesterol is carried in the HDL fraction in the rat, and kinetic studies indicate that HDL cholesterol must be the major substrate for synthesis of rat adrenal hormones (37).

Lipoprotein species differences could have important implications in the interpretation of the study of LDL-receptor interactions. For example, in normal rabbits, the FCR of human LDL is only 64% of the FCR for rabbit LDL, but the FCR of human and rabbit methyl LDL are the same. Therefore, use of human LDL in the rabbit would give lower values for both total and receptor-dependent FCR than would rabbit LDL (24). In addition, there are data suggesting that rat and human LDL receptors differ. A monoclonal antibody against bovine adrenal cortex LDL receptor also binds the human LDL receptor but not the rat adrenal LDL receptor (40). The lesson in all this is, of course, that one must be careful in interpreting data when the sources of tissue and lipoproteins are from different species.

Human Adrenal

Lipoprotein utilization and cholesterol synthesis by the human fetal adrenal gland have been studied extensively (41). Plasma membrane fractions of human fetal adrenal glands contain binding sites for ^{125}I-human LDL which demonstrate high affinity (Kd = 20.8 μg LDL protein/ml), saturable kinetics (1370 ng LDL protein/mg membrane protein), and specificity (competed by human LDL but not human HDL) (42). Heparin pretreatment of membranes increases specific binding of ^{125}I-human LDL, implying heparin displaces endogenous LDL from the LDL receptor. ACTH induces a twofold increase in adrenal membrane LDL receptor number (42).

After culture of human fetal adrenal tissue for 3 days in lipoprotein-poor serum plus ACTH, the uptake of added ^{125}I-human LDL is rapid, and after 1 hour there is degradation to amino acids ([^{125}I] monoiodotyrosine) by lysosomes (43). The similar kinetics of uptake and degradation in relation to ^{125}I-human LDL concentration suggest that these processes are mediated by a common saturable binding site. Heparin, which displaces LDL from its receptor, blocks binding, uptake, and degradation of ^{125}I-human LDL by fetal adrenal tissue. ACTH increases degradation fivefold, an increase that is inhibited only 50% by prior incubation with 500 μg LDL protein/ml. Thus, ACTH markedly increases LDL cholesterol uptake via the LDL receptor, while LDL is relatively ineffective in down-regulating these receptors (43).

In culture, human fetal adrenal tissue secretes dehydroepiandrosterone sulfate (DS) and cortisol (44,45). ACTH stimulates DS and cortisol production two- to threefold more in the presence of lipoprotein than in its absence, which implies that the ability of the adrenal to respond to ACTH is limited if the cell must rely on only de novo cholesterol synthesis (44). ACTH markedly stimulates the activity of HMG-CoA reductase and the conversion of acetate to cholesterol, an effect that is only minimally inhibited by LDL (46). Human HDL and human VLDL have little effect on steroidogenesis (45). These data indicate that ACTH stimulates both de novo cholesterol synthesis and utilization of LDL cholesterol, thus ensuring an adequate supply of cholesterol for steroidogenesis.

In the fetus, the most steroidogenically active portion of the adrenal is the fetal zone, the source of DS. Steroid hormone secretion is an active process in the fetal adrenal in vivo, with its secretory rate greater than that of the basal secretory rate of adult adrenals (41). Although about 43% of the cholesterol in the human fetus is derived from maternal cholesterol pools (47), it is not clear to what degree the fetal intestine and liver are capable of providing de novo synthesis of lipoprotein cholesterol. It has been postulated that fetal levels of LDL are lower than those in adult plasma as a direct consequence of the high rate of LDL-driven human fetal adrenal steroidogenesis. The fact that the fetal zone of the adrenal is a major user of LDL cholesterol in fetal life is also demonstrated by the study of anencephalic fetuses with adrenal atrophy (due to decreased ACTH). These fetuses have markedly decreased circulating DS in association with a fourfold increase in LDL. Presumably, this hypercholesterolemia is due to the decreased fetal adrenal utilization of fetal LDL (48,49).

Adrenal steroidogenesis has been studied in patients whose circulating LDL levels are low (hypobetalipoproteinemia) or very low to absent [abetalipoproteinemia (ABL)]. Patients with ABL have normal basal rates of production of adrenal corticosteroids (i.e., normal rates of excretion of urinary 17-hydroxycorticosteroids, 17-ketosteroids, and free cortisol) (50). However, the patients have an abnormal response to prolonged (24 to 36 hours) ACTH stimulation. Serum cortisol, urinary 17-hydroxycorticosteroids, and 17-ketosteroids in ABL patients given ACTH are one-half normal control values and urinary-free cortisol is one-fourth normal control values (50,51). These data indicate that LDL cholesterol is an important source of cholesterol for steroidogenesis during long-term ACTH stimulation, but in the basal state the adrenal can produce sufficient cholesterol de novo for glucocorticoid production. Mononuclear blood cells isolated from ABL patients have a 5- to 10-fold increase in the rate of synthesis of cholesterol from acetate; it is probable that increased cholesterol synthesis is occurring in the adrenal in an attempt to make up for the lack of LDL cholesterol (52). These mononuclear cells from ABL patients are normal, however, in that LDL added in vitro inhibits this elevated de novo cholesterol synthesis by 85% (52). Patients with heterozygous ABL (LDL cholesterol decreased by 60 to 80%) have normal adrenal steroidogenesis in both the basal and ACTH-stimulated state (51). A possible source of adrenal cholesterol in ABL patients could be HDL_2, a lipoprotein fraction from ABL patients which is relatively rich in apo E and is able to block binding, internalization, and degradation of ^{125}I-LDL by normal fibroblasts (53).

Patients with decreased or absent LDL receptors [familial hypercholesterolemia (FH)] have been similarly studied. In patients with receptor-negative homozygous FH (fibroblasts with no detectable LDL receptors), basal adrenocortical function is normal (54). Acute response to ACTH is normal but on chronic stimulation by ACTH, adrenal steroidogenesis is deficient (urinary free cortisol is 33 to 36% of normal) (54). The normal response to the acute stimulation by ACTH is not unexpected since studies of fetal adrenal cells in culture indicate that de novo synthesized cholesterol is the steroidogenic precursor for this acute response (55). Heterozygous FH patients (LDL receptors diminished by one-half) have normal basal and ACTH-stimulated adrenal steroidogenesis (56). These studies indicate that for maximal response to ACTH, the human adrenal needs both circulating LDL and LDL receptors.

HDL

Mouse Adrenal

Mice treated with 4-APP (to lower circulating lipoprotein levels) demonstrate adrenal uptake of intravenously injected ^{125}I-human HDL. Following intravenous ^{125}I-human HDL, the adrenal accumulates 20-fold more ^{125}I-HDL radioactivity than lung or kidney, and 50- to 200 fold more ^{125}I-human HDL than ^{125}I-albumin (29). The concomitant administration of dexamethasone (which prevents the increase in ACTH, which is stimulated indirectly by 4-APP) inhibits the 4-APP-induced increase in adrenal ^{125}I-human HDL uptake by 80%. ^{125}I-human HDL uptake is saturable, specific (inhibited by human HDL but not human LDL), and associated with increased concentrations of cellular cholesteryl esters and diminished HMG-CoA reductase activity (29). An antibody against the LDL receptor blocks ^{125}I-LDL uptake but has no effect on mouse adrenal ^{125}I-HDL uptake, indicating that HDL uptake is mediated by a mechanism different than the LDL receptor (30). Y-1 mouse adrenal tumor cells do not have mechanisms for HDL uptake.

Rat Adrenal

ACTH stimulates glucocorticoid production by increasing: (1) cholesteryl esterase activity, (2) mitochondrial side chain cleavage activity, and (3) uptake of LDL and HDL cholesterol (57–60)

(Table 1). The importance of lipoproteins for rat adrenal cell steroidogenesis has been studied in detail. The in vivo administration of 4-APP results in: (1) decreased circulating lipoproteins (35,36); (2) 25-fold decrease in adrenal cholesteryl ester content; (3) 42- to 51-fold increase in adrenal sterol synthesis (36,61); (4) 30-fold increase in cholesterol synthesis from acetate (35); (5) 150- to 200-fold increase in HMG-CoA reductase activity (35); (6) decreased plasma corticosterone; and (7) diminished response to ACTH (62). The effects of 4-APP on the adrenal are blocked by the concomitant administration of dexamethasone, implying that ACTH mediates these steroidogenic changes in the adrenal (35). The infusion of rat or human HDL in 4-APP-treated animals causes: (1) 12-fold increase in adrenal cholesteryl ester content; (2) 10-fold decrease in de novo cholesterol synthesis from acetate; (3) decreased HMG-CoA reductase activity; and (4) 12-fold increase in glucocorticoid synthesis (35,36,61) (Table 1). Effects similar to 4-APP are observed when circulating lipoprotein levels are lowered by pharmacological doses of estradiol (38). The changes include a 7-fold decrease in adrenal cholesteryl ester, a 50% decrease in circulating corticosterone, and no response to ACTH. Response to ACTH is restored by a concomitant infusion of HDL (38). These results indicate that human HDL and rat HDL can provide the adrenal with cholesterol in vivo. The kinetics of HDL cholesterol transfer into the adrenal of 4-APP-treated rats are that (1) infused human HDL provides 0.45 mg cholesterol/pair adrenals/hr with a Km of 12 mg human HDL cholesterol/dl, and (2) infused rat HDL provides 0.32 mg cholesterol/pair adrenals/hr with a Km of 7.2 mg rat HDL cholesterol/dl (37). These results suggest a saturable, high-affinity process that mediates HDL cholesterol uptake by the rat adrenal.

In rats injected with rat or human ^{125}I-HDL, the adrenal binds the HDL to a greater extent than any other tissue tested. The specific uptake by the adrenal is 7 times that for liver and 70 times that for spleen (39). The adrenal binding of ^{125}I-rat HDL and ^{125}I-human HDL is approximately equal in vivo (39). Rat adrenocortical cells in culture bind ^{125}I-human HDL_3 (apo E-free) in a saturable and reversible manner (maximum binding = 180 ng human HDL_3 protein/mg cell protein), and with apparent specificity (blocked by human HDL, but less well by human LDL) (63,64). Cell surface binding of ^{125}I-human HDL_3 has been defined as trypsin-releasable radioactivity (63); however, this may be the sum of both specific and nonspecific binding. Heparin, which releases ^{125}I-LDL specifically from its binding site, has no effect on ^{125}I-HDL binding (63). Rat adrenocortical membrane preparations bind ^{125}I-human HDL saturably (binding blocked by 100-fold excess HDL) (65). These membranes also bind rat ^{125}I-HDL with saturable kinetics (maximum binding = 2000 ng rat HDL protein/mg membrane protein) and with high affinity (Kd = 30 μg rat HDL protein/ml) (66). Binding of HDL is followed by internalization (i.e., ^{125}I-human HDL not released by trypsin) and degradation to TCA-soluble radioactivity (monoiodotyrosine) (63,64). Uptake and degradation of ^{125}I-human HDL are blocked by human HDL but less well by human LDL (63,64).

Human HDL containing [^{3}H]cholesterol and rat HDL containing ^{125}I-cholesteryl oleate both transfer cholesterol into the adrenal cells (67,68). Transfer is increased in ACTH-stimulated and hypolipidemic rats, implying that adrenal cholesterol depletion leads to increased HDL cholesterol uptake (67–69). Chronic ACTH simulation of adrenocortical cells in lipoprotein-deficient medium leads to depletion of cellular total cholesterol content, and to a subsequent decrease in steroidogenesis (69). Incubation of rat HDL and human HDL with ACTH-stimulated adrenocortical cells in vitro leads to a concentration-dependent, saturable increase in cellular cholesterol content (Km = 210 μg HDL protein/ml) and glucocorticoid synthesis (Km = 230 μg HDL protein/ml) (69) (Table 1). The similarity of Km values for HDL cholesterol uptake and steroidogenesis suggests that they are linked.

While rat adrenocorticoid cells bind HDL and utilize HDL cholesterol as substrate for steroidogenesis, the mechanism of HDL cholesterol uptake is poorly understood. These cells internalize and degrade HDL but a major discrepancy exists. The ratio of corticosterone production to human HDL protein coat degradation is 10- to 60-fold in excess of the ratio of cholesterol to protein in the human HDL particles used (69). In other words, the amount of cholesterol theoretically made available in association with degradation of the protein coat of HDL (i.e., degradation of the entire HDL particle) can account for only a small portion of the HDL cholesterol supplied to the cell for increased steroidogenesis. Glass et al. (7) addressed this issue by tracing the metabolic fate of rat apo A-I labeled with a nondegradable ^{125}I-tyramine cellobiose tag, while at the same time measuring nondegradable [^{3}H]cholesteryl linoleyl ether uptake from the lipid core of these double-labeled reconstituted rat HDL particles. Since neither of the labels is rapidly exchanged in rat plasma, and both labels are trapped intracellularly in tissues that degrade HDL particles, it is possible to simultaneously evaluate the delivery of HDL surface coat and lipid core into the cell. These experiments show a sevenfold preferential accumulation of the cholesteryl linoleyl ether compared to apo A-I in the rat adrenal. These data validate the original hypothesis of Gwynne and Hess (69) that cholesterol uptake from HDL could be dissociated from whole-particle degradation. The mechanisms that regulate the selective uptake of HDL lipid core await further study of the lipoprotein-receptor interaction. Possible explanations include uptake of cholesteryl esters into the adrenal followed by the selective loss of apoproteins at the cell surface, or by uptake of entire HDL particles with subsequent release of apo A-I from the cells.

These data indicate that the nature and importance of HDL binding to rat adrenal cell membranes are unclear. It is clear that HDL is not binding to the LDL receptor but the components of HDL important for binding to the HDL receptor are unknown. Specific HDL apoproteins, particularly apo A-I (the major HDL apoprotein), have been postulated as important for binding. Gwynne et al. (67) present evidence that added pure apo A-I can enhance adrenal accumulation in vitro of ^{14}C-cholesterol from human HDL. However, added purified apo A-II (a minor component of human HDL) has an even greater enhancing effect, making the characteristics of binding very confusing indeed (67). This is discussed in more detail in the section in this chapter on HDL utilization by the rat ovary.

Human Adrenal

Membrane fractions of fresh fetal adrenocortical tissue contain binding sites for ^{125}I-human HDL that are saturable (316 ng HDL protein/mg membrane protein) and of high affinity (Kd = 108 μg HDL protein/ml) (70). Human HDL competes for ^{125}I-human HDL binding, and human LDL is much less effective. Unlike human LDL binding to this same tissue, the human HDL binding sites are resistant to proteolytic enzymes and specifically bound ^{125}I-human HDL is not released by glucosaminoglycans (70). Calcium ions are required for ^{125}I-human HDL binding. ACTH, which increases human LDL binding site number twofold, has no effect on ^{125}I-human HDL binding. These results suggest that these human HDL binding sites are less important in the acquisition of cholesterol for steroidogenesis than LDL receptors (70) and the HDL binding sites may be present as constitutive, nonregulated receptors to assure maintenance of a basal level of cholesterol flux.

Adrenal Summary

Adrenal membranes and cultured cells contain receptors for LDL that are high affinity, specific for LDL, and saturable. Binding requires Ca^{2+} and proteolytic enzymes destroy the receptor. The bovine adrenal LDL receptor is an acidic glycoprotein with a molecular weight of ∿160,000. Factors that stimulate steroidogenesis, such as ACTH, increase LDL receptor number. Sterols added to cultured adrenal cells down-regulate LDL receptor number by reducing LDL receptor mRNA. After binding, the LDL is internalized and degraded to amino acids and free cholesterol. The cholesterol is stored as cholesteryl ester or converted to glucocorticoids. Added LDL synergizes with ACTH to stimulate glucocorticoid synthesis and blocks de novo cholesterol synthesis by inhibiting HMG-CoA reductase

Table 2 Summary of Characteristics of LDL and HDL Binding Sites

Characteristic	LDL	HDL
Binding affinity (μg protein/ml)	8–35	5–90
Saturable	Yes	Yes
Specific	Yes	Yes
Divalent cations required	Yes	No
Destroyed by proteolytic enzymes	Yes	No
Receptor Stokes radius	53A	?
Receptor sedimentation coefficient	7.3 $S_{20,W}$	?
Receptor isoelectric point	4.6	?
Receptor molecular weight	160,000	?
Heparin displaces ligand from binding site	Yes	No
Lipoprotein degraded by lysosome following internalization	Yes	No
Apoprotein specificity for binding and cholesterol uptake	B/E	A-I, A-II, C's, possibly others

activity. In the absence of the LDL receptor [WHHL rabbit and familial hypercholesterolemic (FH) human], the total amount of cholesterol available to the adrenal is near normal because of increased de novo cholesterol synthesis and increased receptor-independent uptake of LDL due to a greatly increased pool size of LDL. In the human, absence of LDL (abetalipoproteinemia) or the LDL receptor (FH) results in normal basal glucocorticoid synthetic rates but diminished maximum rates of steroidogenesis.

Mouse and rat adrenocortical cells and membranes contain receptors for HDL that are high affinity, specific for HDL, and saturable. Ca^{2+} and heparin have no effect on HDL binding. As opposed to LDL, uptake of HDL cholesterol occurs in excess of HDL particle uptake and apoprotein degradation. HDL provides cholesterol for storage as cholesteryl ester, and for substrate in the synthesis of glucocorticoids. ACTH stimulation increases the uptake of HDL cholesterol. The mechanism of HDL-cholesterol uptake is poorly understood but is clearly different from the mechanism described for LDL. This will be discussed in the summary of the ovary portion of this chapter, and a hypothesis describing the interaction of HDL with steroidogenic cells will be presented in the conclusion. Human adrenal membranes also have HDL binding sites that are high affinity and specific, but ACTH has no effect on binding site number. This suggests that human adrenal HDL receptors have little to do with the acquisition of cholesterol for steroidogenesis. A summary of the characteristics of LDL and HDL binding sites is presented in Table 2.

OVARY

The ovary has two major products: eggs and sex steroids (primarily progestins and estrogen). The control of events that occur throughout the ovarian cycle is a complicated process requiring changes in both pituitary gonadotropin secretion and ovarian steroid hormone synthesis and secretion. The gonadotropins luteinizing hormone (LH) and follicle-stimulating hormone (FSH) are released from the pituitary in a pulsatile manner every 1 to 2 hours under the control of the hypothalamic secretion of gonadotropin-releasing hormone (GnRH). FSH and LH act on the ovary to initiate and maintain the pathways that lead to follicle growth, ovulation, corpus luteum formation, and steroidogenesis. The follicle is composed of granulosa cells and an oocyte within a basal lamina, which is surrounded by layers of theca cells. Theca cells contain receptors that bind LH and human chorionic gonadotropin (hCG), and LH or hCG primarily stimulates thecal androgen production. Granulosa cells possess FSH receptors, and FSH stimulates the aromatization of these androgens to estrogens (71). During follicular development, granulosa cells acquire LH (hCG) receptors and produce primarily progestins in response to LH (hCG). The effect of LH (hCG) and FSH on progestin and androgen synthesis is quite similar to the effect of ACTH on adrenal glucocorticoid synthesis, namely, they bind to specific membrane receptors, stimulate cAMP production, activate cAMP-dependent protein kinase, increase hydrolysis of cellular cholesteryl ester, increase transport of cholesterol to mitochondria, and increase mitochondrial side-chain cleavage activity (71,72) (Fig. 1). The granulosa cells of the preovulatory follicle have no direct access to circulating plasma lipoproteins since there is no vascularization of the follicle at this stage of development, and the basal lamina provides a tight barrier that has selective permeability or filtration characteristics. In 1957, Caravaglios and Cilotti (73) determined the composition of bovine follicular fluid by electrophoretic analysis and demonstrated that β-lipoprotein (LDL) is not detectable although α-lipoprotein (HDL) is present at almost plasma levels. These results on follicular fluid levels of HDL and LDL have been confirmed in the human ovary (74). Following ovulation, the ruptured follicle is extensively vascularized in the process of corpus luteum development, thus establishing a continuous supply of plasma levels of lipoprotein cholesterol for progestin production (Fig. 2). These aspects of ovarian regulation have been reviewed extensively (75,76). On a comparative basis of organ size, the corpus luteum is the most active steroidogenic tissue, with rates of progestin secretion in the range of 25 mg/day in the human ovary (77).

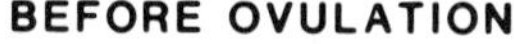

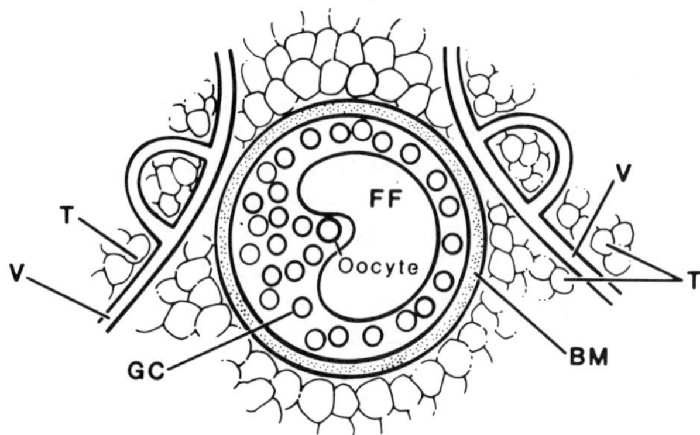

AFTER OVULATION

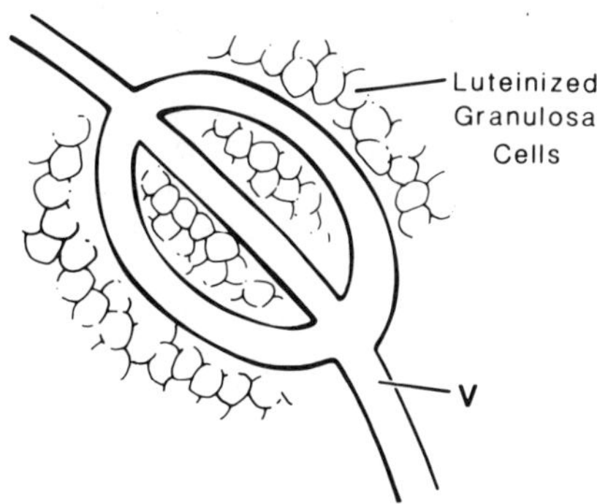

Fig. 2 Vascular supply of the follicle (before ovulation) and corpus luteum (after ovulation) in the ovary. V, blood vessel; T, theca cells; BM, basement membrane; GC, granulosa cell; FF, follicular fluid.

LDL

Bovine Ovary

Membrane preparations of bovine corpora lutea bind ^{125}I-bovine LDL saturably (200 ng bovine LDL/mg membrane protein, a value two-thirds that of adrenal cortex membranes and 4 times that of the ovary interstitial compartment) (17). Cultured bovine granulosa cells bind ^{125}I-human LDL saturably (0.45 μg LDL protein/10^6 cells) and with high affinity (Kd = 0.8×10^{-9} M) (78). Bound ^{125}I-LDL is released from the receptor by dextran sulfate. Binding is followed by internalization and degradation. Chloroquine blocks both degradation and progesterone synthesis, indicating that lysosomal degradation of the LDL particles is required for the cellular utilization of LDL cholesterol for steroidogenesis (78). Dibutyryl-cAMP (Bt_2-cAMP) increases ^{125}I-LDL binding, internalization, degradation, and progesterone synthesis. Human LDL, but not human HDL, inhibits ^{125}I-LDL binding, internalization, and degradation, suggesting that all these processes are linked to a specific LDL receptor (78).

Bovine LDL, human LDL, and to a lesser extent bovine HDL can stimulate progesterone synthesis by cultured bovine granulosa cells (79,80). Bt_2-cAMP induces a two- to threefold increase in HMG-CoA reductase activity, which is suppressed by human LDL and bovine LDL, and to a lesser extent by bovine HDL. Compactin, a competitive inhibitor of HMG-CoA reductase, has little effect on granulosa cell progesterone synthesis in cells exposed to lipoproteins. This indicates that when lipoproteins are available, bovine ovary steroidogenic cells use lipoprotein cholesterol rather than de novo synthesized cholesterol for progesterone synthesis. Bovine follicular fluid, which has concentrations of LDL and HDL that are 24 and 59%, respectively, of those for plasma, supports granulosa cell steroidogenesis 45% as well as bovine plasma. This could be important because, prior to ovulation, the granulosa cells are exposed to only follicular fluid. However, after ovulation, the follicle becomes the highly vascular corpus luteum, and the cells become exposed to plasma levels of lipoproteins at the time of increasing progesterone synthesis (79) (Fig. 2).

Rabbit Ovary

The rabbit corpus luteum has high levels of HMG-CoA reductase activity, the rate-limiting enzyme in de novo cholesterol synthesis, and the activity increases fivefold in the pregnant compared to the nonpregnant animal (81). Feeding the animal enough cholesterol to raise plasma cholesterol levels 30-fold does not inhibit the increase in HMG-CoA reductase activity in pregnancy. These data suggest that exogenous cholesterol, and thus the lipoprotein receptors, may not be important in supplying cholesterol substrate for steroidogenesis (81). In support of this, the rates of synthesis of digitoninprecipitable steroids in vivo and in vitro by ovaries are the same in normal and WHHL (LDL receptor negative) rabbits, suggesting that receptor-mediated LDL cholesterol is not of major importance in rabbit ovary steroidogenesis. By contrast, de novo sterol synthesis in vivo is five times greater in the WHHL rabbit adrenal compared to the normal rabbit adrenal (28).

Hamster Ovary

Using a constant infusion technique, rates of uptake of ^{14}C-labeled sucrose hamster LDL (total LDL uptake) and ^{14}C-labeled sucrose methylated hamster LDL (receptor-independent LDL uptake) were measured in various organs and tissues. [^{14}C]Sucrose is trapped in cells and thus measures total cell uptake of the various lipoproteins. LDL clearance by the ovary is 43 μl/hr/g as compared to the values for adrenal (29 μl/hr/g) and muscle (0.26 μl/hr/g). The rate of uptake of methylated LDL accounts for only 9.3% of total LDL uptake (82). These data suggest that the hamster ovary has a very active LDL receptor-mediated uptake of LDL cholesterol for steroidogenesis. However, hamster lipoproteins (density <1.21 g/ml) do not enhance LH-stimulated progesterone production by either granulosa or luteal cells during short-term (2 to 3 hr) incubations (83). Compactin, an inhibitor of cholesterol synthesis, also has no effect during short-term incubations. These data imply that substrate for acute progesterone synthesis comes from preformed cholesterol (83). The infusion study previously cited would support the idea that these cells would respond to LDL, via the LDL receptor, during longer-term stimulation of steroidogenesis.

Rat Ovary

Rat corpora lutea membrane preparations bind ^{125}I-human LDL specifically (human LDL inhibits binding to a much greater extent than human HDL), saturably, and with high affinity (two sites: Kd = 7.7 and 213 μg LDL protein/ml) (84). Binding is dependent on time (saturates in 2 hr) and temperature (greatest at 37°C). ^{125}I-human LDL binding is destroyed by pronase and trypsin, blocked by EDTA and increasing ionic strength of the incubation buffer, and increased by Ca^{2+}. hCG, which stimulates progesterone secretion, induces a fourfold increase in the number of high-affinity membrane LDL receptors, but has no effect on binding affinity (84). Cultured rat luteal cells bind ^{125}I-human LDL with high affinity (Kd = 37 μg LDL protein/ml). ^{125}I-human LDL binding is inhibited by human LDL, but human HDL (at the same concentration in μg protein/ml) is almost as effective (85). Cultured rat granulosa cells bind ^{125}I-human LDL in a saturable fashion. FSH, which stimulates progestin production, induces a twofold increase in the number of ^{125}I-human LDL binding sites (86). Following binding, ^{125}I-human LDL is internalized. To quantitate the importance of the LDL receptor, ^{14}C-labeled sucrose

LDL (measures total uptake of LDL) and ^{14}C-labeled sucrose methylated LDL (measures receptor-independent uptake of LDL) were infused into rats. Using this method, it was shown that 65% of human LDL uptake by the rat ovary is LDL receptor mediated. Prior infusion of human LDL decreases receptor-mediated uptake (implying that it is saturable) but has no effect on receptor-independent uptake (26). However, in rats given 4-APP to lower circulating cholesterol and pregnant mare serum gonadotropin (PMSG) and human chorionic gonadotropin (hCG) to stimulate steroidogenesis, there is no increase in the in vivo uptake of ^{125}I-human LDL. In contrast, this treatment increases ^{125}I-human HDL uptake by 6- to 10-fold (87). This last observation suggests that LDL uptake by rat ovary cells may not be physiologically important.

^{125}I-human LDL is degraded to monoiodotyrosine by cultured granulosa and luteal cells in a concentration-dependent and saturable manner (Km = 8 to 22 μg human LDL protein/ml) (85,88). Degradation is blocked by pronase, chloroquine, and ammonium chloride, suggesting that lysosomal enzymes degrade the LDL following LDL receptor-mediated uptake (85,88). As was previously observed with ^{125}I-human LDL membrane binding (85), unlabeled human LDL effectively inhibits ^{125}I-human LDL degradation, but human HDL, at high concentrations (⩾100 μg HDL protein/ml), also partially blocks degradation (88). FSH stimulates a 3.5-fold increase in ^{125}I-human LDL degradation by cultured ovary granulosa cells; androgen has no effect; and FSH plus androgen synergistically stimulates both a 6-fold increase in ^{125}I-human LDL degradation and steroid hormone production (89). Therefore, granulosa cell synthesis of progestin from LDL is correlated with LDL binding and degradation.

Pregnant mare serum gonadotropin (PMSG) and human chorionic gonadotropin (hCG) treatment of rats stimulates ovary steroidogenesis. The in vivo administration of 4-APP, which lowers circulating lipoproteins, to PMSG-hCG-treated rats causes a 4- to 10-fold decrease in ovary cholesteryl ester content, but only a slight, if any, decrease in free cholesterol (90,91). In the absence of exogenous cholesterol, the cell utilizes its stored cholesteryl ester for steroidogenesis. In cultured luteinized granulosa cells, added LDL results in increased [^{14}C]oleate incorporation into cholesteryl ester (92). LDL cholesteryl ester is, therefore, internalized, hydrolyzed to cholesterol, and reesterified with oleate.

Administration of 4-APP to PMSG-hCG-treated rats stimulates a 16-fold increase in HMG-CoA reductase activity, indicating that the ovary will synthesize cholesterol in the absence of lipoprotein cholesterol (90). Luteinized granulosa cells grown in medium containing lipoprotein-deficient serum demonstrate increased HMG-CoA reductase activity and increased conversion of acetate to sterols and progestins, all of which are inhibited by the addition of human LDL (90).

Luteinized granulosa cells have decreased progestin production when cultured in medium containing lipoprotein-deficient serum compared to medium with normal serum. Progestin production is restored by addition of human LDL with the maximum effect at a concentration of 150 μg human LDL protein/ml (92). The addition of human LDL, in a concentration-dependent manner, augments the FSH-stimulated production of progesterone and 20α-dihydroprogesterone by granulosa cells cultured in serum-free medium (93). Antibodies to human LDL, but not human HDL, will block LDL-stimulated steroidogenesis, indicating that specific LDL particle surface properties are necessary for the LDL cholesterol transfer into the cell for steroidogenesis (92). Rat luteal cells incubated with reconstituted human LDL particles containing a [^{3}H]cholesteryl linoleate lipid core produce [^{3}H]progesterone, a utilization of LDL cholesteryl ester for steroidogenesis, which is increased by hCG treatment (85,91). Excess unlabeled human LDL blocks human LDL-[^{3}H]cholesteryl linoleate utilization, suggesting that it is a saturable process (85). In addition, excess human HDL and rat HDL also block the conversion of human LDL-[^{3}H]cholesteryl linoleate to [^{3}H]progestin, suggesting that cholesterol from all lipoprotein sources goes to a common cholesterol pool in the cell (94).

The physiological importance of the LDL pathway is not known. In 4-APP-treated rats, the in vivo infusion of human LDL has no effect on ovary sterol synthesis and only one-eighth the effect of infused HDL on steroidogenesis (61,95). It is not known whether rat LDL would behave differently. Since the vast majority of circulating cholesterol is carried by HDL in the rat (96), LDL may have little role in rat ovary steroidogenesis in vivo.

Human Ovary

Membrane preparations from fresh corpora lutea contain binding sites for ^{125}I-human LDL which are high affinity (Kd = 5 to 25 μg LDL protein/ml), specific (human LDL displaces ^{125}I-human LDL more effectively than does human HDL), and saturable (maximum binding = 20 to 500 ng LDL protein/mg membrane protein). The number of LDL receptors (i.e., maximum binding) in membrane fractions obtained from ovaries in mid-luteal phase (the time of maximum progesterone synthesis) is 5- to 12-fold greater than that from tissue obtained at any other phase of the cycle (97). This suggests that LDL receptor number and rate of steroidogenesis are positively correlated. Heparin and pronase prevent ^{125}I-human LDL specific binding (97).

Cultured luteinized granulosa cells internalize ^{125}I-human LDL saturably (Km = 5 to 10 μg human LDL protein/ml) and specifically (blocked by human LDL but not human HDL) (98). Cultured corpus luteum tissue fragments degrade ^{125}I-human LDL to TCA-soluble radioactivity by a saturable mechanism. ^{125}I-human LDL degradation is stimulated by hCG and blocked by preincubation with LDL (99). LDL and hCG or 8-bromo-cAMP synergistically stimulate progesterone synthesis, while HDL is ineffective in supporting progesterone synthesis (99,100). The LDL stimulation of progesterone synthesis and oleate incorporation into cholesteryl oleate are dose dependent and saturable (Km = 5.5 and 10 μg/ml, respectively) (98). In cultured luteinized granulosa cells, hCG and 8-bromo-cAMP stimulate conversion of [^{3}H]-cholesteryl linoleate, which is incorporated in the core of LDL, into [^{3}H]progesterone (100). The similar kinetic parameters for LDL binding, uptake, degradation, cholesteryl oleate synthesis and storage, and progesterone synthesis suggest that all these processes are mediated via the LDL receptor. In the absence of LDL, compactin (which inhibits de novo cholesterol synthesis from acetate) blocks hCG-stimulated progesterone synthesis, an effect that is overcome by added LDL (presumably by providing exogenous cholesterol substrate) (101).

Granulosa cells in the preovulatory follicle are bathed in follicular fluid but are separated from the ovary vasculature by the basal lamina. Human follicular fluid contains little, if any, LDL but contains nearly plasma levels of HDL (74). Since HDL is ineffective in stimulating steroidogenesis, the lack of available LDL would limit progesterone synthesis by ovary granulosa cells prior to ovulation. Following ovulation, the follicle becomes the very vascularized corpus luteum, thus exposing these cells to plasma levels of LDL. Therefore, the rapid rise in ovary progesterone production following ovulation can be explained, at least in part, by the sudden availability of LDL cholesterol as substrate via the LDL receptor (76) (Fig. 2).

HDL

Rat Ovary

Pregnant mare serum gonadotropin (PMSG) and human chorionic gonadotropin (hCG) treatment of rats stimulates ovary corpus luteum formation and progesterone secretion. Membrane preparations of ovaries from rats treated with PMSG-hCG, and rats treated with PMSG-hCG plus 4-APP (which lowers circulating lipoproteins), have high-affinity receptors for ^{125}I-human HDL with Kd values varying from 17.8 to 56 μg human HDL protein/ml (65,84). Binding is specific since both rat and human HDL, but not human LDL, inhibit ^{125}I-human HDL binding (65,84). Binding is saturable, and hCG in vivo stimulates a twofold increase in maximum binding but has no effect on binding affinity (84). In contrast to ^{125}I-human LDL binding, ^{125}I-human HDL binding is not affected by pronase, trypsin, divalent cations, EDTA, ionic strength, or heparin (65,84). Membranes from pregnant rat corpora lutea bind ^{125}I-rat HDL saturably and with high affinity (Kd = 29 to 35 μg rat HDL protein/ml). In hysterectomized, hypophysectomized pregnant rats, both estrogen and testosterone restore progesterone synthesis and induce a threefold increase in maximum ^{125}I-rat HDL binding with no change in affinity (102). Cultured rat luteal cells have high-affinity binding sites for ^{125}I-rat HDL (Kd = 90 μg rat HDL protein/ml) and ^{125}I-human HDL (Kd = 78 μg human HDL protein/ml) (85). Binding is specific since HDL, but not LDL, competes with ^{125}I-HDL binding. Rat and human HDL binding differ, however, since the maximum binding of ^{125}I-human HDL to rat luteal cells is only 15% that of ^{125}I-rat HDL (85).

The issue of rat versus human HDL binding is complex and the physiological significance of the differences is unknown. Human HDL_3 has a possible advantage in HDL specificity studies since it contains predominantly apo A-I and can be prepared essentially free of apo E (103), while rat HDL has apo A-I plus apo E. The apo E in rat HDL complicates matters because the LDL receptor (B/E receptor) can recognize and bind apo E-containing particles (104). However, it has been demonstrated recently that rat ovary granulosa cells synthesize apo E in vitro (105). It is therefore possible that even though apo E-free human HDL_3 is added to the cultures, the ovary cells could alter the HDL by synthesizing and secreting apo E, which then binds to the added lipoprotein.

In 4-APP-treated rats, ^{125}I-rat HDL and ^{125}I-human HDL are taken up by the ovary in vivo, and the amount of uptake is positively correlated with steroidogenesis. PMSG stimulates a slight increase in progestin production and ^{125}I-HDL uptake, while PMSG plus hCG stimulates a 6- to 10-fold increase in both (87). The in situ perfused ovary demonstrates the saturable, specific, and temperature-dependent uptake of ^{125}I-human HDL_3 (i.e., no apo E) since the uptake of human HDL is inhibited by low temperature (4°C) and excess unlabeled human HDL but not human LDL (103). ^{125}I-labeled cholesteryl oleate HDL is taken up by ovary in vivo, and the uptake is increased fourfold in hypolipidemic rats (68). Dispersed corpus luteum cells internalize ^{125}I-human HDL, a process blocked by rat and human HDL but not human LDL (106).

Rat granulosa cells and luteal cells degrade ^{125}I-rat HDL and ^{125}I-human HDL to [^{125}I]monoiodotyrosine. Degradation is specific (inhibited by rat and human HDL but not human LDL) and saturable with half-maximal degradation (Km) of 18 to 21 μg rat HDL protein/ml and 17 to 20 μg human HDL protein/ml (85,88). In contrast to the degradation of LDL, HDL degradation is not inhibited by treatment of the cells with pronase, ammonium chloride, or chloroquine, suggesting that LDL receptors and lysosomes are not involved (85,88, 106). The rate of degradation of ^{125}I-human HDL by rat luteal cells is one-fourth that of ^{125}I-rat HDL (85). With human HDL, there is a major discrepancy between apoprotein degradation and cholesterol conversion to progestin product. The cholesterol theoretically made available due to whole particle degradation of the human HDL particle can account for only 20% or less of the cholesterol needed for progestin synthesis. Human HDL, in contrast to human LDL, seems capable of providing cholesterol in the absence of measurable apoprotein degradation (88). These results are similar to those reported for the rat adrenal, which were mentioned earlier.

Rat luteal tissue from 4-APP-treated rats has decreased cholesteryl ester content, a 10-fold increased de novo cholesterol and progesterone synthesis from [^{14}C]acetate, and relatively unchanged cellular free cholesterol content (107). In 4-APP-treated rats and in cultured granulosa and luteal cells, both human HDL and rat HDL increase ovary cell cholesteryl ester content and the incorporation of oleate into cholesteryl oleate (61). The in vivo infusion of rat and human HDL or the addition of human HDL to cultured granulosa cells decreases de novo cholesterol synthesis (61,95). These data indicate that lack of available lipoprotein cholesterol stimulates increased de novo cholesterol synthesis, increased utilization of cholesteryl ester, and decreased cholesteryl ester synthesis and storage, all of which can be reversed by HDL cholesterol.

The infusion of human HDL in 4-APP-treated rats results in a fourfold increase in progesterone secretion (61), and the infusion of hCG + human HDL into in situ perfused ovaries increases progesterone secretion severalfold (103). The perfused ovaries convert human HDL labeled with [^{3}H]cholesteryl linoleate into [^{3}H]progestin (103). Rat granulosa cells incubated with human HDL reconstituted with both [^{3}H]cholesteryl linoleate and [^{14}C]cholesterol secrete both ^{3}H- and [^{14}C]progestin product. Based on the specific activities of the radioactive sterols in the reconstituted human HDL, twice as much progestin product is synthesized from the free cholesterol component of the HDL particle as compared to the cholesteryl ester component (108).

Rat luteal and granulosa cells in culture produce increased progestin in the presence of human HDL or rat HDL (91,93,94). The effect of rat HDL and human HDL is concentration dependent, and human HDL is slightly more effective than rat HDL (93,94). Concentrations of HDL stimulating half-maximal (Km) progestin synthesis are 19 ± 4 μg rat HDL protein/ml and 32 ± 11 μg human HDL protein/ml (85,88). The Km values for progestin synthesis are similar to the Km values for HDL degradation and the Kd values for binding of HDL, suggesting that they are related. However, the discrepancy between human HDL apoprotein degradation and human HDL cholesterol uptake by these cells exists, and the binding mechanism of HDL and subsequent cholesterol transfer from human HDL into the cell remain unknown. In addition, there are situations where there is a discrepancy between HDL binding and cholesterol transfer. Twelve hours after the injection of a large amount of hCG, the corpus luteum becomes desensitized, i.e., the ovary becomes unresponsive to further stimulation by hCG (109). Interestingly, at that time (12 hours) when progesterone synthesis is decreased by 95% and cellular cholesteryl ester is down by 85%, HDL receptor number is increased 2-fold. Even in the face of increased HDL receptor number, added HDL is still unable to supply cholesterol for cholesteryl ester storage and steroidogenesis (109).

The questions remain: what role does the HDL receptor play in rat steroidogenic tissue and what is the mechanism of cholesterol transfer? To try to answer these questions, several approaches have been attempted. First, certain surface properties of HDL are likely important for cholesterol transfer since an antibody against human HDL, but not against human LDL, blocks human HDL stimulation of progestin synthesis (92). Second, cholesterol, phospholipid, and HDL apoproteins are all necessary for cholesterol transfer since dispersed luteal cells show little increase in progestin production when exposed to either cholesterol-phospholipid dispersions or to human HDL apoprotein-phospholipid dispersions, whereas human HDL apoprotein-phospholipid-cholesterol dispersions markedly increase progestin synthesis (106). In an attempt to learn what surface components are necessary for cholesterol transfer, rat granulosa cells have been incubated with canine HDL (which contains essentially only apo A-I) and several HDL hybrid preparations in which purified apo A-II has displaced apo A-I (hybrid particles with 50 to 95% apo A-II). Hybrid particles containing greater than 95% apo A-II are 30% as effective as canine HDL in stimulating progestin synthesis (110). If apo A-I were absolutely necessary, one would expect the hybrid with greater than 95% apo A-II to be less than 5% as effective as canine HDL in stimulating progestin production. These data indicate that while apo A-I facilitates cholesterol transfer, the delivery of cholesterol from HDL into the cell for steroidogenesis is not strictly dependent on the presence of a specific HDL apoprotein. Hwang and Menon (111) demonstrated that both purified human apo A-I and apo A-II, when complexed with dimyristoyl phosphatidyl choline vesicles, bind saturably and with high affinity to luteinized rat corpus luteum membranes. Consistent with the idea of a relative lack of specificity for particular HDL apoproteins demonstrated in the previously mentioned studies, Phillips and Rothblat (112) demonstrated that all vesicles of egg phosphatidyl choline complexed to either human apo HDL (all apoproteins of HDL), apo A-I, or apo C's remove radiolabeled free cholesterol from cultured rat hepatoma cells equally well. It is clear that much work remains to understand HDL-cell interaction.

Human Ovary

Membrane fractions from fresh corpora lutea bind ^{125}I-human HDL saturably (maximum binding = 278 ng HDL protein/mg membrane protein) and with high affinity (Kd = 136 μg HDL protein/ml). Binding is specific; human HDL competes for ^{125}I-human HDL binding much more effectively than human LDL. Heparin and pronase have no effect on ^{125}I-human HDL binding (97). Cultured luteinized granulosa cells internalize ^{125}I-human HDL in a time- and concentration-dependent manner, but at a much slower rate than ^{125}I-human LDL. After 6 hours of culture, 50 to 100% of cell surface-associated ^{125}I-human LDL is internalized, while only 25% of ^{125}I-human HDL associated with the cell surface is internalized (98). The mechanism and physiological importance of ^{125}I-human HDL binding is unknown, but added HDL does not stimulate human ovary tissue progesterone production (98,99). In fact, the addition of 200 μg/ml human HDL_3 to luteinized granulosa cells cultured in lipoprotein-deficient medium inhibits progesterone production by 60% (101). This inhibition may be important since follicular fluid contains near plasma levels of HDL but no LDL, a combination that would limit follicle progesterone production prior to ovulation (74,76).

Ovary Summary

Ovary cells and membranes bind LDL with high affinity, saturably, and specifically. Binding site number is higher in the granulosa and corpora lutea cells compared to the interstitial compartment. Binding is followed by internalization and degradation of the LDL particle. Ovary LDL receptors have characteristics indistinguishable from those described in the adrenal cortex. Agents that stimulate steroidogenesis, such as LH, hCG, FSH, and Bt_2-cAMP, stimulate increased acquisition of LDL cholesterol via the LDL receptor. LDL cholesterol is stored as cholesteryl ester or is utilized as substrate for steroidogenesis. In the human ovary, compartmentalization of lipoproteins may have a major influence on steroidogenesis. Prior to ovulation, granulosa cells have access to HDL in the follicular fluid, which they cannot use for steroidogenesis, but have little or no access to LDL. Following ovulation, the follicle becomes the vascularized corpus luteum, thus providing the luteinized cells with circulating levels of LDL at the time of rapidly rising progesterone synthesis (Fig. 2).

In the rat, the low level of circulating LDL suggests that the LDL receptor is of little physiological importance. Rat ovary membranes and cultured granulosa cells bind HDL with high affinity, saturably, and specifically. In contrast to LDL binding, HDL binding is unaffected by proteolytic enzymes, divalent cations, EDTA, ionic strength, or heparin (Table 2). Gonadotropins stimulate HDL binding and uptake of HDL cholesterol (Table 1). As was the case with the rat adrenal, HDL cholesterol is taken up by rat ovary cells in excess of apoprotein degradation, and lipoprotein degradation does not seem to involve lysosomes. The mechanisms of HDL cholesterol uptake by rat ovary steroidogenic cells are unclear but certainly different from those described for LDL. Cholesterol transfer into the cell requires cholesterol, phospholipids, and HDL apoproteins. The apoprotein specificity, however, is not particularly stringent, since any of the HDL apoproteins (A-I, A-II, C's) seem capable of mediating cholesterol transfer. This will be discussed in more detail in the conclusion of this chapter. Human ovary membranes also have HDL binding sites, but uptake of HDL cholesterol is very slow and HDL does not stimulate human ovary cell steroidogenesis.

TESTIS

The testis has two major products: sperm cells (spermatozoa), which are produced by the seminiferous tubules; and testosterone, which is produced by Leydig cells in the interstitial compartment of the testis. Androgens are necessary for male sexual differentiation (113) and maintenance of male secondary sex characteristics (114). Locally high levels of testosterone are necessary for spermatogenesis (115). The hormonal control of Leydig cell testosterone production has been studied in great detail. Leydig cell plasma membranes contain receptors that bind LH and hCG specifically and with high affinity (116). LH and hCG stimulate Leydig cell adenylate cyclase activity, cAMP production, cAMP-dependent protein kinase activity, phosphorylation of regulatory proteins, and the conversion of Leydig cell cholesteryl ester and cholesterol to testosterone (117) (Fig. 1). The source of Leydig cell cholesterol has been the subject of numerous studies.

LDL

Pig Testis

Freshly prepared and cultured pig Leydig cells possess specific and high-affinity (Kd = 20 μg LDL protein/ml) binding sites for ^{125}I-human LDL (118). Binding of ^{125}I-human LDL is followed by internalization, and both of these processes are blocked by human LDL but not human HDL (118). hCG increases the receptor number of ^{125}I-human LDL by 1.5- to 2-fold, while incubation of the Leydig cells with 100 μg LDL protein/ml for 24 hours decreases the amount of LDL bound from 18.8 to 4.2 ng/10^6 cells (118). Added human LDL and porcine LDL increase basal testosterone production 8-fold, hCG increases testosterone production 8- to 10-fold, and human LDL and porcine LDL plus hCG increase testosterone production 5-fold over that of hCG alone (118,119). The effect of human LDL on both basal and hCG-stimulated testosterone production is concentration dependent with an ED_{50} of about 4 μg LDL protein/ml, suggesting mediation by the high-affinity LDL receptor (119). De novo synthesis of cholesterol can account for only 25% of maximal testosterone production, emphasizing the importance of LDL cholesterol as substrate for Leydig cell steroidogenesis (119). Human HDL and porcine HDL have little effect on

Leydig cell steroidogenesis and no effect on the interaction of LDL with the Leydig cell (118,119).

Mouse Testis

MA-10 cells, a clonal strain of mouse Leydig tumor cells, respond to LH, hCG, cholera toxin, and cAMP with increased progesterone production (120). These cells bind ^{125}I-human LDL with high affinity and specificity (human LDL blocks ^{125}I-human LDL binding to a much greater extent than does human HDL) (121). At 37°C (but not 4°C), the MA-10 cells internalize and degrade ^{125}I-human LDL. These processes are blocked by human LDL but not human HDL, which suggests mediation by the LDL receptor. Degradation is blocked 60% by NH_4Cl (a lysosomotropic agent), indicating that lysosomal enzymes are involved in the degradation of ^{125}I-human LDL (121). MA-10 cells metabolize reconstituted human LDL, which contains a [^{3}H]cholesteryl linoleate core, to [^{3}H]progesterone (121). Balance studies demonstrate that cholesterol from LDL provides 65% of the substrate for steroidogenesis. In cells grown in lipoprotein-deficient serum, hCG stimulates progesterone synthesis, depletes cellular cholesterol and cholesteryl ester, stimulates HMG-CoA reductase activity, and increases the conversion of acetate to progesterone (122). Human LDL increases progesterone production, decreases HMG-CoA reductase activity by half, and stimulates by twofold the incorporation of oleate into cholesteryl ester (122). hCG-stimulated depletion of cellular cholesterol and cholesteryl ester makes these cells refractory to further hCG stimulation, a process that can be prevented by human LDL (123).

Rat Testis

In enzymatically dissociated testis cells cultured in serum-free medium, the addition of human LDL alone stimulates testosterone production two- to threefold in a concentration-dependent manner (124). hCG alone increases testosterone production 2.5-fold and the combination of human LDL plus hCG is synergistic, stimulating testosterone production sixfold over that of hCG alone at a human LDL concentration of 100 μg protein/ml (124). Human LDL has one-fourth the ability of human HDL, at equal cholesterol concentrations, to stimulate testosterone production by Leydig cells from hCG-treated rats (125). In rats treated with 4-APP (to reduce circulating lipoprotein) and hCG (to stimulate testosterone synthesis), the infusion of human LDL is only one-twelfth as effective as equivalent human HDL cholesterol in stimulating testosterone production in vivo (61). Human LDL also has little effect on testis cholesteryl ester content and de novo cholesterol synthesis (61). In freshly prepared rat testicular membranes, no high-affinity or saturable ^{125}I-rat LDL binding is observed (66). The physiological role, if any, of LDL as a provider of rat testis Leydig cell cholesterol is unknown, since the majority of cholesterol in rat plasma is carried in the HDL fraction (96).

Human Testis

In studies of human fetal testis tissue in culture, human LDL increases testosterone secretion by hCG-treated tissue three- to four-fold. Fetal testis membrane fractions bind ^{125}I-human LDL with high affinity (Kd = 25 μg LDL protein/ml) and saturably (maximum binding = 100 ng LDL/mg membrane protein). During periods of increased testosterone production in fetal life, testis preparations contain both increased LDL receptor content and an increased rate of de novo cholesterol synthesis (126). These data suggest that human testis utilizes LDL cholesterol, via the LDL receptor pathway, as substrate for testosterone synthesis.

HDL

Rat Testis

Freshly prepared rat testis membranes bind ^{125}I-rat HDL with high affinity (Kd at 37°C = 32 μg rat HDL protein/ml) (66). ^{125}I-rat HDL binding is specific; rat HDL but not rat LDL displaces ^{125}I-rat HDL. ^{125}I-rat HDL binding is saturable and localized primarily in the interstitial compartment, which contains the testosterone-producing Leydig cells. Maximum binding is 3200 ng rat HDL protein/mg interstitial membrane protein and 1250 ng rat HDL protein/mg seminiferous tubule membrane protein. hCG treatment in vivo increases ^{125}I-rat HDL binding 220%. Unlike ^{125}I-human LDL binding to human fibroblast LDL receptors, ^{125}I-rat HDL binding to rat testis membrane receptors is not affected by Ca^{2+} or EDTA (66,127). The rat membrane HDL receptors are also insensitive to the proteolytic enzymes pronase and trypsin [unlike LDL receptors, which are destroyed by these enzymes (66,127)]. Chacko (128) has studied the binding of ^{125}I-HDL_3 to purified rat testis membranes and reported that 50 to 65% of total HDL binding was abolished by 1% bovine serum albumin in the incubation medium. The remaining albumin-insensitive HDL_3 binding sites were specific for HDL, were high affinity (Kd = 12.7 μg protein/ml), and were saturable (maximum binding = 1.3 μg protein/mg membrane protein). Egg phosphatidylcholine (PC) vesicles had no effect on ^{125}I-HDL_3 binding, but egg PC vesicles complexed with either apo A-I or apo C's competed equally well for the HDL binding sites as did HDL_3. Chemical modification of lysine and arginine residues of HDL apoproteins had no effect on HDL_3 binding (128). Therefore, the testis HDL binding sites do not appear specific for apo A-I, but may have important physiological roles in lipid transport since they appear to recognize apoprotein-phospholipid complexes (128).

Both human HDL and rat HDL stimulate testosterone production by cultured rat testis cells. Human HDL and rat HDL synergistically augment hCG-stimulated testis cell testosterone production to levels two- to fourfold greater than with hCG stimulation alone (124). The HDL effect is concentration-dependent with an ED_{50} of 25 μg rat HDL protein/ml, a value that suggests the involvement of the HDL receptors in the provision of cholesterol for testosterone synthesis (66,124). In rats made lipoprotein deficient with 4-APP, hCG increases testis sterol synthesis 10-fold, while the concomitant infusion of HDL inhibits cellular sterol synthesis, increases cellular content of cholesterol and cholesteryl ester, and increases circulating testosterone from 8.8 to 20.5 ng/ml (61). As noted before, infused LDL has little effect, suggesting that the main source of cholesterol substrate for rat testis testosterone production is circulating HDL (61). HDL cholesterol uptake seems to be mediated by an HDL binding site that has characteristics quite distinct from LDL receptors.

Testis Summary

Testis Leydig cells contain LDL receptors with characteristics similar to those described for adrenal and ovary. hCG (LH) stimulates LDL binding, uptake, degradation, and cholesterol storage conversion to testosterone. In the human, LDL cholesterol appears to be the major source of substrate for testis steroidogenesis.

In the rat, LDL is probably not a major source of cholesterol for the testis since the majority of circulating cholesterol is carried by HDL. Rat testis contains HDL binding sites, localized primarily to the interstitial compartment (i.e., Leydig cells), which have the same characteristics as HDL binding sites described in the ovary and adrenal. As was previously described for the rat ovary, binding of HDL to its membrane receptor does not seem to be dependent on a particular HDL apoprotein.

PLACENTA

The human placenta is a very active steroidogenic endocrine organ, producing 250 mg or more progesterone per day at term (129–131). This rate of progesterone synthesis requires the utilization of one-fourth to one-third of the daily cholesterol turnover observed in non-pregnant adults (132). The capacity of the placenta to synthesize cholesterol de novo is low (133), and evidence indicates that the majority of cholesterol used for progesterone synthesis comes from the maternal blood (134,135). Detailed examinations of the interaction of LDL and HDL with both normal placental tissue and choriocarcinoma (placental tumor) cells have been performed.

LDL

Human Placenta

Specific and high affinity receptors for human LDL have been identified and characterized in membrane fractions of human placenta (136). In membranes pretreated with heparin to displace endogenous human LDL, the specific binding capacity is 107 ng human LDL protein/mg membrane protein and the Kd of binding is 77 μg LDL protein/ml. ^{125}I-LDL is displaced by human LDL but not human HDL. Heparin displaces human LDL from the binding site, and preincubation of membranes with trypsin or pronase destroys the receptor (136). Similar binding sites are found in primary cell cultures of placenta (136). In studies of microvillous membrane preparations of term human placenta, ^{125}I-human LDL binds with high affinity (Kd = 6.12 μg protein/ml) and limited capacity (130 ng/mg membrane protein) (137). After binding, the cellular uptake of ^{125}I-human LDL is immediate, and after a lag period of 30 min to 1 hr, primary cultures of both normal placenta cells and placenta tumor choriocarcinoma cells degrade the protein coat of ^{125}I-human LDL to monoiodotyrosine (138,139). Studies of uptake and degradation of ^{125}I-human LDL as a function of substrate concentration reveal Kd values of 3 to 8 μg protein/ml, suggesting that these processes are mediated by a high-affinity LDL receptor (138,139). Human LDL but not human HDL blocks ^{125}I-human LDL uptake and degradation. Lysosomal proteolytic enzymes degrade ^{125}I-human LDL since degradation is blocked by chloroquine and the protease inhibitors TPCK and TLCK (138,139). Human LDL, but not human HDL, increases [^{14}C]oleate incorporation into cellular cholesteryl ester (140,141), inhibits the synthesis of endogenous cholesterol from acetate (141), inhibits HMG-CoA reductase activity (142), increases significantly progesterone synthesis (143), and decreases the number of functional LDL receptors (141). These data suggest that human placenta utilizes human LDL cholesterol for progesterone synthesis via the LDL receptor pathway.

HDL

Human Placenta

Human placental membrane fractions and trophoblastic cells maintained in culture bind ^{125}I-human HDL with high affinity (Kd = 152 μg HDL protein/ml) and saturably (323 ng HDL protein/mg membrane protein). ^{125}I-human HDL is displaced from the placental membrane binding site by human HDL but not human LDL. In contrast to ^{125}I-human LDL, ^{125}I-human HDL specific binding is not affected by heparin, pronase, or trypsin (136). ^{125}I-human HDL uptake by human trophoblastic cells increases in a linear fashion as the concentration of ^{125}I-human HDL increases to 1000 μg protein/ml, but degradation of ^{125}I-human HDL is negligible (139). Since added human HDL has no effect on placental cell cholesterol metabolism and progesterone synthesis, the physiological role of ^{125}I-human HDL binding and uptake, if any, is unknown. The primary source of cholesterol for progesterone synthesis is circulating maternal human LDL.

CONCLUSION

Even though many species differences have been identified, the data reviewed in this chapter do demonstrate several common themes in the interaction of lipoproteins with steroidogenic tissue. Steroidogenic cells need cholesterol as substrate for steroid hormone production. The utilization of cellular cholesterol is increased by all factors that stimulate steroidogenesis, and lipoproteins provide the majority of the cholesterol to these stimulated cells.

Most species examined, including the human, utilize predominantly LDL cholesterol for steroidogenesis. The majority of LDL cholesterol is taken up by the cell via the LDL membrane receptor. LDL receptor binding is a process characterized by high affinity, saturability, and specificity for LDL. Binding requires divalent cations, is destroyed by pronase, and LDL is displaced from the LDL receptor by polyanionic compounds such as heparin and dextran sulfate. The LDL receptor, at least in the bovine adrenal, is a single-chain acidic protein. Trophic agents that stimulate steroidogenesis, and thus the tissue's requirement for cholesterol, increase the LDL receptor number via augmented receptor synthesis. Increased LDL receptor synthesis is mediated by elevated levels of receptor mRNA. After the binding of LDL to its receptor, the cell obtains the LDL cholesterol via the now classic LDL pathway, described by Brown, Goldstein, and co-workers, in the cultured human fibroblast (2). The steps of this pathway include internalization, degradation, and storage of the cholesterol as cholesteryl ester. Trophic agents stimulate all these processes, plus the hydrolysis of cellular cholesteryl ester and the transport of cholesterol to the mitochondria for pregnenolone production. Maximum steroidogenesis requires the presence of both circulating LDL and cell surface LDL receptors. Absence of LDL (either spontaneous as in abetalipoproteinemia or induced as with 4-APP) causes an increase in both LDL receptor number and de novo cholesterol synthesis by the cell, but the cells are unable to meet the cholesterol requirement for maximum steroidogenesis. In addition, human ovarian follicular fluid lacks LDL, which should limit progesterone synthesis by ovary follicle granulosa cells prior to ovulation. In the absence of LDL receptors (familial hypercholesterolemia), there is a large increase in nonreceptor-mediated LDL uptake due to the greatly increased concentration of circulating LDL, although maximum steroidogenesis is still limited.

A summary of the interaction of steroidogenic cells with LDL is presented in Fig. 3.

Mouse and rat steroidogenic cells utilize primarily HDL cholesterol as substrate for hormone production. These tissues bind HDL saturably, specifically, and with high affinity. In contrast to LDL binding, HDL binding is not affected by proteolytic enzymes, divalent cations, or heparin. Agents that stimulate steroidogenesis also stimulate HDL binding, degradation, cholesterol and cholesteryl ester uptake, and conversion of cholesterol to steroid hormone products. The mechanism of HDL interaction with the cell is poorly understood. What is known is that HDL apoproteins seem to be required for HDL membrane binding and cholesterol transfer, but the apoprotein specificity is not very rigid. In various in vitro model systems, apo A-II and apo C can substitute for apo A-I, the predominant HDL apoprotein. In addition, free cholesterol in the HDL particle is taken up by the steroidogenic cell and more readily converted to hormone products than cholesteryl ester. Finally, cholesterol uptake from the HDL particle occurs greatly in excess of the degradation of the

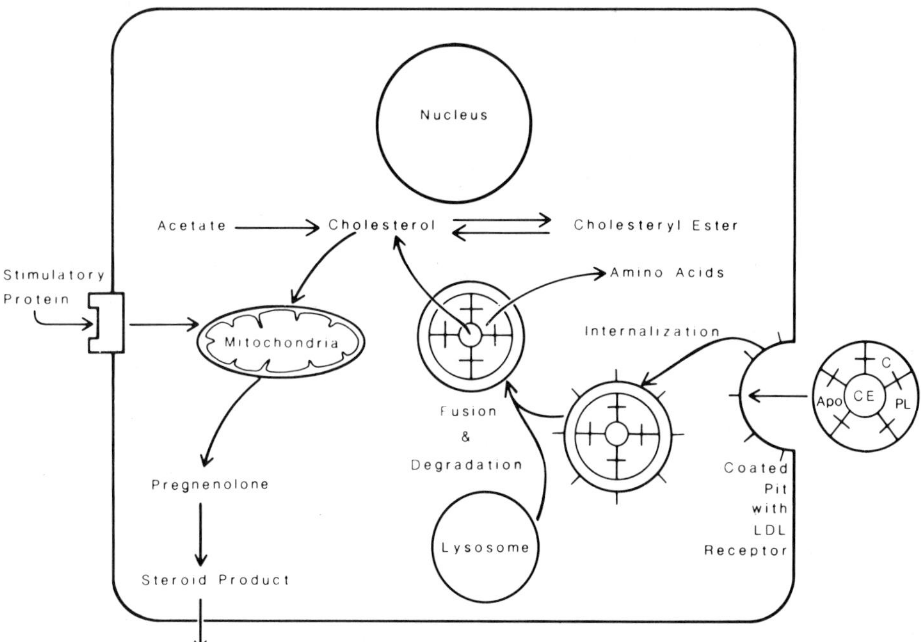

Fig. 3 Model of LDL uptake by a steroidogenic cell via the LDL receptor. C, cholesterol; CE, cholesteryl ester; PL, phospholipid; Apo, apolipoprotein.

HDL apoprotein coat. These separate pieces of information suggest the following series of events: (1) the amphiphilic surface of HDL (apoproteins and phospholipids) stabilizes the HDL particles at specific regions on the cell surface; (2) cholesterol, and to a lesser extent cholesteryl ester, move from the HDL particle into the cell membrane and then into the cell proper where they become part of the cholesterol pool available to the cell for various functions including steroidogenesis; and (3) the HDL particle is released from the cells. Apoprotein degradation could occur at the cell surface, in the medium due to secreted proteolytic enzymes (144), or within the cell due to nonlysosomal enzymes. Partial proteolysis of the HDL surface coat could destabilize the particle and facilitate cholesterol transfer. The

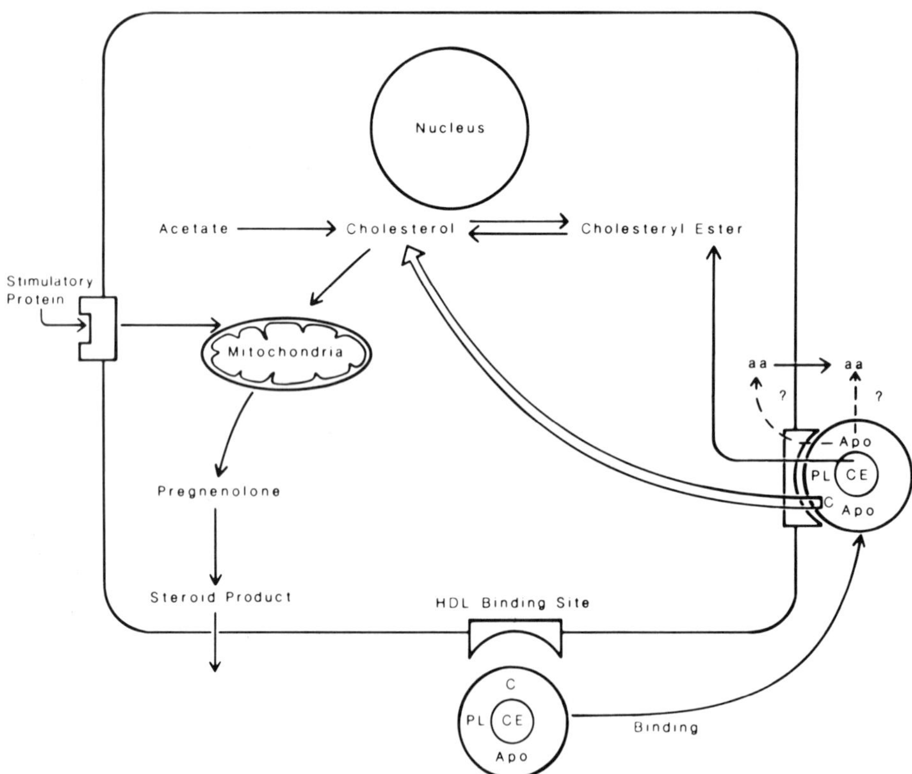

Fig. 4 Model of HDL cholesterol uptake by steroidogenic cells that can use HDL cholesterol (i.e., rat steroidogenic cells). C, cholesterol; CE, cholesteryl ester; PL, phospholipid; Apo, apolipoprotein; aa, amino acids.

phospholipid component of the HDL surface could also be degraded by cell-surface-associated lipases, such as the salt-resistant, hepatic-like lipases (145). These cell-induced changes in the HDL particle could lead to increased cholesterol transfer into the cell. Whether apoproteins function just to stabilize the HDL particle at the cell surface, or can act as a cholesterol carrier into the cell, is unknown. Many questions remain to be answered. A proposed model of HDL-steroidogenic cell interaction is presented in Fig. 4.

Human steroidogenic cells have HDL binding sites, but their function is uncertain. Unlike rat steroidogenic cells, the number of HDL binding sites does not vary with the rate of steroidogenesis and HDL does not stimulate steroidogenesis. These nonregulated receptors may serve to assure the maintenance of a basal level of cholesterol flux, but their role remains unknown.

Many studies have demonstrated that an elevated HDL to LDL ratio is associated with a decreased risk of atherosclerosis (3). The mechanism of this HDL action is unknown, but it is possible that insights gained from the study of the interaction of HDL with steroidogenic cells will lead to a better understanding of HDL interaction with cells in general.

REFERENCES

1. Brown, M., Kovanen, P., and Goldstein, J., *Science, 212*:628 (1981).
2. Brown, M., Kovanen, P., and Goldstein, J., *Rec. Prog. Horm. Res., 35*:215 (1979).
3. Lewis, B., *Br. Med. J., 287*:1161 (1983).
4. Dietschy, J., Spady, D., and Stange, E., *Biochem. Soc. Trans., 11*:639 (1983).
5. Steinberg, D., *Arteriosclerosis, 3*:283 (1983).
6. Stein, O., Halperin, G., and Stein, Y., *Biochim. Biophys. Acta, 620*:247 (1980).
7. Glass, C., Pittman, R., Weinstein, D., and Steinberg, D., *Proc. Natl. Acad. Sci. U.S.A., 80*:5435 (1983).
8. Gwynne, J., and Strauss, J., III, *Endocrine Rev., 3*:299 (1982).
9. Ways, D., Zimmerman, C., and Ontjes, D., *Mol. Pharmacol., 12*:789 (1976).
10. Grahame-Smith, D., Butcher, R., Ney, R., and Sutherland, E., *J. Biol. Chem., 242*:5535 (1967).

11. Gill, G., and Garren, L., *Biochem. Biophys. Res. Commun.*, *39*:335 (1970).

12. Boyd, G., and Trzeciak, W., *Ann. N.Y. Acad. Sci.*, *212*:361 (1973).

13. Mikami, K., Nishikawa, T., Saito, Y., Tamura, Y., Matsuoka, N., Kumagai, A., and Yoshida, S., *Endocrinology, 114*:136 (1984).

14. Shima, S., Mitsunaga, M., and Nakao, T., *Endocrinology, 90*: 808 (1972).

15. Brownie, A., Simpson, E., Jefcoate, C., Boyd, G., Orme-Johnson, W., and Beinert, H., *Biochem. Biophys. Res. Commun.*, *46*:483 (1972).

16. Purvis, J., Canick, J., Mason, J., Estabrook, R., and McCarthy, R., *Ann. N.Y. Acad. Sci.*, *212*:319 (1973).

17. Kovanen, P., Basu, S., Goldstein, J., and Brown, M., *Endocrinology, 104*:610 (1979).

18. Schneider, W., Goldstein, J., and Brown, M., *J. Biol. Chem.*, *255*:11,442 (1980).

19. Schneider, W., Beisiegel, U., Goldstein, J., and Brown, M., *J. Biol. Chem.*, *257*:2664 (1982).

20. Russell, D., Yamamoto, T., Schneider, W., Slaughter, C., Brown, M., and Goldstein, J., *Proc. Natl. Acad. Sci. U.S.A.*, *80*:7501 (1983).

21. Kovanen, P., Faust, J., Brown, M., and Goldstein, J., *Endocrinology, 104*:599 (1979).

22. Kondo, T., and Watanabe, Y., *Exp. Anim.*, *24*:89 (1976).

23. Tanzawa, K., Shimada, Y., Kuroda, M., Tsujita, Y., Arai, M., and Watanabe, Y., *FEBS Lett.*, *118*:81 (1980).

24. Bilheimer, D., Watanabe, Y., and Kita, T., *Proc. Natl. Acad. Sci. U.S.A.*, *79*:3305 (1982).

25. Kita, T., Brown, M., Watanabe, Y., and Goldstein, J., *Proc. Natl. Acad. Sci. U.S.A.*, *78*:2268 (1981).

26. Carew, T., Pittman, R., and Steinberg, D., *J. Biol. Chem.*, *257*:8001 (1982).

27. Pittman, R., Carew, T., Attie, A., Witztum, J., Watanabe, Y., and Steinberg, D., *J. Biol. Chem.*, *257*:7994 (1982).

28. Dietschy, J., Kita, T., Suckling, K., Goldstein, J., and Brown, M., *J. Lipid Res.*, *24*:469 (1983).

29. Kovanen, P., Schneider, W., Hillman, G., Goldstein, J., and Brown, M., *J. Biol. Chem.*, *254*:5498 (1979).

30. Kita, T., Beisiegel, U., Goldstein, J., Schneider, W., and Brown, M., *J. Biol. Chem.*, *256*:4701 (1981).

31. Kovanen, P., Goldstein, J., Chappell, D., and Brown, M., *J. Biol. Chem.*, *255*:5591 (1980).

32. Faust, J., Goldstein, J., and Brown, M., *J. Biol. Chem.*, *252*:4861 (1977).

33. Hall, P., and Nakamura, M., *J. Biol. Chem.*, *254*:12,547 (1979).

34. Stein, Y., Halperin, G., and Stein, O., *Biochim. Biophys. Acta*, *663*:569 (1981).

35. Balasubramaniam, S., Goldstein, J., Faust, J., Brunschede, G., and Brown, M., *J. Biol. Chem.*, *252*:1771 (1977).

36. Andersen, J., and Dietschy, J., *Biochem. Biophys. Res. Commun.*, *72*:880 (1976).

37. Andersen, J., and Dietschy, J., *J. Biol. Chem.*, *256*:7362 (1981).

38. Verschoor-Klootwyk, A., Verschoor, L., Azhar, S., and Reaven, G., *J. Biol. Chem.*, *257*:7666 (1982).

39. Koelz, H., Sherrill, B., Turley, S., and Dietschy, J., *J. Biol. Chem.*, *257*:8061 (1982).

40. Beisiegel, U., Schneider, W., Goldstein, J., Anderson, R., and Brown, M., *J. Biol. Chem.*, *256*:11,923 (1981).

41. Carr, B., and Simpson, E., *Endocrine Rev.*, *2*:306 (1981).

42. Ohashi, M., Carr, B., and Simpson, E., *Endocrinology*, *108*:1237 (1981).

43. Carr, B., Porter, J., MacDonald, P., and Simpson, E., *Endocrinology*, *107*:1034 (1980).

44. Simpson, E., Carr, B., Parker, C., Jr., Milewich, L., Porter, J., and MacDonald, P., *J. Clin. Endocrinol. Metab.*, *49*:146 (1979).

45. Carr, B., Parker, C., Jr., Milewich, L., Porter, J., MacDonald, P., and Simpson, E., *Endocrinology*, *106*:1854 (1980).

46. Carr, B., MacDonald, P., and Simpson, E., *Endocrinology*, *107*:1000 (1980).

47. Pitkin, R., Conner, W., and Lin, D., *J. Clin. Invest.*, *51*:2584 (1972).

48. Parker, C., Jr., Carr, B., Winkel, C., Casey, M., Simpson, E., and MacDonald, P., *J. Clin. Endocrinol. Metab.*, *57*:37 (1983).

49. Carr, B., Ohashi, M., and Simpson, E., *Endocrinology*, *110*: 1994 (1982).

50. Illingworth, D., Kenny, T., Connor, W., and Orwoll, E., *J. Lab. Clin. Med.*, *100*:115 (1982).

51. Illingworth, D., Kenny, T., and Orwoll, E., *J. Clin. Endocrinol. Metab.*, *54*:27 (1982).

52. Illingworth, D., Alam, N., and Sundberg, E., in *Atherosclerosis* (Schettler, F., Gotto, A., Middelhoff, G., Habenicht, A., Jurutka, K., eds.), Vol. 6, Springer-Verlag, Berlin, 1983.

53. Illingworth, D., Alam, N., Sundberg, E., Hagemenas, F., and Layman, D., *Proc. Natl. Acad. Sci. U.S.A.*, *80*:3475 (1983).

54. Illingworth, D., Lees, A., and Lees, R., *Metabolism*, *32*:1045 (1983).

55. Mason, J., Hemsell, P., and Korte, K., *J. Clin. Endocrinol. Metab.*, *56*:1057 (1983).

56. Illingworth, D., Alam, N., and Lindsey, S., *J. Clin. Endocrinol. Metab.*, *58*:206 (1984).

57. Dexter, R., Fishman, L., and Ney, R., *Endocrinology*, *87*:836 (1970).

58. Stone, D., and Hechter, O., *Arch. Biochem.*, *51*:457 (1954).

59. Bolte, E., Coudert, S., and Lefebvre, Y., *J. Clin. Endocrinol. Metab.*, *38*:394 (1974).

60. Simpson, E., *Mol. Cell. Endocrinol.*, *13*:213 (1979).

61. Andersen, J., and Dietschy, J., *J. Biol. Chem.*, *253*:9024 (1978).

62. Brecher, P., and Hyun, Y., *Endocrinology*, *102*:1404 (1978).

63. Fidge, N., Nestel, P., and Suzuki, N., *Biochim. Biophys. Acta*, *753*:14 (1983).

64. Gwynne, J., and Hess, B., *Metabolism*, *27*:1593 (1978).

65. Christie, M., Gwynne, J., and Strauss, J., III, *J. Steroid Biochem.*, *14*:671 (1981).

66. Chen, Y., Kraemer, F., Reaven, G., *J. Biol. Chem.*, *255*: 9162 (1980).

67. Gwynne, J., Mahaffee, D., Brewer, H., Jr., and Ney, R., *Proc. Natl. Acad. Sci. U.S.A.*, *73*:4329 (1976).

68. Counsell, R., Korn, N., Pohland, R., Schwendner, S., and Seevers, R., *Biochim. Biophys. Acta*, *750*:497 (1983).

69. Gwynne, J., and Hess, B., *J. Biol. Chem.*, *255*:10,875 (1980).

70. Ohashi, M., Carr, B., and Simpson, E., *Endocrinology*, *109*: 783 (1981).

71. Hsueh, A., Adashi, E., Jones, P., and Welsh, T., Jr., *Endocrine Rev.*, *5*:76 (1984).

72. Armstrong, D., *Rec. Prog. Horm. Res.*, *24*:255 (1968).

73. Caravaglios, R., and Cilotti, R., *J. Endocrinol.*, *15*:273 (1957).

74. Simpson, E., Rochelle, D., Carr, B., and MacDonald, P., *J. Clin. Endocrinol. Metab.*, *51*:1469 (1980).

75. Goodman, A., and Hodgen, G., *Rec. Prog. Horm. Res.*, *39*:1 (1983).

76. Carr, B., MacDonald, P., and Simpson, E., *Fertil. Steril.*, *38*:303 (1982).

77. Lipsett, M., in *Reproductive Endocrinology* (Yen, S., and Jaffee, R., eds.), W. B. Saunders, Philadelphia, 1978.

78. Savion, N., Laherty, R., Lui, G., and Gospodarowicz, D., *J. Biol. Chem.*, *256*:12,817 (1981).

79. Savion, N., Laherty, R., Cohen, D., Lui, G., and Gospodarowicz, D., *Endocrinology*, *110*:13 (1982).

80. Pate, J., and Condon, W., *Mol. Cell. Endocrinol.*, *28*:551 (1982).

81. Kovanen, P., Goldstein, J., and Brown, M., *J. Biol. Chem.*, *253*:5126 (1978).

82. Spady, D., Bilheimer, D., and Dietschy, J., *Proc. Natl. Acad. Sci. U.S.A.*, *80*:3499 (1983).

83. Silavin, S., and Strauss, J., III, *Biol. Reprod.*, *29*:1163 (1983).

84. Hwang, J., and Menon, K., *J. Biol. Chem.*, *258*:8020 (1983).

85. Rajendran, K., Hwang, J., and Menon, K., *Endocrinology*, *112*: 1746 (1983).

86. Schreiber, J., Nakamura, K., and Weinstein, D., in *Factors Regulating Ovarian Function* (Greenwald, G., and Terranova, P., eds.), Raven Press, New York, 1983.

87. Strauss, J., III, MacGregor, L., and Gwynne, J., *J. Steroid Biochem.*, *16*:525 (1982).

88. Schreiber, J., Nakamura, K., and Weinstein, D., *Endocrinology, 110*:55 (1982).

89. Schreiber, J., Nakamura, K., Schmit, V., and Weinstein, D., *Steroids, 43*:25 (1984).

90. Schuler, L., Scavo, L., Kirsch, T., Flickinger, G., and Strauss, J., III, *J. Biol. Chem., 254*:8662 (1979).

91. Azhar, S., and Menon, K., *J. Biol. Chem., 256*:6548 (1981).

92. Rosenblum, M., Huttler, C., and Strauss, J., III, *Endocrinology, 109*:1518 (1981).

93. Schreiber, J., Hsueh, A., Weinstein, D., and Erickson, G., *J. Steroid Biochem., 13*:1009 (1980).

94. Azhar, S., Menon, M., and Menon, K., *Biochim. Biophys. Acta, 665*:362 (1981).

95. Andersen, J., and Dietschy, J., *J. Biol. Chem., 252*:3652 (1977).

96. Lasser, N., Roheim, P., Edelstein, D., and Eder, H., *J. Lipid Res., 14*:1 (1973).

97. Ohashi, M., Carr, B., and Simpson, E., *Endocrinology, 110*:1477 (1982).

98. Tureck, R., Wilburn, A., Gwynne, J., Paavola, L., and Strauss, J., III, *J. Steroid Biochem., 19*:1033 (1983).

99. Carr, B., Sadler, R., Rochelle, D., Stalmach, M., MacDonald, P., and Simpson, E., *J. Clin. Endocrinol. Metab., 52*:875 (1981).

100. Soto, E., Silavin, S., Tureck, R., and Strauss, J., III, *J. Clin. Endocrinol. Metab., 58*:831 (1984).

101. Tureck, R., and Strauss, J., III, *J. Clin. Endocrinol. Metab., 54*:367 (1982).

102. Gibori, G., Chen, Y., Khan, I., Azhar, S., and Reaven, G., *Endocrinology, 114*:609 (1984).

103. Paavola, L., and Strauss, J., III, *J. Cell Biol., 97*:593 (1983).

104. Mahley, R., Weisgraber, K., and Innerarity, T., *Biochim. Biophys. Acta, 575*:81 (1979).

105. Driscoll, D., Schreiber, J., Schmit, V., and Getz, G., *J. Biol. Chem., 260*:9031 (1985).

106. Schuler, L., Langenberg, K., Gwynne, J., and Strauss, J., III, *Biochim. Biophys. Acta, 664*:583 (1981).

107. Christie, M., Strauss, J., III, and Flickinger, G., *Endocrinology, 105*:92 (1979).

108. Nestler, J., Bamberger, M., Rothblat, G., and Strauss, J., III, in *Proceedings of the Symposium on Lipoproteins and Cholesterol Metabolism in Steroidogenic Tissues* (Strauss, J., and Menon, K., eds.), G. Strickley Co., Philadelphia, 1984.

109. Azhar, S., Chen, Y., and Reaven, G., *J. Biol. Chem., 258*:3735 (1983).

110. Schreiber, J., Edelstein, C., and Scanu, A., in *Proceedings of the Symposium on Lipoprotein and Cholesterol Metabolism in Steroidogenic Tissue* (Strauss, J., and Menon, K., eds.), G. Strickley Co., Philadelphia, 1984.

111. Hwang, J., and Menon, K., in *Proceedings of the Symposium on Lipoprotein and Cholesterol Metabolism in Steroidogenic Tissues* (Strauss, J., and Menon, K., eds.), G. Strickley Co., Philadelphia, 1984.

112. Phillips, M., and Rothblat, G., in *Proceedings of the Symposium on Lipoprotein and Cholesterol Metabolism in Steroidogenic Tissues* (Strauss, J., and Menon, K., eds.), G. Strickley Co., Philadelphia, 1984.

113. Jost, A., *Philos. Trans. Roy. Soc. London (Biol.), 259*:119 (1970).

114. Bardin, C., in *Reproductive Endocrinology* (Jaffe, R., and Yen, S., eds.), W. B. Saunders, Philadelphia, 1978.

115. Steinberger, E., *Physiol. Rev., 51*:1 (1971).

116. Christensen, A., in *Handbook of Physiology* (Greep, R., and Astwood, E., eds.), Williams & Wilkins, Baltimore, 1975.

117. Catt, K., Harwood, J., Clayton, R., Davies, T., Chan, V., Katikineni, M., Nozu, K., and Dufau, M., *Rec. Prog. Horm. Res., 36*:557 (1980).

118. Benahmed, M., Dellamonica, C., Haour, F., and Saez, J., *Biochem. Biophys. Res. Commun., 99*:1123 (1981).

119. Benahmed, M., Reventos, J., and Saez, J., *Endocrinology, 112*:1952 (1983).

120. Ascoli, M., *Endocrinology, 108*:88 (1981).

121. Freeman, D., and Ascoli, M., *Biochim. Biophys. Acta, 754*:72 (1983).

122. Freeman, D., and Ascoli, M., *J. Biol. Chem., 257*:14,231 (1982).

123. Freeman, D., and Ascoli, M., *Proc. Natl. Acad. Sci. U.S.A.*, *79*:7796 (1982).

124. Schreiber, J., Weinstein, D., and Hsueh, A., *J. Steroid Biochem.*, *16*:39 (1982).

125. Quinn, P., Dombrausky, L., Chen, Y., and Payne, A., *Endocrinology*, *109*:1790 (1981).

126. Carr, B., Parker, C., Jr., Ohashi, M., MacDonald, P., and Simpson, E., *Am. J. Obstet. Gynecol.*, *146*:241 (1983).

127. Basu, S., Goldstein, J., and Brown, M., *J. Biol. Chem.*, *253*:3852 (1978).

128. Chacko, G., *Biochim. Biophys. Acta*, *795*:417 (1984).

129. Pearlman, W., *Biochem. J.*, *65*:7P (1957).

130. Lin, T., Lin, S., Erlenmeyer, F., Kline, I., Underwood, R., Billiar, R., and Little, B., *J. Clin. Endocrinol. Metab.*, *34*:287 (1972).

131. Lurie, A., Reid, D., and Villee, C., *Am. J. Obstet. Gynecol.*, *96*:670 (1966).

132. Grundy, S., and Ahrens, E., *J. Lipid Res.*, *10*:91 (1969).

133. Zelewski, L., and Villee, C., *Biochemistry*, *5*:1805 (1966).

134. Bloch, K., *J. Biol. Chem.*, *157*:661 (1945).

135. Hellig, H., Gottereau, D., Lefebvre, Y., and Bolte, E., *J. Clin. Endocrinol. Metab.*, *30*:624 (1970).

136. Cummings, S., Hatley, W., Simpson, E., and Ohashi, M., *J. Clin. Endocrinol. Metab.*, *54*:903 (1982).

137. Alsat, E., Bouali, Y., Goldstein, S., Malassine, A., Laudat, M., and Cedard, L., *Mol. Cell. Endocrinol.*, *28*:439 (1982).

138. Simpson, E., Bilheimer, D., MacDonald, P., and Porter, J., *Endocrinology*, *104*:8 (1979).

139. Winkel, C., Gilmore, J., MacDonald, P., and Simpson, E., *Endocrinology*, *107*:1892 (1980).

140. Simpson, E., and Burkhart, M., *Arch. Biochem. Biophys.*, *200*:86 (1980).

141. Winkel, C., MacDonald, P., Hemsell, P., and Simpson, E., *Endocrinology*, *109*:1084 (1981).

142. Simpson, E., Porter, J., Milewich, L., Bilheimer, D., and MacDonald, P., *J. Clin. Endocrinol. Metab.*, *47*:1099 (1978).

143. Winkel, C., Snyder, J., MacDonald, P., and Simpson, E., *Endocrinology, 106*:1054 (1980).

144. Ritter, M., and Scanu, A., *J. Biol. Chem., 255*:3763 (1980).

145. Jansen, H., and DeGreef, W., *Biochem. J., 196*:739 (1981).

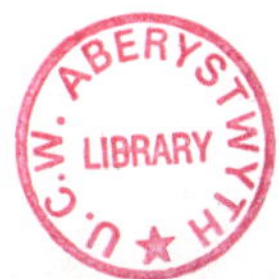

15

Immunoregulation by Plasma Lipoproteins

JUDITH A. K. HARMONY, ANN L. AKESON, BECKY M. McCARTHY, RANDALL E. MORRIS, DAVID W. SCUPHAM, AND STEPHAN A. GRUPP
University of Cincinnati College of Medicine, Cincinnati, Ohio

GOALS

We shall develop a hypothetical model, consistent with available data, that accounts for suppression by plasma lipoproteins of mitogen-induced proliferation of lymphocytes in vitro and employ the model to evaluate the potential for regulation of the cell cycle by plasma lipoproteins in vivo. According to the model, plasma lipoproteins block progression of activated lymphocytes through the cycle at three locations. One control point regulates the entry of nonproliferating cells into the G_1 phase of the cycle, one regulates the maintenance of the G_1 state, and one regulates the progression of cycle-competent cells through G_1 and into S. The suppressive potencies of "conventional" plasma lipoproteins, isolated from the peripheral circulation, of hydrated densities ≤ 1.21 g/ml will be emphasized; these are chylomicrons (d ≤ 1.006 g/ml), very-low-density (VLDL d 1.006 g/ml), intermediate-density (IDL; d 1.006 to 1.019 g/ml), low-density (LDL; d 1.019 to 1.063 g/ml), and high-density (HDL; 1.063 to 1.21 g/ml) lipoproteins (1). In addition, suppression by purified apolipoproteins will be contrasted with suppression by intact lipoproteins. The term "immunosuppression" here refers to the inhibition of lymphocyte activation and proliferation rather than to the inhibition of lymphocyte function (e.g., antibody secretion, cytotoxicity).

INTRODUCTION

The roles of circulating plasma lipoproteins in lipid catalysis and lipid mobilization (1–3) and in regulation of cholesterol homeostasis (4,5) are well appreciated. In recent years, additional functions of these macromolecular complexes have been suggested, including alteration of membrane protein activities (5–7), neutralization of xenotropic type C viruses (8), inhibition of virus hemagglutination (9,10), lysis of trypanosomes (11), both induction and suppression of expression of cellular procoagulant activity (12,13), stimulation of prothrombin activation (14), and inhibition of plasmin activity (15), complement-mediated cell lysis (16), and urate crystal-induced neutrophil luminol-dependent chemiluminescence (17). Plasma lipoproteins also have selective but profound effects on lymphoid cell proliferation. The lipoprotein influence on lymphoid cell function thus becomes evident when T- or B-lymphocyte proliferation is a prerequisite for expression of function.

Intensive investigation of lipoprotein suppression of lymphocyte proliferation by lipoproteins was initiated when Chisari and Edgington (18) isolated and described the bioactivity of an immunosuppressive subpopulation of LDL, designated rosette-inhibitory factor (RIF). In succeeding years, a number of investigators have made substantial contributions to this field of research. Understanding the detailed molecular basis of lipoprotein suppression has been impeded by three barriers: the heterogeneity of the plasma lipoproteins, the complexity of the lymphocyte response to mitogens, and the sensitivity of in vitro experimental systems of lymphocyte activation to culture conditions. Our approach and that of other investigators has been to focus on four major questions; none of these questions has been answered completely.

1. Which landmarks along the pathway of lymphocyte activation-proliferation are susceptible to suppression by lipoproteins?
2. Which lipoprotein constituents are responsible for this suppression?
3. Is the direct target of the lipoprotein a lymphocyte, an accessory cell, or both?
4. What is the molecular mechanism of suppression?

CLONAL SELECTION AND EXPANSION: THE BASIS OF CELL-MEDIATED AND HUMORAL IMMUNE RESPONSES

Lymphoid cells originate from pluripotent stem cells located in the bone marrow. The stem cells undergo a controlled program of differentiation during which they become immunocompetent. Mature, immunocompetent T and B lymphocytes are small, relatively inactive cells arrested out of the cell cycle in a phase termed G_0. Lymphocyte proliferation occurs when specific cells reactive against foreign antigens are activated and amplified. Since the number of cells specific for any single antigen is small, the sequence of activation responses that trigger the stimulated G_0 cells to enter and progress through the cell cycle has been investigated with nonspecific polyclonal activators such as phytohemagglutinin (PHA), concanavalin A (conA), neuraminidase-galactose oxidase (NAGO) for T cells, and anti-IgM and lipopolysaccharide (LPS) for B cells. The mitogenicity of these activators is not dependent on their antigenicity. Studies of suppression by lipoproteins have emphasized the in vitro activation of lymphocytes, particularly of T cells, by polyclonal mitogens.

Any hypotheses concerning the mechanisms of lipoprotein-mediated immunosuppression must be understood in the context of the cascade of biochemical and physiological events initiated by the mitogen-lymphocyte interaction. This program of metabolic processes involves events dependent upon both the action of mitogen binding alone and the presence of immunoregulators external to the cell being activated. The independent immunoregulators include T-cell help, soluble mediator proteins [such as the interleukins and B-cell growth factor (BCGF)], and accessory cells. Accessory cells include monocytes, dendritic cells, and other such cells in the front line of antigen contact.

Lymphocyte Activation

The program of metabolic processes important in lymphocyte activation and proliferation is incompletely understood, and the conclusions of different investigators are often mutually exclusive. We briefly present here some aspects of current thought concerning the sequence of T- and B-lymphocyte activation events, with special reference to T lymphocytes and to those events through which lipoproteins may achieve their suppressive effect. The sequence of activation events in B cells has not been as well characterized as that in T cells.

The lymphocyte cell cycle is depicted in Fig. 1, and some of the associated activation events are listed in Table 1. Activation of lymphocytes by mitogen signals the cells to leave G_0 and enter G_0* (or early G_1). This process is often referred to as "commitment" of the resting cell to entry into the cell cycle. A continuous activation signal may be necessary to sustain progress along the cell cycle, especially in its earliest phases. In addition, contributions from accesory cells are required. Having lost the activation signal, lymphocytes may halt in G_0*-G_1, or even drop back into G_0. The activation signal has been observed to have several different components (Table 1), depending on the stage of cellular activation.

As a consequence of antigen or mitogen binding, lymphocytes follow a sequence of early metabolic changes, including membrane

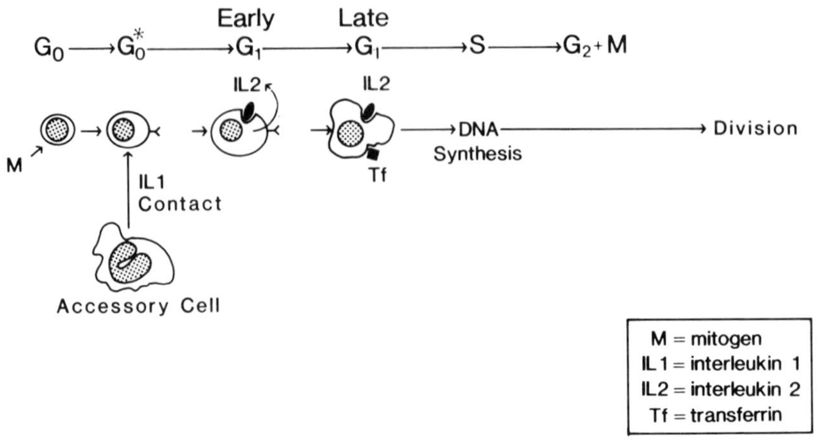

Early Late

$G_0 \longrightarrow G_0^* \longrightarrow G_1 \longrightarrow G_1 \longrightarrow S \longrightarrow G_2 + M$

IL2 IL2

M → DNA Synthesis → Division

IL1 Contact Tf

Accessory Cell

M = mitogen
IL1 = interleukin 1
IL2 = interleukin 2
Tf = transferrin

Fig. 1 Schematic representation of the lymphocyte cell cycle. This diagram represents some landmark events that occur when a T lymphocyte is activated by a polyclonal mitogen (M). The mitogen alters the surface of the lymphocyte in G_0, and activates the cell to G_0*, from which it can receive signals from accessory cells. Accessory cell signals include soluble mediators such as IL1 and undefined mediators provided by direct cell contact. Fully activated T cells enter G_1, enlarge, express membrane receptors for IL2, and synthesize and secrete IL2. Progression through G_1 is driven by the utilization of IL2 and culminates in the expression of membrane receptors for transferrin (Tf), Late G_1 is also indicated by a further enlargement of the activated cell. S, the phase of DNA replication, is followed by G_2 and mitosis-cytokinesis.

depolarization (19), stimulated phosphatidylinositol (PI) metabolism (20–22), increased levels of cellular Ca^{2+} (23), and stimulated uptake of other ions and small molecules. The events that occur early in mitogen-stimulated lymphocytes are common to other receptor-mediated activation systems, such as activation by epidermal growth factor or platelet- or fibroblast-derived growth factor.

With few exceptions, not one of the signaling processes is sufficient in and of itself to allow lymphocyte proliferation. The simplest interpretation of the sequence of activation signaling events is that each allows a step along the activation pathway, with a previous event setting the stage for the next event. The evidence available to date in this area is more phenomenological than mechanistic, however, and it may turn out that these events will be sorted into separate and parallel pathways, each of which addresses an aspect of activation and all of which together result in cell cycle progression, proliferation, and terminally differentiated cell function (24,25).

Table 1 Events Occurring During the Multisignal Activation of Lymphocytes[a]

Signal	Time	Event	Cell cycle phase
Mitogen or antigen	sec–min	Membrane depolarization Ca^{2+} increases PI response $Na^{+}K^{+}$-ATPase cGMP increase	$G_0 \rightarrow G_0^*$ and/or $G_0^* \rightarrow G_1$
Accessory cells and IL1; BCGF	1–24 hours	PI → PIP → PIP_2[b] Protein phosphorylation RNA synthesis IL2-specific mRNA Other specific mRNA Protein synthesis IL2-R Tf-R IL2 General PL synthesis Cell enlargement	G_1 progression
IL2 and transferrin	6–96 hours	RNA synthesis Protein synthesis Cell and nuclear enlargement DNA replication Mitosis Cytokinesis	$G_1 \rightarrow S$ and $S \rightarrow G_2 \rightarrow M$

[a]BCGF, B-cell growth factor; IL1, interleukin 1, IL2, interleukin 2; IL2-R, IL2 receptor; Tf-R, transferrin receptor; PI, phosphatidylinositol; PIP, phosphatidylinositol-4-phosphate; PIP_2, phosphatidylinositol-4-5-bis-phosphate.

[b]Increased incorporation of PI, PIP, and PIP_2 found on interaction of lymphocyte and accessory cell. The PI metabolism of either or both cell types may be affected (79).

Progression of activated lymphocytes through the cell cycle depends on signals from accessory cells. Accessory cells bind, process, and present antigen to lymphocytes, as well as produce the nonspecific growth factor interleukin 1 (IL1) (26,27). IL1 is necessary for further progression of the T cell through G_1, in large part by prompting the synthesis and secretion of the T-cell-derived T-cell growth factor interleukin 2 (IL2) from cells that have been activated previously by antigen. IL1 may also regulate a variety of lymphocyte surface receptors involved in maturation and functional activation. While IL1 is important for lymphocyte activation, direct contact between T cells and accessory cells is required for optimal stimulation by mitogen (28–31).

The final signaling event between mitogen activation and DNA synthesis in T cells is the interaction of IL2 with its receptor (IL2-R). This interaction triggers subsequent events necessary to release activated lymphocytes from G_1 into S. IL2 is the essential T-cell proliferation factor, although it functions as a differentiation-inducing factor as well (32). While it is clear that the production of IL2 is dependent on both mitogen and accessory cells (33,34), there is controversy over the dependence of IL2-R expression on the presence of accessory cells or IL1. Some reports (35,36) suggest that IL2-R expression on the surface of the T cell depends solely on mitogen binding. Others (33,34,37) see IL2-R expression as IL1 and accessory cell dependent. Requirement for accessory cell help in IL2-R expression may depend on the state of differentiation of the responding lymphocyte.

Transferrin Required for Lymphocyte Proliferation

Additional growth factors, and particularly transferrin, are needed for T- and B-lymphocyte proliferation (38–42). Transferrin, the predominant serum iron-binding and transporting glycoprotein, is required for cell growth in general (43), presumably because it provides iron essential for cofactors and enzymes that participate in oxidative respiration, and for enzymes such as ribonucleotide reductase, which is involved in DNA synthesis. In serum, transferrin levels are 3 to 4 mg/ml (44). Uptake of iron by eukaryotic cells is mediated by the tight binding of transferrin to transferrin receptors (Tf-R) (45). The human Tf-R is an integral membrane protein of Mr 190K and is comprised of two identical subunits. The receptor is both phosphorylated (46) and acylated (47,48), although no functional roles have been definitively assigned to these posttranslational modifications. Diferric-transferrin is internalized by Tf-R-mediated endocytosis, and iron dissociates in the acidic endosome compartment while apotransferrin remains bound to the Tf-R to recycle to the cell surface (49–51).

Resting lymphocytes do not have detectable (high-affinity) cell surface Tf-R, but express them when activated (52–55). The molecular signal for Tf-R induction in lymphocytes is unknown. Neckers and Cossman (56) suggested that, in the case of T-cell activation, the binding of IL2 to the IL2-R results in Tf-R expression. They found that anti-TAC, a monoclonal antibody against the IL2-R that blocks IL2 binding (57), blocks expression of Tf-R and inhibits DNA synthesis.

LIPOPROTEIN SUPPRESSION OF MITOGEN-INDUCED LYMPHOCYTE ACTIVATION AND PROLIFERATION

Structural Features of Suppressive Lipoproteins

Suppressive lipoproteins are constitutive or are induced by nutritional, hormonal, or disease states. Proliferation-suppressing plasma lipoproteins are those of hydrated densities ≤ 1.063 g/ml: the chylomicrons, VLDL, IDL, and LDL (23,58–60). In general, HDL are not suppressive, although HDL_c, an abnormal HDL isolated from dogs fed a semisynthetic diet of cholesterol and hydrogenated coconut oil, are potent suppressors of lymphocyte activation (61). Suppressive lipoproteins have been isolated from plasma by ultracentrifugal flotation in KBr and by gel filtration in the absence of a high-salt concentration. Of the suppressive lipoproteins, IDL are the most suppressive and LDL the least. The suppressive potency of VLDL is variable from donor to donor. This variability probably depends on the relative contamination of VLDL with chylomicrons and IDL. A minor but highly suppressive subfraction of LDL, termed LDL-In by Curtiss and Edgington (58), is an IDL (62). Suppressive lipoproteins contain the same lipid constituents as the nonsuppressive HDL, although the relative ratio of lipids and of lipid to protein distinguishes each lipoprotein class. The major difference (apart from size) between suppressive and nonsuppressive lipoproteins is the protein constituents. Present in chylomicrons, VLDL, IDL, and LDL but absent in normal HDL are the apolipoproteins E and B. These apolipoproteins are important in the binding of lipoproteins of d ≤ 1.063 g/ml to glycosaminoglycans (63–65).

Apo E-rich lipoproteins are the most suppressive of the lipoproteins (66,67). For example, the capacity of lipoproteins to suppress mitogen-induced phospholipid (PI) metabolism correlates directly with their apo E content (66). No similar correlation exists for suppressive potency versus the major lipoprotein-lipids (triglyceride, cholesteryl ester, cholesterol, phospholipid) or versus other apolipoproteins (apo B, apo C-II, apo C-III). In addition, Curtiss and collaborators (67) found a strong correlation between inhibitory activity and the apo E content of cord blood lipoproteins. Plasma levels of apo E are proportional to the levels of both triglyceride and cholesterol (68). However, in cord blood, the apo E levels are elevated relative to those predicted by the amounts of triglyceride and cholesterol. Based on results of a careful study (61) in which the suppressive potencies of two lipoproteins of nearly identical sizes and chemical compositions but distinct protein constituents (apo B versus apo E) were compared, apo E lipoproteins are three to four times more effective on a molar basis than apo B lipoproteins in suppressing the early inductive event of Ca^{2+} accumulation, as well as the later synthesis of DNA.

The most compelling evidence for the key role of apo E in immunoregulation is that purified, delipidated apo E suppresses both mitogen-induced early events and DNA replication (66,69). The four major isoforms of apo E appear to be equally suppressive. Apo B (both B-100 and B-48) is also suppressive (69), whereas other apolipoproteins (apo A-I, C-II, C-III) are not. While apolipoproteins clearly suppress early activation events in the absence of lipid, their suppression of DNA replication in mitogen-induced lymphocytes in the absence of serum has not been tested. Thus, an apolipoprotein-bound lipid may be important in suppressing lymphocyte proliferation. Apo E may be one of the important immunomodulatory products secreted by cells of the immune system. Monocyte-macrophages synthesize and secrete apo E (70–72). Apo E synthesis by these cells is developmentally regulated (73–75). Since monocyte-macrophages can suppress B- and T-lymphocyte proliferation (76,77), Werb and Chin (78) have proposed that apo E is important in this suppression.

Activation Events Sensitive to Lipoprotein Suppression

Considering the number of events important in lymphocyte activation that utilize cellular energy (Table 1) and the economy of cell cycle control mechanisms in general, suppression by lipoproteins might logically be directed toward processes that occur relatively early, such as mitogen signaling, accessory cell to lymphocyte signaling, growth factor production or utilization by activated lymphocytes, or some combination of these processes. Suppression of T-lymphocyte responses by plasma lipoproteins in vitro has been investigated at the levels of inductive, intermediate, and terminal events to identify the positions of cell cycle control. Table 2 summarizes landmark activation events that are and are not influenced by plasma lipoproteins. In summarizing these data, we have, guided by the principle of Occam's razor, assumed that suppressive lipoproteins of all classes suppress lymphocyte activation and proliferation by the same mechanism(s). The cells used to investigate mid-cycle and late events are, in general, cultured at low density (typically 10^5 cells per microtiter

Table 2 Plasma Lipoproteins Suppress Some but Not All of the Activation Events in T Lymphocytes

Activation event	Suppressed		Mitogen	Ref.
	Cells cultured in			
Early events (⩽6 hours)	Serum	SFM[a]		
Ca^{2+} accumulation	NA	Yes	PHA	23
PI response	Yes	Yes	PHA, NAGO	20,21
Cyclic nucleotide increase	Yes	Yes	PHA	7,89
Mid-cycle events (6–48 hours)				
Cell enlargement				
24 hours (250–330 μm^3)	No	No	PHA, NAGO	84,87
⩾48 hours (331–400 μm^3)	Yes	Yes	PHA, NAGO	87
Sterol biosynthesis	NA[b]	NA		
RNA synthesis	No	NA	PHA	84
Protein synthesis	No[c]	NA	PHA	84
IL2-R expression	No	Yes[d]	PHA, NAGO	84,87
Tf-R expression	No	Yes[d]	PHA, NAGO	84,87
Growth factor secretion	NA	NA		
Late events (60–120 hours)				
DNA replication	Yes	Yes	PHA, NAGO	7,84,87
Cell division	Yes	NA	PHA, conA	86

[a]SFM, serum-free medium.
[b]NA, not assessed.
[c]Chisari (85) reported that VLDL do inhibit PHA-stimulated protein synthesis.
[d]Depends on the amount of transferrin in the culture (see text).

well in 0.2 to 0.25 ml) for an optimum proliferative response. These cell populations have consisted of peripheral blood mononuclear cells, nonadherent lymphocytes, or T cells plus accessory cells (85% glass-adherent monocytes) in a 10:1 ratio. Although early activation events such as the PI response occur under these conditions (79), their measurement requires higher cell numbers most easily satisfied by higher cell densities, 1×10^6 to 5×10^7 cells/ml. Since lymphocyte responses are influenced profoundly by cell density, the relationship between early events and mid-cycle/late events is complicated. No data addressing the dose dependence of lipoprotein suppression of the PI response, the blastogenic response, the autocrine cycle response, and the DNA synthetic response under *identical* culture conditions are yet available.

The striking aspect of the summary in Table 2 is that not all events in the activation pathway are suppressed by lipoproteins. Furthermore, the sensitivity of several of the processes to suppression by lipoproteins depends on whether the cells are cultured in serum-free (SFM) or in serum-containing medium. The early inductive metabolic changes—enhanced PI metabolism, Ca^{2+} accumulation, and cGMP elevation—are inhibited in both SFM and serum-containing medium. (Suppression of these events by lipoproteins will be discussed in more detail later.) In contrast, there are a number of events that occur to the same extent in serum-containing medium in the absence and presence of lipoproteins, even at high lipoprotein concentrations. These include initial T-cell enlargement (a volume increase from 180 to 250 to 330 μm^3 at <24 to 48 hr), general synthesis of the macromolecules RNA and protein (measured at 24 hr), and expression of the cell surface receptors for IL2 and transferrin. The appearance of large lymphoblasts (331 to 400 μm^3 at 48 hr and later) and DNA replication are suppressed by lipoproteins in SFM and in serum-containing medium. Whether mitogen-induced expression of T-cell receptors for IL2 and for transferrin is suppressed by lipoproteins when the cultures are maintained in SFM depends on the amount of transferrin present. Transferrin levels of less than about 50 μg/ml allow suppression, whereas higher levels of transferrin favor receptor expression in the presence of suppressive lipoproteins. Ideally, all of this information should be useful in defining the position(s) in the cell cycle where lipoprotein-suppressed lymphocytes accumulate. Identification of the block position, in turn, should lead to an understanding of the suppressive mechanism(s).

Initial cell enlargement in the absence of appreciable nuclear enlargement, which we believe to be indicative of the G_0* or early G_1 stage, occurs at a time (4 to 24 hr) when cellular metabolism of all phospholipids increases (21). The timing coincidence suggests that net synthesis of lipids is required for the cells to enlarge. A general lipid synthesis requirement has been demonstrated to exist for G_1

progression (80), but not yet for entry into G_1. Although lipoproteins do not suppress this initial blastogenesis, their effect on lipid synthesis at these intermediate times remains to be determined. Unfortunately, little is known regarding the requirements for the second phase of cell enlargement (48 hr), a phase characterized by significant increase in nuclear volume. We tentatively assign this enlargement process to late G_1 or entry into S. Correlative data (81) link cell and nuclear volume (size or critical cell mass) to eukaryotic cell cycle progression, and unequivocal data implicate size control in sporulation and division of yeast (82,83). Mitogen induction of lymphocyte receptors for growth factors, including IL2 and transferrin, is not by itself sufficient for cell and nuclear enlargement. Lipoproteins suppress the secondary phase of cell enlargement, but not the initial phase, regardless of whether or not expression of these growth factor receptors is suppressed (Table 2).

Lipoproteins do not decrease overall RNA and protein synthesis that occur in mitogen-activated lymphocytes within the first 24 hr following mitogen stimulation. (However, cf. Refs. 84 and 85.) No inhibition of RNA synthesis was detected by Cuthbert and Lipsky (84) at any concentration of LDL, suggesting that the major part of RNA synthesis in stimulated cells continues regardless of where lipoproteins actually block cell cycle progression. There may be, however, proteins that are minor in mass or translated from low copy number mRNAs, but which at the same time are required for critical phases of the cell cycle, such as secondary cell and nuclear enlargement, DNA replication, or completion of the post-S phase of the cell cycle and cell division. These proteins could be suppressed by lipoproteins, an effect that would be hard to detect. Alternatively, lipoproteins may reduce transcription/translation of cell cycle-promoting proteins that occurs after the first 24 hr of the activation period. The effect of lipoproteins on RNA and protein synthetic behavior has not been characterized for this period.

The expression of receptors for growth factors indicates that activated lymphocytes have definitively entered G_1 and are competent to cycle. Cuthbert and Lipsky (86) and Scupham (87) reported that IL2-R and Tf-R expression are uninfluenced by LDL when activated lymphocytes are cultured in serum. Their experimental systems were quite different, supporting the validity of this result. Cuthbert and Lipsky (86) stimulated peripheral blood mononuclear cells or nonadherent cells with PHA, and cultured the stimulated cells in serum-containing medium prior to receptor measurement. Scupham (87) stimulated T cells with the oxidative enzymes NAGO, and cultured the stimulated cells with accessory cells (10:1 ratio). In SFM, lipoproteins can influence receptor expression. Scupham (87) correlated suppression by LDL of mitogen-induced DNA replication with suppression of IL2-R and Tf-R expression when the cells were cultured in

SFM containing low-transferrin concentrations (<50 μg/ml). This suppression by LDL was the same when IL-2 and transferrin receptors were measured at intervals between starting at 24 hr and ending at 96 hours after stimulation, indicating that the appearance of receptor-positive cells is not simply delayed by the presence of LDL.* The combined results of the two groups suggest that a factor in serum exists that somehow modulates the suppressive effects of lipoproteins.

DNA synthesis is the accepted indicator of the S phase of the cell cycle, although the transition of a lymphocyte from G_0 to S may require considerable expansion of the mitochondrial compartment (hence, replication of mitochondrial DNA). DNA replication induced by polyclonal mitogens is most sensitive to lipoprotein suppression at 72 hr and beyond (84,87). The early phase of DNA synthesis measurable between 48 and 60 hr—putatively corresponding to the first round of replication—is not as sensitive to lipoproteins and, in fact, is insensitive to relatively low concentrations of LDL. High concentrations of LDL, however, block DNA synthesis at 48 hr and at later times. These results and the kinetic analysis of PHA activation by Cuthbert and Lipsky (84) can suggest that stimulated lymphocytes exposed to low amounts of suppressive lipoproteins enter G_1 and traverse the G_1-S boundary and arrest at G_2M, whereas stimulated cells exposed to high amounts of lipoproteins arrest in G_0 or G_1 and do not reach the G_1-S transition point. We believe that this conclusion is premature and subject to modification, pending a careful cell cycle kinetics study in which the progression of individual cells is monitored as a function of time. The DNA synthesis measured at 48 hr is typically 10% of that at 72 hr. This low level of replication is consistent with the possibility that it occurs in an extranuclear compartment (i.e., mitochondrial). It is also possible that the more "activated" cells in the population are less susceptible to suppression by lipoproteins, and simply escape suppression in their first pass through the cycle. The most "activated" cells should reach S relatively early.

Important information is missing from Table 2. Immunosuppressive lipoproteins are those with the potential to suppress the synthesis of 3-hydroxy-3-methylglutaryl coenzyme A (HMGCoA) reductase, the enzyme controlling the flow of intermediates through the sterol biosynthetic pathway (88). However, the influence of lipoproteins on

---

*It should be noted that receptor expression is quantitated by binding of specific monoclonal antibodies, and the extent of binding of the antibodies to functional and nonfunctional receptors is probably equivalent. Thus, the results do not address the issue of the expression of *functional* receptors. Moreover, the density of expressed receptors per cell has not been determined.

HMGCoA reductase activity has not been correlated with suppression of lymphocyte proliferation. Furthermore, and in view of the crucial role of the IL2-IL2-R interaction in lymphocyte proliferation, regulation of IL2 production and utilization by lipoproteins should also be investigated.

Suppression of Early Activation Events Mediated by an Immunoregulatory Receptor

Chylomicrons (from rat mesenteric lymph), VLDL, IDL, and LDL suppress the events that occur in mitogen-induced lymphocytes within the first hr following mitogen stimulation and for as long as 6 hr thereafter. These events are enhanced cellular Ca^{2+} accumulation (23), enhanced metabolic labeling of PI (20,21), and enhanced accumulation of cyclic nucleotides (7,89). All three of these mitogen-stimulated biochemical events are suppressed to the same extent at the same lipoprotein dose (90). To investigate the early suppressive effect of lipoproteins, we have therefore used these three events interchangeably, and will henceforth refer to these biochemical processes collectively as the early activation events. When DNA replication and the early events are assayed under the same conditions (high cell density), DNA replication measured at 72 hr postmitogen is also inhibited by LDL, and the dose-dependent profile for its inhibition is roughly superimposable on that for inhibition of early events. Suppression of the early events by LDL is not due to a change in optimum conditions for mitogenic stimulation or in the timing at which a particular event occurs. Extracellular, ionized Ca^{2+} is required for the early activation events to occur, but suppression by lipoproteins does not decrease available Ca^{2+} since suppression is not prevented by the addition of excess Ca^{2+} to the medium. Although dibutyryl-cAMP also inhibits mitogen-activated early events, LDL do not elevate cellular cAMP (89) and therefore do not suppress via cAMP-dependent processes. Pairault et al. (91) reported that LDL activate liver membrane adenylate cyclase. The mechanism by which lipoproteins suppress the early events is not known. In the case of PHA mitogenesis, Hui and Harmony (20) suggested that LDL prevent mitogen-accelerated PI metabolism by inhibiting the PI-specific phospholipase C_2, which catalyzes hydrolysis of PI to DAG and inositol phosphate.

Suppression by lipoproteins of the mitogen-induced early events appears to be the result of the binding of lipoproteins to the lymphocyte surface. Internalization of bound lipoprotein from these binding sites is inefficient, suggesting that they are not situated in coated pits. The binding sites are referred to as the immunoregulatory receptors (61). These receptors recognize apo E (all isoforms), apo B-100 and apo B-48 (61,66,69), classifying them as apo E,B receptors as are the extrahepatic LDL receptors (92–94) and one class of the hepatic lipoprotein receptors (95,96). Suppression of the early events by lipoproteins is contingent on occupancy of the immunoregulatory receptors. This conclusion is supported by five lines of evidence:

1. Arginine-derivatized LDL do not bind to lymphocytes and are not suppressive (65). This result indicates that a suppressive constituent is not transferred to the cells from the lipoproteins.
2. The extent to which the receptors are occupied by lipoproteins correlates directly with the extent to which the mitogen-triggered early events are inhibited (97).
3. LDL-Sepharose complexes are as suppressive as uncomplexed LDL. Since the complexed forms of LDL cannot be internalized (97), internalization and degradation of lipoproteins are not required for suppression of mitogen-triggered early events.
4. The relative suppressive potencies of LDL and HDL_c correlate with their relative abilities to bind to the immunoregulatory receptors (61).
5. Heparin "rescues" the cellular response to mitogen, and rescue correlates with the removal of radiolabeled lipoproteins from the cell surface (97).

Important features of the immunoregulatory receptors were identified by studying the binding of LDL (human) that contain only apo B (B-100) and of HDL_c (cholesterol-induced dogs) that contain only apo E as protein constituents (61). Both classes of lipoproteins suppress PHA-induced lymphocyte activation by inhibiting the early activation events (e.g., Ca^{2+} accumulation) and the late event of DNA replication. On a molar basis, HDL_c are 3.5 times more effective than LDL in suppressing Ca^{2+} accumulation and 3.8 times more effective than LDL in suppressing DNA synthesis. These two classes of lipoproteins compete for the same receptors. The immunoregulatory receptors comprise a homogeneous class of binding sites that do not act cooperatively. The equilibrium binding parameters determined for LDL and HDL_c are presented in Table 3. Binding is essentially temperature independent, and the K_d for LDL is 2.0×10^{-7} M while that for HDL_c is 7.0 to 9.3×10^{-8} M. At saturation, 16,000 to 20,000 LDL particles and 5,500 to 6,700 HDL_c particles are bound per cell.

Since the extent of suppression of early events correlates with the extent of receptor occupancy, the increased effectiveness of HDL_c in suppressing the PHA-induced events is explained by the capacity of each HDL_c particle to bind simultaneously to more cell surface receptors than each LDL particle. Each HDL_c particle can occupy receptors at a ratio of roughly 4:1 relative to LDL. The slightly enhanced affinity of HDL_c for the receptors relative to that

Table 3 Plasma Lipoproteins Bind to Lymphocytes

	Cells[a]	K_d (*M*)		Number of sites occupied at saturation		Ref.
		4°C	37°C	4°C	37°C	
LDL (apo B-100)	NAC	2×10^{-7}	2×10^{-7}	15,800	20,000	61
HDL_c (apo E)	NAC	9×10^{-8}	7×10^{-8}	6,700	5,500	61
LDL-In	PBM	7×10^{-8}	ND[b]	4,900	ND	99,170
VLDL	Spleen[c]	1×10^{-8}	ND	31,000[d]	ND	105
	PBM	1×10^{-8}	ND	28,000[d]	ND	104

[a]Different human lymphocyte populations were used: NAC, non-adherent lymphocytes (about 95% lymphocytes); PBM, peripheral blood mononuclear cells (about 85% lymphocytes).
[b]ND, not determined.
[c]Rat spleen lymphocytes.
[d]Prior to binding, the cells were incubated at 37°C for 48 hours in lipoprotein-deficient serum. Binding of VLDL was not altered by preincubation.

of LDL is attributed to this multiple receptor occupancy. Simultaneous occupancy of multiple receptors by HDL_c can be explained by the fact that approximately 16 apo E molecules per HDL_c are available to bind to receptors.

The binding sites on the lymphocyte that are responsible for suppression of mitogen-triggered early events are clearly not the classic LDL receptors (LDL-R) responsible for cholesterol transport into cells and for maintenance of cholesterol homeostasis (4,5). There are, however, striking similarities. Most notable among these is the feature of multiple receptor occupancy of receptors by HDL_c relative to LDL (93,94). Also, the binding of lipoproteins to immunoregulatory and cholesterol transport receptors is facilitated by Ca^{2+} (97–99). Binding of lipoproteins to both classes of receptors is prevented or reversed by heparin (61,100) and prevented by modification of the basic amino acid residues of the lipoprotein-protein (65,101,102).

Significant differences between the cholesterol transport receptors and the immunoregulatory receptors exist, however, leaving no doubt about their separate identities. Lymphocytes from patients with the homozygous form of familial hypercholesterolemia (FH or type II hypercholesterolemia) lack classic LDL-R (4) but have immunoregulatory receptors since lymphocytes from these subjects are responsive to regulation of mitogen-induced biochemical alterations and DNA replication by lipoproteins (90,99,103). The number of immunoregulatory receptors is not regulated by cholesterol or oxysterol (99), whereas the biosynthesis of the LDL-R is tightly controlled by cholesterol-oxysterol (4). There is a difference of nearly two orders of magnitude between the strength of the interaction of the lipoproteins LDL and HDL_c with the cholesterol transport receptors (93) and with the lymphocyte receptors (61), the lymphocyte receptors having the lower affinity for lipoproteins. In addition, multiple occupancy of receptors by HDL_c increases the affinity of HDL_c binding to the classic LDL-R by a factor of 23 (93), but only increases that of HDL_c binding to the lymphocyte receptors by a factor of 2 relative to LDL (61). Finally, purified, delipidated apolipoproteins do not bind to the LDL-R but do bind to the immunoregulatory receptors (66). Binding parameters have not been determined for the apolipoproteins.

The number of receptors for LDL and HDL_c per cell is somewhat greater than that determined for LDL-In (Table 3), an apo E-containing IDL, but about 50% of that for VLDL. The differences in receptor number are not considered significant since the cell preparations used were different. Curtiss and Edgington (99) utilized human peripheral blood mononuclear cells (consisting of an appreciable number of monocytes); Yi et al. (104,105) studied both human peripheral blood mononuclear cells and rat splenocytes (consisting of macrophages in addition to lymphocytes). Monocytes also have membrane receptors for lipoproteins (106–110). In our studies (61), the binding of LDL and HDL_c to nonadherent lymphocytes (>98%) was investigated. Since suppression by lipoproteins is not species specific, the receptors on cells from different species are most likely identical or quite similar in structure. The conclusion of Curtiss and Edgington (99) that lymphocytes have distinct receptors for LDL-In and for LDL, both of which are immunosuppressive, does not contradict the assumption that there is one class of immunoregulatory receptors. These investigators measured the binding of lipoproteins to peripheral blood mononuclear cells preincubated for 48 hr in lipoprotein-deficient serum, conditions that amplify the number of LDL-R on leukocytes (111). Probably the cells used in their binding studies simultaneously expressed both receptors, a possibility supported by their finding that binding of LDL but not LDL-In is greatly reduced by inclusion of cholesterol or 25-hydroxycholesterol in the preincubation medium. Thus, LDL may bind with higher affinity to the LDL-R, while LDL-In bind with higher affinity to the immunoregulatory receptors.

The role of the immunoregulatory receptors in the suppression of mid-cycle and late activation events by lipoproteins has not been clearly established. Certainly, the lipoproteins that are the most potent in suppressing mitogen-induced early events are those that most effectively suppress DNA replication and proliferation. There is, however, uncertainty regarding the role of early biochemical changes in stimulated lymphocyte proliferation. This uncertainty is compounded by our failure thus far to study suppression of early, mid-cycle, and late events under the same conditions, thereby deriving cause-effect relationships. In addition, mitogen stimulation induces the high-affinity LDL-R (103), allowing the balance of different types of lipoprotein-cell interactions to shift as the activated cells traverse the cycle. Meaningful approaches to the question of the role of immunoregulatory receptors in control of the lymphocyte cell cycle by lipoproteins mandate knowledge of both the structure of the immunoregulatory receptors and the development of reagents that interfere specifically with the lipoprotein-receptor interaction.

Suppression of Mid-Cycle and Late Events by Lipoproteins Relieved by Accessory Cells and Transferrin

The identification of situations in which lipoproteins are not suppressive or in which the suppression is reversed is an alternative to characterizing suppression by assessment of the influence of lipoproteins on lymphocyte activation landmarks. At least two such situations exist: suppression by lipoproteins can be decreased by increasing the number of accessory cells and by increasing the concentration of transferrin in the culture.

Modulation by accessory cells: Accessory cells, isolated by glass adherence or by counterflow centrifugation, are >85% monocytes based on monoclonal antibody staining (112). Suppression of mitogen-induced T-cell activation by lipoproteins decreases dramatically as the ratio of accessory cells to T cells in the cultures is increased to 1:1 (110,113). Suppression by lipoproteins is reduced regardless of mitogen concentration and type, e.g., plant lectins or oxidative enzymes over a wide dose range. To influence the extent of suppression by lipoproteins of T-cell proliferation, the accessory cells must be viable and present during the 24 hr immediately following mitogen addition. It is within this same time period that lipoproteins exert their inhibitory action (58,85) and accessory cell function is most important (114). Accessory cells also decrease the extent of suppression by apolipoproteins (110). Accessory cells isolated from normal subjects and those isolated from subjects with the homozygous form of FH are equally effective in modulating suppression by lipoproteins, suggesting that the phenomenon is independent of the high-affinity, sterol-regulated LDL-R.

The accessory cells bind, endocytize, and degrade too little lipoprotein to account for reduced suppression by a decrease in the effective concentration of the suppressors. Okano et al. (110) found that only 0.3 to 1.1% of the ^{125}I-VLDL (30 μg as protein) incubated with 1.25 × 10^6 cells at a T cell:accessory cell ratio of 1:1 is degraded in 72 hr. Furthermore, paraformaldehyde-fixed and -unfixed accessory cells bind the same amount of lipoproteins, but the fixed cells do not reduce lipoprotein suppression. Although the suppressive potency of lipoproteins is occasionally reduced by their preincubation with accessory cells or with activated T cells plus accessory cells, direct chemical modification of the lipoproteins cannot be the major mechanism whereby suppression by lipoproteins is reduced. Medium conditioned by oxidative enzyme-stimulated cells can also reduce the extent of suppression by lipoproteins, suggesting the importance of a soluble lymphokine or monokine in the accessory cell effect. Neither the active factor (although IL1 and IL2 have been eliminated from the list of candidates) nor the cell that secretes this factor has been identified. The soluble factor, like the accessory cells from which it may be secreted, does not directly alter the structure of the suppressive lipoproteins. It may alter the cell surface to prevent a deleterious lipoprotein-cell interaction, prevent or reverse the lipoprotein block of a key cellular process or pathway, or, if the lipoproteins complex with the soluble factor, competitively reverse the effect of the lipoproteins. Lymphokines have been reported (108,115) to reduce the interaction of lipoproteins with receptors on monocyte-macrophages.

It is intriguing that accessory cells can also reduce the extent to which lipoproteins suppress proliferation of cells of the IL2-dependent murine cytotoxic T-cell line, CTLL-2 (Macy, McCarthy, and Harmony, unpublished). Proliferation of CTLL-2 cells cultured in the absence of lipoproteins is not influenced by accessory cells, a result consistent with their progression through the cell cycle from G_1 through M and back to G_1 again without entering G_0. Modulation of suppression of CTLL-2 proliferation by accessory cells occurs over the same range of accessory cell number as does modulation of suppression of activated peripheral blood T cells. Erythrocytes have no similar modulatory properties on suppression by lipoproteins. Suppression of IL2-dependent CTLL-2 proliferation by lipoproteins can, in addition, be reduced by medium conditioned by oxidative enzyme-stimulated T cells cultured with accessory cells (116).

Modulation by transferrin: Lipoprotein suppression of IL2-R and Tf-R expression by stimulated lymphocytes occurs in SFM but not in serum-containing medium. One difference is the transferrin level of the medium. Our SFM typically contains 10 μg/ml transferrin, sufficient to support cell proliferation, while serum-supplemented medium contains about 75 μg/ml transferrin. Consequently, we investigated the effect of transferrin on suppression and discovered that this growth factor has a profound influence on both mitogenesis and suppression of mitogenesis by plasma lipoproteins.

In SFM in the absence of lipoproteins, an increase in the concentration of transferrin enhances lymphocyte activation as determined by an increase in the number of Tf-R-positive cells and in the number of cells reaching S phase (87). Transferrin, at concentrations greater than 10 μg/ml, has no similar influence on the number of cells expressing IL2-R, which implies that the Tf-R is subject to regulation by factors other than IL2. In addition, increased transferrin prevents or reverses suppression of lymphocyte activation and proliferation by lipoproteins, regardless of whether the cells are stimulated by PHA (86) or NAGO (87). Increasing the level of transferrin prevents suppression by LDL of both the secondary phase of cell enlargement and DNA synthesis (87). Transferrin protection against LDL suppression of these two responses correlates well with transferrin prevention of suppression of the number of cells expressing the Tf-R. When lymphocyte proliferation is suppressed by 25-hydroxycholesterol, increasing the amount of transferrin has no similar influence on suppression. LDL also suppress expression of the IL2-R when low but not high concentrations of transferrin are included in the SFM.

Serum concentrations of transferrin, around 75 μg/ml, are just sufficient to relieve LDL suppression of the IL2-R and the Tf-R. Thus, there is no effect of LDL on Tf-R expression in serum-containing medium. In contrast, LDL do suppress the later blastogenic and DNA synthesis responses in both serum-free and serum-supplemented cultures. Further increases in transferrin levels are protective against these later suppressive effects under *both* culture conditions. Using these data, a gradient of transferrin effects along the events of G_1 is established. A low level (10 μg/ml) of transferrin is sufficient to permit cell proliferation. At this level, lipoproteins suppress Tf-R expression as well as later events. A higher level of transferrin (50 to 75 μg/ml), equivalent to that found in serum-containing cultures, moves the suppressive effect forward along G_1. Suppression of Tf-R expression is relieved, but the later events of blastogenesis and entry into S are still suppressed. Finally, a still higher concentration of transferrin (100 to 200 μg/ml) will protect against lipoprotein suppression of these later events. Therefore, we conclude that a critical difference between lipoprotein suppression in serum-free and serum-supplemented medium lies in transferrin concentration. The role of transferrin in modulating lipoprotein suppression will be of critical importance in developing the model.

When lymphocytes isolated from most donors are stimulated by mitogen, the proliferation of cells in cultures established in the presence of *low* LDL concentration and high transferrin concentration is enhanced relative to that of cells maintained in control cultures lacking LDL. Thus, LDL under appropriate conditions can actually have a growth-*promoting* effect. Suppression by LDL is prevented when lymphocytes from donors with homozygous FH are stimulated under comparable conditions (103), but there is no similar enhancement of growth. These results indicate that the LDL-R is required for augmentation of activation and proliferation by LDL at high transferrin concentrations, but is not required for transferrin prevention against suppression. The increase in proliferation that occurs when cells are cultured with low levels of LDL and high levels of transferrin is most certainly due to an increase in the number of responding cells in the population. The component of LDL responsible for augmented proliferation has not been identified; it may be cholesterol functioning as mevalonate diversion to a product(s) essential for the proliferative pathway (88).

Lipoprotein suppression of IL2-induced proliferation of the mouse cytotoxic CTLL-2 cells is also prevented by high concentrations of transferrin (McCarthy, Macy, and Harmony, unpublished). As is the case for NAGO-stimulated peripheral blood T lymphocytes, lipoproteins suppress DNA replication in CTLL-2 cells when transferrin levels are below 50 μg/ml. No suppression, and often augmentation, of the DNA synthetic response occurs when transferrin is present at a concentration of 100 μg/ml and greater. The CTLL-2 cell proliferation that occurs at the higher transferrin levels in the presence of lipoproteins remains dependent on IL2. Moreover, high concentrations of transferrin have a growth-enhancing effect on CTLL-2 lymphocytes that is independent of lipoproteins. This effect of transferrin is evident when CTLL-2 cells are cultured in SFM containing purified IL2 or conditioned medium (crude IL2). The transferrin-induced increase in the cellular response is most pronounced when the amount of transferrin present is limiting (10 μg/ml).

Possible mechanisms for the transferrin effect include chelation by transferrin of a metal ion instrumental in the suppressive mechanism; interference by lipoproteins with transferrin (or iron) utilization when transferrin levels are low; interference by transferrin with the binding and processing of LDL via the immunoregulatory receptors; direct correction by transferrin of the key lipoprotein-inhibited cellular process; or a transferrin-induced switch in the state of the system from one dependent on a lipoprotein-suppressed reaction or product to one independent of the same. With regard to the latter possibility, transferrin is proposed (117,118) to be directly mitogenic in some systems. Furthermore, a transforming gene associated with uncontrolled lymphocyte proliferation has been isolated recently from DNA from chicken lymphoma cells, and the nucleotide sequence of this gene indicates that it encodes a protein that is homologous to the amino-terminal sequence of transferrin (119).

Suppressive Lipoprotein Constituents

A large number of naturally occurring compounds with diverse structures modulate the immune system, including glycolipids, phospholipids, oxidized sterols, $\beta(1\rightarrow3)$glucans, retinoids, thymic hormones, proteins such as interferon and α-fetoprotein, proteolytic cleavage fragments of plasma and dietary proteins such as albumin, complement, and casein, and certain viruses. The plasma lipoproteins fall within this broad category of suppressors and, in fact, contain some of the other compounds cited above (e.g., glycolipids, phospholipids, oxidized sterols).

In predicting a suppressive mechanism, down-regulation of the cellular sterol pathway by lipoproteins is an attractive hypothesis. A functioning sterol biosynthetic pathway is required for cell proliferation, and cholesterol biosynthesis and HMGCoA reductase activity are elevated in proliferating cells including lymphocytes (80,88, 120–124). Lipoproteins can contain oxysterols that are potent regulators of sterol biosynthesis (125). The oxysterols may be present as a result of autooxidation (25-hydroxycholesterol) or enzymatic metabolism (16-hydroxycholesterol, 7-α-hydroxycholesterol, 32-hydroxycholesterol, etc.). The elegant and seminal investigations of Brown and Goldstein (4,88) have led to an understanding of the cellular path by which LDL, and specifically LDL-sterols, down-regulate the synthesis of HMGCoA reductase and suppress squalene synthetase. This path is contingent on the presence and function of the LDL-R. The LDL-R pathway does exist in lymphocytes, and it is regulated by LDL (111). However, since lymphocytes isolated from donors with homozygous FH and stimulated with mitogens are suppressed by lipoproteins (90,99,103), suppression is not dependent on the delivery of lipoproteins by the LDL-R pathway.

A great deal of work has focused on what "the" suppressive component of lipoproteins might be. Results have pointed in both directions—toward a protein component and toward a lipid component. As indicated above, the amount of apo E on a lipoprotein particle is correlated with its suppressive potency. On the other hand, sterol (i.e., oxysterol) inactivation of HMGCoA reductase has been implicated in blocking the cell's progress through G_1, although the sterol effect perhaps cannot be attributed solely to inhibition of the cholesterol biosynthetic pathway. It is premature to conclude that the protein constituents contribute more (or less) than the lipids to the establishment of the suppressed state. The weight of the evidence does, however, favor the importance of a lipoprotein-lipid, particularly when the culture conditions are optimum for the responses of DNA replication and proliferation (low cell density). Nonetheless, apo E and apo B must direct the relevant interaction of the lipoproteins with the cells. Apolipoproteins are capable of suppressing lymphocyte proliferation, although their suppressive potency has not been assessed in the absence of serum lipids. Interestingly, apo E suppression cannot be reversed by increasing the transferrin concentration (86).

If a lipoprotein-lipid is involved in suppression of mid-cycle and late activation events in proliferation-optimized cultures, which lipid is it? Yachnin and Hsu (126) speculated that oxysterols account for the suppressive potency of plasma lipoproteins. Circumstantial evidence is on their side; certainly no one has demonstrated conclusively that oxysterols are not involved. Curtiss and Edgington (127–129) concluded that the suppressive lipid is not an oxysterol, an unesterified fatty acid, or a neutral lipid. Their evidence against a suppressive lipoprotein-oxysterol is indirect: the lack of protection by mevalonate, the absence of inhibition of E-rosette formation, and no loss of suppressive potency following starch-heptane extraction. Cuthbert and Lipsky (86) have argued that, since transferrin prevents suppression by both cholesterol and LDL, and since they have not identified any suppressive LDL from which lymphocytes cannot be protected by transferrin, "cholesterol" is the major lipoprotein suppressive constituent. We (87) and others (130,131) have not observed suppression by cholesterol of lymphocyte activation, suggesting that the cholesterol employed by Cuthbert and Lipsky was contaminated with oxysterols. The oxysterol explanation satisfactorily accounts for one of the unexplained characteristics of suppression by lipoproteins, namely the variability of lipoprotein suppressive potency. Lipoproteins of the same density class isolated from different donors, as well as those isolated from the same donor at different times, vary in ability to suppress mid-cycle and late activation events by as much as an order of magnitude, in spite of the great similarity in their chemical composition (84,116).

The oxysterol explanation is, however, not without its flaws. Transferrin does not prevent 25-hydroxycholesterol from suppressing NAGO-activated lymphocyte enlargement and DNA replication (87), whereas it does prevent suppression by lipoproteins of these events. In addition, mevalonate not only fails to prevent lipoprotein suppression of DNA synthesis in activated peripheral blood T cells (84,127), but also of the mid-cycle event of blastogenesis (87). On the other hand, mevalonate protection should not be taken as an absolute indication of oxysterol-induced suppression. In none of the studies was the actual activity of the sterol pathway measured, so it is not known whether it was suppressed by lipoproteins. Nor is it known whether, if suppressed, synthesis of cholesterol and nonsterol products was restored by mevalonate. When suppression of lymphocyte proliferation by oxysterols is tested for mevalonate protection, the extent of protection ranges from partial but significant (126,127) to none (87). The concentrations of oxysterols in these experiments were comparable. Variability in the outcome of these experiments may be due to differences in cell composition, cell density, and serum concentration, all of which influence oxysterol suppression (126). Oxysterol structure is also important, and distinct oxysterols differentially influence cellular processes (132–134). To summarize, any hypothesis that accounts for suppression by lipoproteins cannot ignore the probability of a suppressive lipoprotein-oxysterol.

The Lipoprotein Target: Mitogen-Responsive Lymphocyte or Accessory Cell?

Is lymphocyte activation suppressed by plasma lipoproteins because the stimulated, cycling lymphocytes are incapable of progressing through the cell cycle, or because the accessory cells are incapable of delivering crucial signals required for cell cycle progression, or both? Lymphocytes are certainly one cellular target for suppression by lipoproteins. Suppression by lipoproteins of mitogen-induced early events such as the PI response appears to be a direct result of the interaction of lipoproteins and apolipoproteins with lymphocytes. In addition to evidence presented above indicating that the extent of suppression correlates with the extent to which lipoproteins occupy the immunoregulatory receptors, other lines of evidence support this view. The PI response occurs in T cells, and is independent of accessory cells (79). This T-cell response is suppressed in populations of highly purified T lymphocytes ($\sim$99%) to the same extent as it is suppressed in peripheral blood mononuclear cells ($\sim$85% T cells) (Macy and Harmony, unpublished data). In addition, the proliferation of lymphocyte cell lines, such as the IL2-dependent CTLL-2 line, is suppressed by lipoproteins.

Curtiss and Edgington (135) also concluded that the potentially responsive lymphocyte is the cell that is directly suppressed by lipoproteins. They, and later Fugii and Edgington (62), found that LDL-In, depending on their concentration, irreversibly suppress the DNA synthetic response of mitogen- and allogeneic cell-stimulated lymphocytes. The suppressed state is achieved by a 24-hr preincubation of peripheral blood mononuclear cells or lymphocyte-enriched cell populations with lipoproteins in the absence of stimuli. Raskova and Raska (163), studying VLDL obtained from patients with uremia, reached the same conclusion. Their VLDL are distinguished from LDL-In on the basis of adsorption to conA-Sepharose. Irreversible suppression is reported to occur without cytotoxicity. However, in contrast to the results of Curtiss and Edgington (135) and Fugii and Edgington (62), Cuthbert and Lipsky (84) as well as Nakayasu et al. (136) failed to find evidence for a permanently suppressed state induced by preincubation of LDL or VLDL with either peripheral blood mononuclear cells or lymphocyte-enriched cell populations. Therefore, the situation is confused: do or do not lipoproteins inactivate cells in the absence of mitogen?

We approached the lipoprotein cell target problem with a strategy similar to that of Curtiss and Edgington (135). However, we reached a different conclusion. The accessory cell, or at least a cell type within the accessory cell population, is suppressed by lipoproteins (136). Accessory cells (>85% monocytes) were isolated from peripheral blood mononuclear cells by a 1-hr glass adherence step or by counterflow centrifugation, and their functional capacity was determined by their ability to facilitate the activation and proliferation of T lymphocytes stimulated by polyclonal mitogens PHA, conA, and NAGO. Preincubation of accessory cells with VLDL or LDL for 24 hr inactivates accessory cell function without killing the cells and without altering the cell phenotypic distribution (including the percent of cells that is DR-positive). Accessory cell function remains suppressed when the cells are preincubated an additional 24 hr after the lipoproteins are removed and prior to their addition to stimulated T lymphocytes. Lipoprotein-preincubated accessory cells remain viable during this entire 48-hr period, indicating that cell death does not explain the loss of cell function. The extent to which accessory cell function is suppressed depends on the amounts of serum and lipoproteins included in the preincubation. Increasing the serum concentration protects accessory cell function. The inability of lipoprotein-exposed accessory cells to facilitate T-cell activation is not due to suppressed IL1 production since control- and lipoprotein-preincubated cells produce identical quantities of IL1 and since the addition of partially purified IL1 does not restore lymphocyte responses. In contrast, preincubation of T lymphocytes (>99% OKT3-positive cells) with lipoproteins does not influence their responsive capacity.

To determine what type of accessory function is lost, mid-cycle and late events were compared in mitogen-activated lymphocytes cultured with control- and lipoprotein-preincubated accessory cells (McCarthy and Harmony, unpublished). The initial blastogenic response at 24 hr is not suppressed. However, the number of cells expressing I12-R and Tf-R is significantly reduced as is the number that have undergone the secondary blastogenic response by 72 hr. Suppression of accessory cell function is attributed to a decrease in IL2 production or utilization by cultures containing VLDL-preincubated accessory cells since exogenous medium conditioned by activated cells containing IL2 and purified IL2 bypass the block along the activation pathway and allows control levels of T-cell activation. The conditioned medium is *not* effective in enhancing the T-cell responses induced by mitogen if *no* VLDL-preincubated accessory cells are added, however. Since IL2 enhances the expression of the IL2-R (137) and since IL2 utilization precedes Tf-R expression (56), the responsiveness of the lymphocytes to factors in conditioned medium indicates that the lymphocytes incubated with VLDL-treated accessory cells have the potential to express IL2-R. The results suggest, therefore, that there is more than one type of accessory cell help in this system, and lipoproteins inactivate only one of the required functions. The medium conditioned by activated cells may provide additional IL2 or an IL2 utilization-promoting factor, or both, whereas the VLDL-preincubated accessory cells provide sufficient signal to establish the IL2-dependent state in the mitogen-stimulated lymphocytes. A very exciting recent finding (McCarthy and Harmony, unpublished) is that transferrin, included in the lipoprotein-accessory cell preincubation, not only protects accessory cell function in the presence of lipoproteins, but enhances it in the absence of lipoproteins.

Based on our results, it is tempting to speculate that the primary target of suppression by lipoproteins in mixed cell cultures of responding lymphocytes plus accessory cells is an accessory cell. Levy and co-workers (12) found that LDL suppress the expression of procoagulant activity by monocytes, substantiating the possibility of a lipoprotein-accessory cell interaction that alters the function of the cell. This interpretation is also consistent with the capacity of accessory cells to reduce the extent of suppression by lipoproteins. Lipoproteins are most suppressive when the number of accessory cells per culture is low, and become progressively less effective as the number of accessory cells increases. It is possible that, in systems in which polyclonal mitogens are used, accessory cells are constitutively capable of delivering certain signals (e.g., those for IL2-R and IL2 induction) to activated lymphocytes, but must respond to lymphokines before they deliver other signals (e.g., those for facilitating IL2 utilization). Therefore, the lipoprotein-suppressed accessory cells may fail to differentiate sufficiently to offer this latter type of help in response to signals from mitogen-activated lymphocytes.

Why do our results, which implicate the accessory cell as the lipoprotein target, seemingly contradict those of Curtiss and Edgington (135) and Fujii and Edgington (62), which implicate the responding lymphocyte? And why do we and others fail to obtain significant irreversible suppression when peripheral blood mononuclear cells are preincubated with lipoproteins? First, the second question. Achievement of a permanently suppressed state will depend on the suppressive potency of the lipoproteins. Lipoproteins of d $\leqslant 1.063$ g/ml isolated from certain donors are highly suppressive, while those from other donors are hardly suppressive. Nakayasu and colleagues (136) found that accessory cell function is readily inactivated during a preincubation with lipoproteins only when the lipoproteins are highly suppressive. Achievement of a permanently suppressed state will also depend on the cellular composition of the preincubated mononuclear population. When the number of accessory cells is relatively high (5 to 20%), the chance that accessory function will be suppressed is low, since only a few accessory cells are required for an optimum lymphocyte response to a polyclonal mitogen such as PHA.

The first issue, the apparent disagreement between our results and those of Curtiss and Edgington, is more difficult to explain satisfactorily. It is easy and probably incorrect to conclude that VLDL and LDL irreversibly ablate an important accessory cell function, whereas LDL-In irreversibly suppress mitogen-responsive lymphocytes. Rather, the real difference may be in the definition of the cell populations. As with accessory cells, Curtiss and Edgington (135) use adherent macrophages derived from blood monocytes during a 6-day incubation in vitro. Their responding cells are nonadherent and nonphagocytic lymphocytes, a population that no doubt includes some accessory cells. The nonadherent cells are permanently suppressed by preincubation with LDL-In, whereas the macrophages are indifferent to preincubation with lipoproteins. The number of accessory cells in their lymphocyte-enriched population is low so that mitogen-induced lymphocyte DNA replication is enhanced—particularly at low mitogen concentration—by addition of macrophages. However, the accessory cells contaminating the lymphocytes may be uniquely sensitive to lipoproteins. These accessory cells may be more effective than macrophages in facilitating IL2 utilization, the function we suggest to be suppressed by lipoproteins. The macrophages, on the other hand, are insensitive to lipoproteins, but may provide help that is unrelated to IL2 utilization but nonetheless important.

To summarize, both lymphocytes and accessory cells are susceptible to suppression by lipoproteins. In in vitro systems reconstituted from lymphocytes and accessory cells it will be difficult to assign relative degrees of susceptibility of accessory cells versus lymphocytes to suppression. The contribution from each type of suppressed cell to the overall level of suppression in the culture will surely depend on the culture conditions. The presence of lymphocytes that enlarge in response to mitogenic challenge but express few receptors for IL2 and transferrin suggests a block in signal transmission from accessory cells. The presence of lymphocytes that enlarge in response to mitogen and express growth factor receptors suggests a block in progression of the lymphocytes through the latter stages of the cell cycle.

MECHANISM OF SUPPRESSION OF LYMPHOCYTE ACTIVATION BY LIPOPROTEINS: AN HYPOTHESIS

We propose a model to account for suppression of lymphocyte activation by plasma lipoproteins. This model, illustrated in Fig. 2, considers suppression of early accessory cell-independent activation processes, and relates suppression of accessory cell-dependent processes to the effects of plasma lipoproteins on late events occurring in the activated lymphocytes. The model is proposed to provide a conceptual framework for further experiment, not to suggest that solutions to many of the fundamental problems in this system have been found. Cause and effect have not been adequately distinguished to validate this model. For example, the expression of IL2-R and Tf-R is considered indicative of the entry of activated lymphocytes into the G_1 phase of the cycle and therefore of the receipt of accessory cell help by activated lymphocytes. Accessory cells may indeed be required to induce IL2-R expression, but the maintenance of the

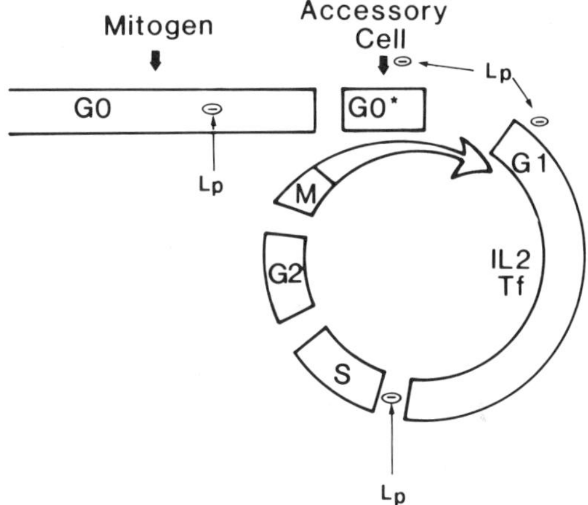

Fig. 2 Control of the lymphocyte cell cycle by lipoproteins (Lp). Plasma lipoproteins and their apoliproteins, E and B, regulate the transduction of activation signals by cells in G_0; interfere with the communication from accessory cells which is necessary for cells to progress through G_1; and prevent cells from crossing the G_1/S boundary.

receptor at the cell membrane depends on other processes occurring in the activation system, and notably on the induction and utilization of IL2 (137). Induction of IL2 biosynthesis and secretion also requires accessory cell help. Little definitive molecular information is therefore available from a static measurement of presence versus absence of a particular activation event or marker.

The Model

The model proposes three distinct control points at which lipoproteins (or their suppressive constituents) act: (1) at G_0, (2) between G_0* and G_1 or early in G_1, and (3) during G_1 to prevent entry into S. This rich regulatory capacity of plasma lipoproteins is unique in cell biology. The first and third control points result from inhibition by lipoproteins of the responsive lymphocyte, while the second control point results from inhibition by lipoproteins of the accessory cell. A reasonable and consistent explanation of suppression by lipoproteins at the second and third points is that the lipoproteins interfere with transferrin utilization. For control point 2, lipoproteins interfere with transferrin utilization by accessory cells; at control point 3, by activated lymphocytes. Thus, the lipoproteins' target is the accessory cell, the responding lymphocyte, or both, depending on the conditions of the culture. Transferrin is suggested to play two distinct roles in this system: provider of essential iron and maintainer of the autocrine loop of growth stimulation.

The Supporting Evidence

Lipoproteins and apolipoproteins suppress recruitment of activated lymphocytes (control point 1). This $G_0 \rightarrow G_0^*$ block is the direct result of the binding of lipoproteins to immunoregulatory receptors on the lymphocytes. The evidence for this conclusion has been summarized above. The fact that lipoproteins suppress the early events that are stimulated in lymphocytes by the oxidative enzymes prior to the addition of lipoproteins indicates that it is the transduction of the mitogenic signal that is inhibited. The signal delivered by the oxidative enzymes is a covalent modification of the lymphocyte cell membrane. Measurement of signal transduction requires special conditions that are not conducive to progression of the activated lymphocytes through the cell cycle. Therefore, an understanding of the relative significance of this block requires additional new information about the precise roles played by these early biochemical processes in progression of lymphocytes through the cell cycle.

In a second control mechanism, lipoproteins prevent the accessory cell from delivering a signal(s) essential for further progression of activated lymphocytes. A cell in G_0^* (or early in G_1) not receiving this additional information will return to G_0. The signal that is missing is possibly a secreted soluble factor, but it is not IL1. This control point seems to be the primary block by lipoproteins operating when cells are cultured in serum-free medium containing low amounts of transferrin, and also in SFM and in serum-containing medium when the cultures of T cells contain few accessory cells. Five pieces of evidence support a lipoprotein-imposed block directed against the accessory cell:

1. To suppress lymphocyte activation, lipoproteins must be present in culture during that time period following mitogenic stimulation in which accessory cell help is required.
2. Few mitogen-activated lymphoblasts, indicative, we believe, of the G_0 to G_0^* (or early G_1) transition, express receptors for either IL2 or transferrin in SFM-low transferrin. This result suggests that the activated cells did not receive an important signal from accessory cells in the population.
3. The activated lymphoblasts are capable of receiving signals from accessory cells. Addition of more accessory cells to the population significantly reduces the extent of suppression by lipoproteins. The added accessory cells are effective even when the lymphoblasts have had nearly 24 hr to interact with suppressive lipoproteins. Furthermore, the magnitude of the

DNA synthetic response at 72 hr, assessed after a short thymidine pulse to produce a measurement proportional to the number of responding cells (138), is the same regardless of whether the additional accessory cells are added at 1, 12, or 24 hr. This result suggests that the cells are activated and remain activated for at least 24 hr. The number of accessory cells necessary to reduce the suppression by lipoproteins significantly is in excess of that required for optimum cell proliferation when PHA but not NAGO is the activator.

4. The accessory cells can be directly inactivated by lipoproteins. Preincubation of the accessory cells with plasma lipoproteins suppresses one of their important functions, and this function remains suppressed after the lipoproteins are removed.
5. Increasing the transferrin concentration ablates suppression by lipoproteins of IL2-R and Tf-R expression by lymphoblasts, indicative of restoration of complete accessory cell-lymphocyte communication. Transferrin also protects accessory cells from suppression by lipoproteins during a preincubation period. By implication, accessory cell function may be dependent on transferrin utilization, and lipoproteins may interfere with this utilization.

Control point 3 is just preceding entry of fully activated cells into S. The evidence for block 3 is the presence in the culture of activated cells, by the criteria of size and activation markers (IL2-R, Tf-R, and by inference IL2), which do not divide. When mitogen-activated peripheral blood T cells are cultured with accessory cells (ratio of T cells to accessory cells of at least 10:1) in serum-containing medium, block 3 is relatively more important than block 2. Block 3 also occurs when IL2-dependent lymphocytes are cultured with crude IL2 in the presence of lipoproteins. IL-2 dependent CTLL-2 cells respond reasonably synchronously to IL2 through the first two turns of the cell cycle (116). The cells incubated with lipoproteins do not reach the first S phase. Transferrin also prevents or reverses the lipoprotein-imposed block at position 3. Thus, utilization of transferrin by activated T lymphocytes may also be inhibited by lipoproteins.

The Interrelationship Between Cells, Lipoproteins, and Transferrin

A complex interrelationship between cells, transferrin, and lipoproteins determines whether the response of the cells is suppressed, unaltered, or augmented by the lipoproteins in the culture. Table 4 lists experimental situations that tend to favor suppression by lipoproteins. Suppression by lipoproteins depends on a number of factors,

Table 4 Conditions That Favor Suppression by Lipoproteins

Low cell density
Limited number of accessory cells
Serum-free medium
Low concentrations of transferrin
High concentrations of lipoproteins
High inherent lipoprotein suppressive potency

including the composition of the lipoproteins and the susceptibility of the cells in the culture. The former issue has been dealt with above, both in terms of the oxidized sterol effect and the correlation of the presence of apolipoprotein E with suppressive potential of the lipoprotein. The latter issue has been alluded to, however, the issue in its entirety is quite complex. There are several points to consider.

Transferrin

High concentrations of transferrin can double the number of lymphocytes responding in SFM to polyclonal activators. This is also true of CTLL-2 cells responding to IL2 in SFM. Increasing amounts of transferrin push the events suppressed by lipoproteins further and further along the cell cycle, up to the point (100 to 200 μg/ml) where suppression is entirely prevented. Transferrin does not ablate suppression by lipoproteins by interacting with them in culture to remove or neutralize a suppressive lipoprotein component (86,87).

Cell Density

Cells cultured at low density are suppressed by lipoproteins, whereas those cultured at high density are much less subject to this suppression. This is the case even when the number of lipoprotein particles per cell is held constant. High cell density encourages cell-cell interactions, especially for cells that prefer communal living such as activated lymphocytes. Soluble mediators can transfer directly from one cell to another in a multicell cluster without diffusing into the medium to be diluted. This type of metabolic cooperation is predicted to lessen the need for any comitogens, and consequently to reduce the susceptibility of the system to suppression by lipoproteins.

Other Serum Factors

There are at least two functionally identifiable factors in serum or conditioned medium that modulate the growth responses of cells in culture. One allows lipoproteins to manifest their suppressive effect (a permissive factor). The other, possibly acting as a comitogen, allows for optimal growth, perhaps through the mechanism of enhancing IL2 utilization. The permissive factor is probably a glycosaminoglycan. Activated lymphocytes produce and secrete glycosaminoglycans (139) as well as a heparan sulfate endoglycosidase (140).

In the light of this information, we propose a speculative set of interactions to account for the complex effects of lipoproteins, transferrin, IL2, cell density, and various serum factors including a possible comitogen and a lipoprotein-suppression permissive factor. These interactions revolve around the transferrin receptor. Cells will grow at fairly low doses of transferrin, although transferrin at higher doses has a profound effect on recruitment of cells into the cycle and on lipoprotein suppression of cell activation. This argues for the existence of a low-affinity transferrin receptor (Tf-R'), which we further argue acts as the immunoregulatory receptor in this system. The proliferation-enhancing and antisuppressive effects of transferrin may therefore be explained by the interaction of these growth-regulating substances with the same receptors. We thus propose that the receptors for transferrin on lymphoid cells can exist in two states: low and high affinity (Fig. 3). A high-affinity Tf-R is responsible for delivering iron to the cells through a well-characterized mechanism. Transferrin binds to the Tf-R, is relocated to specialized regions of the membrane known as coated pits, is endocytized while bound to the Tf-R, and is recycled back to the cell surface with the Tf-R after its iron dissociates in the acidic environment of the endosome. This is the established high-affinity transferrin pathway of iron delivery. It appears to be relatively unimportant in freshly isolated accessory cells and in nonproliferating lymphocytes, but important in differentiated macrophages and in proliferating lymphocytes.

The Physiological Importance of High Concentrations of Transferrin

What then is the proposed function of the low-affinity Tf-R'? The Tf-R' may be requisite for production of a comitogen as suggested in Fig. 3. Transferrin bound to the Tf-R' may also enter by means of coated pits, but its fate is different. The transferrin that is internalized by the low-affinity pathway is routed to the endosomal compartment as well, but instead of being carried back to the cell surface as are transferrin and the Tf-R, it dissociates from the Tf-R'. Dissociation occurs because the affinity of transferrin for the Tf-R' is

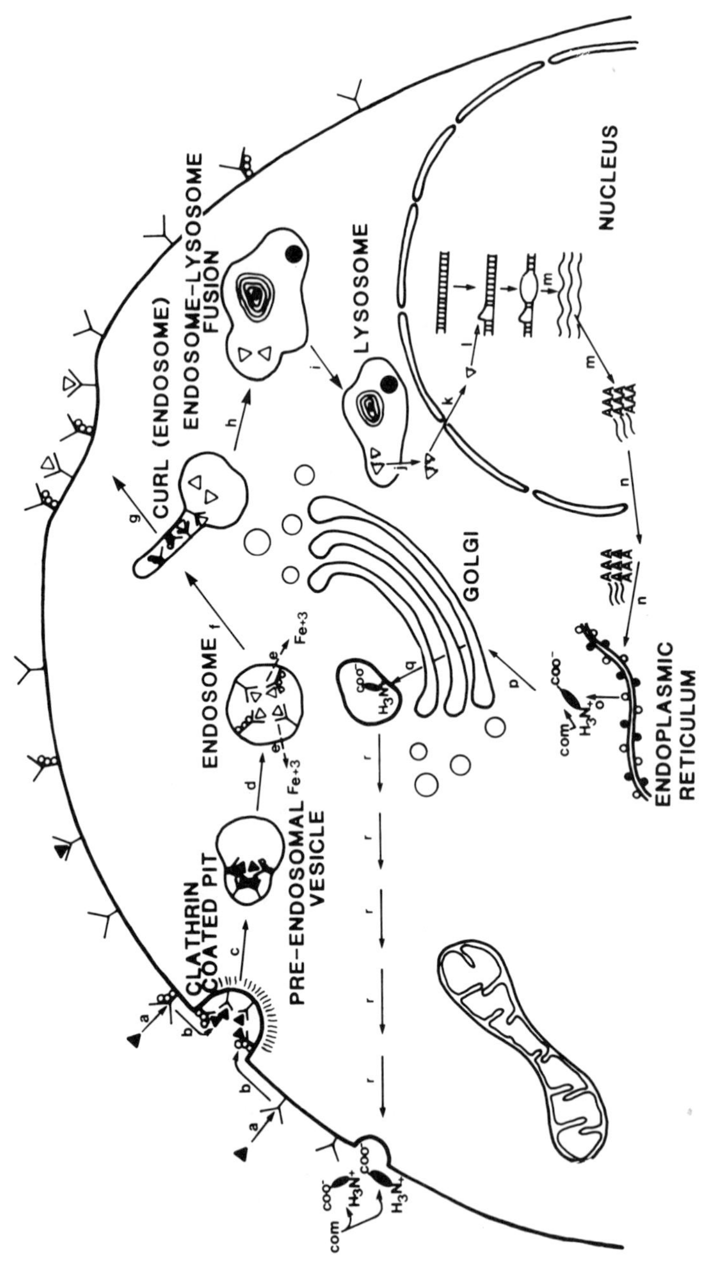
CLATHRIN COATED PIT
PRE-ENDOSOMAL VESICLE
ENDOSOME
CURL (ENDOSOME)
ENDOSOME-LYSOSOME FUSION
LYSOSOME
GOLGI
NUCLEUS
ENDOPLASMIC RETICULUM

Fig. 3 Transferrin regulates the production of a comitogen (COM) by activated cells. For the purposes of this model, high- and low-affinity receptors for Tf are shown in about equal numbers. In fact, this ratio is probably dynamic, depending on the cell's demand for iron. ▲, diferric-transferrin; △, apotransferrin; Y, high-affinity Tf receptor; Y, heparan-sulfinated, low-affinity Tf receptor. (a) diferric-Tf binds to cell surface receptors; (b) receptor-ligand complexes cluster into clathrin-coated pits; (c) receptor-ligand complexes are internalized; (d) transfer into an endosome; (e) low pH of endosome causes release of Fe^{+3} with concomitant conversion of transferrin to apotransferrin (apotransferrin binds tightly to the high-affinity receptor at low pH, and loosely to the low-affinity heparan-sulfinated receptor; (f) formation of the CURL where the membrane-bound receptors are segregated from the luminal contents; (g) membrane-bound receptors are recycled back to the cell surface; (h) luminal contents of endosome and lysosome are mixed by fusion; (i) lysosomal degradation of Tf, yielding a growth-promoting peptide; (j) lysosomal release of the growth-promoting peptide; (k) transport of growth-promoting peptide to the nucleus; (l) binding of the growth-promoting peptide to DNA; (m) transcription of comitogen mRNA; (n) transport of comitogen mRNA to membrane-bound ribosomes of the endoplasmic reticulum; (o) translation of comitogen mRNA; (p) transport of comitogen to the Golgi; (q) Golgi modification of comitogen; (r) secretion of comitogen.

considerably less than its affinity for the Tf-R. The dissociated transferrin (or a fragment of it) is released inside the cell and signals the cell to produce a comitogen.

The suggestion of low- (Tf-R') and high-affinity (Tf-R) receptors for transferrin is entirely consistent with the report (141) that the receptors for transferrin on confluent human skin fibroblasts are complexed at the cell surface with proteoheparan sulfate molecules. The complexed receptors are not recognized by a variety of monoclonal antibodies specific for the Tf-R, but bind these antibodies after the heparan sulfate is removed. The isolated Tf-R-proteoheparan sulfate complex does bind transferrin, although the binding capacity of the complex at the cell surface has not been tested. At least one other cell surface receptor is complexed with a proteoglycan. Anderson and Fambrough (142) reported that the acetylcholine receptors of muscle are invariably associated with heparan sulfate proteoglycan plaques. They suggested that this association is important in localizing the receptor at sites of adhesion in the development of the neuromuscular junction. The formation of receptor-proteoglycan complexes may be a common cellular mechanism for achieving nonrandom receptor distribution. A two-state transferrin receptor is also suggested by the finding of Hunt et al. (143) that the distribution of Tf-R on uninduced and differentiating K562 erythroleukemia cells is different. On uninduced cells, receptors are both localized in coated pits and distributed, apparently randomly, on the cell surface. More receptors are recruited into coated pits as differentiation proceeds. Differentiation in this system is induced by heme, and it appears to mimic the normal erythropoietic process in that the cell's need for iron increases during the early stages of differentiation. Further evidence is the difference in the pattern of reactivity of various monoclonal antibodies against the transferrin receptor with different cell lines (144).

Is the transferrin or the iron it carries (or both) important in transferrin's proliferation-enhancing and antisuppressive effects? Our speculative model would argue for transferrin's primary importance when internalized via the Tf-R', and for iron's importance when internalized via the Tf-R. In an effort to demonstrate specificity for transferrin in preventing suppression by lipoproteins, Cuthbert and Lipsky (86) determined that denatured transferrin is ineffective in reducing lipoprotein suppression and that other proteins such as bovine serum albumin, ovalbumin, catalase, ferritin, and lactoferrin cannot substitute for transferrin. Moreover, other iron carriers such as ferric chloride and nitrilotriacetate do not influence lipoprotein suppression. Our work (87) confirmed and extended these observations: ferric pyridoxal isonicotinoylhydrazone, a lipophilic iron carrier shown to provide essential iron to some cultured cell lines (145), does not influence lipoprotein suppression of lymphocyte activation-proliferation. Nor, however, do any of the alternative sources of iron enhance mitogen-induced lymphocyte proliferation, which occurs with increasing concentrations of transferrin in the absence of lipoproteins. Since iron transport was not measured in any of these studies, the issue of whether transferrin itself or its iron hitchhiker provides the essential enhancement or antisuppressive signal has not been definitely resolved.

What is the function of the putative comitogen? The comitogen (com in Fig. 3) is a protein required to maintain the autocrine loop of cell proliferation. This is the factor in conditioned medium, and perhaps in serum, which allows for optimal cell growth. This autocrine loop is suggested to be the IL2 autocrine loop. Lipoproteins suppress proliferation of both T and B cells, and both cell types utilize this growth factor. However, if the comitogen is nonspecific, it may be able to facilitate autocrine enhancement of growth in a number of cell types and for different (but related in some fundamental way) autocrine growth factors. According to our model, a transferrin-derived peptide directly or indirectly influences comitogen production. Comitogen expression can be induced in accessory cells appropriately "activated" by lymphokines. Once the stimulated lymphocytes have differentiated sufficiently, they can also become capable of responding to transferrin by producing the comitogen. Only cells that remain "activated" have the capacity to produce the comitogen. To maintain the autocrine growth loop, the comitogen is suggested to facilitate the utilization of IL2. Its effect should be most pronounced when IL2 is present in limiting amounts (e.g., during the initial phases of cell activation). The system is, therefore, self-perpetuating if the requisite transferrin signal can be received: a little IL2 keeps lymphocytes sufficiently activated to produce the comitogen, and the comitogen ensures that a little more of the IL2 is utilized, and so forth.

A role of transferrin in autocrine growth control was previously suggested by Symonds and Sachs (146). Myeloid leukemic cells constitutively produce and utilize their own growth factor so long as transferrin is maintained in the medium. Deletion of transferrin induces the cells to cease cycling and to differentiate. The idea that a transferrin degradation product plays a key role in gene expression is in keeping with the report (119) that a 7.8K-transforming peptide (Blym-1) with sequence homology to the N-terminal region of transferrin is present in a continuously proliferating chicken B-lymphoma cell line. An activated transforming gene that appears to be the homolog of chicken Blym-1 has been detected in the DNAs of Burkitt's human B-lymphoma cell lines (147). Moreover, many human melanomas contain a cell surface glycoprotein that is structurally and functionally related to transferrin (148).

How might the comitogen work to maintain the IL2 autocrine loop? It may bind directly to the IL2 receptor at a site distinct from that which recognizes IL2 with resultant stabilization of the receptor.

A precedent exists for this mechanism: serum β_2-microglobulin is reported (149) to bind to and to stabilize expression of a T-cell leukemia differentiation antigen that shares structural features with class I MHC products. Alternatively, the comitogen may bind to a membrane antigen distinct from the IL2-R but required for IL2 utilization via the IL2-R. The work of Malek and colleagues (150) suggests that the IL2-R may be complexed with an effector antigen at the cell membrane. The absence of comitogenlike product and effector antigen have been extended (151) as possible explanations for the inability of cyclosporin A-treated, IL2-R-positive lymphocytes to respond to IL2. Alternatively, the comitogen may bind and transport IL2 into IL2-responsive cells, catalytically process IL2 extracellularly to a form with high biological activity, or catalytically unmask a nonfunctional IL2-R.

The Molecular Basis of Suppression

Suppression by lipoproteins. How do lipoproteins and a possible suppression permissive factor fit into this picture? It is proposed that the suppressive effect of lipoproteins is caused by their ability to interfere with the transferrin/Tf-R' interaction and thereby reduce comitogen production. Competition for binding at the Tf-R' would account for transferrin's dose-dependent relief of lipoprotein suppression. We believe that the relevant structural feature of the suppressive lipoproteins and apolipoproteins is their ability to bind certain glycosaminoglycans such as heparin and heparan sulfate. Tf-R, which binds a proteoheparan sulfate, becomes the Tf-R', which is in turn a likely candidate for the immunoregulatory receptor. The immunoregulatory receptor is certainly important in suppression by lipoproteins of early activation events and is, by inference, also important in suppression of mid-cycle and late activation events. The suppressive lipoproteins and apolipoproteins can bind to a site on the receptor complex distal to the site at which transferrin binds, as is illustrated in Fig. 4. A plasma lipoprotein is sufficiently large to prevent the binding of transferrin by steric hindrance, and these two ligands will therefore compete for receptor occupancy.

Suppression by apolipoproteins. Suppression of lymphocyte activation by apolipoproteins such as apo E has a number of special characteristics that are potentially interesting in the light of our model. As indicated above, transferrin does not protect against suppression by apo E (86). Apo E may be small enough that it can occupy concurrently the Tf-R' with transferrin (Fig. 4). Thus, it is clear that the suppressive effect of apo E cannot be ascribed simply to physical interference with transferrin binding. How, then, is the suppression achieved? Also, since the growth-enhancing property of transferrin delivered via Tf-R' is not absolutely required (e.g., the cells do cycle, albeit less efficiently, if their needs for growth factors, including

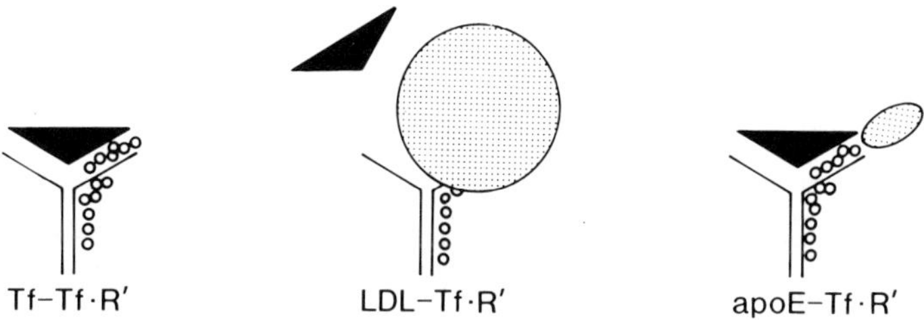

Fig. 4 Lipoproteins—but not apolipoproteins—compete with transferrin for binding to its low-affinity receptor, Tf-R'. A lipoprotein and apo E and apo B bind to the heparan sulfate constituent of the low-affinity Tf-R' distal to the site at which transferrin binds. The lipoprotein and transferrin compete for occupancy of the receptor, while the apolipoprotein and transferrin are able to simultaneously occupy the receptor.

transferrin at low concentrations, are met), how can apo E completely suppress lymphocyte activation? Finally, when activated cells can obtain sufficient transferrin and its iron via the high-affinity Tf-R, why can the intact lipoprotein completely suppress activation via the Tf-R'? The answer to these questions is probably the same: the low- and high-affinity receptors for transferrin migrate to the same coated pits to enter cells together. This possibility is depicted in Fig. 3. The lipoprotein or apolipoprotein can inhibit the consequent internalization process (step c) or the fusion of the initial internalized coated vesicle with an endosome (step not shown in Fig. 3). Or, once inside the endosome bound to Tf-R', the lipoprotein or the apolipoprotein can interfere with the proper processing of all the transferrin contained within that endosome (steps e and f). The results of Cuthbert and Lipsky (86) favor this latter possibility. The result, regardless of mechanism, is complete suppression of lymphocyte activation: transferrin scheduled to deliver its iron is prevented from doing so; transferrin destined for the lysosome is halted along its route.

What are the chemical details by which lipoproteins/apolipoproteins might achieve the inhibition of the internalization of the receptor-bound ligands or the inhibition of transferrin trafficking and processing? The important lipoprotein ingredient is either apo E or an oxidized sterol or a combination of both. Our apo E suppression studies were performed with peripheral blood cells cultured in medium containing serum (69). The actual active ingredient, therefore, could be an apo E-associated lipid. Likewise, Cuthbert and Lipsky's (86) finding that suppression by "cholesterol" is prevented by transferrin is based on a result of an experiment in which the culture medium contains lipoprotein-deficient serum, and therefore also apo E (152).

It is intriguing that apo E is the only apolipoprotein reported thus far to interact with cholesterol (153). Further evidence for a bioactive lipid is the loss of suppressive potency of lipoproteins incubated with high concentrations of albumin (116). If the important lipid is a sterol or oxysterol, its intercalation into membranes (154) may influence membrane properties and membrane-associated enzymes by altering the microenvironment in functional regions of the membrane. The sterol content of the membrane does influence binding of transferrin to cells (155) and to the receptor reconstituted into lipid vesicles (156). Moreover, the membrane sterols presumed to be located in coated pits (157) appear to have different properties than sterols located in other regions of the membrane based on their inability to complex with filipin (158). Thus, a potent sterol delivered directly to the relevant coated pit could have profound consequences for receptor-mediated endocytosis. It could also influence the requisite acidification of the primary endosome by inhibiting the proton pump, thereby preventing iron-transferrin dissociation as well as transferrin-receptor dissociation.

Summary of the Model

Occupying the pivotal position in the model is the immunoregulatory receptor, which is the low-affinity receptor for transferrin. The presence of this receptor on responding lymphocytes and accessory cells is not essential for lymphocyte activation. However, its presence is essential for regulation of that activation by transferrin and plasma lipoproteins. Transferrin exerts positive control, while lipoproteins exert negative control of activation through their interactions with this receptor (Fig. 5). Transferrin utilized through the immunoregulatory receptor pathway results in the production of a factor

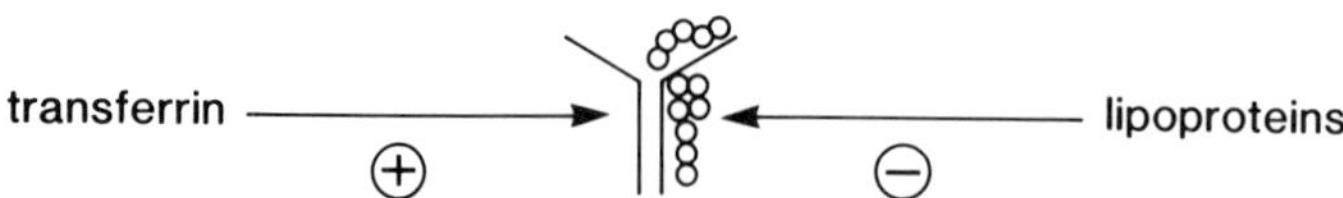

Fig. 5 The immunoregulatory receptor transmits growth-promoting and growth-inhibiting signals. The immunoregulatory receptor, the low-affinity receptor for transferrin, regulates the proliferation of the activated lymphocyte. Transferrin, the positive effector, recruits more cells into the cycle and facilitates their progression through the cycle. The lipoprotein, the negative effector, restrains the cells from entering and progressing through the cycle.

that recruits more cells into the cell cycle. This factor is particularly important when the amount of IL2 is limiting. Lipoproteins prevent this positive transferrin effect by binding to the immunoregulatory receptors and competing against transferrin binding. Through the mechanism of apolipoprotein E binding to cholesterol, lipoproteins may also interfere with the metabolically essential pathway of iron delivery.

IMMUNOREGULATION BY LIPOPROTEINS IN VIVO

Knowledge of the factors that regulate the functional capacity of the immune system is fundamental to an understanding of the diseases associated with impaired host immune competence. Lymphocyte activation is an exceedingly complex process. The entry of lymphocytes into the cell cycle requires the correct presentation of antigen and contributions from accessory cells and T-cell subsets. Signals are continuously transmitted between cells in the system, and the cells are receptive to chemical modulators in their immediate environment. If the balance of signals is positive, the system is activated; if negative, the system is suppressed. The possibility that plasma lipoproteins are natural modulators of immunity deserves close attention. The plasma lipoproteins circulate in the appropriate milieu, the blood and lymph, to modulate the immune system. Diet profoundly influences immune status (159), and variations in the diet have direct influence on the quality and quantity of the various classes of plasma lipoproteins.

The in vitro evidence for the role of certain classes of lipoproteins in regulating the proliferative response that underlies the development of the immune state is overwhelming. If our model proves to be correct, lipoproteins can control the population of antigen-specific lymphocytes in vivo—at two points very early in the cell cycle—by blocking the transduction of the initial activation signals and by preventing the transmission of information from accessory cells to activated lymphocytes. In addition, lipoproteins can inhibit the entry of responding lymphocytes into the terminal phases of the cell cycle. Whether or not plasma lipoproteins can provide a negative signal that restrains the entry of activated cells into the cycle and their progression through it in vivo will depend on a number of factors. In the plasma, where most lymphocytes are in the resting state, both lipoproteins and transferrin are in very high concentration with respect to experiments performed in vitro. Further in vivo experimentation is required to determine if lipoproteins in plasma aid in maintaining circulating lymphocytes in G_0 and, more importantly, to determine what effect *variations* in lipoproteins might have on this immunomodulatory effect. In the tissues, where the immune response takes place in vast aggregations of activated and resting lymphocytes and accessory cells, a possible lipoprotein immunoregulatory effect would depend on the density of the cells in the lymphoid aggregate, the ratio of responding cells to accessory cells, and the local concentrations of lipoprotein and transferrin in the microenvironment. These are unknowns. While tissue concentrations of lipoproteins and transferrin have not been measured accurately, the lipoprotein concentration is at least one-tenth that of plasma (160). In the normal situation, it is therefore unlikely that plasma lipoproteins exert much immunoregulation in the tissues. However, in subjects with hyperlipidemia, and particularly hypercholesterolemia, the tissue concentration of immunoregulatory lipoproteins will increase to a level at which the lipoproteins may indeed be effective immunomodulators. Hypercholesterolemia does correlate with decreased resistance to transplantable tumors (161), implying immunosuppression. Also, the suppressive potency of the lipoproteins is certainly increased in disease states such as uremia (162,163).

The bioregulatory properties of plasma lipoproteins have been shown to be expressed in vivo (164). The work of Curtiss and Edgington provides compelling support for an important immunoregulatory role of lipoproteins. Administration of 500 to 600 μg human LDL-In protein intravenously to mice, markedly increasing their serum cholesterol concentration, suppresses the anti-sheep erythrocyte hemagglutination response (165) and reduces the number of splenic plaque-forming cells, the mean lytic plaque volume, the number of splenic T- and B-antigen-binding cells, and the serum hemagglutination titers (166). These results indicate that LDL-In suppress the clonal expansion of antigen-specific T and B cells. LDL-In do not block B-cell differentiation to antibody-secreting cells. Maximal suppression occurs when LDL-In are injected 1 to 2 days prior to antigen administration. LDL-In also suppress the generation of cytolytic T cells specific for P815 mastocytoma cells in C57BL/6 mice in vivo (167). LDL-In was infused prior to immunization and, after 10 days, the cytotoxic splenic T-cell activity was reduced 70% compared to controls. In vitro, LDL-In had no effect on the cytotoxic activity of previously primed T-killer cells or on the differentiation of memory cells to T-killer cells.

Is proliferation of cells other than those important in the immune response sensitive to lipoprotein regulation? Perhaps, but only if the immunoregulatory receptor is present and active. The corollary to this requirement is the prediction that lipoprotein-suppressible cells will be under autocrine growth control, with transferrin participating in maintenance of the autocrine growth loop. Our model to account for lipoprotein suppression emphasizes transferrin, with inhibition directed at both its receptor expression and its utilization. The focus is particularly intriguing in regard to the reports (168,169) that natural killer cells—cells that are directly cytotoxic to proliferating target cells—may select these targets from a mixed population on the basis of their Tf-R expression. Perhaps the body has developed general strategies of cell birth control which involve transferrin.

Since circulating levels of transferrin in adults are high—3 to 4 mg/ml—lipoprotein control mechanisms must ordinarily operate during development or in tissues in which the ratio of lipoproteins to transferrin is high.

ACKNOWLEDGMENTS

The authors thank Ms. Susan Eder and Ms. Janet Simons for preparing the manuscript, and Drs. Frank Chisari, Jennifer Cuthbert, and Linda Curtiss for preprints of manuscripts submitted for publication. The editorial assistance of Ms. Maria Davila is gratefully acknowledged. J. A. K. Harmony was an Established Investigator of the American Heart Association, and is supported by grants HL 27333 from the National Institutes of Health, BC-434 from the American Cancer Society, and 82-704 from the American Heart Association. A. L. Akeson and S. A. Grupp are supported by NIH Molecular and Cellular Biology Training grant HL 07527.

REFERENCES

1. Morrisett, J. D., Jackson, R. L., and Gotto, A. M., Jr., *Biochim. Biophys. Acta, 472*:93–133 (1977).
2. Jackson, R. L., Morrisett, J. D., and Gotto, A. M., Jr., *Physiol. Rev., 56*:259–316 (1976).
3. Owen, J. S., and McIntyre, N., *Trends Biochem. Sci., 7*: 95–98 (1982).
4. Goldstein, J. L., and Brown, M. S., *Ann. Rev. Biochem., 46*: 897–930 (1977).
5. Mahley, R. W., and Innerarity, T. L., *Biochim. Biophys. Acta, 737*:197–222 (1983).
6. Hui, D. Y., and Harmony, J. A. K., *Biochim. Biophys. Acta, 550*:425–434 (1979).
7. Chisari, F. V., and Curtiss, L. K., *Cell. Immunol., 65*:325–336 (1981).
8. Kane, J. P., Hardman, D. A., Dimpfl, J. D., and Levy, J. A., *Proc. Natl. Acad. Sci. U.S.A., 76*:5957–5961 (1979).
9. Ho, W. K. K., and Shortridge, K. F., *Lipids, 12*:85–91 (1977).
10. Seganti, L., Mastromarino, P., DeStasio, A., Sinibaldi, L., Valenti, P., and Orsi, N., *Acta Virol., 24*:311–316 (1980).

11. Rifkin, M. R., *Proc. Natl. Acad. Sci. U.S.A.*, *75*:3450–3454 (1978).

12. Levy, G. A., Schwartz, B. S., Curtiss, L. K., and Edgington, T. S., *J. Clin. Invest.*, *67*:1614–1622 (1981).

13. Schwartz, B. S., Levy, G. A., Curtiss, L. K., Fair, D. S., and Edgington, T. S., *J. Clin. Invest.*, *67*:1650–1658 (1981).

14. Bajaj, S. P., Harmony, J. A. K., Martinez-Carrion, M., and Castellino, F. J., *J. Biol. Chem.*, *251*:5233–5236 (1976).

15. Riding, I. M., and Ellis, D., *J. Atherosclerosis Res.*, *4*:189–193 (1964).

16. Lint, T. F., Behrends, C. L., and Gewurz, H., *J. Immunol.*, *119*:883–888 (1977).

17. Terkeltaub, R., Curtiss, L. K., Tenner, A. J., and Ginsberg, M. H., *J. Clin. Invest.*, *73*:1719–1730 (1984).

18. Chisari, F. V., and Edgington, T. S., *J. Exp. Med.*, *142*:1092–1107 (1975).

19. Cambier, J., and Monroe, J., *J. Immunol.*, *133*:576–581 (1984).

20. Hui, D. Y., and Harmony, J. A. K., *Biochem. J.*, *192*:91–98 (1980).

21. Akeson, A. L., Scupham, D. W., and Harmony, J. A. K., *J. Lipid Res.*, *25*:1195–1205 (1984).

22. Grupp, S. A., and Harmony, J. A. K., *J. Immunol.*, *134*:4087–4094 (1985).

23. Hui, D. Y., Berebitsky, G. L., and Harmony, J. A. K., *J. Biol. Chem.*, *254*:4666–4673 (1979).

24. Hume, D. A., and Weidemann, M. J., *Mitogenic Lymphocyte Transformation: A General Model for the Control of Mammalian Cell Proliferation and Differentiation*, Elsevier/North-Holland, Amsterdam, 1980.

25. Ashman, R. F., in *Fundamental Immunology* (Paul, W. E., ed.), Raven Press, New York, 1984, pp. 267–300.

26. Oppenheim, J. J., Stadler, B. M., Siraganian, R. P., Mage, M., and Mathieson, B., *Fed. Proc.*, *41*:257–262 (1982).

27. Lachman, L. B., *Fed. Proc.*, *42*:2639–2645 (1983).

28. Rosenstreich, D. L., Farrar, J. J., and Dougherty, S., *J. Immunol.*, *116*:131–139 (1976).

29. Kondracki, E., and Milgrom, F., *J. Immunol.*, *118*:381–387 (1977).

30. Bell, G. I., *Immunol. Today, 4*:237–240 (1983).

31. Hünig, T., *Eur. J. Immunol., 13*:596–601 (1983).

32. Robb, R. J., *Immunol. Today, 5*:203–209 (1984).

33. Hünig, T., Loos, M., and Schimpl, A., *Eur. J. Immunol., 13*: 1–6 (1983).

34. Williams, J. M., Ransil, B. J., Shapiro, H. M., and Strom, T. B., *J. Immunol., 133*:2986–2995 (1984).

35. Lipkowitz, S., Greene, W. C., Rubin, A. L., Novogrodsky, A., and Stenzel, K., *J. Immunol., 132*:31–37 (1984).

36. Roffman, E., Sredni, B., Smolinsky, A., and Wilchek, M., *Proc. Natl. Acad. Sci. U.S.A., 81*:5209–5213 (1984).

37. Kaye, J., Gillis, S., Mizel, Shevach, E. M., Malek, T. R., Dinarello, C. A., Lachman, L. B., and Janeway, C. A., Jr., *J. Immunol., 133*:1339–1345 (1984).

38. Iscove, N. N., and Melchers, F., *J. Exp. Med., 147*:923–933 (1978).

39. Dillner-Centerlind, M.-L., Hammarstrom, S., and Perlmann, P., *Eur. J. Immunol., 9*:942–948 (1979).

40. Sutherland, R., Delia, D., Schneider, C., Newman, R., Kemshead, J., and Greaves, M., *Proc. Natl. Acad. Sci. U.S.A., 78*:4515–4519 (1981).

41. Trowbridge, I. S., and Omary, M. B., *Proc. Natl. Acad. Sci. U.S.A., 78*:3039–3043 (1981).

42. Trowbridge, I. S., and Lopez, F., *Proc. Natl. Acad. Sci. U.S.A., 79*:1175–1179 (1982).

43. Barnes, D., and Sato, G., *Anal. Biochem., 102*:255–270 (1980).

44. Bezkorovainy, A., and Zschocke, R. H., *Arzneim.-Forsch./ Drug Res., 24*:476–485 (1974).

45. Newman, R., Schneider, C., Sutherland, R., Vodinelich, L., and Greaves, M., *Trends Biochem. Sci., 1*:397–400 (1982).

46. May, W. S., Jacobs, S., and Cuatrecasas, P., *Proc. Natl. Acad. Sci. U.S.A., 81*:2016–2020 (1984).

47. Omary, M. B., and Trowbridge, I. S., *J. Biol. Chem., 256*: 12,888–12,892 (1981).

48. Adam, M., Rodriguez, A., Turbide, C., Larrick, J., Meighen, E., and Johnstone, R. M., *J. Biol. Chem., 259*: 15,460–15,463 (1984).

49. Dautry-Varsat, A., Ciechanover, A., and Lodish, H. F., *Proc. Natl. Acad. Sci. U.S.A.*, *80*:2258–2262 (1983).

50. Klausner, R. D., Ashwell, G., van Renswoude, J., Harford, J. B., and Bridges, K. R., *Proc. Natl. Acad. Sci. U.S.A.*, *80*:2263–2266 (1983).

51. Yamashiro, D. J., Tycko, B., Fluss, S. R., and Maxfield, F. R., *Cell*, *37*:789–800 (1984).

52. Hamilton, T. A., *J. Cell. Phys.*, *113*:40–46 (1982).

53. Weiel, J. E., and Hamilton, T. A., *Biochem. Biophys. Res. Commun.*, *119*:598–602 (1984).

54. Neckers, L. M., Yenokida, G., and James, S. P., *J. Immunol.*, *133*:2437–2441 (1984).

55. Brock, J. H., and Mainou-Fowler, T., *Immunol. Today*, *4*: 347–351 (1983).

56. Neckers, L. M., and Cossman, J., *Proc. Natl. Acad. Sci. U.S.A.*, *80*:3494–3498 (1983).

57. Leonard, W. J., Depper, J. M., Uchiyama, T., Smith, K. A., Waldmann, T. A., and Greene, W. C., *Nature (London)*, *300*: 267–269 (1982).

58. Curtiss, L. K., and Edgington, T. S., *J. Immunol.*, *116*: 1452–1458 (1976).

59. Waddell, C. C., Taunton, O. D., and Twomey, J. J., *J. Clin. Invest.*, *58*:950–954 (1976).

60. Morse, J. H., Witte, L. D., and Goodman, D. S., *J. Exp. Med.*, *146*:1791–1803 (1977).

61. Hui, D. Y., Harmony, J. A. K., Innerarity, T. L., and Mahley, R. W., *J. Biol. Chem.*, *255*:11,775–11,781 (1980).

62. Fujii, D. K., and Edgington, T. S., *J. Immunol.*, *124*:156–160 (1980).

63. Shelburne, F. A., and Quarfordt, S. H., *J. Clin. Invest.*, *60*: 944–950 (1977).

64. Warnick, G. R., and Albers, J. J., *J. Lipid Res.*, *19*:65–76 (1978).

65. Noel, J. G., Hui, D. Y., Blankenship, D. T., and Harmony, J. A. K., *Biochim. Biophys. Acta*, *665*:519–530 (1981).

66. Avila, E. M., Holdsworth, G., Sasaki, N., Jackson, R. L., and Harmony, J. A. K., *J. Biol. Chem.*, *257*:5900–5909 (1982).

67. Curtiss, L. K., Forte, T. M., and Davis, P. A., *J. Immunol.*, *133*:1379–1384 (1984).

68. Blum, C. B., Aron, L., and Sciacca, R., *J. Clin. Invest.*, *66*: 1240–1250 (1980).

69. Macy, M., Okano, Y., Cardin, A. D., Avila, E. M., and Harmony, J. A. K., *Cancer Res.*, *43*:2496s–2502s (1983).

70. Basu, S. K., Brown, M. S., Ho, Y. K., Havel, R. J., and Goldstein, J. L., *Proc. Natl. Acad. Sci. U.S.A.*, *78*:7545–7549 (1981).

71. Basu, S. K., Ho, Y. K., Brown, M. S., Bilheimer, D. W., Anderson, R. G. W., and Goldstein, J. L., *J. Biol. Chem.*, *257*:9788–9795 (1982).

72. Basu, S. K., Goldstein, J. L., and Brown, M. S., *Science*, *219*:871–873 (1983).

73. Werb, Z., and Chin, J. R., *J. Biol. Chem.*, *258*:10,642–10,648 (1983).

74. Werb, Z., and Chin, J. R., *J. Cell Biol.*, *97*:1113–1118 (1983).

75. Takemura, R., and Werb, Z., *J. Exp. Med.*, *159*:167–178 (1984).

76. Stobo, J. D., *J. Immunol.*, *199*:918–924 (1977).

77. Gmelig-Meyling, F., and Waldmann, T. A., *J. Immunol.*, *126*: 529–537 (1981).

78. Werb, Z., and Chin, J. R., *J. Exp. Med.*, *158*:1272–1293 (1983).

79. Akeson, A. L., Ph.D. dissertation, University of Cincinnati, Cincinnati, Ohio, 1985.

80. Cornell, R., Grove, G. L., Rothblat, G. H., and Horwitz, A. F., *Exp. Cell Res.*, *109*:299–307 (1977).

81. Killander, D., and Zetterberg, A., *Exp. Cell Res.*, *40*:12–20 (1965).

82. Johnston, G. C., Pringle, J. R., and Hartwell, L. H., *Exp. Cell Res.*, *105*:79–98 (1977).

83. Calvert, G. R., and Dawes, I. W., *Nature (London)*, *312*:61–63 (1984).

84. Cuthbert, J. A., and Lipsky, P. E., *J. Lipid Res.*, *24*:1512–1524 (1983).

85. Chisari, F. V., *J. Immunol.*, *119*:2129–2136 (1977).

86. Cuthbert, J. A., and Lipsky, P. E., *J. Clin. Invest.*, *73*: 992–1003 (1984).

87. Scupham, D. W., Ph.D. dissertation, Indiana University, Bloomington, Indiana, 1985.

88. Brown, M. S., and Goldstein, J. L., *J. Lipid Res.*, *21*: 505–517 (1980).

89. Hui, D. Y., and Harmony, J. A. K., *J. Biol. Chem.*, *255*: 1413–1419 (1980).

90. Harmony, J. A. K., and Hui, D. Y., *Cancer Res.*, *41*: 3799–3802 (1981).

91. Pairault, J., Levillier, J., and Chapman, M. J., *Nature (London)*, *269*:607–609 (1977).

92. Innerarity, T. L., and Mahley, R. W., *Biochemistry*, *17*: 1440–1447 (1978).

93. Pitas, R. E., Innerarity, T. L., Arnold, K. S., and Mahley, R. W., *Proc. Natl. Acad. Sci. U.S.A.*, *76*:2311–2315 (1979).

94. Pitas, R. E., Innerarity, T. L., and Mahley, R. W., *J. Biol. Chem.*, *255*:5454–5460 (1980).

95. Mahley, R. W., Hui, D. Y., Innerarity, T. L., and Weisgraber, K. H., *J. Clin. Invest.*, *68*:1197–1206 (1981).

96. Hui, D. Y., Innerarity, T. L., and Mahley, R. W., *J. Biol. Chem.*, *256*:5646–5655 (1981).

97. Hui, D. Y., and Harmony, J. A. K., *Proc. Natl. Acad. Sci. U.S.A.*, *77*:4764–4768 (1980).

98. Goldstein, J. L., and Brown, M. S., *J. Biol. Chem.*, *249*: 5153–5162 (1974).

99. Curtiss, L. K., and Edgington, T. S., *J. Clin. Invest.*, *61*: 1298–1308 (1978).

100. Goldstein, J. L., Basu, S. K., Brunschede, G. Y., and Brown, M. S., *Cell*, *7*:85–95 (1976).

101. Mahley, R. W., Innerarity, T. L., Pitas, R. E., Weisgraber, K. H., Brown, J. H., and Gross, E., *J. Biol. Chem.*, *252*: 7279–7287 (1977).

102. Weisgraber, K. H., Innerarity, T. L., and Mahley, R. W., *J. Biol. Chem.*, *253*:9053–9062 (1978).

103. Cuthbert, J. A., and Lipsky, P. E., *Proc. Natl. Acad. Sci. U.S.A.*, *81*:4539–4543 (1984).

104. Yi, P. I., Beck, G., and Zucker, S., *Blood*, *57*:1055–1064 (1981).

105. Yi, P. I., Beck, G., and Zucker, S., *Int. Archs. Allergy Appl. Immunol.*, *65*:8–14 (1981).

106. Fogelman, A. M., Seager, J., Edwards, P. A., Hokom, M., and Popjak, G., *Biochem. Biophys. Res. Commun.*, *76*:167–173 (1977).

107. Fogelman, A. M., Haberland, M. E., Seager, J., Hokom, M., and Edwards, P. A., *J. Lipid. Res.*, *22*:1131–1141 (1981).

108. Fogelman, A. M., Hokom, M. M., Haberland, M. E., Tanaka, R. D., and Edwards, P. A., *J. Biol. Chem.*, *257*:14,081–14,086 (1982).

109. Chait, A., Henze, K., Mazzone, T. Jensen, M., and Hammond, W., *Metabolism, 31*, 721–727 (1982).

110. Okano, Y., Macy, M., and Harmony, J. A. K., *Biochim. Biophys. Acta, 845*:68–80 (1985).

111. Ho, Y. K., Brown, M. S., Bilheimer, D. W., and Goldstein, J. L., *J. Clin. Invest.*, *58*:1465–1474 (1976).

112. Rosenberg, S. A., Ligler, F. S., Ugolini, V., and Lipsky, P. E., *J. Immunol.*, *126*:1473–1477 (1981).

113. Okano, Y., Macy, M., Cardin, A. D., and Harmony, J. A. K., *Exp. Cell Biol.*, *53*:199–212 (1985).

114. Thiele, D. L., and Lipsky, P. E., *J. Immunol.*, *129*:1033–1040 (1982).

115. Fogelman, A. M., Seager, J., Groopman, J. E., Berliner, J. A., Haberland, M. E., Edwards, P. A., and Golde, D. W., *J. Immunol.*, *131*:2368–2373 (1983).

116. Okano, Y., McCarthy, B. M., Macy, M., Nakayasu, T., Watson, S. R., and Harmony, J. A. K., *J. Lipid Res.*, in press.

117. Ii, I., Kimura, I., and Ozawa, E., *Dev. Biol.*, *94*:366–377 (1982).

118. Popiela, H., Taylor, D., Ellis, S., Beach, R., and Festoff, B., *J. Cell Physiol.*, *119*:234–240 (1984).

119. Goubin, G., Goldman, D. S., Luce, J., Neiman, P. E., and Cooper, G. M., *Nature (London)*, *302*:114–119 (1983).

120. Chen, H. W., Heiniger, H.-J., and Kandutsch, A. A., *Proc. Natl. Acad. Sci. U.S.A.*, *72*:1950–1954 (1975).

121. Heiniger, H. J., *Cancer Res.*, *41*:3792–3794 (1981).

122. Witte, L. D., Cornicelli, J. A., Miller, R. W., and Goodman, D. S., *J. Biol. Chem.*, *257*:5392–5401 (1982).

123. Cuthbert, J. A., and Lipsky, P. E., *J. Immunol.*, *124*: 2240–2246 (1980).

124. Cuthbert, J. A., and Lipsky, P. E., *J. Immunol.*, *126*: 2093–2099 (1981).

125. Javitt, N. B., Kok, E., Burstein, S., Cohen, B., and Kutscher, J., *J. Biol. Chem.*, *256*:12,644–12,646 (1981).

126. Yachnin, S., and Hsu, R., *Cell. Immunol.*, *51*:42–54 (1980).

127. Curtiss, L. K., and Edgington, T. S., *J. Immunol.*, *125*: 1470–1474 (1980).

128. Curtiss, L. K., and Edgington, T. S., *J. Immunol.*, *126*: 1382–1386 (1981).

129. Curtiss, L. K., and Edgington, T. S., *J. Immunol.*, *126*: 1008–1012 (1981).

130. Kandutsch, A. A., and Chen, H. W., *J. Biol. Chem.*, *252*: 409–415 (1977).

131. Chen, H. W., Cavenee, W. C., and Kandutsch, A. A., *J. Biol. Chem.*, *254*:715–720 (1979).

132. Kandutsch, A. A., Chen, H. W., and Heiniger, J. H., *Science*, *201*:498–501 (1978).

133. Streuli, R. A., Chung, J., Scanu, A. M., and Yachnin, S., *J. Immunol.*, *123*:2897–2902 (1979).

134. Defay, R., Astruc, M. E., Roussillon, S., Descomps, B., and Crastes de Paulet, A., *Biochem. Biophys. Res. Commun.*, *106*:362–372 (1982).

135. Curtiss, L. K., and Edgington, T. S., *J. Immunol.*, *118*: 1966–1970 (1977).

136. Nakayasu, T., Macy, M., Okano, Y., McCarthy, B. M., and Harmony, J. A. K., *Exp. Cell Res.*, *163*:247–260 (1986).

137. Reem, G. H., and Yeh, N.-H., *Science*, *225*:429–430 (1984).

138. Hall, D. J., O'Leary, J. J., and Rosenberg, A., *J. Cell Physiol.*, *112*:157–161 (1982).

139. Hart, G. W., *Biochemistry*, *21*:6088–6096 (1982).

140. Naparstek, Y., Cohen, I. R., Fuks, Z., and Vlodavsky, I., *Nature (London)*, *310*:241–244 (1984).

141. Fransson, L.-A., Carlstedt, I., Coster, L., and Malmstrom, A., *Proc. Natl. Acad. Sci. U.S.A.*, *81*:5657–5661 (1984).

142. Anderson, M. J., and Fambrough, D. M., *J. Cell Biol.*, *97*: 1396–1411 (1983).

143. Hunt, R. C., Ruffin, R., and Yang, Y.-S., *J. Biol. Chem.*, *259*:9944–9952 (1984).

144. Lebman, D., Trucco, M., Bottero, L., Lange, B., Pessano, S., and Rovera, G., *Blood*, *59*:671–678 (1982).

145. Landschulz, W., Thesleff, I., and Ekbloom, P., *J. Cell Biol.*, *98*:596–601 (1984).

146. Symonds, G., and Sachs, L., *EMBO J.*, *1*:1343–1346 (1982).

147. Diamond, A., Cooper, G. M., Ritz, J., and Lane, M.-A., *Nature (London)*, *305*:112–116 (1983).

148. Brown, J. P., Hewick, R. M., Hellstrom, I., Hellstrom, K. E., Doolittle, R. F., and Dreyer, W. J., *Nature (London)*, *296*: 171–173 (1982).

149. Kefford, R. F., Calabi, F., Fearnley, I. M., Burrone, O. R., and Milstein, C., *Nature (London)*, *308*:641–645 (1984).

150. Malek, T. R., Robb, R. J., and Shevach, E. M., *J. Immunol.*, *130*:747–755 (1983).

151. Lillehoj, H. S., Malek, T. R., and Shevach, E. M., *J. Immunol.*, *133*:244–250 (1984).

152. Castro, G. R., and Fielding, C. J., *J. Lipid Res.*, *25*:58–67 (1984).

153. Demel, R. A., Louwers, H., Jackson, R. L., and Wirtz, K. W. A., *J. Colloid Sci.*, *10*:301–311 (1984).

154. Yachnin, S., Streuli, R. A., Gordon, L. I., and Hsu, R. C., *Curr. Topics Hematol.*, *2*:245–271 (1979).

155. Muller, C., and Shinitzky, M., *Br. J. Haematol.*, *42*:355–362 (1979).

156. Nunez, M. T., and Glass, J., *Biochemistry*, *21*:4139–4143 (1982).

157. Marsh, M., Bolzau, E., and Helenius, A., *Cell*, *32*:931–940 (1983).

158. McGookey, D. J., Fagerberg, K., and Anderson, R. G. W., *J. Cell Biol.*, *96*:1273–1279 (1983).

159. Chandra, R. K., *Nutr. Rev.*, *39*:225–231 (1981).

160. Reichl, D., Myant, N. B., Brown, M. S., and Goldstein, J. L., *J. Clin. Invest.*, *61*:64–71 (1978).

161. Newberne, P. M., and Thurman, G. B., *Cancer Res.*, *41*, 3803–3804 (1981).

162. Raska, K., Morrison, A. B., and Raskova, J., *Lab. Invest.*, *42*:636–642 (1980).

163. Raskova, J., and Raska, K., *Lab. Invest.*, *45*:410–417 (1981).

164. Edgington, T. S., and Curtiss, L. K., *Cancer Res.*, *41*: 3786–3788 (1981).

165. Curtiss, L. K., DeHeer, D. H., and Edgington, T. S., *J. Immunol.*, *118*:648–652 (1977).

166. Curtiss, L. K., DeHeer, D. H., and Edgington, T. S., *Cell Immunol.*, *49*:1–11 (1980).

167. Edgington, T. S., Henney, C. S., and Curtiss, L. K., in *Regulatory Mechanisms of Lymphocyte Activation* (Lucas, D. O., ed.), Academic Press, New York, 1977, pp. 736–738.

168. Brieva, J. A., and Stevens, R. H., *J. Immunol.*, *133*:1288–1292 (1984).

169. Newman, R. A., Warner, J. F., and Dennert, G., *J. Immunol.*, *133*:1841–1845 (1984).

16

Lipoprotein Disorders: Defects of Apolipoproteins, Enzymes, and Receptors

ANGELO M. SCANU and VENERACION CABANA The Pritzker School of Medicine, The University of Chicago, Chicago, Illinois

ARTHUR A. SPECTOR College of Medicine, University of Iowa, Iowa City, Iowa

CAUSES OF ABNORMAL PLASMA LIPID LEVELS

Many factors can cause an abnormal distribution of lipoproteins in the plasma. In general, lipoprotein disorders can be classified as primary and secondary (1–3). An early classification of the lipoprotein disorders developed by Fredrickson et al. (2) comprised the six phenotypes listed in Table 1. Although useful from the descriptive aspect, this classification proved to be of limited value from the biochemical and genetic aspects since it is now known that one phenotype may express more than one genotype.

The primary hyperlipidemias are hereditary and taken together appear to have an incidence of 1 to 2/100. The secondary hyperlipidemias are higher in occurrence and their pathogenesis varies from case to case, as is indicated by the many different causes listed in Table 2. Also, their expression can be influenced by age, sex, and severity and length of exposure to the determining factor(s). Secondary hyperlipidemias must be ruled out any time the study of a hyperlipoproteinemic patient is undertaken.

The correction of the underlying disease or the elimination of the causative factor produces normalization of the plasma lipid levels in all cases except when a familial component is also present.

FAMILIAL DISORDERS

The genetic disorders known today all recognize a defect at a protein level; these involve either apolipoproteins, lipolytic enzymes, or membrane receptors.

Table 1 Lipoprotein Phenotypes According to Fredrickson et al. (2)

Phenotype	Appearance of fasting serum	Serum (mg/dl)		Lipoprotein electrophoresis
		Cholesterol	Triglycerides	
Type I	Milky	260	1000	
Type IIa	Clear	300	150	
Type IIb	Clear or turbid	300	150–300	
Type III	Turbid	350–500	350–500	
Type IV	Turbid to milky	260	200–1000	
Type V	Milky	300	1000	O β preβ

Table 2 Causes of Secondary Hyperlipidemia

Alcohol intake	Obesity
Calcium and beta-blockers	Pancreatitis
Cigarette smoking	Pregnancy
Diabetes mellitus	Progestational agents
High calorie diets rich in carbohydrates or fats	Renal dialysis
Diuretics	Renal insufficiency
Gout	Steroid hormones
Hypothyroidism	Lipid storage diseases (sphingolipidoses)
Nephrotic syndrome	

Apolipoprotein Defects

Several plasma apolipoprotein variants have been identified, as indicated in Table 3, and others are likely to be uncovered through ongoing screening techniques employing either uni- or two-dimensional electrophoretic techniques (4,5). Therefore, apolipoproteins already have acquired an important position in lipoprotein disorders. More genetic disorders of this kind also are likely to be uncovered as techniques in cell and molecular biology are systematically applied in their study. In some cases, the amino acid substitution does not lead to a charge shift and only amino acid sequence analyses can detect the structural variant. From Table 3, however, it is also apparent that apolipoprotein structural changes are not necessarily attended by pathology.

In the older nomenclature, the apo E-2/E-2 genotype was encompassed in the hyperlipoproteinemia variously designated type III, dysbetalipoproteinemia, broad beta-disease, or floating beta-disease.

Enzyme Defects

Three lipid-modifying enzymes are known to affect the metabolism of lipoproteins during their presence in plasma: lipoprotein lipase, hepatic lipase, and lecithin-cholesterol acyltransferase (LCAT) (1). For each of them, deficiency states attended by important lipid abnormalities have been described (see Table 4). In the older nomenclature classifying dyslipoproteinemias, the familial form involving lipoprotein lipase deficiency was designated type I (Table 1).

The frequency of these genetic defects has been estimated to be about 1 in 100,000. As indicated in Table 4, an absence of apo C-II in plasma can have the same clinical manifestations as those seen in lipoprotein lipase deficiency.

Table 3 Apolipoprotein Defects

Apolipoprotein	Nature of defect	Mechanism	Mode of transmission	Main clinical presentation
Apo B	Abetalipoproteinemia, absence of plasma apo B-100 and apo B-48, low cholesterol, no chylomicrons	Unknown	Autosomal recessive	Abetalipoproteinemia, defective fat absorption, acanthocytosis, retinitis pigmentosa, Friedreich ataxia; parents of proband have normal LDL levels
	Hypobetalipoproteinemia (homozygous)	Unknown	Autosomal dominant	Parents of proband have low LDL cholesterol levels; same clinical presentation as recessive form
	Abetalipoproteinemia with normotriglyceridemia; apo B-100 absent, apo B-48 present	Unknown	Unknown	Only one case reported
Apo C-II	Absence of apo C-II from plasma; deficiency in the lipoprotein lipase system	Unknown	Autosomal recessive	Severe hyperchylomicronemia, lipemia retinals, hepatosplenomegaly; propensity for pancreatitis
Apo A-I Tangier disease	Low levels of apo A-I approximately equally distributed between proapo A-I and apo A-I	Unknown	Autosomal recessive	Low plasma cholesterol, low HDL, normal triglycerides, yellow-orange tonsils, splenomegaly, neuropathy

Apo A-I Milano	High plasma triglycerides, low HDL cholesterol; presence of disulfide-linked apo A-I dimers	$Arg_{173} \rightarrow Cys$	Autosomal recessive	No evidence of atherosclerosis; defect in activation of LCAT by apo A-I
Apo A-I Marburg	No evidence of lipoprotein abnormalities	$Lys_{107} \rightarrow O$	Autosomal recessive	No clinical abnormalities
Apo A-I Munster	No evidence of lipoprotein abnormalities	$Asp_{103} \rightarrow Asn$ $Pro_4 \rightarrow Arg$ $Pro_3 \rightarrow His$	Autosomal recessive	No clinical abnormalities
Apo A-I Giessen	No evidence of lipoprotein abnormalities	$Pro_{145} \rightarrow Arg$	Unknown	No clinical abnormalities
Apo A-I/C-III	Absence of apo A-I and apo C-III in plasma	Abnormal apo A-I gene	Autosomal codominant	Onset of severe atherosclerosis in early age (see Table 7)
Apo E-2/E-2	Homozygosity for this isoform is associated with impaired binding to the apo E receptor	$Arg_{158} \rightarrow Cys$	Polygenic	Xanthomas and atherosclerosis; present in type III hyperlipoproteinemia (see Table 8)

Table 4 Enzyme Defects

Enzyme deficiency	Plasma abnormalities	Mechanism of deficiency	Mode of transmission	Main clinical features
Lipoprotein lipase	Creamy appearance; high triglycerides and chylomicron levels	Unknown	Autosomal recessive	Upper abdominal pain, hepatosplenomegaly, lipemia retinalis eruptive xanthomas; present in type I hyperlipoproteinemia; usually occurs first during childhood
Hepatic lipase (6)	Elevated plasma cholesterol, triglyceride, and VLDL; LDL and HDL enriched in triglycerides; reduced postheparin lipoprotein lipase activity; elevation of apo B, apo C-II, and apo E	Unknown	Unknown	Angina pectoris, eruptive skin xanthomas responsive to diet; arcus corneae
LCAT	Low levels of cholesteryl esters with relatively high unesterified cholesterol and phospholipids; low levels of abnormal HDL species	Unknown	Autosomal recessive	Anemia, proteinuria, corneal infiltration, abnormality in the cholesterol and physiological content of erythrocytes (target cells)

Receptor Defects

Through the brilliant studies of Goldstein and Brown it is now established that the LDL or apo B,E receptor plays a key role in cholesterol metabolism (see Chapter 13). This is dramatically documented by the disorder familial hypercholesterolemia in either its hetero- or homozygous form. In the older Fredrickson nomenclature classifying hyperlipoproteinemias (Table 1), this disorder encountered the type IIa category. Based on receptor functional studies, three types of patients have been identified: those with absence of LDL receptors, those with defective LDL receptors, and those with receptor internalization defects. With the acquisition of a better knowledge about the receptor structure and biosynthesis (see Table 5 and Chapter 13), it is recognized that the gene for the LDL receptor has four main classes of mutations, each of which affects a different region in the gene (7). This leads to an interference with the various steps involved in normal receptor synthesis, passage through the Golgi complex and transport to coated pits in the plasma membrane where it binds to LDL (see Table 6). Each of the three common alleles, R → O, R 120, and R 120 → 160, are genetically

Table 5 Structure of Apo B,E Receptor (839 Amino Acids)

Domains	Properties
First	NH_2-terminal 322-amino-acid domain composed of eight 40-amino-acid sequence repeats; each repeat contains 6 cysteine residues (last repeat contains only 5) for a total of 47 cysteine residues linked by disulfide bonds causing high structural rigidity; this region is likely involved in apo B or apo E binding
Second	350-amino-acid domain with a strong homology with the polyprotein precursor of epidermal growth factor (33% identity over a segment of 350 amino acids), suggesting that both this growth factor and the apo B,E receptor are derived from a common ancestral gene
Third	Stretch of 48 amino acids, 18 of which are serine and threonine residues containing carbohydrates attached in o-glycosidic linkage; this domain is external to the plasma membrane
Fourth	Membrane-spanning region of 22 amino acids
Fifth	Sequence of 50 amino acids at the COOH-terminal end of the receptor projecting into the cytoplasm; this sequence may bind clathrin

Table 6 Apo B,E Receptor: Mutant Alleles

Class of mutation	Nature of mutation	Allele	Mol wt by SDS gels		Frequency
			Precursor	Mature	
1	Not detectable precursor	R-0	Not detected	Not detected	Common
2	Precursor not processed	R-100	100,000	100,000	Rare
		R-120	120,000	120,000	Common
		R-135	135,000	135,000	Rare
3	Precursor processed at abnormally low rate	R-120–160	120,000	160,000	Rare, found in South African patients and WHHL rabbits
4	Precursor processed normally, but does not bind LDL	R^{b}-100–140	100,000	140,000	Rare
		R^{b}-120–160	120,000	160,000	Common
		R^{b}-170–210	170,000	210,000	Rare
5	Precursor processed normally and binds LDL normally, but fails to cluster into coated pits	R^{b+io}, 110–150	110,000	150,000	Rare
		R^{b+io}, 120–160	120,000	160,000	Rare

Table 7 Features of Familial Hypercholesterolemia

Plasma		Frequency of genetic defect	Mode of transmission	Clinical manifestation
Heterozygous	Chol,[a] 600 mg/dl; LDL chol, 500 mg/dl; apo B, 280 mg/dl; HDL chol, normal or low; apo A-I, normal or low	1/1000; 50% reduction of apo B,E receptor	Autosomal dominant	Tendinous and tuberous xanthomas; arcus corneae
Homozygous	Chol, 600 mg/dl; LDL chol, 500 mg/dl; apo B, 280 mg/dl; HDL chol, low; apo A-I, low	1/1,000,000; absent or defective apo B,E receptor (see Table 5)	Autosomal dominant	Same as heterozygous, but more severe

[a]Chol, cholesterol.

Table 8 Familial Disorders of HDL Metabolism of Unknown Etiology Associated with Coronary Heart Disease or Xanthomatosis

Disease	Cholesterol (mg/dl)			Triglycerides (mg/dl)	Apo A-I	Mode of transmission	Clinical findings
	Total	LDL	HDL				
Hypoalphalipoproteinemia							
Familial hypoalphalipoproteinemia	165 ± 38	115 ± 35	26 ± 4	113 ± 29	55 ± 5	Autosomal dominant	Early myocardial infarction
Fish-eye disease							
Heterozygote	238 ± 61	186 ± 51	33 ± 5	132 ± 63	22 ± 4	Unknown	Corneal opacity; coronary disease
Homozygote	207 ± 36	199 ± 27	7 ± 1	424 ± 97	12 ± 2	Unknown	
Apo A-I/apo C-III deficiency (9)	177	173	4	62	Trace	Autosomal codominant	Onset of severe atherosclerosis at an early age
Hyperalphalipoproteinemia							
Johannesburg	208	103	85	59	193	Unknown	Single case, diffuse xanthomatosis

heterogeneous and likely to be subdivided into additional alleles as more DNA sequence data become available.

The salient features of familial hypercholesterolemia are presented in Table 7.

Familial Hypo- and Hyperalphalipoproteinemias

A number of familial disorders associated with low or high levels of HDL have been described. They have been referred to as hypo- and hyper-alphalipoproteinemia (1,8).

Hypoalphalipoproteinemias

These include various disorders: familial hypoalphalipoproteinemia, fish-eye disease, familial apo A-I/apo C-III deficiency, Tangier disease, and those associated with apo A-I variants (see Tables 3 and 8). Whereas no important clinical abnormalities are associated with the apo A-I variants, other cases have been associated with either corneal opacification or premature coronary disease. The precise relationships between these HDL deficiencies and atherosclerosis have not been established but could be related to a defective removal of cholesterol from the cells, although other factors may also play a role.

Hyperalphalipoproteinemias

Familial hyperalphalipoproteinemias, with levels of HDL cholesterol between 70 and 90 mg/dl affecting several family members, have been described (see Table 8). This polygenic disorder of metabolism is associated with an increased life expectancy and low incidence of coronary heart disease. However, this may not be true in all cases. The patient reported in Table 7 presented with HDL cholesterol levels of 160 mg/dl and apo A-I of 200 mg/dl, and had diffuse xanthomatosis sufficient to justify treatment with hypocholesterolemic agents (H. Seftel, personal communication). Additional cases with marked elevation of HDL and peripheral vascular disease were seen in the Lipid Clinic at the University of Chicago. The biochemical basis for these complications is not known, but one may speculate that in these cases the high levels of HDL in the plasma may cause a gradient favoring the entry of cholesterol into the tissues.

LIPOPROTEIN DISORDERS WITH HIGH TRIGLYCERIDE LEVELS BUT UNCERTAIN FAMILIAL DETERMINATION (Table 9)

Except for familial hyperchylomicronemia, also referred to as type I hyperlipidemia (Table 1), where the biochemical defect is the absence of either lipoprotein lipase (Table 3) or its activator apo C-II (Table 2), the other forms of hypertriglyceridemias or mixed hyperlipidemias

Table 9 Disorders of Unknown or Partially Known Familial Determination

Phenotype	Frequencies	Appearance of serum	Serum (mg/dl)	
			Cholesterol	Triglyceride
Type III	2–3/10,000	Turbid	350–500	350–500
Familial combined hyperlipidemia; phenotypes IIa, IIb, and IV expressed in the same family	3–5/1000	Clear or turbid	Elevation of either cholesterol, triglycerides, or both	
Familial hypertriglyceridemia	2–3/1000	Turbid	Cholesterol normal or slightly elevated; triglycerides markedly elevated	
Type V	1/5000	Creamy	Triglycerides, 1000; cholesterol, 300	

Lipoprotein abnormalities	Chemical features	Biochemical defect	Mode of transmission
Floating β-VLDL by ultracentrifugation; broad beta-band by electrophoresis	Xanthomas in palmar creases, coronary atherosclerosis, and peripheral vascular disease; often associated with other diseases such as diabetes mellitus and hyperuricemia	Apo E-1/E-2 homozygosity associated with primary and secondary hyperlipidemias; defective uptake of chylomicrons and VLDL remnants by the hepatic apo E receptor	Polygenic
Phenotype IIa: (elevated LDL cholesterol), phenotypes IIb and IV (elevation of LDL cholesterol and VLDL triglycerides)	Associated with high risk of myocardial infarction; within the same family the phenotype changes; hypertriglyceridemia expressed after age 30	Unknown Polygenic?	Autosomal dominant?
Normal LDL cholesterol; marked elevation of VLDL triglycerides	Expressed in middle age; can be associated with diabetes mellitus and obesity	Unknown	Autosomal dominant
Marked elevation of chylomicrons and VLDL; reduced HDL	Eruptive xanthomas; lipemia retinalis, hepatosplenomegaly, pancreatitis	Not clearly defined	Unknown

(elevation of both plasma cholesterol and triglycerides) are not well defined in biochemical and genetic terms. Some are rare phenotypes such as types III and V (Table 1); others are relatively more frequent such as types IIb and IV (Table 1), which may be seen in family members of patients with familial combined hyperlipidemia. The biochemical defect and mode of inheritance of these forms of hyperlipidemias are not yet clearly established. The biochemical defect in familial hypertriglyceridemia also is undefined.

APPENDIX

The segregation of the lipid disorders into major classes as outlined in this chapter, although in keeping with current concepts in lipoprotein metabolism, does not take into account the wide variability in the expression of plasma lipoprotein distribution among individuals either in the normo- or dyslipoproteinemic state. We are presently unable to explain this class heterogeneity, which is likely to be the resultant of the complex interplay between the genetic make-up of each individual and environmental factors. The examples reported were selected from about 1500 plasma lipoprotein profiles examined using a single-step isopycnic density gradient ultracentrifugal procedure requiring only 0.4 ml of plasma. Each profile represents a continuous 280-nm recording of the effluents after the ultracentrifugal run. Whenever necessary, 0.2-ml fractions were collected at the points indicated by the event markers to permit the physicochemical and immunological characterization of each fraction. Of particular interest are the profiles of normolipidemic subjects with comparable levels of total cholesterol: important differences in the peak position of each lipoprotein fraction are evident. Since ultracentrifugation was carried to equilibrium, this indicates that there were differences in the hydrated density of the lipoprotein fractions under consideration.

NORMOLIPIDEMIC SUBJECTS

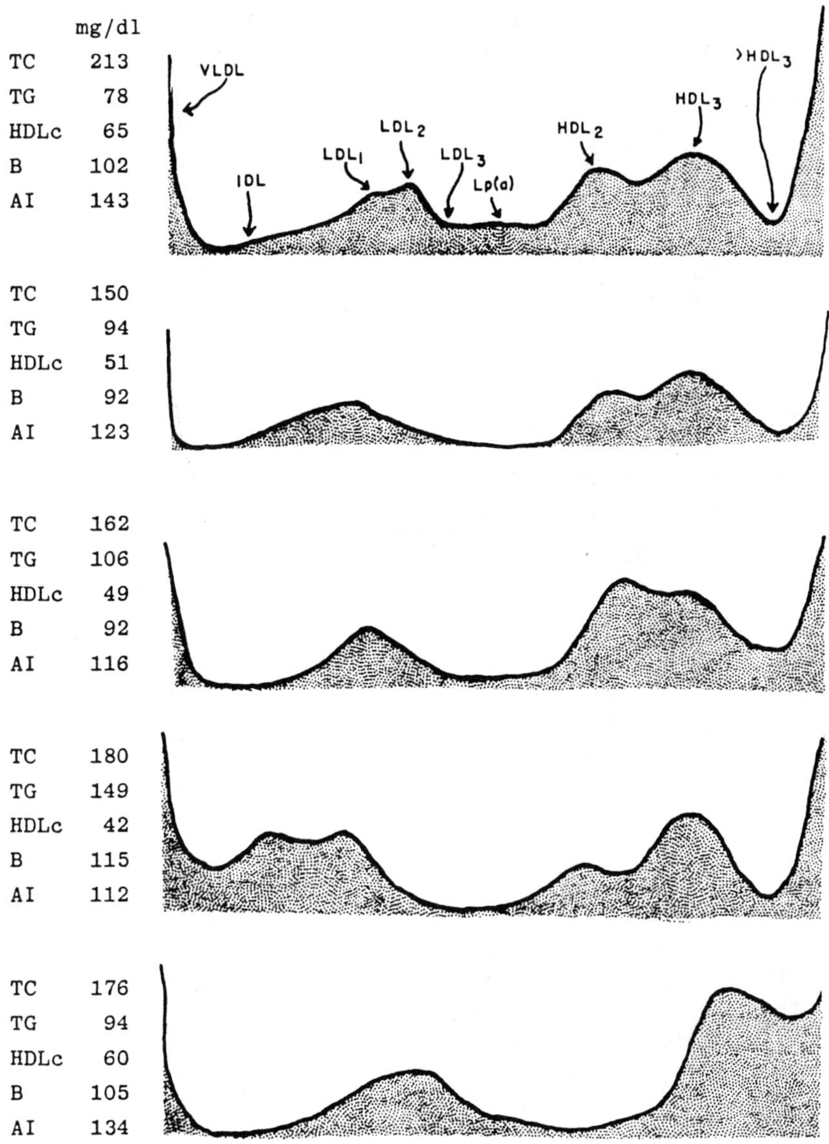

Fig. 1

FAMILIAL HYPERCHOLESTEROLEMIA
VLDL
IDL
LDL1
LDL2
LDL3
Lp(a)
HDL2
HDL3
>HDL3
mg/dl
TC 712
TG 85
B 1710
AI 54
HOMOZYGOUS
TC 732
TG 82
B 532
AI 63
HOMOZYGOUS
TC 506
TG 68
B 470
AI 67
HETEROZYGOUS
TC 380
TG 170
B 332
AI 100
HETEROZYGOUS
TC 332
TG 130
B 306
AI 140
HETEROZYGOUS

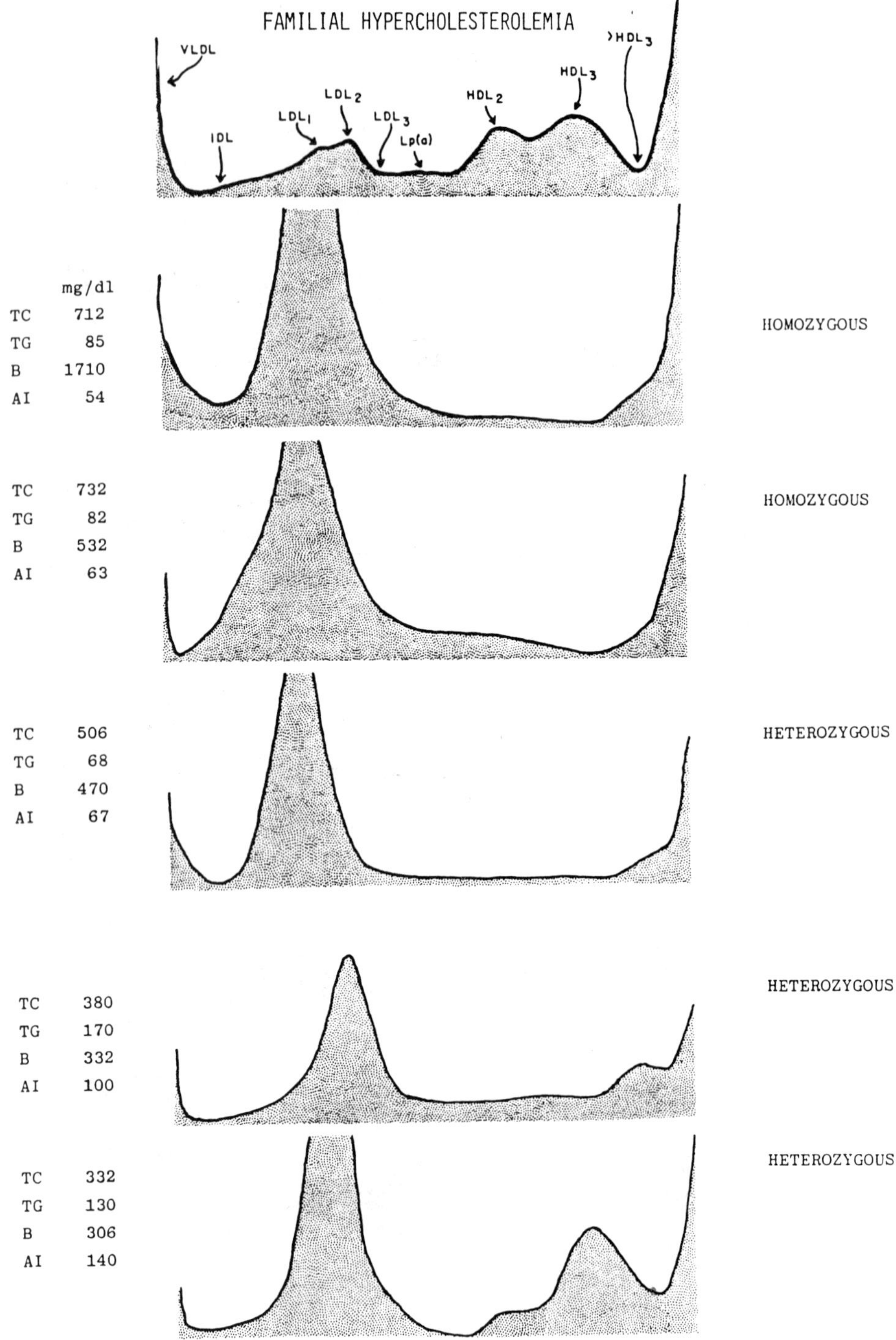

Fig. 2

HYPER-HDLEMIA
VLDL
IDL
LDL1
LDL2
LDL3
Lp(a)
HDL2
HDL3
>HDL3
mg/dl
TC 386
TG 108
HDLc 170
B 95
AI 288
TC 199
TG 146
HDLc 98
B 98
AI 211
TC 270
TG 138
HDLc 108
B 128
AI 236
TC 208
TG 59
HDLc 98
B 128
AI 201
TC 186
TG 91
HDLc 91
B 97
AI 194

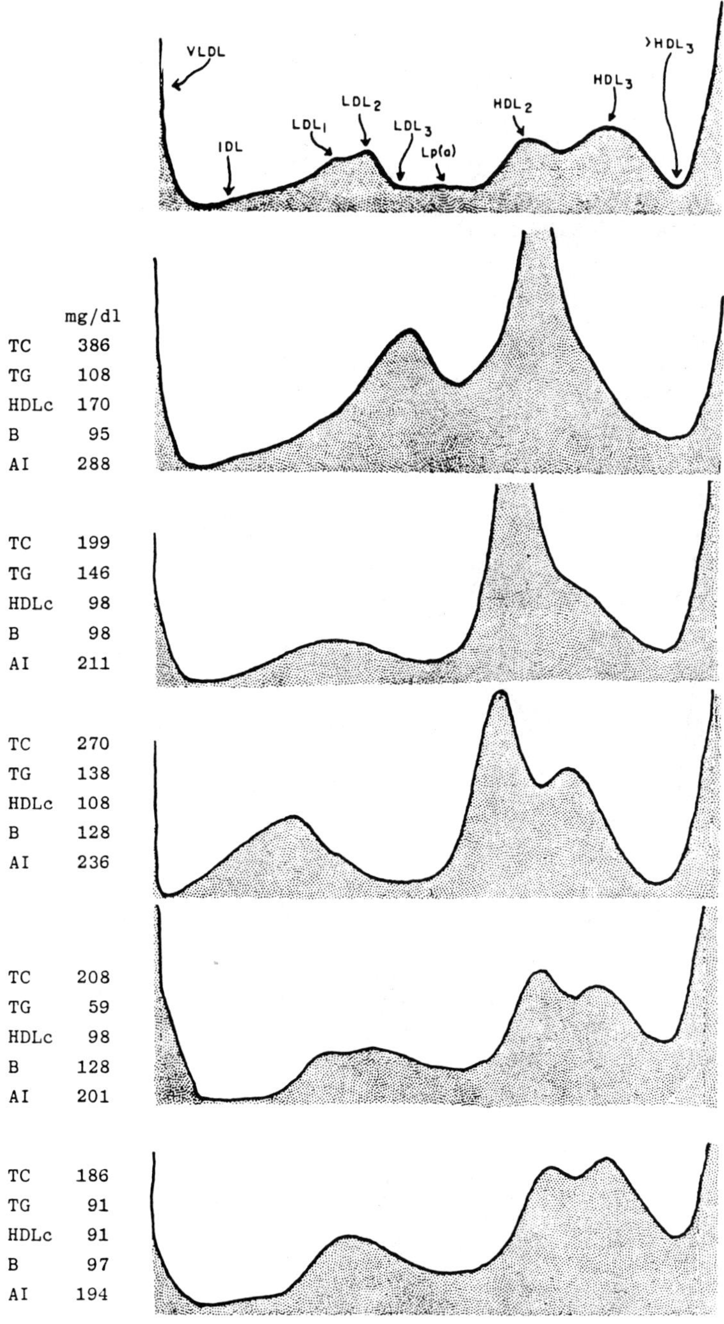

Fig. 3

SUBJECTS WITH Lp(a)

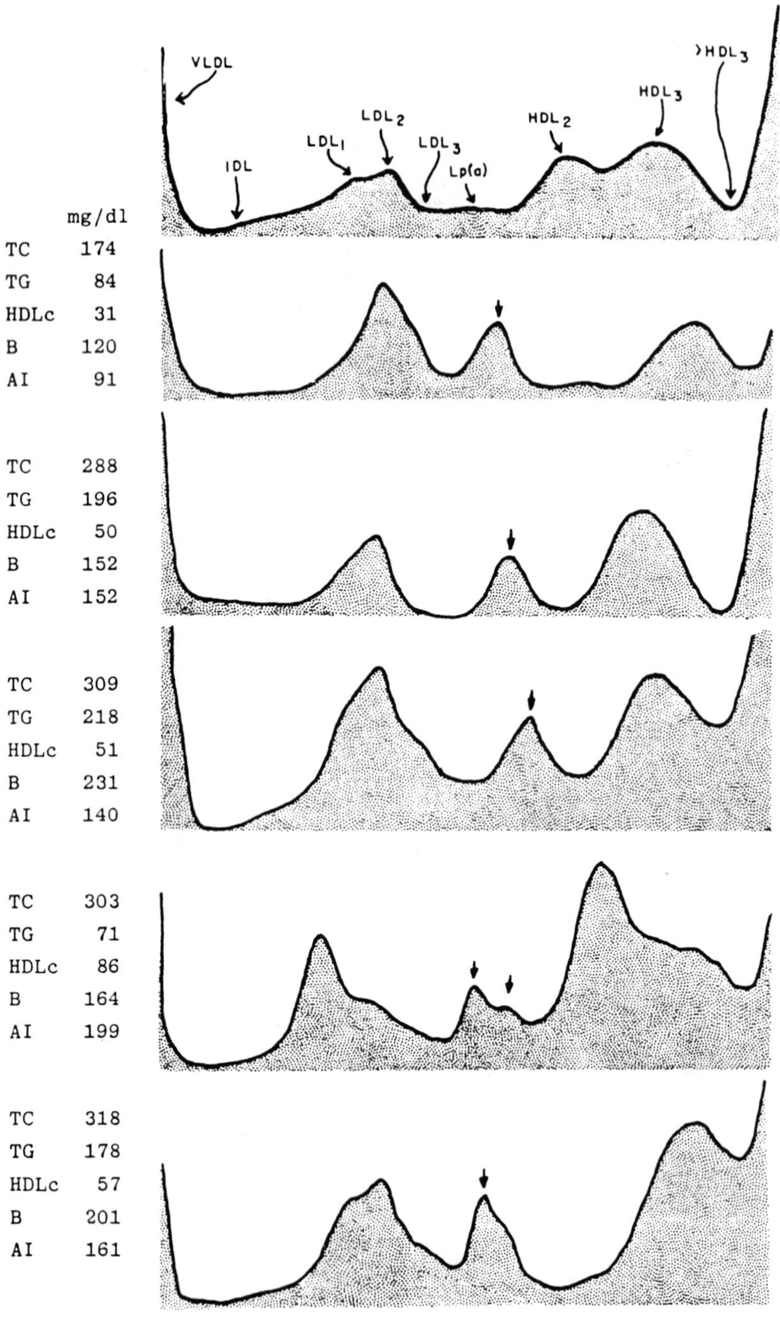

Fig. 4

HYPO-LDLEMIA

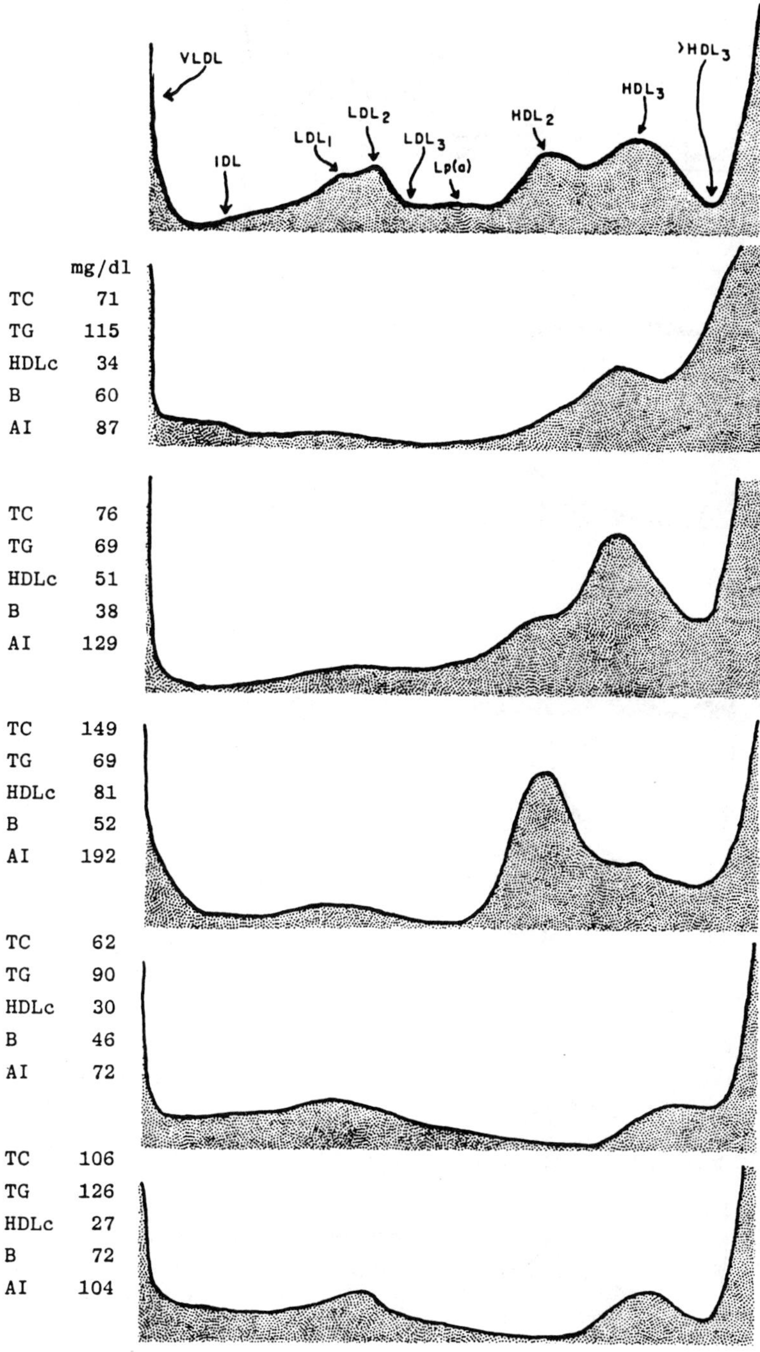

Fig. 5

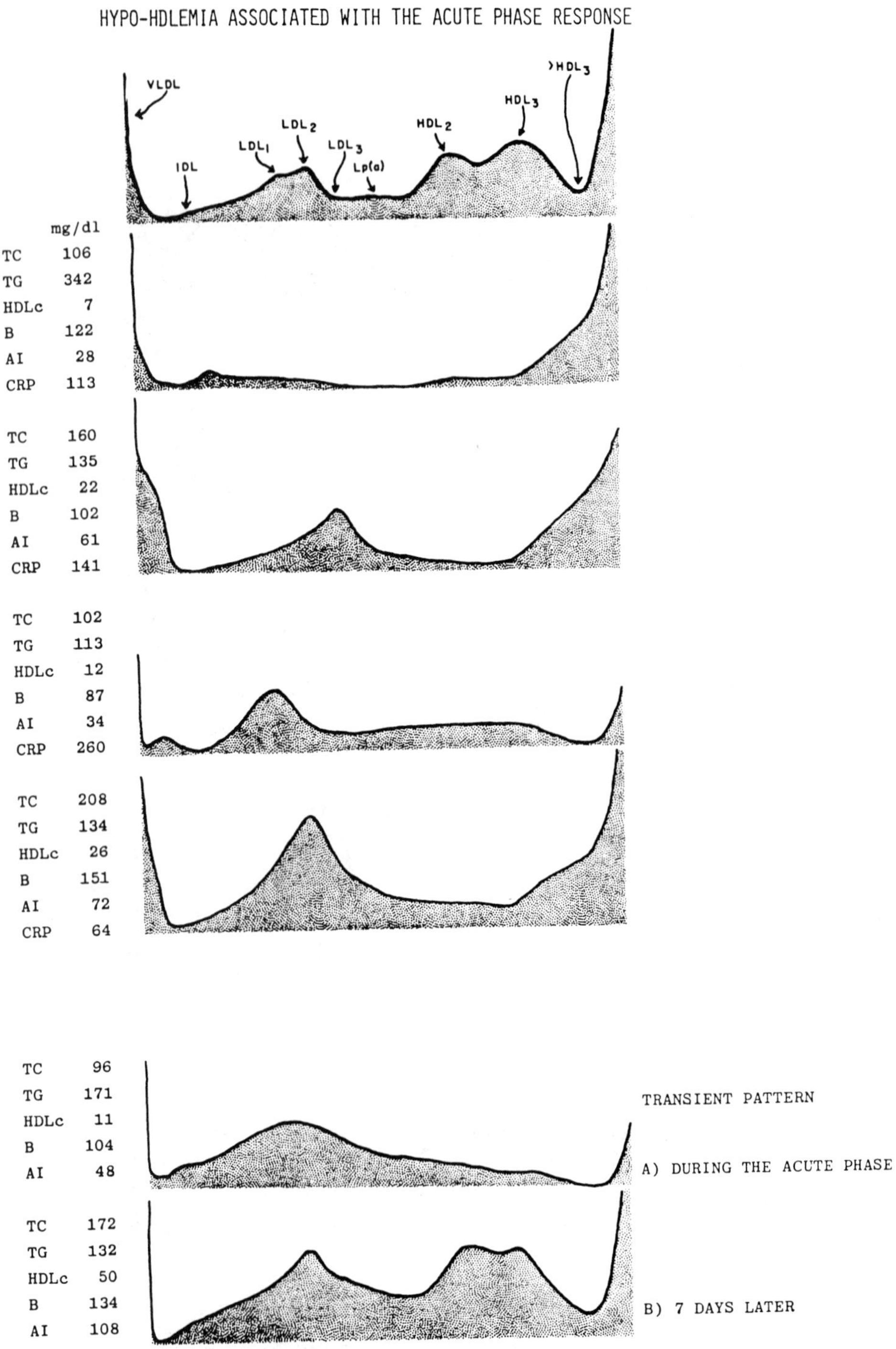

HYPO-HDLEMIA ASSOCIATED WITH THE ACUTE PHASE RESPONSE
VLDL
IDL
LDL_1
LDL_2
LDL_3
Lp(a)
HDL_2
HDL_3
$>HDL_3$
mg/dl
TC 106
TG 342
HDLc 7
B 122
AI 28
CRP 113
TC 160
TG 135
HDLc 22
B 102
AI 61
CRP 141
TC 102
TG 113
HDLc 12
B 87
AI 34
CRP 260
TC 208
TG 134
HDLc 26
B 151
AI 72
CRP 64
TC 96
TG 171
HDLc 11
B 104
AI 48
TRANSIENT PATTERN
A) DURING THE ACUTE PHASE
TC 172
TG 132
HDLc 50
B 134
AI 108
B) 7 DAYS LATER

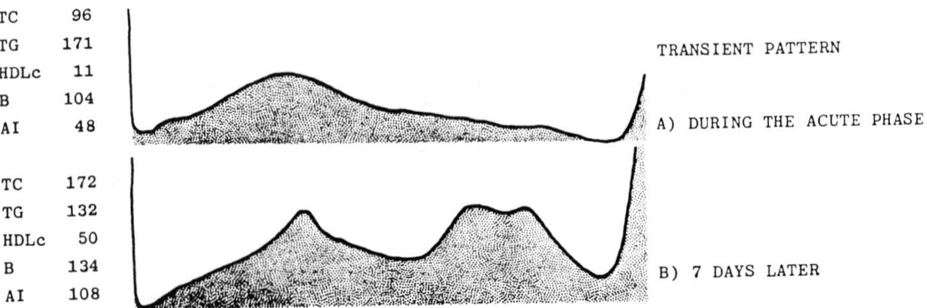

Fig. 6

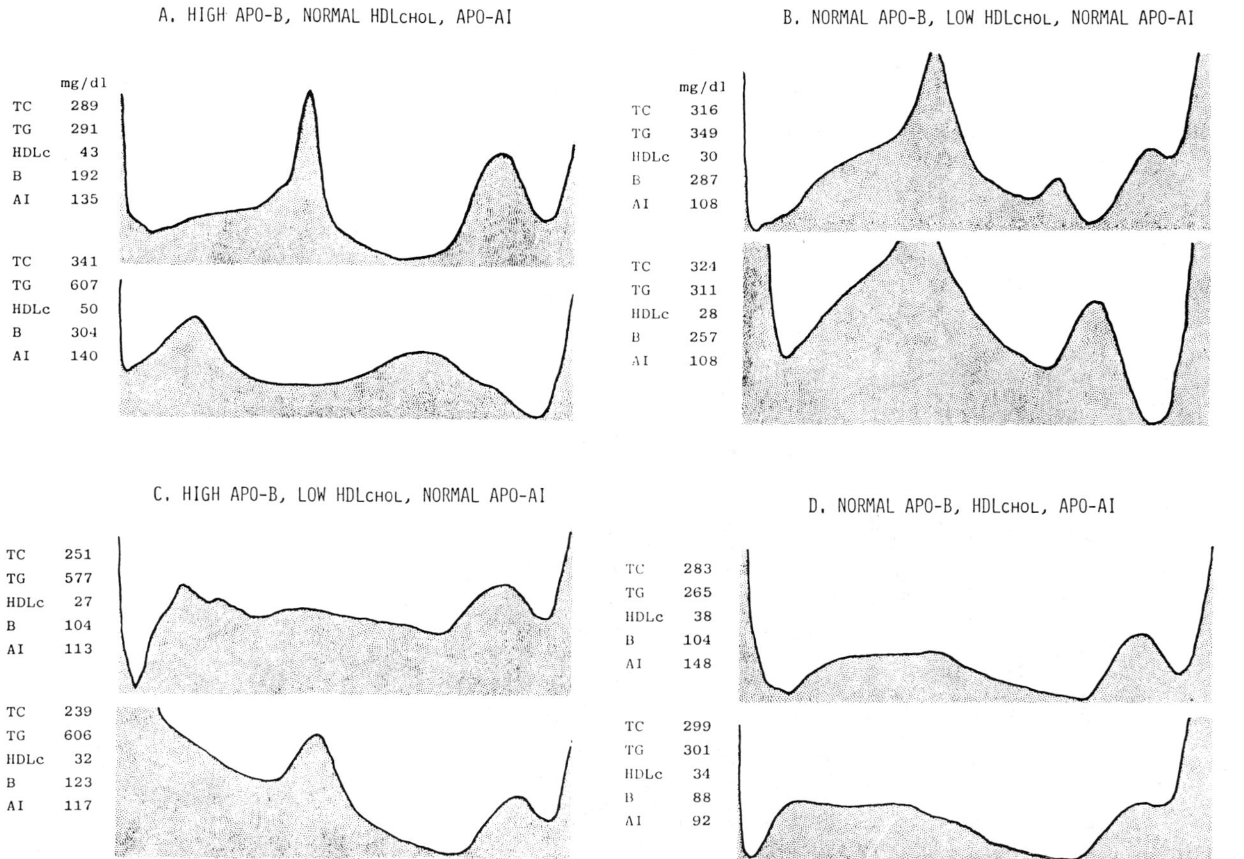

Fig. 7 Mixed hyperlipidemias.

REFERENCES

1. Assmann, G., *Lipid Metabolism and Atherosclerosis*, Schattauer Verlag, Stuttgart, 1982, pp. 101–148.

2. Fredrickson, D. S., Levy, R. I., and Lees, R. S., *New Engl. J. Med.*, *276*:34 (1967).

3. Grundy, S. M., *J. Lipid Res.*, *25*:1611–1618 (1984).

4. Mahley, R. W., Innerarity, T. L., Rall, S. C., and Weisgraber, K. H., *J. Lipid Res.*, *25*:1277–1294 (1984).

5. Sprecher, D. L., Taam, L., and Brewer, H. B., Jr., *Clin. Chem.*, *30*:2084–2092 (1984).

6. Breckenridge, W. C., Little, J. A., Alaupovic, P., Wang, C.-S., Xuksis, A., Lindgren, F., and Gardiner, G., *Atherosclerosis*, *45*:161–179 (1982).

7. Goldstein, J. L., and Brown, M. S., *J. Lipid Res.*, *25*:1415–1461 (1984).

8. Schaefer, E. J., *Atherosclerosis*, *4*:303–322 (1984).

9. Norum, R. A., Lakier, J. B., Goldstein, S., Angel, A., Goldberg, R. B., Block, W. D., Noffee, D. K., Dolphin, P. J., Edelglass, J., Borograd, D. D., and Alaupovic, P., *New Engl. J. Med.*, *306*:1513 (1982).

Appendix 1

Nucleotide and Corresponding Amino Acid Sequences of Human Apo A-I, Apo A-II, Apo C-I, Apo C-II, Apo C-III, and Apo E cDNA Clones

SOTIRIOS K. KARATHANASIS and ISSAM A. HADDAD Children's Hospital, Medical School, Boston, Massachusetts

ELIZABETH SALMON and VASSILIS I. ZANNIS Boston University Medical Center, Boston, Massachusetts

INTRODUCTION

Apolipoproteins are the protein moieties of lipoproteins, the macromolecules involved in the transport of lipids (cholesterol, triglycerides, and phospholipids) from one tissue to another (1). Following the nomenclature system proposed by Alaupovic, the apolipoproteins have been designated apo A-I, apo A-II, apo A-IV, apo B, apo C-I, apo C-II, apo C-III, apo D, and apo E (2). With the exception of apo A-IV, apo B, and apo D, the primary amino acid sequence of the plasma forms of the remaining apolipoproteins has been determined (3–9). Our current knowledge of the structure and function of apolipoproteins is reviewed in references 10 to 12.

The isolation and characterization of several apolipoprotein cDNA clones have provided new insights into the structure of apolipoproteins and their corresponding genes. In addition, it offers new tools for a systematic study of the genetic variations of apolipoprotein genes and their flanking regions as they relate to human disease, as well as for studies of the regulation of expression of the apolipoprotein genes. In this appendix we have compiled the cDNA and the corresponding amino acid sequences of human apo A-I, apo A-II, apo C-I, apo C-II, apo C-III, and apo E that have been reported by various laboratories. The cDNA-derived amino acid sequences provide the complete sequence of the primary translation product of apoprotein mRNA and in some instances modify the currently available protein sequences. The observed differences in the apoprotein sequences may represent true allelic variations in the apolipoprotein genes; alternatively, they may represent corrections of the previously published amino acid sequences of apolipoprotein molecules.

APO A-I

The nucleotide sequences of human apo A-I cDNA clones have been reported recently by four independent research groups (13–16). Table I is a composite of the nucleotide sequences and the corresponding amino acid sequence of two overlapping apo A-I cDNA clones described in reference 13. The nucleotide sequences of apo A-I cDNA clones described in references 14 to 16 are identical to the sequences 62 to 954, 97 to 900, and 97 to 183 of Table I, respectively.

Sharpe et al. have presented evidence suggesting that the nucleotides 1 through 61 of Table I are absent from the major species of

Table I Nucleotide and Corresponding Amino Acid Sequences Derived from the Analysis of Two Overlapping Human Apo A-I cDNA Clones[a,b]

								27									54
CCT	CCC	AGC	CCA	GAC	CCT	GGC	TGC	AGA	CAT	AAA	TAG	GCC	CTG	CAA	GAG	CTG	GCT
								81									108
GCT	TAG	AGA	CTG	CGA	GAA	GGA	GGT	CCC	CCA	CGG	CCC	TTC	AGG	ATG	AAA	GCT	GCG
														MET	Lys	Ala	Ala
								135									162
GTG	CTG	ACC	TTG	GCC	GTG	CTC	TTC	CTG	ACG	GGG	AGC	CAG	GCT	CGG	CAT	TTC	TGG
Val	Leu	Thr	Leu	Ala	Val	Leu	Phe	Leu	Thr	Gly	Ser	Gln	Ala	Arg	His	Phe	Trp
-20										-10							
								189									216
CAG	CAA	GAT	GAA	CCC	CCC	CAG	AGC	CCC	TGG	GAT	CGA	GTG	AAG	GAC	CTG	GCC	ACT
Gln	Gln	Asp	Glu	Pro	Pro	Gln	Ser	Pro	Trp	Asp	Arg	Val	Lys	Asp	Leu	Ala	Thr
	-1	+1									10						
								243									270
GTG	TAC	GTG	GAT	GTG	CTC	AAA	GAC	AGC	GGC	AGA	GAC	TAT	GTG	TCC	CAG	TTT	GAA
Val	Tyr	Val	Asp	Val	Leu	Lys	Asp	Ser	Gly	Arg	Asp	Tyr	Val	Ser	Gln	Phe	Glu
			20										30				*
								297									324
GGC	TCC	GCC	TTG	GGA	AAA	CAG	CTA	AAC	CTA	AAG	CTC	CTT	GAC	AAC	TGG	GAC	AGC
Gly	Ser	Ala	Leu	Gly	Lys	Gln	Leu	Asn	Leu	Lys	Leu	Leu	Asp	Asn	Trp	Asp	Ser
					40										50		
								351									378
GTG	ACC	TCC	ACC	TTC	AGC	AAG	CTG	CGC	GAA	CAG	CTC	GGC	CCT	GTG	ACC	CAG	GAG
Val	Thr	Ser	Thr	Phe	Ser	Lys	Leu	Arg	Glu	Gln	Leu	Gly	Pro	Val	Thr	Gln	Glu
							60										70
								405									432
TTC	TGG	GAT	AAC	CTG	GAA	AAG	GAG	ACA	GAG	GGC	CTG	AGG	CAG	GAG	ATG	AGC	AAG
Phe	Trp	Asp	Asn	Leu	Glu	Lys	Glu	Thr	Glu	Gly	Leu	Arg	Gln	Glu	MET	Ser	Lys
									80								

Table I (continued)

								459									486
GAT	CTG	GAG	GAG	GTG	AAG	GCC	AAG	GTG	CAG	CCC	TAC	CTG	GAC	GAC	TTC	CAG	AAG
Asp	Leu	Glu	Glu	Val	Lys	Ala	Lys	Val	Gln	Pro	Tyr	Leu	Asp	Asp	Phe	Gln	Lys
	90										100						
								513									540
AAG	TGG	CAG	GAG	GAG	ATG	GAG	CTC	TAC	CGC	CAG	AAG	GTG	GAG	CCG	CTG	CGC	GCA
Lys	Trp	Gln	Glu	Glu	MET	Glu	Leu	Tyr	Arg	Gln	Lys	Val	Glu	Pro	Leu	Arg	Ala
			110										120				
								567									594
GAG	CTC	CAA	GAG	GGC	GCG	CGC	CAG	AAG	CTG	CAC	GAG	CTG	CAA	GAG	AAG	CTG	AGC
Glu	Leu	Gln	Glu	Gly	Ala	Arg	Gln	Lys	Leu	His	Glu	Leu	Gln	Glu	Lys	Leu	Ser
					130										140		
								621									648
CCA	CTG	GGC	GAG	GAG	ATG	CGC	GAC	CGC	GCG	CGC	GCC	CAT	GTG	GAC	GCG	CTG	CGC
Pro	Leu	Gly	Glu	Glu	MET	Arg	Asp	Arg	Ala	Arg	Ala	His	Val	Asp	Ala	Leu	Arg
			*	*			150										160
								675									702
ACG	CAT	CTG	GCC	CCC	TAC	AGC	GAC	GAG	CTG	CGC	CAG	CGC	TTG	GCC	GCG	CGC	CTT
Thr	His	Leu	Ala	Pro	Tyr	Ser	Asp	Glu	Leu	Arg	Gln	Arg	Leu	Ala	Ala	Arg	Leu
									170								
								729									756
GAG	GCT	CTC	AAG	GAG	AAC	GGC	GGC	GCC	AGA	CTG	GCC	GAG	TAC	CAC	GCC	AAG	GCC
Glu	Ala	Leu	Lys	Glu	Asn	Gly	Gly	Ala	Arg	Leu	Ala	Glu	Tyr	His	Ala	Lys	Ala
	180										190						
								783									810
ACC	GAG	CAT	CTG	AGC	ACG	CTC	AGC	GAG	AAG	GCC	AAG	CCC	GCG	CTC	GAG	GAC	CTC
Thr	Glu	His	Leu	Ser	Thr	Leu	Ser	Glu	Lys	Ala	Lys	Pro	Ala	Leu	Glu	Asp	Leu
			200										210				
								837									864
CGC	CAA	GGC	CTG	CTG	CCC	GTG	CTG	GAG	AGC	TTC	AAG	GTC	AGC	TTC	CTG	AGC	GCT
Arg	Gln	Gly	Leu	Leu	Pro	Val	Leu	Glu	Ser	Phe	Lys	Val	Ser	Phe	Leu	Ser	Ala
					220										230		
								891									918
CTC	GAG	GAG	TAC	ACT	AAG	AAG	CTC	AAC	ACC	CAG	TGA	GGC	GCC	CGC	CGC	CGC	CCC
Leu	Glu	Glu	Tyr	Thr	Lys	Lys	Leu	Asn	Thr	Gln	**END**						
							240										

[a] Data from Ref. 13.

[b] In this and the subsequent Tables II through VI, numbers on the top of each row identify the nucleotide sequences. Numbers underneath each row identify the amino acid sequences. Negative numbers correspond to signal (and propeptide) sequences. Positive numbers correspond to mature protein sequences. *indicates amino acid differences between the cDNA-derived sequences (13–15) and that derived by protein sequencing techniques (6). The latter sequence has Gln at the indicated positions.

human liver apo A-I mRNA and thus may represent sequences present in only minor liver apo A-I mRNA transcripts (14).

The cDNA-derived amino acid sequence showed that the primary translation product of apo A-I mRNA consists of 267 amino acids. The first 18 N-terminal amino acids comprise the signal peptide, which is cleaved intracellularly by the signal peptidase of the rough endoplasmic reticulum (17–20). The next six N-terminal amino acids comprise a prosegment, which is cleaved extracellularly by a protease present in plasma, lymph (21,22), and possibly in other cellular compartments. At the protein level the cDNA-derived amino acid sequence of apo A-I agrees, with three exceptions, with the most recently reported protein sequence of plasma apo A-I (6). The difference occurs at residues +34, +146, and +147 where the cDNA-derived amino acid sequence predicts Glu and the protein sequence specifies Gln.

APO A-II

The nucleotide sequence of three independently isolated human apo A-II cDNA clones have been reported recently (14,23,24). The longest of these DNA sequences (23) and the corresponding amino acid sequence are shown in Table II. The apo A-II cDNA sequences described in references 14 through 24 correspond to nucleotide sequences 25 through 428 and 30 through 467 of Table II, respectively. Both sequences described in references 14 and 24 lack the nucleotide C, which is present at residue position 364 of Table II. In addition, the sequence described in reference 24 contains the nucleotide A instead of G at residue position 150 of Table II. The cDNA-derived amino acid sequence of apo A-II agrees, with one exception, with the protein sequence of plasma apo A-II. The difference occurs at residue 37 where the cDNA-derived amino acid sequence predicts Glu and the protein sequence specifies Gln (3). The cDNA-derived amino acid sequence showed that the primary translation product of apo A-II mRNA consists of 100 amino acids. The first 18 N-terminal amino acids comprise the signal peptide, which is cleaved intracellularly by the signal peptidase of the rough endoplasmic reticulum (17,18,25). The next five N-terminal amino acids comprise a prosegment, which is cleaved extracellularly by a thiol protease (26).

APO C-I

The nucleotide sequence and the corresponding amino acid sequence of a human apo C-I cDNA clone have been reported recently (27) and are shown in Table III. The cDNA-derived amino acid sequence showed that the primary translation product of apo C-I mRNA consists of 83 amino acids, including a 26-amino-acid-long N-terminal signal peptide.

Table II Nucleotide and Corresponding Amino Acid Sequences of a Full-Length Human Apo A-II cDNA Clone[a,b]

```
                                27                                  54
ATA CCC GAG GAC AGA GAT GTT GGT TAG GCC GCC CTC CCC ACT GTT ACC AAC ATG
                                                                    MET

                                81                                  108
AAG CTG CTC GCA GCA ACT GTG CTA CTC CTC ACC ATC TGC AGC CTT GAA GGA GCT
Lys Leu Leu Ala Ala Thr Val Leu Leu Leu Thr Ile Cys Ser Leu Glu Gly Ala
    -20                                         -10

                                                    α
                                135                 ↓               162
TTG GTT CGG AGA CAG GCA AAG GAG CCA TGT GTG GAG AGC CTG GTT TCT CAG TAC
Leu Val Arg Arg Gln Ala Lys Glu Pro Cys Val Glu Ser Leu Val Ser Gln Tyr
            -1  +1                                  10

                                189                                 216
TTC CAG ACC GTG ACT GAC TAT GGC AAG GAC CTG ATG GAG AAG GTC AAG AGC CCA
Phe Gln Thr Val Thr Asp Tyr Gly Lys Asp Leu MET Glu Lys Val Lys Ser Pro
                    20                              30

                                243                                 270
GAG CTT CAG GCC GAG GCC AAG TCT TAC TTT GAA AAG TCA AAG GAG CAG CTG ACA
Glu Leu Gln Ala Glu Ala Lys Ser Tyr Phe Glu Lys Ser Lys Glu Gln Leu Thr
                *           40                                      50

                                297                                 324
CCC CTG ATC AAG AAG GCT GGA ACG GAA CTG GTT AAC TTC TTG AGC TAT TTC GTG
Pro Leu Ile Lys Lys Ala Gly Thr Glu Leu Val Asn Phe Leu Ser Tyr Phe Val
                                    60

                                                    β
                                351                 ↓               378
GAA CTT GGA ACA CAG CCT GCC ACC CAG TGA AGT GTC CAG CAC CAT TGT CTT CCA
Glu Leu Gly Thr Gln Pro Ala Thr·Gln END
    70

                                405                                 432
ACC CCA GCT GGC CTC TAG AAC ACC CAC TGG CCA GTC CTA GAG CTC CTG TCC CTA

                                459
CCC ACT CTT TGC TAC AAT AAA TGC TGA ATG AAT CC
```

[a]Described in Reference 23.
[b]α indicates substitution of A for G (24). β indicates deletion of C (14,24). * indicates amino acid differences between the cDNA-derived sequences (14,23,24) and that derived by protein sequencing techniques (3). The latter sequence has Gln at this position.

Table III Nucleotide and Corresponding Amino Acid Sequences of a Full-length Human Apo C-I cDNA Clone (27)

								27									54
CC	CGC	AGC	TCA	GCC	ACG	GCA	CAG	ATC	AGC	ACC	ACG	ACC	CCT	CCC	TCG	GGC	CTC
								81									108
GCC	ATG	AGG	CTC	TTC	CTG	TCG	CTC	CCG	GTC	CTG	GTG	GTG	GTT	CTG	TCG	ATC	GTC
	MET	Arg	Leu	Phe	Leu	Ser	Leu	Pro	Val	Leu	Val	Val	Val	Leu	Ser	Ile	Val
							-20										-10
								135									162
TTG	GAA	GGC	CCA	GCC	CCA	GCC	CAG	GGG	ACC	CCA	GAC	GTC	TCC	AGT	GCC	TTG	GAT
Leu	Glu	Gly	Pro	Ala	Pro	Ala	Gln	Gly	Thr	Pro	Asp	Val	Ser	Ser	Ala	Leu	Asp
								-1	+1								
								189									216
AAG	CTG	AAG	GAG	TTT	GGA	AAC	ACA	CTG	GAG	GAC	AAG	GCT	CGG	GAA	CTC	ATC	AGC
Lys	Leu	Lys	Glu	Phe	Gly	Asn	Thr	Leu	Glu	Asp	Lys	Ala	Arg	Glu	Leu	Ile	Ser
10										20							
								243									270
CGC	ATC	AAA	CAG	AGT	GAA	CTT	TCT	GCC	AAG	ATG	CGG	GAG	TGG	TTT	TCA	GAG	ACA
Arg	Ile	Lys	Gln	Ser	Glu	Leu	Ser	Ala	Lys	MET	Arg	Glu	Trp	Phe	Ser	Glu	Thr
		30										40					
								297									324
TTT	CAG	AAA	GTG	AAG	GAG	AAA	CTC	AAG	ATT	GAC	TCA	TGA	GGA	CCT	GAA	GGG	TGA
Phe	Gln	Lys	Val	Lys	Glu	Lys	Leu	Lys	Ile	Asp	Ser	END					
				50													
								351									378
CAT	CCA	GGA	GGG	GCC	TCT	GAA	ATT	TCC	CAC	ACC	CCA	GCG	CCT	GTG	CTG	AGG	ACT
								405									432
CCC	GCC	ATG	TGG	CCC	CAG	GTG	CCA	CCA	ATA	AAA	ATC	CTA	CCG				

Furthermore, the predicted sequence of the 57-amino-acid-long mature protein agrees completely with the previously published protein sequence of plasma apo C-I (5)

APO C-II

The nucleotide sequences of four independently isolated human apo C-II cDNA clones have been reported recently (14,28–30). A composite of cDNA sequences and the corresponding amino acid sequence are shown in Table IV. Nucleotide sequences 1 through 312, 7 through 450, 20 through 456, and 37 through 456 correspond to apo

Table IV Composite Nucleotide and Corresponding Amino Acid Sequences of Three Overlapping Human Apo C-II cDNA Clones[a]

								27									54
GAC	ACT	ATG	GGC	ACA	CGA	CTC	CTC	CCA	GCT	CTG	TTT	CTT	GTC	CTC	CTG	GTA	TTG
		MET	Gly	Thr	Arg	Leu	Leu	Pro	Ala	Leu	Phe	Leu	Val	Leu	Leu	Val	Leu
				-20										**-10**			

								81									108
GGA	TTT	GAG	GTC	CAG	GGG	ACC	CAA	CAG	CCC	CAG	CAA	GAT	GAG	ATG	CCT	AGC	CCG
Gly	Phe	Glu	Val	Gln	Gly	Thr	Gln	Gln	Pro	Gln	Gln	Asp	Glu	MET	Pro	Ser	Pro
					-1	**+1**									**10**		

								135									162
ACC	TTC	CTC	ACC	CAG	GTG	AAG	GAA	TCT	CTC	TCC	AGT	TAC	TGG	GAG	TCA	GCA	AAG
Thr	Phe	Leu	Thr	Gln	Val	Lys	Glu	Ser	Leu	Ser	Ser	Tyr	Trp	Glu	Ser	Ala	Lys
							20										**30**

								189									216
ACA	GCC	GCC	CAG	AAC	CTG	TAC	GAG	AAG	ACA	TAC	CTG	CCC	GCT	GTA	GAT	GAG	AAA
Thr	Ala	Ala	Gln	Asn	Leu	Tyr	Glu	Lys	Thr	Tyr	Leu	Pro	Ala	Val	Asp	Glu	Lys
									40								

								243									270
CTC	AGG	GAC	TTG	TAC	AGC	AAA	AGC	ACA	GCA	GCC	ATG	AGC	ACT	TAC	ACA	GGC	ATT
Leu	Arg	Asp	Leu	Tyr	Ser	Lys	Ser	Thr	Ala	Ala	MET	Ser	Thr	Tyr	Thr	Gly	Ile
	50										**60**						

								297									324
TTT	ACT	GAC	CAA	GTT	CTT	TCT	GTG	CTG	AAG	GGA	GAG	GAG	TAA	CAG	CCA	GAC	CCC
Phe	Thr	Asp	Gln	Val	Leu	Ser	Val	Leu	Lys	Gly	Glu	Glu	**END**				
			70														

								351									378
CCA	TCA	GTG	GAC	AAG	GGG	AGA	GTC	CCC	TAC	TCC	CCT	GAT	CCC	CCA	GGT	TCA	GAC

					α ↓	β ↓		405									432
TGA	GCT	CCC	CCT	TCC	CAG	TAG	CTC	TTG	CAT	CCT	CCT	CCC	AAC	TCT	AGC	CTG	AAT

								459
TCT	TTT	CAA	TAA	AAA	ATA	CAA	TTC	

[a]Data from refs. 14,28, and 30. α and β indicate insertion of C at both positions (29).

C-II cDNA clones described in references 28, 14, 29, and 30, respectively. There was no difference in the nucleotide sequence of three of these clones (14,28,30); however, the sequence of the clone described in reference 29 has insertions of the nucleotide C between residues 395 and 396 and between 398 and 399 compared to the sequences of references 14 and 30. The cDNA-derived amino acid sequence showed that the primary translation product of apo C-II mRNA consists of 101 amino acids, including a 22-amino-acid-long N-terminal signal peptide (14,28). Furthermore, the predicted sequence of the 79-amino-acid-long mature protein agrees completely with the previously published sequence of plasma apo C-II (9).

APO C-III

The nucleotide sequences of three independently isolated human apo C-III cDNA clones have been reported recently (14,31). Two of these sequences correspond to different apo C-III gene alleles isolated from a cDNA library that was prepared from liver mRNA of an apparently heterozygous human subject (31). The nucleotide sequence of one of these apo C-III alleles and the corresponding amino acid sequence are shown in Table V. The presence of G at residue position 370 generates the recognition sequence, G*AGCTC (* indicates residue 370), for the restriction endonuclease SacI, and the allele shown in

Table V Nucleotide and Corresponding Amino Acid Sequences of a Full-length Human Apo C-III cDNA Clone (Sac^{+} Allele)

								27									54
GAG	GCG	GGC	TGC	TCC	AGG	AAC	AGA	GGT	GCC	ATG	CAG	CCC	CGG	GTA	CTC	[illegible]T	GTT
										MET	Gln	Pro	Arg	Val	Leu	Leu	Val
										-20							
								81									108
GTT	GCC	CTC	CTG	GCG	CTC	CTG	GCC	TCT	GCC	CGA	GCT	TCA	GAG	GCC	GAG	GAT	GCC
Val	Ala	Leu	Leu	Ala	Leu	Leu	Ala	Ser	Ala	Arg	Ala	Ser	Glu	Ala	Glu	Asp	Ala
		-10									-1	+1					
							a ↓	135									162
TCC	CTT	CTC	AGC	TTC	ATG	CAG	GGT	TAC	ATG	AAG	CAC	GCC	ACC	AAG	ACC	GCC	AAG
Ser	Leu	Leu	Ser	Phe	MET	Gln	Gly	Tyr	MET	Lys	His	Ala	Thr	Lys	Thr	Ala	Lys
			10										20				
								189									216
GAT	GCA	CTG	AGC	AGC	GTG	CAG	GAG	TCC	CAG	GTG	GCC	CAG	CAG	GCC	AGG	GGC	TGG
Asp	Ala	Leu	Ser	Ser	Val	Gln	Glu	Ser	Gln	Val	Ala	Gln	Gln	Ala	Arg	Gly	Trp
					30		*	*				*		*	40		

Table V (continued)

								243									270
GTG	ACC	GAT	GGC	TTC	AGT	TCC	CTG	AAA	GAC	TAC	TGG	AGC	ACC	GTT	AAG	GAC	AAG
Val	Thr	Asp	Gly	Phe	Ser	Ser	Leu	Lys	Asp	Tyr	Trp	Ser	Thr	Val	Lys	Asp	Lys
							50										60
								297									324
TTC	TCT	GAG	TTC	TGG	GAT	TTG	GAC	CCT	GAG	GTC	AGA	CCA	ACT	TCA	GCC	GTG	GCT
Phe	Ser	Glu	Phe	Trp	Asp	Leu	Asp	Pro	Glu	Val	Arg	Pro	Thr	Ser	Ala	Val	Ala
									70								
															α β ↓		
								351									378
GCC	TGA	GAC	CTC	AAT	ACC	CCA	AGT	CCA	CCT	GCC	TAT	CCA	TCC	TGC	GAG	CTC	CTT
Ala	END																
							α ↓										
								405									432
GGG	TCC	TGC	AAT	CTC	CAG	GGC	TGC	CCC	TGT	AGG	TTG	CTT	AAA	AGG	GAC	AGT	AT[illegible]
								459									486
CTC	AGT	GCT	CTC	CTA	CCC	CAC	CTC	ATG	CCT	GGC	CCC	CCT	CCA	GGC	ATG	CTG	GCC
								513									
TCC	CAA	TAA	AGC	TGG	ACA	AGA	AGC	TGC	TAT	GAG							

α indicates differences between the sac$^+$ and sac$^-$ allele isolated from the same cDNA library. The sac$^-$ allele has C, C, T at residue positions 132, 370, and 401, respectively. β indicates differences between the sac$^+$ allele and an independently isolated sac$^-$ allele. The sac$^-$ allele has C at residue 370. * indicates amino acid differences between the cDNA-derived sequences (14,31) and that derived by protein sequencing techniques (4). The latter sequence contains Ser, Gln, Ala, and Gln at amino acid residues 32, 33, 37, and 39, respectively.

Table V has been designated Sac$^+$. The second allele of reference 31 contains the nucleotides C, C, and T at residue positions 132, 370, and 401, respectively, and has been designated Sac$^-$. An independently isolated Sac$^-$ clone (14) corresponds to sequence 31 through 517 of Table V. This Sac$^-$ allele differs from the Sac$^+$ allele of Table V at residue position 370 where it contains C instead of G.

The cDNA-derived amino acid sequence showed that the primary translation product of apo C-III mRNA consists of 99 amino acids, including a 20-amino-acid-long N-terminal signal peptide. The cDNA-derived amino acid sequence differs at four amino acid residues from the previously reported protein sequence (4). More specifically, at residues +32, +33, +37, and +39 the cDNA sequence predicts Glu, Ser, Gln, and Ala, respectively, while the previously reported sequence specifies Ser, Gln, Ala, and Gln, respectively (14,31).

Table VI Nucleotide and Corresponding Amino Acid Sequences of a Full-length Human Apo E3 cDNA Clone[a]

α β ↓																	
								27									54
CGC	AGC	GGA	GGT	GAA	GGA	CGT	CCT	TCC	CCA	GGA	GCC	GAC	TGG	CCA	ATC	ACA	GGC
								81									108
AGG	AAG	ATG	AAG	GTT	CTG	TGG	GCT	GCG	TTG	CTG	GTC	ACA	TTC	CTG	GCA	GGA	TGC
		MET	Lys	Val	Leu	Trp	Ala	Ala	Leu	Leu	Val	Thr	Phe	Leu	Ala	Gly	Cys
										-10							
								135									162
CAG	GCC	AAG	GTG	GAG	CAA	GCG	GTG	GAG	ACA	GAG	CCG	GAG	CCC	GAG	CTG	CGC	CAG
Gln	Ala	Lys	Val	Glu	Gln	Ala	Val	Glu	Thr	Glu	Pro	Glu	Pro	Glu	Leu	Arg	Gln
	-1	+1									10						
								189									216
CAG	ACC	GAG	TGG	CAG	AGC	GGC	CAG	CGC	TGG	GAA	CTG	GCA	CTG	GGT	CGC	TTT	TGG
Gln	Thr	Glu	Trp	Gln	Ser	Gly	Gln	Arg	Trp	Glu	Leu	Ala	Leu	Gly	Arg	Phe	Trp
			20										30				
								243									270
GAT	TAC	CTG	CGC	TGG	GTG	CAG	ACA	CTG	TCT	GAG	CAG	GTG	CAG	GAG	GAG	CTG	CTC
Asp	Tyr	Leu	Arg	Trp	Val	Gln	Thr	Leu	Ser	Glu	Gln	Val	Gln	Glu	Glu	Leu	Leu
					40										50		
		α β ↓			α β ↓												
								297									324
AGC	TCC	CAG	GTC	ACC	CAG	GAA	CTG	AGG	GCG	CTG	ATG	GAC	GAG	ACC	ATG	AAG	GAG
Ser	Ser	Gln	Val	Thr	Gln	Glu	Leu	Arg	Ala	Leu	MET	Asp	Glu	Thr	MET	Lys	Glu
							60										70
														β ↓			
								351									378
TTG	AAG	GCC	TAC	AAA	TCG	GAA	CTG	GAG	GAA	CAA	CTG	ACC	CCG	GTG	GCG	GAG	GAG
Leu	Lys	Ala	Tyr	Lys	Ser	Glu	Leu	Glu	Glu	Gln	Leu	Thr	Pro	Val	Ala	Glu	Glu
									80								
										β ↓							
								405									432
ACG	CGG	GCA	CGG	CTG	TCC	AAG	GAG	CTG	CAG	GCG	GCG	CAG	GCC	CGG	CTG	GGC	GCG
Thr	Arg	Ala	Arg	Leu	Ser	Lys	Glu	Leu	Gln	Ala	Ala	Gln	Ala	Arg	Leu	Gly	Ala
	90									*	100						
								459									486
GAC	ATG	GAG	GAC	GTG	TGC	GGC	CGC	CTG	GTG	CAG	TAC	CGC	GGC	GAG	GTG	CAG	GCC
Asp	MET	Glu	Asp	Val	Cys	Gly	Arg	Leu	Val	Gln	Tyr	Arg	Gly	Glu	Val	Gln	Ala
			110										120				
								513									540
ATG	CTC	GGC	CAG	AGC	ACC	GAG	GAG	CTG	CGG	GTG	CGC	CTC	GCC	TCC	CAC	CTG	CGC
MET	Leu	Gly	Gln	Ser	Thr	Glu	Glu	Leu	Arg	Val	Arg	Leu	Ala	Ser	His	Leu	Arg
					130										140		
									β ↓								
								567									594
AAG	CTG	CGT	AAG	CGG	CTC	CTC	CGC	GAT	GCC	GAT	GAC	CTG	CAG	AAG	CGC	CTG	GCA
Lys	Leu	Arg	Lys	Arg	Leu	Leu	Arg	Asp	Ala	Asp	Asp	Leu	Gln	Lys	Arg	Leu	Ala
							150		*								160
								621									648
GTG	TAC	CAG	GCC	GGG	GCC	CGC	GAG	GGC	GCC	GAG	CGC	GGC	CTC	AGC	GCC	ATC	CGC
Val	Tyr	Gln	Ala	Gly	Ala	Arg	Glu	Gly	Ala	Glu	Arg	Gly	Leu	Ser	Ala	Ile	Arg
									170								

Table VI (continued)

675 702
GAG CGC CTG GGG CCC CTG GTG GAA CAG GGC CGC GTG CGG GCC GCC ACT GTG GGC
Glu Arg Leu Gly Pro Leu Val Glu Gln Gly Arg Val Arg Ala Ala Thr Val Gly
180 190

729 756
TCC CTG GCC GGC CAG CCG CTA CAG GAG CGG GCC CAG GCC TGG GGC GAG CGG CTG
Ser Leu Ala Gly Gln Pro Leu Gln Glu Arg Ala Gln Ala Trp Gly Glu Arg Leu
200 210

β
↓
783 810
CGC GCG CGG ATG GAG GAG ATG GGC AGC CGG ACC CGC GAC CGC CTG GAC GAG GTG
Arg Ala Arg MET Glu Glu MET Gly Ser Arg Thr Arg Asp Arg Leu Asp Glu Val
220 230

α
↓
837 864
AAG GAG CAG GTG GCG GAG GTG CGC GCC AAG CTG GAG GAG CAG GCC CAG CAG ATA
Lys Glu Gln Val Ala Glu Val Arg Ala Lys Leu Glu Glu Gln Ala Gln Gln Ile
240 250

891 918
CGC CTG CAG GCC GAG GCA TTC CAG GCC CGC CTC AAG AGC TGG TTC GAG CCC CTG
Arg Leu Gln Ala Glu Ala Phe Gln Ala Arg Leu Lys Ser Trp Phe Glu Pro Leu
260

945 972
GTG GAA GAC ATG CAG CGC CAG TGG GCC GGG CTG GTG GAG AAG GTG CAG GCT GCC
Val Glu Asp MET Gln Arg Gln Trp Ala Gly Leu Val Glu Lys Val Gln Ala Ala
270 280

999 1026
GTG GGC ACC AGC GCC GCC CCT GTG CCC AGC GAC AAT CAC TGA ACG CCG AAG CCT
Val Gly Thr Ser Ala Ala Pro Val Pro Ser Asp Asn His END
290

1053 1080
GCA GCC ATG CGA CCC CAC GCC ACC CCG TGC CTC CTG CCT CCG CGC AGC CTG CAG

1107 1134
CGG GAG ACC CTG TCC CCG CCC CAG CCG TCC TCC TGG GGT GGA CCC TAG TTT AAT

1161
AAA GAT TCA CCA AGT TTC ACG C

[a]Data from reference 32.
α indicates differences between this clone and the normal apo E3 clone of reference 33. The latter clone has C, A, A, A at residue positions 2, 279, 288, and 858, respectively. β indicates differences between the normal apo E3 clone of reference 32 and a variant apo E3 clone of reference 33. The latter clone has C, A, A, A, A, C, T at residue positions, 2, 279, 288, 369, 409, 568, and 783, respectively. * indicates amino acid substitutions in the variant apo E3 clone (33). The substitutions are Thr and Pro at amino acid residues 99 and 152, respectively.

APO E

The nucleotide sequence of three independently derived full-length apo E cDNA clones has been reported recently (32,33). The nucleotide sequence and the corresponding amino acid sequence of the clone described in reference 32 are shown in Table VI. All three clones code for a protein that gives an E3/3 phenotype. Two of these clones code for a normal apo E3 (32,33) and the third for a variant apo E (33).

Compared to the sequence of Table VI and reference 32, the normal E3 clone described in reference 33 has C, A, A, A instead of G, G, G, G at residue positions 2, 279, 288, and 858, respectively. These nucleotide substitutions are silent and thus do not lead to amino acid substitution. The variant apo E3 clone of reference 33 has C, A, A, A, A, C, T instead of G, G, G, G, G, G, C at residue positions 2, 279, 288, 369, 409, 568, and 783, respectively (Table VI and references 32 and 33). The nucleotide substitutions at residues 2, 279, 288, 369, and 783 are conservative, whereas the nucleotide substitutions at residues 409 and 568 result in amino acid substitutions of the normal Ala-99 and Ala-152 for Thr-99 and Pro-152, respectively.

The cDNA-derived amino acid sequence showed that the primary translation product of apo E mRNA consists of 317 amino acids, in-

Table VII Amino Acid and Inferred Nucleotide Substitutions Corresponding to Different Human Apo E Alleles

Allele	Codon at the polymorphic site					Expected base substitution relative to ε3 allele	Amino acid substitution relative to E3/3 phenotype
	112	127	145	146	158		
ε3	TGC	GGC	CGT	AAG	CGC	None	None
ε4	CGC	Same	Same	Same	Same	T C	112 Cys→Arg
ε2	Same	Same	Same	Same	TGC	C T	158 Arg→Cys
ε2*	Same	Same	TGT	Same	Same	C T	145 Arg→Cys
ε2**	Same	Same	Same	CAG	Same	A C	146 Lys→Gln
ε1	Same	GAC	Same	Same	TGC	{G A {C T	{127 Gly→Asp {158 Arg→Cys

Table VIII The Signal Peptide and Propeptide Sequences of Human Apolipoproteins

Apolipoproteins		Ref.
A-I	Met Lys Ala Ala Val Leu Thr Leu Ala Val Leu Phe Leu Thr Gly Ser Gln Ala Arg His Phe Try Gln Gln	14-16
A-II	Met Lys Leu Leu Ala Ala Thr Val Leu Leu Leu Thr Ile Cys Ser Leu Glu Gly Ala Leu Val Arg Arg	14,23,24
A-IV	Met $\overset{+}{\text{Phe}}$ Leu $\overset{+}{\text{Lys}}$ Ala Val Val Leu $\overset{+}{\text{Thr}}$ Leu Ala Leu Val Ala Val Ala $\overset{*}{\text{Gly}}$ $\overset{+}{\text{Ala}}$ $\overset{+}{\text{Arg}}$ Ala	39, α
C-I	Met Arg Leu Phe Leu Ser Leu Pro Val Leu Val Val Val Leu Ser Ile Val Leu Glu Gly Pro Ala Pro Ala Gln Gly	27
C-II	Met Gly Thr Arg Leu Leu Pro Ala Leu Phe Leu Val Leu Leu Val Leu Gly Phe Glu Val Gln Gly	14,28
C-III	Met Gln Pro Arg Val Leu Leu Val Val Ala Leu Leu Ala Leu Leu Ala Ser Ala Arg Ala	14,31
E	Met Lys Val Leu Trp Ala Ala Leu Leu Val Thr Phe Leu Ala Gly Cys Gln Ala	32,33

The amino acid sequences are inferred from the nucleotide sequences of full-length apolipoprotein cDNA clones. The propeptide sequences are enclosed in boxes. (+) Unidentified residues by protein sequence analysis (39). (*) Protein sequence analysis showed Leu rather than Gly at this position (39).
(α) Karathanasis, Yunis, and Zannis, unpublished.

cluding an 18-amino-acid-long N-terminal signal peptide (32,33). The predicted sequence of the 299-amino-acid-long mature apo E3 protein agrees completely with the recently reported sequence of plasma apo E3 (7,8).

Previous studies have shown extensive genetic variation in human apo E (34,35). This variation results from structural mutations in the apo E gene (36–38). Three common (ε3, ε4, and ε2) and three rare (ε2*, ε2**, and ε1) apo E alleles have been described at the protein level (36–38). The observed differences of these alleles at the protein level and the predicted changes at the nucleotide level are shown in Table VII.

THE SIGNAL PEPTIDE AND PROPEPTIDE SEQUENCES OF HUMAN APOLIPOPROTEINS

The cDNA-derived amino acid sequence shows that all apolipoproteins studied contain an N-terminal signal peptide, which ranges from 18 to 26 amino acids in length. The signal peptide is cleaved intracellularly by the signal peptidase of the rough endoplasmic reticulum (17,18). Furthermore, apo A-I and apo A-II contain six- and five-amino-acid-long N-terminal prosegments, respectively, which are cleaved extracellularly by two different proteases (19–22,25,26). The currently known signal peptide and propeptide sequences of human apolipoproteins are shown in Table VIII.

SUMMARY

Tables I through VI provide the nucleotide and the corresponding amino acid sequences of cDNA clones for human apo A-I, apo A-II, apo C-I, apo C-II, apo C-III, and apo E. The differences of the corresponding clones at the nucleotide and amino acid level are discussed. In addition, the cDNA-derived amino acid sequences are compared with corresponding sequences of plasma apolipoproteins that were published previously.

The cDNA-derived amino acid sequence confirmed the presence of signal peptides in all apolipoproteins studied, as well as the presence of propeptides in human apo A-I and apo A-II.

The various apolipoprotein cDNA clones provide new tools which will promote new studies pertinent to the structure, function, and regulation of expression of apolipoprotein genes and their corresponding proteins. In addition, they will facilitate the study of the molecular basis of human diseases associated with mutations in apolipoproteins.

ACKNOWLEDGMENTS

This work was supported by grants from the National Institutes of Health (HL 32032), The National Science Foundation (DCB-8400173), the March of Dimes Birth Defects Foundation (1-817), and the Massachusetts Affiliate of the American Heart Association (13-517-845). V. I. Zannis and S. K. Karathanasis are Established Investigators of the American Heart Association. The research by the authors cited in this review was performed at Housman Medical Research Center of the Boston University Medical School and the Department of Cardiology of Children's Hospital at Harvard Medical School. S. K. Karathanasis is a Syntex Scholar.

REFERENCES

1. Morrisett, J. D., Jackson, R. L., and Gotto, A. M., Jr., Lipoproteins: Structure and function, *Annu. Rev. Biochem.*, *44*:183–207 (1975).

2. Alaupovic, P., Conceptual development of the classification systems of plasma lipoproteins, in *Protides of the Biological Fluids* (Peeters, H., ed.), Pergamon Press, Oxford, 1971, pp. 9–20.

3. Brewer, H. B., Jr., Lux, S. E., Ronan, R., and John, K. M., Amino acid sequence of human apo Lp-Gln-II (apo A-II), an apolipoprotein isolated from the high density lipoprotein complex, *Proc. Natl. Acad. Sci. U.S.A.*, *69*:1304–1308 (1972).

4. Brewer, H. B., Jr., Shulman, R., Herbert, P., Ronan, R., and Wehrly, R., The complete amino acid sequence of alanine apolipoprotein (apo C-III), an apolipoprotein from human plasma very low density lipoproteins, *J. Biol. Chem.*, *249*:4975–4984 (1974).

5. Shulman, R. S., Herbert, P. N., Wehrly, K., and Fredrickson, D. S., The complete amino acid sequence of C-I (apo lp-ser), an apolipoprotein from human very low density lipoproteins, *J. Biol. Chem.*, *250*:182–190 (1975).

6. Brewer, H. B., Fairwell, T., LaRue, A., Ronan, R., Houser, A., and Bronzert, T. J., The amino acid sequence of human apo-I, an apolipoprotein isolated from high density lipoproteins, *Biochem. Biophys. Res. Commun.*, *80*:623–630 (1978).

7. Weisgraber, K. H., Rall, S. C., Jr., and Mahley, R. W., Human E apoprotein heterogeneity. Cystein-argining interchanges in the amino acid sequence of the apo E isoforms, *J. Biol. Chem.*, *256*:9077–9083 (1981).

8. Rall, S. C., Weisgraber, K. H., and Mahley, R. W., Human apolipoprotein E. The complete amino acid sequence, *J. Biol. Chem.*, *257*:4171–4178 (1981).

9. Hospattankar, A. V., Fairwell, T., Ronan, R., and Brewer, H. B., Jr., Amino acid sequence of human plasma apolipoprotein C-II from normal and hyperlipoproteinemic subjects, *J. Biol. Chem.*, *259*:318–322 (1984).

10. Herbert, P. M., Assmann, G., Gotto, A. M., Jr., and Fredrickson, D. S., Familial lipoprotein deficiency: Abetalipoproteinemia, hypobetalipoproteinemia, and Tangier disease, in *The Metabolic Basis of Inherited Disease*, (Stanbury, J. B., Wyngaarden, J. B., Fredrickson, D. S., Goldstein, J. L., and Brown, M. D., eds.), 5th ed., McGraw-Hill, New York, 1982, pp. 489–651.

11. Zannis, V. I., and Breslow, J. L., Genetic, mutation affecting human lipoprotein metabolism, *Adv. Hum. Genet.*, *14*:125–215 (1984).

12. Mahley, R. W., Innerarity, T. L., Rall, S. C., Jr., and Weisgraber, K. H., Plasma lipoproteins: Apolipoprotein structure and function, *J. Lipid Res.*, *25*:1277–1294 (1984).

13. Karathanasis, S. K., Zannis, V. I., and Breslow, J. L., Isolation and characterization of the human apolipoprotein A-I gene, *Proc. Natl. Acad. Sci. U.S.A.*, *80*:6147–6151 (1983).

14. Sharpe, C. R., Sidoli, A., Shelley, C. S., Lucero, M. A., Shoulders, C. C., and Baralle, F. E., Human apolipoproteins AI, AII, CII. cDNA sequences and mRNA abundance, *Nucleic Acids Res.*, *12*:3917–3932 (1984).

15. Cheung, P., and Chan, L., Nucleotide sequence of cloned cDNA of human apolipoprotein A-I, *Nucleic Acids Res.*, *11*:3703–3715 (1983).

16. Law, S. W., Gray, G., and Brewer, H. B., Jr., cDNA cloning of human apo A-I: Amino acid sequence of preproapo A-I, *Biochem. Biophys. Res. Commun.*, *112*:257–264 (1983).

17. Blobel, G., Walter, P., Chang, C. N., Goldman, B., Erickson, A. H., and Lingappa, V. R., Translocation of proteins across

membranes: The signal hypothesis and beyond, in *Symposium of the Society of Experimental Biology (Great Britain)*, (Hopkins, C. R., and Duncan, C. J., eds.), Vol. 33, Cambridge University Press, London, 1979.

18. Blobel, G., and Dobberstein, B., Transfer of proteins across membranes. II. Reconstitution of functional rough microsomes from heterologous components, *J. Cell Biol.*, *67*:852–862 (1975).

19. Zannis, V. I., Karathanasis, S. K., Keutmann, H. T., Goldberger, G., and Breslow, J. L., Intracellular and extracellular processing of human apolipoprotein A-I: Secreted apolipoprotein A-I isoprotein 2 is a propeptide, *Proc. Natl. Acad. Sci. U.S.A.*, *80*:2574–2578 (1983).

20. Gordon, J. I., Sims, H. F., Lentz, S. R., Edelstein, C., Scanu, A. M., and Strauss, A. W., Proteolytic processing of human preproapolipoprotein A-I. A proposed defect in the conversion of pro A-I to A-I in Tangier disease, *J. Biol. Chem.*, *258*:4037–4044 (1983).

21. Edelstein, C., Gordon, J. I., Toscas, K., Sims, H. F., Strauss, A. W., and Scanu, A. M., In vitro conversion of proapoprotein A-I to apoprotein A-I, *J. Biol. Chem.*, *258*:11,430–11,433 (1984).

22. Bojanovski, D., Gregg, R. E., and Brewer, H. B., Jr., In vitro conversion of proapo $A\text{-}I_{Tangier}$ to mature apo $A\text{-}I_{Tangier}$, *J. Biol. Chem.*, *259*:6049–6051 (1984).

23. Knott, R. J., Priestley, L. M., Urdea, M., and Scott, J., Isolation and characterization of a cDNA encoding the precursor for human apolipoprotein AII, *Biochem. Biophys. Res. Commun.*, *120*:734–740 (1984).

24. Lackner, K. J., Simon, W. L., and Brewer, H. B., Jr., Human apolipoprotein A-II: Complete nucleic acid sequence of preproapo A-II, *FEBS Lett.*, *175*:159–164 (1984).

25. Gordon, J. I., Budelier, K. A., Sims, H. F., Edelstein, C., Scanu, A. M., and Strauss, A. W., Biosynthesis of human preproapolipoprotein A-II, *J. Biol. Chem.*, *258*:14,054–14,059 (1983).

26. Gordon, J. I., Sims, H. F., Edelstein, C., Scanu, A. M., and Strauss, A. W., Human proapolipoprotein A-II is cleaved following secretion from HepG2 cells by a thiol protease, *J. Biol. Chem.*, *259*:15,556–15,563 (1984).

27. Knott, T. J., Robertson, M. E., Priestley, L. M., Urdea, M., Wallis, S., and Scott, J., Characterisation of mRNAs encoding

the precursor for human apolipoprotein CI, *Nucleic Acids Res.*, *12*:3909–3915 (1984).

28. Fojo, S. S., Law, S. W., and Brewer, H. B., Jr., Human apolipoprotein C-II: Complete nucleic acid sequence of preapolipoprotein C-II, *Proc. Natl. Acad. Sci. USA*, *81*:6354–6357 (1984).

29. Myklebost, O., Williamson, B., Markham, A. F., Myklebost, S. R., Rogers, J., Woods, D. E., and Humphries, S. E., The isolation and characterization of cDNA clones for human apolipoprotein CII, *J. Biol. Chem.*, *259*:4401–4404 (1984).

30. Jackson, C. L., Bruns, G. A. P., and Breslow, J. L., Isolation and sequence of a human apolipoprotein CII cDNA clone and its use to isolate and map to human chromosome 19 the gene for apolipoprotein CII, *Proc. Natl. Acad. Sci. USA*, *81*:2945–2949 (1984).

31. Karathanasis, S. K., Zannis, V. I., and Breslow, J. L., Isolation and sequence of human apo CIII cDNA clones specifying two different alleles, *J. Lipid Res.*, *26*:451–456 (1985).

32. Zannis, V. I., McPherson, J., Goldberger, G., Karathanasis, S. K., and Breslow, J. L., Synthesis, intracellular processing and signal peptide of human apo E, *J. Biol. Chem.*, *259*: 5495–5499 (1984).

33. McLean, J. W., Elshourbagy, N. A., Chang, D. J., Mahley, R. W., and Taylor, J. M., Human apolipoprotein E mRNA. cDNA cloning and nucleotide sequencing of a new variant, *J. Biol. Chem.*, *259*:6498–7504 (1984).

34. Utermann, G., Langenback, U., Beisiegel, U., and Weber, W., Genetics of the apolipoprotein E system in man, *Am. J. Hum. Genet.*, *32*:339–342 (1980).

35. Zannis, V. I., and Breslow, J. L., Human VLDL apo E isoprotein polymorphism is explained by genetic variation and post-translational modification, *Biochemistry*, *20*:1033–1041 (1981).

36. Rall, S. C., Jr., Weisgraber, K. H., Innerarity, T. L., and Mahley, R. W., Structural basis for receptor binding heterogeneity of apolipoprotein E from type III hyperlipoproteinemic subjects, *Proc. Natl. Acad. Sci. U.S.A.*, *79*:4696–4700 (1982).

37. Rall, S. C., Jr., Weisgraber, K. H., Innerarity, T. L., Bersot, T. P., Mahley, R. W., and Blum, C. B., Identification of a new structural variant of human apolipoprotein E, E2(Lys_{146}–Gln), in a type III hyperlipoproteinemic subject with the E3/2 phenotype, *J. Clin. Invest.*, *72*:1288–1287 (1983).

38. Weisgraber, K. H., Rall, S. C., Jr., Innerarity, T. L., and Mahley, R. W., A novel electrophoretic variant of human apolipoprotein E: Identification and characterization of apolipoprotein E1, *J. Clin. Invest.*, *73*:1024–1033 (1984).

39. Gordon, J. I., Bisgaier, C. L., Sims, H. F., Sachder, O. P., Glickman, R. M., and Strauss, A. W., Biosynthesis of human proapolipoprotein A-IV, *J. Biol. Chem.*, *259*:468–474 (1984).

Appendix 2

General Properties of Plasma Lipoproteins and Apolipoproteins

CELINA EDELSTEIN The Pritzker School of Medicine, The University of Chicago, Chicago, Illinois

The following tables summarize some of the properties of the plasma lipoproteins and apolipoproteins of human subjects. The data must be considered averages in that they do not take into account factors such as age, sex, and nutritional status of the subject analyzed. Systematic studies examining these variables in terms of plasma lipoprotein and apolipoprotein distribution have not been carried out. More specifically in terms of apolipoproteins, it is likely that additional isoforms will be detected whether or not associated with pathology. In terms of lipid species, the more detailed applications of advanced techniques are now available to lipids extracted from the whole serum. These techniques are being applied to the study of plasma lipoproteins; however, at this time the information is not sufficiently exhaustive to be included into this account.

Table I Physicochemical Properties of Human Serum Lipoproteins[a]

Characteristic	Chylomicrons	VLDL	LDL	HDL_2	HDL_3
Solvent density (g/ml)	0.93–1.006	0.95–1.006	1.019–1.063	1.063–1.125	1.125–1.21
Flotation rate					
$S_f(1.063)$[b]	400–15,000	20–400	0–12	Sediments	Sediments
$S_f(1.21)$[b]	—	—	—	3.5–9	0–3.5
Molecular weight	$0.4–30 \times 10^6$	$5–10 \times 10^6$	$2–3 \times 10^6$	3.6×10^5	1.75×10^5
Diameter (Å)	750–6,000	250–750	170–260	60–140	40–100
Hydrated density (g/ml)	0.93	0.97	1.034	1.14	1.19
Electrophoretic mobility	Origin	Pre-β	β	α_1	α_2

[a]Average values.
[b]S_f = Svedberg unit, x 10^{-13}s. The numbers in parentheses indicate the density at which flotation was measured.
Source: Refs. 1–3 and 6.

Table II Composition of Human Serum Lipoproteins

	Wt % of total lipoproteins				
Component	Chylomicrons	VLDL	LDL	HDL_2	HDL_3
Phospholipid	6–9	16–20	24–30	24–30	22–25
Free cholesterol	1–3	4–8	9–12	2–5	2–3
Cholesteryl esters	3–6	9–13	28–30	16–20	10–13
Triglycerides	82–86	50–60	7–11	4–5	4–5
Protein	1–2	8–11	20–22	41–50	55–58

Source: Refs. 1–6.

Table III Phospholipid Composition of Human Serum Lipoproteins

	Wt % of total phospholipids				
Phospholipid	Chylomicrons	VLDL	LDL	HDL_2	HDL_3
Phosphatidylcholine	78.5	59.7	63.7	73.8	77.1
Lysophosphatidylcholine	4.2	5.0	2.7	2.0	4.0
Sphingomyelin	11.7	14.8	25.9	14.5	9.2
Phosphatidylethanolamine	5.6	4.6	2.2	3.3	2.5
Phosphatidylserine	ND[a]	1.5	0.8	0.9	0.6
Phosphatidylinositol	ND	3.6	1.6	2.4	2.4
Polyglycerophosphatides and phosphatidic acid	ND	7.6	2.0	2.2	2.0

[a]ND, not determined.
Source: Refs. 3 and 6.

Table IV Fatty Acid Composition of Lipids from Normal Human Serum

Fatty acid	Wt % of lipids							
	Phospholipids		Free fatty acids		Triglycerides		Cholesteryl esters	
	Mean	SEM	Mean	SEM	Mean	SEM	Mean	SEM
6:0	0.00	0.00	0.00	0.00	0.00	0.00	0.00	0.00
8:0	0.00	0.00	0.00	0.00	0.00	0.00	0.00	0.00
10:0	0.00	0.00	0.00	0.00	0.00	0.00	0.00	0.00
12:0	0.02	0.01	0.16	0.04	0.22	0.05	0.02	0.01
14:0	0.45	0.05	1.99	0.24	2.11	0.14	0.91	0.07
14:1-T	0.00	0.00	0.00	0.00	0.00	0.00	0.00	0.00
14:1-C	0.05	0.02	0.24	0.04	0.30	0.04	0.14	0.02
15:0	0.21	0.01	0.17	0.07	0.10	0.03	0.06	0.02
16:0-B	0.48	0.04	0.04	0.04	0.58	0.56	0.05	0.02
16:0	26.73	0.43	24.85	0.83	23.61	0.88	11.48	0.34
16:1-T	0.00	0.00	0.00	0.00	0.21	0.21	0.00	0.00
16:1W7	1.09	0.06	4.64	0.28	5.83	0.24	4.28	0.33
16:2	0.00	0.00	0.00	0.00	0.00	0.00	0.00	0.00
17:0-B	0.64	0.09	0.00	0.00	0.02	0.02	0.00	0.00

17:0	0.46	0.05	0.01	0.01	0.01	0.01	0.00	0.00
18:0-B	0.64	0.07	0.01	0.01	0.25	0.04	0.18	0.03
18:0	11.30	0.41	10.23	0.45	3.29	0.18	1.07	0.07
18:1-T	0.00	0.00	0.00	0.00	0.00	0.00	0.00	0.00
18:1-C	8.80	0.25	38.90	0.77	38.20	0.53	19.96	0.67
18:1-I	3.23	0.13	0.02	0.02	0.09	0.05	0.00	0.00
18:2-TT	0.00	0.00	0.00	0.00	0.00	0.00	0.00	0.00
18:2-CT	0.00	0.00	0.00	0.00	0.00	0.00	0.00	0.00
18:2W6	22.94	0.57	15.60	0.63	19.54	0.84	49.82	1.79
18:3W6	0.13	0.01	0.04	0.02	0.48	0.04	1.07	0.07
18:3W3	0.21	0.03	0.71	0.11	1.18	0.08	0.50	0.06
19:0	0.00	0.00	0.00	0.00	0.00	0.00	0.00	0.00
20:0	0.19	0.01	0.03	0.02	0.10	0.04	0.00	0.00
20:1W9	0.09	0.01	0.04	0.04	0.05	0.02	0.00	0.00
20:2W9	0.00	0.00	0.00	0.00	0.00	0.00	0.00	0.00
20:2W6	0.33	0.02	0.22	0.04	0.35	0.04	0.09	0.02
20:3W9	0.15	0.01	0.06	0.02	0.16	0.03	0.03	0.01
20:3W6	3.11	0.12	0.14	0.04	0.36	0.05	0.91	0.06
20:4-T	0.00	0.00	0.00	0.00	0.00	0.00	0.00	0.00
20:4W7	0.00	0.00	0.00	0.00	0.00	0.00	0.00	0.00

Table IV (continued)

Fatty acid	Wt % of lipids							
	Phospholipids		Free fatty acids		Triglycerides		Cholesteryl esters	
	Mean	SEM	Mean	SEM	Mean	SEM	Mean	SEM
20:4W6	10.95	0.45	1.25	0.17	1.64	0.14	8.08	0.39
20:4W3	0.00	0.00	0.00	0.00	0.00	0.00	0.00	0.00
20:5W3	0.65	0.08	0.02	0.01	0.14	0.02	0.70	0.10
22:0	0.51	0.05	0.00	0.00	0.00	0.00	0.00	0.00
22:1	0.00	0.00	0.00	0.00	0.00	0.00	0.00	0.00
22:3W6	0.00	0.00	0.00	0.00	0.00	0.00	0.00	0.00
23:0	0.31	0.04	0.00	0.00	0.00	0.00	0.00	0.00

22:4W6	0.42	0.02	0.02	0.01	0.22	0.02	0.01	0.01
22:4W3	0.00	0.00	0.00	0.00	0.00	0.00	0.00	0.00
22:5W6	0.41	0.03	0.03	0.01	0.17	0.02	0.05	0.02
22:5W3	0.77	0.03	0.12	0.05	0.29	0.03	0.04	0.01
24:0	0.56	0.05	0.00	0.00	0.02	0.01	0.00	0.00
22:6W3	2.23	0.14	0.34	0.06	0.35	0.04	0.49	0.08
24:1	0.56	0.06	0.00	0.00	0.02	0.01	0.00	0.00
Saturated acids	40.73	0.52	37.45	1.27	29.46	1.09	13.55	0.44
Branched acids	1.76	0.15	0.06	0.04	0.86	0.55	0.23	0.04
Monoenoic acids	13.83	0.31	43.84	0.83	44.70	0.51	24.38	0.96
Odd chain acids	0.97	0.08	0.19	0.07	0.11	0.03	0.06	0.02

SEM, standard error of the mean. T, trans; TT, trans, trans; C, cis; CT, cis, trans; B, branched chain; I, isomer.
Source: Ref. 12 and R. T. Holman and S. B. Johnson, personal communication.

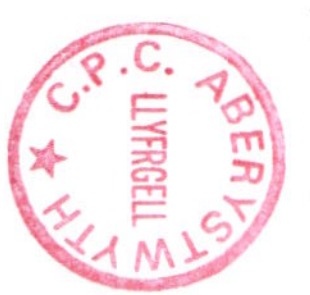

Table V Apoprotein Composition of Human Serum Lipoproteins

	g/100 g protein				
Apoprotein	Chylomicrons	VLDL	LDL	HDL_2	HDL_3
A-I	33.0	0.9	0.8	58.7	64.9
A-II	Trace	0.2	0.4	10.0	25.6
A-IV	14.0	ND[a]	ND	ND	Trace
B-48	5.0	Absent	Absent	Absent	Absent
B-100	Absent	25.0	95.0	3.0	Absent
C	32.0	55.0	2.0	13.0	5.0
D	ND	ND	Trace	2.0	4.0
E	10.0	15.0	3.2	3.0	1.0

[a]ND, not determined.
Source: Refs. 1–3.

Table VI Properties of Human Serum Apolipoproteins

Apolipo-protein	M_r	No. of amino acids	Chromosome	pl of major isoform	Concentration in plasma (mg/dl)
A-I	28,016	243	11	5.6	100–150
A-II	17,414	154	1	4.9	50–70
A-IV	46,000	393	11	5.5	4–15
B-100	500,000	—	1[a]	—	80–120
B-48	250,000	—	—	—	50
C-I	6,630	57	—	8.0	5–10
C-II	8,824	79	19	4.7	3–5
C-III	8,764	79	11	4.9	7–12
D	32,000	—	—	5.3	7–12
E	34,145	299	19	5.9	4–14
H	43,000	—	—	9.5	70

[a]A. Lusis, personal communication.
Source: Refs. 1, 7, and 8.

Table VII Human Apo A-I Isoforms

Isoform	$pI_{apparent}$	Charge relative to isoform 4
1	≥6.50	ND[a]
2	5.85	+2
3	5.74	+1
4	5.64	0
5	5.52	−1
6	5.40	−2

[a]ND, not determined.
Source: Ref. 9.

Table VIII Human Apo A-I Genetic Variants

Variant	Amino acid substitution
Milano	Arg_{173} → Cys
Münster-2(A)(Marburg)	Lys_{107} → deletion
Münster-3(A)	Asp_{103} → Asn
Münster-3(B)	Pro_{4} → Arg
Münster-3(C)	Pro_{3} → His
Münster-3(D)	Asp_{213} → Gly
Münster-4	Glu_{198} → Lys
Giessen	Pro_{143} → Arg
Norway	Glu_{136} → Lys

Source: Ref. 10.

Table IX Human Apo A-II Isoforms

Isoform	$pI_{apparent}$	Charge relative to isoform $A\text{-}II_0$
$A\text{-}II_{+1}$	5.17	+1
$A\text{-}II_0$	4.90	0
$A\text{-}II_{-1}$[a]	4.68	−1
$A\text{-}II_{-2}$[a]	4.42	−2
$A\text{-}II_{-3}$[a]	4.20	−3

[a]Apo $A\text{-}II_{-1}$, apo $A\text{-}II_{-2}$, and $A\text{-}II_{-3}$ contain one and two sialic acid residues.
Source: Ref. 11.

Table X Human Apo E Genetic Variants

Variant	Amino acid substitution(s)	Charge relative to E3
E1	$Gly_{127} \rightarrow Asp$, $Arg_{158} \rightarrow Cys$	−2
E2	$Arg_{158} \rightarrow Cys$	−1
E2	$Arg_{145} \rightarrow Cys$	−1
E2	$Lys_{146} \rightarrow Gln$	−1
E3	$Cys_{112} \rightarrow Arg$, $Arg_{142} \rightarrow Cys$	0
E3	$Ala_{gg} \rightarrow Thr$, $Ala_{152} \rightarrow Pro$	0
E4	$Cys_{112} \rightarrow Arg$	+1

Source: Ref. 10.

REFERENCES

1. Assmann, G., in *Lipid Metabolism and Atherosclerosis*, Schattauer, New York, 1982.
2. Scanu, A. M., Edelstein, C., and Keim, P., in *The Plasma Proteins* (Putnam, F. W., ed.), Academic Press, New York, 1975, pp. 318–391.
3. Scanu, A. M., Edelstein, C., and Shen, B. W., in *Lipid-Protein Interactions* (Jost, P. C., and Griffith, O. H., eds.), Wiley-Interscience, New York, 1982, pp. 259–328.
4. Kuksis, A., Myher, J. J., Geher, K., Breckenridge, W. C., Jones, G. J. L., and Little, J. A., *J. Chromatogr.*, *224*:1–23 (1981).
5. Blaton, V. H., and Peeters, H., in *Blood Lipids and Lipoproteins: Quantitation, Composition, and Metabolism* (Nelson, G. J., ed.), 1972, pp. 275–313.
6. Skipski, V. P., in *Blood Lipids and Lipoproteins: Quantitation, Composition, and Metabolism* (Nelson, G. J., ed), Wiley-Interscience, New York, 1972, pp. 275–313.
7. Alaupovic, P., McConathy, W. J., and Fesmire, J. D., in *Proceedings of the Workshop on Apolipoprotein Quantification* (Lippel, K., ed.), NIH Pub. No. 83–1266, 1983.
8. Sprecher, D. L., Taam, L., and Brewer, H. B., Jr., Two-dimensional electrophoresis of human plasma apolipoproteins, *Clin. Chem.*, *30*:2084–2092 (1984).
9. Zannis, V. I., Breslow, J. L., and Katz, A. J., Isoproteins of human apolipoprotein A-I demonstrated in plasma and intestinal organ culture, *J. Biol. Chem.*, *255*:8612–8617 (1980).
10. Mahley, R. W., Innerarity, T. L., Rall, S. C., and Weisgraber, K. H., Plasma lipoproteins: Apolipoprotein structure and function, *J. Lipid Res.*, *25*:1277–1294 (1984).
11. Lackner, K. J., Edge, S. B., Gregg, R. E., Hoeg, J. M., and Brewer, H. B., Jr., Isoforms of apolipoprotein A-II in human plasma and thoracic duct lymph, *J. Biol. Chem.*, *260*:703–706 (1985).
12. Johnson, S. B., Gordon, E., McClain, C., Low, G., and Holman, R. T., Abnormal polyunsaturated fatty acid patterns of serum lipids in alcoholism and cirrhosis: Arachidonic acid deficiency in cirrhosis, *Proc. Natl. Acad. Sci. U.S.A.*, *82*, 1815–1818 (1985).

Index

Abetalipoproteinemia, 109
Acylcoenzyme A:cholesterol
acyltransferase (ACAT),
18, 288, 342–343, 345,
350, 361
Adrenal gland, 360–374
Amino acid sequences, 476–477
apo A-I, 476–478
apo A-II, 478–479
apo C-I, 478, 480
apo C-II, 480–482
apo C-III, 482–483
apo E, 484–488
Apo B,E receptor, 81
Apolipoproteins, 53–67, 85–134
apolipoprotein(a) (apo(a))
intrinsic viscosity, 81
isolation frame Lp(a), 80
molecular weight, 80
surface binding, 80
apolipoprotein A-I, 23, 85–100
association with human
diseases (table), 86–87
cDNA, 88–96
nucleotide sequence (table),
90, 476–477
DNA repeats (table), 92

[Apolipoproteins]
exons, 97
gene, 94–98
location, 98
rearrangement, 121
genetic variants (table), 99,
503
Giessen, 99
Marburg, 99
Milano, 99
Münster, 99
isoforms (table), 503
mutations, 98–100
prepeptide, 91
propeptide, 91
protein variant, 108
cosegragation with apo A-IV,
108
apolipoprotein A-II, 100–102
cDNA, 102
nucleotide sequence (table),
104–105, 479
DNA repeats (table), 106
gene, 107–108
genetic variants, 107–108
(table), 504
human chromosome, 11, 108

[Apolipoproteins]
isoforms (table), 504
protein variant, 108
cosegregation with apo A-I, 108
22 amino acid repetitions, 103
apolipoprotein B, 28, 108–110
genetic properties, 108–109
genetic variation, 109–110
Ag variants, 109
Lp variants, 109
variants, 28
apo B,E receptor, 307–312
apolipoprotein C-I, 110–112
cDNA, 112
nucleotide sequence (table), 111
genetic properties, 110–111
apolipoprotein C-II, 112–116
cDNA, 113
nucleotide sequence (table), 114, 481
chromosome 19 gene mapping, 115
deficiency, 116
gene structure and variants, 113–116
mapping of gene in chromosome, 19, 115
genetic properties, 112
apolipoprotein C-III, 116–123
association with hypertriglyceridemia, 120
cDNA, 117–119
nucleotide sequence (table), 118, 482–483
gene rearrangement, 121
gene structure and variants, 119–120
genetic variants and hypertriglyceridemias, 120
general properties, 116–117
prepeptide, 117
apolipoprotein E, 123–134
alleles, 130–134
allelic variations (table), 486

[Apolipoproteins]
and cholesterol metabolism, 301–329
cDNA, 125–128
nucleotide sequence (table), 124, 484–485
DNA repeats (table), 126
gene
locus, 129
structure and mapping, 128–129
general properties, 123–124, 304–307
genetics, 85–143
HDLc, 308–310
interaction with apo B,E (LDL) receptors, 307–312
isoforms, 304–307
metabolism, 314–318
chylomicrons, remnants, clearance, 314–315
intracellular regulation, 314
reverse cholesterol transport, 315–318
mutations, 129–134
nomenclature of alleles and phenotypes (figure), 130
phenotypes, 130–134
receptors, liver, 312–314
binding domain, 321–324
chemical modification, 312
regulation of expression (table), 313
22 amino acid repetitions, 125
type III HLP, 129–134
variants (table), 308
variants, clinically relevant, 318–321
type III hyperlipoproteinemia, 318–321
composition (table), 502
extracellular processing, 53–67
general properties, 495–504

[Apolipoproteins]
polymorphism, 115
prepeptide,
apo A-I, 91
apo A-II, 102
apo C-III, 117
proapo A-I, processing, 58–61
proapo A-II, processing, 58–61
propeptide
apo A-I, 91
apo A-II, 102
properties (table), 502
protein processing, 54–58
extracellular, 55–58
intracellular, 54–55
signal peptide and propeptide sequences, 487–488
(table), 487

Cholesterol, 37–40, 281–283
agents affecting biosynthesis (table), 286
apo B-dependent and -independent homeostasis in cells, 281
functions in vertebrates, 281
biosynthesis, 284–296
oxysterol binding protein, 295
regulation by oxysterol metabolites, 291–296
5-alpha-cholestan-3-beta-OL, 292
32-hydroxylanosterol, 292
sites of regulation, 284
tissue rates of cholesterol synthesis (table), 284
biosynthetic pathway, 282–283
regulation, 283–284
cellular homeostasis, 291–296
functions in vertebrates, 281
HMG-CoA reductase, 283–287
apo B (apo E)-dependent regulation, 287
regulation by reversible

[Cholesterol]
phosphorylation, 297
synthesis/degradation regulation, 287, 292
metabolism, 301–304
homeostasis, 301, 316, 324
overview, 301–304
transport scheme (figure), 302
oxysterols, 285, 291–296
binding protein, 295
HMG-CoA reductase synthesis, 292
responses in experimental animals, 38–40
Cholesteryl ester exchange/transfer protein, 232–234, 239
intracellular lipid transfer protein, 234
localization of, 234
mode of action of, 233
plasma lipid transfer protein, 235
purification and properties, 234–237
(table), 236–237
Cholestyramine, 285, 292
Chromatofocusing, 77
Clathrin, 333–334, 338
Coated pits, 332–333, 335–338, 345, 352–353
Compactin, 285, 292

Familial combined hyperlipidemia, 110
Familial hypercholesterolemia, 110
Fatty acid composition of lipids (table), 498–501

Glycolipids, 201–219
atherogenesis, 218
chemistry, 201–208
composition (table), 206–207
demyelination, 218

[Glycolipids]
disease states, 217–219
distribution in serum, 210–211
dynamics, 212–217
catabolism, 214–216
exchange, 216–217
synthetic vesicles, 216
synthesis, 212–214
gangliosides, 208
glycosphingolipids, 201–210
hyperlipoproteinemias, 218
hypolipoproteinemias, 218–219
physical properties, 209–210
storage diseases, 217–218
structure, 208–209
synthetic vesicles, 216

HMG-CoA reductase, 342–343, 345–347, 349–350, 355
Homozygous hypobetalipoproteinemia, 110
Hormones, 40–41
Hyperapobetalipoproteinemia, 110
Hypertriglyceridemia, 120

Intestinal lipoproteins, 15

Lecithin cholesterol acyl transferase (LCAT), 24, 223–226, 228–232, 238–239
activators and inhibitors of, 226–229
apolipoproteins, and, 225–228
deficiency of, 238–239
enzyme regulation, 232
general properties of, 229–231
immunological properties of, 232
properties (table), 230–231
reaction of, 224
source of, 223
stability of, 226

Lipoprotein disorders, 453–474
familial, 453–463
apo B,E receptor mutant alleles (table), 460
apolipoprotein defects, 455
(table), 456–457
enzyme defects, 455
(table), 458
HDL metabolism (table), 462
hyperalphalipoproteinemias, 463
hypercholesterolemia features (table), 461
hypoalphalipoproteinemias, 463
lipoprotein phenotypes (table), 454
receptor defects, 459
(table), 459
with unknown or partially known familial determination, 464–465
Low-density lipoprotein (LDL) receptors, 331–356
biological and clinical implications, 331–356
biosynthesis, scheme (figure), 336
clustering and internalization, 338
degradation, 341–342
synthesis/degradation (figure), 338
independent uptake of cholesterol-rich lipoproteins, 344–345
life cycle, 332–335
modulation by factors other than cholesterol, 345–346
molecular weight, 333
pathway to cell surface, 335–337
regulation and function in cultured cells, 342

[Low-density lipoprotein (LDL) receptors]
cholesterol homeostasis
in cultured skin fibroblasts, 342–344
in living organisms, 347–348
role in lipid metabolism, 346–356
of LDL metabolism in vivo, 351–352
schematic representation of various domains (figure), 334
tissue localization, 344
Lp(a) lipoprotein, 21

Membranes, 145–177
amphipathy, 147
bilayer, 148–152
biogenesis, 170–174
complex carbohydrates, 171
lipids, 170–171
membranes and organelles, 170–174
proteins, 171–184
biological, 145–174
channels, 159–161
coupled transport, 162
reciprocating transporters, 161–162
redox-driven transport, 163
transport ATPases, 162–163
cholesterol, 179–195
cellular, 190–192
diffusion, 183, 185, 191
distribution with the cell, 188
plasma lipoproteins, 188–190
effect on membrane permeability and fluidity, 181–182
function, 180–183
in plasma membrane, 190–191, 193
intracellular movement, 192–195
phospholipid–cholesterol complex, 180
sterol carrier proteins, 194
structure, 179
phospholipid-cholesterol complex in bilayers, 180
transbilayer distribution, 189
transfer, 183–185, 193
transfer between membranes and lipoproteins, 183–185
collision mechanism, 183, 185
diffusion mechanism, 183, 185
transmembrane movement, 185–188
cytoskeleton, 168
extracellular matrix, 168–170
fission, 152–153
fusion, 152–153
glycerolipids, 146
hydrophobic effect, 147
lipid(s), 145–152
asymmetry, 151
composition, 146
motion, 148–152
melting temperatures of selected phospholipids (table), 150
organelles, biosynthesis, 170–174
phase behavior, 148–152
proteins, 153–157
membrane assoication, 153–154
integral or intrinsic, 153
peripheral or extrinsic, 154
receptors, 164–167
receptor-mediated membrane transduction (table), 166
reconstitution, 157–158
sphingolipids, 146
sterols, 146
transport, 158–159

Nascent lipoproteins, 13–140

Plasma albumin, 247–274
free fatty acid, 248–252
albumin-bound fatty acid, 267–272
binding sites, 255–256
structural requirements, 256–257
binding to albumin, 257–267
effect of fatty acid chain modification (table), 258
effect of fatty acid chain length (table), 258
rates, 259
structure of fatty acids, 257–259
unbound fatty acid, 260
composition, 250
(table), 498–501
concentration, 249–250
metabolism, 251–252
solubility, 251
turnover, 251–252
functions, 247–248
structure, 252–257
Plasma lipoproteins, 1–10
acylcoenzyme A:cholesterol acyltransferase (ACAT), 18
agarose gel electrophoresis, 3
apolipoproteins
apolipoprotein A-I, 23
apolipoprotein B, 28
variants, 28
biosynthesis regulation, 35–36
synthesis and secretion, general considerations, 25–29
synthesis in peripheral tissue, 29–30
beta-VLDL, 37
biogenesis, 11–42
cholesterol, 37–40
responses in experimental animals, 38–40
[Plasma lipoproteins]
chylomicrons, 4, 15–18
metabolism, scheme, 5
postsecretory transformations of chylomicrons, 17
properties, 4
cotranslational modifications, 26
extrahepatic synthesis, 25
fat adsorption, 15
fatty acid, 37
general properties, 3, 495–504
hepatic lipoproteins, 18
HDL maturation, 22
high-density lipoproteins (HDL), 8, 18, 85–88
ACAT, 18
composition, 78–79
fate, 24
properties, 8
subclasses, 37
HDL_1, 37
HDL_c, 37
high density Lp(a), 77
hormones, 40–41
and estrogens, 40
follicle-stimulating, 41
and lipoprotein regulation, 40
sex, 40
immunoregulation, 403–452
basis of cell-mediated and humoral immune response, 404–409
lymphocyte activation, 405–408
transferrin independence of lymphocyte proliferation, 408–409
lipoprotein suppression, 409–443
activation events, 410–415
immunoregulatory receptor mediation, 415–419
target cells, 425–428
role of lipoproteins in mid-cycle and late events, 419–422

[Plasma lipoproteins]
modulation by accessory cells, 419–420
modulation by trans- ferring, 420–422
immunoregulation in vivo, 441–443
lipoprotein constituents, 422–424
mechanism of suppression of lymphocyte activation, 428–441
molecular basis of suppres- sion, 438–440
structural features, 409–410
intestinal lipoproteins, 15
intracellular formation, 30–35
lecithin cholesterol acyl transferase (LCAT), 24
familial deficiency, 24
lipoprotein(a) (Lp(a)), 73–82
biochemistry and biology, 73–82
chemical composition, 78
clinical considerations
atherosclerosis, and, 82
coronary heart disease, relation to, 82
risk factor for cardio- vascular disease, 82
comparative properties, 78–80
density, 78–79
dietary manipulation, effects on, 81–82
fractional catabolic rate, 81
function, 81
heterogeneity, 73
isolation, 73
chromatofocusing, 77
gel filtration, 77
heparin sepharose chromatography, 77
lipid content, 81
rate zonal flotation, 77
low-density lipoproteins (LDL), relationship with composition, 78–79

[Plasma lipoproteins]
fractional catabolic rate, 81
function, 81
lipid content, 81
viscosity, 79
low-density Lp(a), 77
molar composition (table), 79
molecular weight, 78–79
origin, 81
pharmacological agents, action of, 82
physiological considerations, 81–82
receptor-independent uptake, 81
receptors in steroidogenesis, 359–393
adrenal gland, 360–362
high-density lipoprotein (HDL) receptor, 369–372, 380–385, 391–392
adrenal membranes:
human, 372
mouse, 369
rat, 369–372
ovary:
human, 383–384
rat, 380–383
testis: rat, 387–388
low-density lipoprotein (LDL) receptor, 362–369, 390–391
adrenal membranes:
bovine cortex, 362–364
human, 367–369
mouse, 365
rabbit, 364–365
rat, 365–367
ovary:
bovine, 376
hamster, 377
human, 379–380
rabbit, 376–377
rat, 377–379
placenta: human, 389–390

[Plasma lipoproteins]
testis:
human, 387
mouse, 386
pig, 385–386
rat, 386–387
ovary, 374–385
placenta, 388–390
testis, 385–388
synthetic rate, 81
viscosity, 79
water–lipoprotein interface, behavior at, 78
packing of protein and phospholipid, 78
low-density lipoproteins (LDL), 6, 18
de novo production, 21
metabolism, scheme, 7
properties, 6
Lp(a) lipoprotein, 21
nascent lipoproteins, 13–14
high-density lipoproteins, 18, 21–25
N-glycosylation, 27
overview, 1–10
regulation, 35–38, 40
dietary factors, 36
and estrogen in birds, 40–41
follicle-stimulating hormone and cyclic AMP in ovary, 41
genetic factors, 36
hormones, 40–41
structural model of HDL_3, 2

[Plasma lipoproteins]
ultracentrifugal profile, 4
very low-density lipoproteins (VLDL), 5, 18–20
composition, 78–79
conversion to LDL, 19–20
metabolism, scheme, 6
modification by dietary treatment, 19
properties, 5

Serum lipoproteins
apoprotein composition (table), 502
composition (table), 497
phospholipid composition (table), 497
physicochemical properties (table), 496
Steroid hormones, precursor, 283
Sterol synthesis, 290
regulation by oxysterol metabolites, 291–296
Structural sterol, 291

Tangier disease, 100

Ultracentrifugation, 73

WHHL rabbits, 290